To David Southgate
with compliments and
appreciation of many years
of stimulating contacts

Nik

Iron Nutrition in Health and Disease

The Swedish Nutrition Foundation
20th International Symposium

The Swedish Society of Medicine
Berzelius Symposium XXXI

Iron Nutrition in Health and Disease

The Swedish Nutrition Foundation
20th International Symposium

The Swedish Society of Medicine
Berzelius Symposium XXXI

Edited by
Leif Hallberg and Nils-Georg Asp

British Library Cataloguing in Publication Data

Hallberg, L.,
Iron Nutrition in Health and Disease
1. Iron - Physiological effect 2. Iron deficiency disease
3. Iron in the body
I. Title II. Asp, N.
612.3'924

ISBN: 0 86196 5442

Published by

John Libbey & Company Ltd, 13 Smiths Yard, Summerley Street, London SW18 4HR, England.
Telephone: 0181-947 2777 Fax: 0181-947 2664 E-mail: LIBBEY@Earlsfield.Win-UK.Net.
John Libbey & Company Pty Ltd, Level 10, 15/17 Young Street, Sydney, NSW 2000, Australia
John Libbey Eurotext Ltd, 127 Avenue de la République, 92120 Montrouge, France.
John Libbey - C.I.C. s.r.l., via Lazzaro Spallanzani 11, 00161 Rome, Italy.

Printed in Great Britain by WBC Bookbinders Ltd, Unit 5, Waterton Industrial Estate, Bridgend, Mid Glamorgan CF13 3YN.

Proceedings

Iron Nutrition in Health and Disease
The Swedish Nutrition Foundation's
20th International Symposium
and
The Swedish Society of Medicine
Berzelius Symposium XXXI

August 24–27, 1995 Saltsjöbaden, Stockholm, Sweden

Editors

Leif Hallberg
University of Göteborg, Sweden

Nils-Georg Asp
University of Lund and the Swedish Nutrition Foundation, Sweden

Assistance

Anita Laser Reutersward
The Swedish Nutrition Foundation, Sweden

Sponsors

The Cerealia Foundation R&D

The Swedish Dairies' Association

The Swedish Meat Information Institute

Semper AB

Svenska Nestlé AB

Van den Bergh Foods AB

Swedish Council for Forestry and Agricultural Research

Contents

Preface

In 1967, The Swedish Nutrition Foundation (SNF) arranged one of its first international symposia on iron deficiency – "Occurrence, causes and prevention of nutritional anaemias". Since then, research in this field has expanded at an unforeseen rate. Iron deficiency is still the most frequent nutritional deficiency disorder in the world and much research has been performed in all fields related to iron metabolism, iron absorption, epidemiology of iron deficiency, negative effects, prevention, etc.

In recent years, increased interest in iron overload has also been shown – its prevalence and negative effects. The possibility that even mild degrees of iron overload might have adverse effects has been suggested.

A new international symposium – "Iron Nutrition in Health and Disease" – was arranged in August 24–27 1995, by the SNF, together with the Swedish Society of Medicine, as the Berzelius Symposium XXXI, in Saltsjöbaden, Sweden. The purpose was to update present knowledge on iron metabolism, creating a platform for optimism in iron nutrition. Scientists from all over the world were invited to present and discuss in depth recent findings related to the physiology and pathology of iron metabolism, iron deficiency and iron overload. Another aim was to identify areas where most research is needed.

The present volume contains 35 chapters covering both basic research and its practical application in clinical and public health work. The last section includes two papers concerning the role of the food industry in iron nutrition *i.e.* iron intake from industrial products and the effect of food processing on iron bioavailability.

The Editors would like to express sincere thanks to the authors of this book for their excellent contributions and to our colleagues in the Scientific and Organizing Committee, Prof. Göran Hallmans, Dept. of Nutritional Research, University of Umeå, Prof. Stephan Rössner, the Swedish Society of Medicine, Prof. Gösta Samuelson, Dept. of Clinical Physiology, University of Uppsala and Anita Laser Reuterswärd, the Swedish Nutrition Foundation, for fruitful cooperation during the planning and performance of the symposium.

Leif Hallberg
Göteborg, Sweden

Nils-Georg Asp
Lund, Sweden

June, 1996

Iron Nutrition in Health and Disease, edited by Leif Hallberg and Nils-Georg Asp

Chapter 1

Iron balance and the capacity of regulatory systems to prevent the development of iron deficiency and overload

T.H. Bothwell

Department of Medicine, University of the Witwatersrand Medical School, 7 York Road, Parktown 2193, Johannesburg, South Africa

Summary

The 3–4 g iron in the body of an adult is complexed in a number of proteins which maintain it in the non-toxic yet bioavailable forms involved in vital functions, such as oxygen and electron transport and the activation of oxygen. In addition there is a reserve of variable size in which iron is sequestered in storage proteins. The major internal circuit is the one involving red cell metabolism, with most of the iron involved in this circuit being conserved and re-utilized.

Although external iron exchange is very small in relation to the body iron content, it is small variations in the balance between iron losses and dietary iron absorption that are responsible for the major disturbances of iron metabolism, namely iron deficiency and iron overload. While the rate of iron absorption is regulated to match body needs, the range within which this occurs is limited by the bioavailability of iron in the diet, with an upper limit of about 4–5 mg daily. However, there are many cereal-based diets consumed in developing countries in which the figure is a good deal lower, because of the presence of potent inhibitors of iron absorption in the diet. As a result, iron deficiency anaemia remains a major problem in many parts of the world, with infants and women during their reproductive lives being particularly vulnerable, and its prevention, through supplementation and fortification programmes, remains an urgent priority. The situation in industrialized countries is more complex. Although there is persuasive evidence that the prevalence of iron deficiency has declined, it is not clear what the relative contributions of preventative programmes, changes in life style and dietary habits have been. Whatever the reasons, the end result is a situation in which adult males have an average storage surplus of about 1 g which may even be greater in certain meat eating populations. In iron replete populations storage iron concentrations tend to stabilize in later adult life, which reflects the gastrointestinal mucosa's capacity to regulate the body iron content. Unresolved at the present time are the effects of improved iron nutrition on the phenotypic expression of iron loading disorders nor is there clarity on possible deleterious associations between iron stores in the upper normal range, as assessed by serum ferritin concentrations, and other diseases, including ischaemic heart disease and malignancy.

Introduction

Iron is the fourth most abundant element and the second most abundant metal in the earth's crust[1]. It is, however, almost exclusively in the oxidized state which greatly reduces its accessibility. In examining the exchange between man and the environment it has become clear that the body has a unique capacity to conserve iron but a very limited capacity to absorb it from many contemporary diets. For optimal iron status to be achieved the body iron content must be steadily increased during infancy and childhood, and thereafter iron balance must be maintained by an absorption rate which meets physiological body losses and thus ensures an optimal body iron content.

In the discussion that follows, attention will first be directed briefly to the various body iron compartments and to internal iron exchange. Thereafter the discussion will consider how iron balance is maintained, with special emphasis on the source and extent of iron losses and the mechanisms by which these losses are matched by absorption from the gut in different dietary settings. The final section will review the degree to which the body's regulatory mechanisms can protect it from developing iron deficiency and iron overload. Throughout, the focus will be on adults rather than infants and children, since it is their iron status that is the centre of current controversies.

Internal iron exchange

Iron has an inexorable tendency to hydrolyse and polymerize, with the formation of insoluble amorphous iron(III) hydroxide hydrates[2]. It is not, therefore, surprising that nature has evolved protein-dependent systems for both the transport and the intracellular storage of iron in tightly complexed, soluble, non-toxic yet bioavailable forms. The complexing of iron in such compounds has a second advantage in that it prevents the potential toxicity associated with iron's capacity to produce the extremely reactive hydroxyl radical[2]. Of iron's diverse reactions the most important is the reversible one-electron oxidation-reduction reaction that takes iron between its two common oxidation states, the ferrous and ferric forms. The many roles in which iron is involved in the body include oxygen carriage (e.g. haemoglobin and myoglobin), the activation of molecular oxygen (e.g. peroxidases and catalases) and electron transport (e.g. cytochromes and iron-sulfur proteins)[2].

Body iron compartments

The major portion of body iron is found in a number of *functional compounds*[1]. There are several iron porphyrin complexes. They include haemoglobin (30 mg/kg), myoglobin (4 mg/kg) and various haem- containing enzymes (1 mg/kg). There are also a number of other iron enzymes (1 mg/kg) that are found in tissues. They include metallo- flavoproteins and a variety of enzymes in which iron is a cofactor. In addition, there is a small but extremely important transport compartment (± 3 mg), in which iron is shuttled between tissues attached to transferrin. Iron in excess of functional needs is present in a *storage compartment* in which it is held in a relatively non-reactive form in the compounds ferritin and haemosiderin. Altogether the body contains a complement of 35–40 mg/kg of functional iron and a reserve of between 0 and 20 mg/kg of storage iron.

The functional compartment

Transferrin plays a central role in iron metabolism[3]. Not only does it maintain extracellular iron in a soluble form suitable for cellular uptake, but it also regulates the supply of iron to cells by influencing its distribution within the body and its availability to individual cells. Uptake of transferrin iron, in its turn, is determined largely by the cell's complement of transferrin receptors. Although such receptors are present in nearly all types of cell, they vary greatly in number depending on the cell type and its functional state. In this way the adequate supply of iron to meet individual needs is ensured and the uncontrolled entry of excessive amounts of iron into cells is prevented. Because of their large iron requirements for haemoglobin synthesis, transferrin receptors are particularly abundant on erythroid precursors and, as a result, the major iron circuit within the body is one involving the production and destruction of red cells.

There are normally only about 3 mg of transferrin-bound iron in the plasma of an adult, and the plasma iron turnover rate is approximately 30–40 mg per day[1]. This means that the plasma pool of transport iron turns over more than 10 times daily. Approximately 80 per cent of this iron is directed towards the erythroid bone marrow for haemoglobin synthesis. Once the red cells have lived out their life span they are phagocytosed in the reticuloendothelial system and the iron is returned to the plasma. Exchange with other tissues is at a much lower level. There is a limited bidirectional exchange between plasma transferrin and the liver, while exchange with other tissues is even less, with many retaining iron for relatively long periods and hence taking up very little iron from transferrin. The capacity to increase iron turnover through the plasma is large, with figures rising up to 10 times normal in chronic haemolytic states[1]. However, when iron deficiency is present, iron supply is not sufficient to supply the normal needs of the erythroid marrow, with the result that haemoglobin production decreases. In addition, the iron supply to all other tissues is similarly decreased.

The storage iron compartment

In normal subjects a variable quantity of iron is deposited in tissues in two forms which are closely related both structurally and functionally[1]. The diffuse soluble fraction is known as ferritin and the aggregated insoluble fraction as haemosiderin. These two compounds act as repositories for the storage of iron which is surplus to immediate body needs, with the level of stores in a particular individual reflecting the previous iron nutrition.

Changes in storage iron status can most conveniently be gauged by measuring the levels of serum ferritin, since they mirror the size of the iron stores, with each μg/l being equivalent to between 8 and 10 mg of storage iron[1]. The level is low at between 20 and 30 μg/l during late infancy, childhood and adolescence since most of the absorbed iron is needed for growth and an expanding red cell mass[4]. An appreciable increase occurs in males between the ages of 15 and 30 years, which is a reflection of the more favourable balance once growth has ceased. Thereafter a more gradual increase occurs, with a tendency to plateau after the age of 40–50 years[4,5]. The level at which this plateau occurs is usually around 100 μg/l[4], although higher figures have recently been reported from Australia[5]. The possible reasons for these differences will be discussed in a later section. In adult females the serum ferritin remains around 30 μg/l until after the menopause when it starts rising and eventually it nearly reaches the levels in males[4]. Variations in the iron status of different populations are reflected in their serum ferritin concentrations at different ages. For example, in Indian women, in whom iron deficiency is common, the expected rise does not occur after the menopause[6].

The measurement of serum ferritin levels has provided an invaluable tool for defining the two major disturbances of iron metabolism, iron deficiency and iron overload. It has proved particularly useful as a method for detecting the mildest stage of iron deficiency, which is storage iron depletion (serum ferritin < 12 μg/l), in epidemiological studies[1]. It is also helpful in detecting storage iron excess. However, the interpretation of a raised serum ferritin level is complicated by the fact that it is not specific for iron overload. Levels are also raised when hepatic disease is present and in acute and chronic inflammatory states[7]. In epidemiological studies excessive alcohol consumption creates special problems, since levels of serum ferritin can be raised without any other biochemical evidence of liver disease[5].

Definitions of iron status

Later sections include a discussion of iron balance and the regulatory mechanisms that exist in order to maintain the body iron content within physiological limits. To understand this discussion it is important to have an understanding of the different levels of iron status.

Normal iron status is present when the functional needs of the erythroid mass and all other tissues are satisfied. For such a state to be maintained it is helpful to have a reserve store of iron to meet any increase in iron requirements, such as occurs in pregnancy. In iron replete subjects living on a varied Western-type diet the average store in males is about 1000 mg, with a figure of about 300 mg in females, but there are considerable individual variations[1].

Iron depletion is the state when there is no storage iron present in the body. Although there is no evidence that an absence of iron stores has any adverse consequences, it does indicate that iron nutrition is borderline, since any further reduction in body iron is associated with a decrease in the level of functional compounds, such as haemoglobin.

Iron deficient erythropoiesis is the stage when the needs of the erythroid marrow for iron are no longer fully met and these unmet needs are associated with a rise in erythrocyte protoporphyrin and serum transferrin receptor levels. The haemoglobin level may still be above the arbitrary cut-off point for anaemia at this stage but with time, frank anaemia develops.

Iron deficiency anaemia is the most severe degree of iron deficiency. At this stage the restriction in haemoglobin production is severe enough to lead to distortion of red cells, with microcytosis and hypochromia.

Iron overload is the term usually reserved for situations in which the storage iron compartment is many times normal and the iron deposits are large enough to cause direct tissue damage[1]. Whether iron stores of much more limited degree, and indeed within the upper range of what has been regarded as normal, can be associated with pathology is a matter of current debate. The debate centres around whether or not subjects with such stores are at greater risk of developing cancer and ischaemic heart disease[8,9].

External iron exchange

Although external iron exchange is extremely limited in relation to the total body iron content, it is small variations in the balance between iron losses and dietary iron absorption that are responsible for the major disturbances of iron metabolism, namely iron deficiency and iron overload. The present section addresses the two sides of this equation, namely iron losses and iron absorption.

Quantitative aspects of iron losses

There are several sources of iron losses. These include basal obligatory losses, menstrual losses, losses incurred through pregnancy and, finally, pathological losses. Each will be considered separately.

Basal losses

Obligatory losses of iron in the adult male are derived from two main sources - the desquamation of surface cells from the skin, gastrointestinal and urinary tracts and the small amounts of gastrointestinal blood loss which occur even in normal individuals. The daily loss is less than 0.1 mg in the urine, 0.2–0.3 mg from the skin and 0.6 mg in faeces. Most of the iron in faeces represents blood loss, with only about 0.14 mg being derived from bile and desquamated cells[10]. Total iron losses in males therefore amount to about 0.9–1.0 mg daily (12–14 ng/kg/day). Because of smaller body surface areas, the losses in women would be expected to be correspondingly less and can be assumed to be in the range of 0.7–0.8 mg daily. Iron losses vary in relation to the iron content but within a narrow range which varies between 0.5 mg daily in iron deficiency[11] and 2–3 mg when iron overload is present[10]. While such variations may be the result of a regulatory process, it seems more likely that they merely reflect variations in the iron content of desquamated cells.

Menstrual losses

Median monthly menstrual blood loss in the adult female is between 20 and 30 mg. This loss increases daily requirements from a basal figure of about 0.8 mg to 1.47 mg, with a 90th percentile of 2.30[12]. Methods of contraception markedly influence iron losses. Oral contraceptives reduce losses by about 50 per cent, whereas intrauterine devices increase them by up to 100 per cent[13].

Pregnancy

Approximately 1000 mg iron is needed by a 55 kg woman during a normal pregnancy. This requirement includes 230 mg for basal losses, 450 mg for an increased red cell mass, 270–300 mg for the fetus, and 50–90 mg for the placenta. Since the greatest increase in fetal and erythropoietic requirements occurs late in gestation, the major requirements (5–6 mg per day) are in the second and third trimesters[1]. The iron present in the expanded red cell mass is returned to stores postpartum but this recovery is partially nullified by iron lost with peripartum blood loss. A period of amenorrhoea occurs postpartum, but iron losses via lactation are roughly equivalent to losses incurred via menstruation.

Pathological losses

Epidemiologically, the most important pathological losses of iron occur with hookworm infestation, which affects as many as 450 million people. It has been calculated that infestation with *Necator americanus* (± 5000 eggs per gram of faeces) increases the daily iron requirement by 3–4 mg[14]. It should, however, by emphasized that the hookworm load is small in the majority of subjects living in endemic areas and that other factors, such as the poor bioavailability of dietary iron, contribute to the widespread prevalence of iron deficiency anaemia in endemic areas.

Dietary iron absorption

The amount of iron absorbed from the diet at any one time is dependent on three factors: the quantity of iron, the composition of the diet and the behaviour of the mucosa of the upper small bowel.

Dietary iron content

Typical Western diets usually contain about 6 mg iron per 1000 kcal, with surprisingly little variation from meal to meal[15]. In certain circumstances the iron content is appreciably increased by extrinsic iron, either in the form of dirt or from the surface of containers or cooking vessels. The former is usually of very low bioavailability[16] but iron derived from pans or containers can add significantly to the absorbable iron intake, especially when the pH of the food being prepared in them is low[1]. This is strikingly illustrated by the traditional alcoholic beverages brewed in iron containers by Southern African blacks, whose daily iron intake may be increased from about 15 mg to as much as 100 mg[17].

Bioavailability of dietary iron

Variations in the bioavailability of food iron are of greater importance for iron nutrition than is the amount of iron in the diet. The haem iron in meat, poultry and fish is easily absorbed whatever the dietary composition[1], whereas non-haem iron is markedly influenced by other ingredients in the diet[15,18,19]. Haem iron is taken up by mucosal cells as such and the iron within it is therefore not exposed to the effects of the many ligands in the diet which inhibit non-haem iron absorption. In addition to containing haem, meat is a *promoter* of the absorption of the various forms of non-haem iron present in a mixed diet, possibly due to the release during digestion of amino acids which form stable complexes with iron[20]. The other single most important promoter of the absorption of non-haem iron is ascorbic acid, which not only is a powerful reductant, but also binds iron in equimolar fashion. Its action is dose dependent and it is effective in a number of dietary settings[15,18,21]. A number of *inhibitors* of iron absorption have also been identified. These include phytates present in bran[22,23], polyphenols in tea, coffee and certain vegetables[24], calcium salts,[12] and factors in soy protein.[26,27]. The bioavailability of the iron in any particular diet ultimately depends on the relative quantities of promoters and inhibitors of iron absorption present in that diet.

In addition to exogenous dietary ligands, the secretions of the upper intestinal tract influence non-haem iron absorption[1]. During peptic digestion a proportion of the non-haem iron in food is rendered ionizable, whereas haem is split from its globin bond. Gastric hydrochloric acid plays a key role in this regard and has been shown to be necessary for the adequate absorption of ferric iron salts and of non-haem food iron[1]. This is presumably because polymeric iron complexes are less likely to form at low pH. Although other components of the gastrointestinal secretions must obviously be relevant to iron absorption, in that they promote digestion with release of iron from food, they do not appear to contain a specific carrier.

Mucosal behaviour

Two major factors affect iron absorption, the body iron content and the rate of erythropoiesis. They will be considered separately.

Effect of body iron content: The size of the iron stores in the body has a major influence on iron absorption. This inverse relationship, which has been demonstrated in both animal experiments and in human studies, holds true over a wide range of iron stores[28–30]. In initial studies, stores were measured directly but in more recent ones the serum ferritin level which, as previously discussed, closely mirrors iron stores, has shown the same inverse relationship with iron absorption[28]. There are two distinct components. Absorption rises slowly when stores decline from high levels to lower levels, but a steep rise occurs when they approach depletion and iron supply to the erythroid marrow starts becoming compromised[30].

Although the rate of iron absorption is inversely related to the size of the body's iron stores, the limits within which this regulatory control is exercised are small. For example, the rate of reconstitution of iron stores in subjects with storage iron depletion suggests the increase occurs at less than 1 mg daily[31]. This is in agreement with the observation that the prevalence of anaemia increases in women with menstrual losses equivalent to more than 1 mg daily[32] and is also in agreement with the slow rate at which stores increase in women after the menopause[4,5]. In contrast, the rate rises to 4–5 mg daily when the needs of the erythroid marrow are not met[30]. This has led to the suggestion that there are two regulators of iron absorption, a store regulator and an erythroid regulator[31].

Effect of erythropoietic rate: When erythropoiesis is stimulated acutely there is a prompt rise in the absorption rate[33]. The relative importance of increased erythropoietic activity and the concomitant reduction in iron stores has been dissected out in experiments in human volunteers in which the erythroid marrow was stimulated by the injection of recombinant human erythropoietin and storage iron status was assessed by the levels of serum ferritin[34]. The brisk increase in erythropoiesis was accompanied by a fivefold increase in the absorption of dietary non-haem iron and when these data were adjusted to a common serum ferritin level the increase was still 2.5-fold, indicating a significant and independent erythropoietic effect. However, in chronic haemolytic states, such as congenital spherocytosis, the absorption rate is usually normal or close to normal[35]. In contrast, iron absorption is inappropriately increased in thalassaemia major and other anaemias associated with markedly increased but ineffective erythropoiesis. As a result, iron overload is a major complication of such anaemias.

The major differences in iron absorption patterns in different haemolytic states indicate that it is not the erythropoietic rate *per se* that affects absorption but rather some other component of erythropoietic activity[31]. In this context, it is noteworthy that the red cell protoporphyrin, which is a sensitive indicator of a deficient supply of iron to the marrow, is raised in thalassaemia major, which indicates that the large amounts of iron being delivered to the marrow via the plasma are still not sufficient to supply the needs of a markedly expanded erythroid mass[31]. Presumably the signal to the absorbing mucosa is the same one that increases the rate of iron absorption when there is an absolute decrease in the supply of iron to the erythroid marrow, as occurs with iron deficiency.

Regulatory control of iron absorption at a cellular level: Although the effects on iron absorption of the body iron content and of erythropoietic activity have been known for a long time, there is still no clear understanding of how control is mediated at a cellular level. At the same time, a good deal of information has accumulated on the various steps in the absorptive process.

The most active site of iron absorption is the duodenum and upper jejunum. There are two components of the absorptive mechanism, mucosal uptake and intracellular transport, with some regulation occurring at both phases[1].

Within the cell there are two major pathways. Iron is either transported within minutes into the portal circulation or is stored in the cell as ferritin[36]. The relative amounts following these alternate pathways depend on body demands for iron. When demand is high a large proportion of the iron entering the mucosal cell is transported rapidly into the body. As iron stores expand, an increasing proportion of the iron taken up by the cell is deposited in mucosal ferritin and is subsequently lost to the body at the end of the cell's 2–3 day life span[1]. Regulation of iron absorption may therefore occur at the point where iron entering from the lumen is directed along one or other of the two alternative pathways. Concentrations of mucosal ferritin are closely related to the absorptive process, with the intestinal concentrations of both L- and H-type ferritins being inversely correlated with iron absorption[37]. Whether mucosal cell ferritin plays an active or a passive role in iron absorption is not clear, but it seems likely that ferritin iron uptake is a passive response to the iron which accumulates within the cell rather than an active means of reducing the amount available for transporting to the circulation[36]. A proposal that mucosal transferrin may function as an active carrier in the absorptive process[38] has not been confirmed. No evidence of transferrin mRNA has been found in mucosal cells and transferrin concentrations have not been found to correlate with absorption rates[39]. The possibility that other proteins may be involved in the absorptive process must also be considered. Two such proteins have recently been described. The one is an iron-binding protein (*m* approximately 56 kDa) has been identified in the apical cytoplasm of proximal small intestinal cells in both rats and man[40]. The other is a glycoprotein, assembled as a trimer composed of 54 kDa monomers, which has been found in brush border plasma membranes[41].

The mechanisms involved in the control of iron absorption have not been elucidated. It has been suggested that the regulation is a local one, perhaps mediated by changes in the luminal secretions, the brush border receptors for iron, the intracellular transport protein, or the cells' ability to sequester ferritin, but no definitive evidence particularly favours any of these possibilities[1]. Attempts to demonstrate that the plasma iron transport system regulates iron absorption have been equally unsuccessful, as have searches for some humoral controlling mechanism[42]. Perhaps the most plausible of current hypotheses is that the iron content of individual tissues is itself a regulating factor[43]. A labile pool of iron available to transferrin is assumed to be present in all body tissues, the size of the pool in each tissue reflecting that tissue's iron stores. Iron uptake from transferrin is determined by the requirements of the erythroid marrow, and each tissue supplies iron to transferrin in proportion to its iron pool. Thus a decrease in tissue iron content results in an increased entrance of iron from the gut, whereas a rise in plasma iron turnover due to enhanced erythropoietic activity also results in increased iron absorption. Some experimental evidence supporting the hypothesis has been obtained in rats[44] but the exact nature of the mechanism by which the output of iron by donor tissues is regulated to match requirements still eludes explanation. In this connection, the discovery that a truncated form of the transferrin receptor circulates in the plasma, with the concentration correlating with the number of tissue receptors, has excited some interest. Whereas the concentration of the fragment increases sharply with enhanced or iron deficient erythropoiesis, there is no evidence that this has any direct effect on iron absorption[45].

One final point merits comment. In seeking to define normal regulatory control it may be particularly helpful to look at genetic disorders in which control is deranged. In this context, there are several in which different phases of the absorptive process are affected. Examples include two mutant strains of mice, one known as *mk* in which mucosal uptake is defective but cellular transfer is normal, and the other *sla* in which the reverse is the case[18]. Then there is hereditary haemochromatosis in which absorption is inappropriately raised due to increased mucosal iron transfer[7]. Finally, severe iron overload has recently been reported in three Japanese families with a mutation in the caeruloplasmin gene[46].

Quantitative aspects of dietary iron absorption

As discussed in the previous section, the mucosa of the gut has the ability to adjust its behaviour according to the body's need for iron. The capacity to increase iron absorption when the need arises is a large one and subjects with iron deficiency anaemia can absorb 20–40 mg of medicinal iron daily as long as the anaemia is present[47]. Thereafter there is sharp decline in the rate of absorption and iron stores are reconstituted at a slow rate. Insofar as iron absorption from the diet is concerned, the range of absorption is much less, with the ceiling being set by the relative bioavailability of iron in different foodstuffs. In quantitative terms, figures from balance studies in anaemic phlebotomized subjects indicate that they are able to replace as much as 3–4 mg of the iron loss daily, in addition to their normal excretory losses[48]. This is equivalent to a total absorption of 4–5 mg daily. These results were, however, obtained in subjects consuming a varied Western-type diet and lesser figures would be anticipated with diets of lower bioavailability. Unlike the mixed and varied diets consumed in industrialized countries, such diets tend to be cereal based and to contain large amounts of inhibitors of iron absorption, with little in the way of promoters.

Overall bioavailability of iron in different diets: Diets can be divided into those of low, intermediate and high iron bioavailability. These correspond to absorptions of about 5 per cent, 10 per cent and 15 per cent in subjects with depleted iron stores[49,50]. A diet of low bioavailability (< 5 per cent) has a high inhibitor content. It contains cereals, beans and tubers but negligible quantities of meat, fish, or ascorbic acid and is typically consumed in many developing countries. Such a diet supplies only about 0.7 mg of iron daily, which is insufficient to meet normal physiological requirements in females and in many males. A diet of intermediate bioavailability (± 10 per cent) is similar but includes limited amounts of food which promote iron absorption (meat, fish and/or ascorbic acid) and supplies enough iron (± 1.5 mg) to meet the needs of more than 50 per cent of women. The promoters in such diets may only be present during certain seasons. A diversified diet of high bioavailability (> 15 per cent) contains generous quantities of meat, poultry, or fish, together with ascorbic acid-containing vegetables and fruit and supplies at least 2.1 mg iron daily. It is typically eaten by many people in industrialized countries, where there is a low prevalence of iron deficiency anaemia. While such diets meet the needs of most adult members of the population, they cannot match the daily amounts required in the second half of pregnancy.

Limits of regulatory control of iron absorption

There is general agreement that it is the low bioavailability of iron in cereal-based diets that accounts for the high prevalence of iron deficiency in many developing countries and, as a result, a major focus of research interest has been on the development of methodologies, such as iron supplementation and fortification, to combat the problem. It is important that this research should be carried forward and expanded into implementation programmes, since iron deficiency has a number of adverse sequelae, apart from the anaemia, and it still represents a major challenge in the developing world. In this context, it is infants and women during these reproductive lives who are most vulnerable[51]. What is much more debatable is the need for the untargeted iron fortification programmes which are in place in many industrialized countries where iron deficiency is both less prevalent and usually of mild degree. It has been argued that such programmes, which are primarily directed at vulnerable groups, such as women during their reproductive years, may put at risk individuals with a genetic propensity to accumulate iron even in normal iron replete ones. At particular potential risk are individuals with the HLA-linked iron-loading disorder, hereditary haemochromatosis, and, to a lesser degree, those with iron-loading anaemias[52]. In addition, as previously mentioned, there have been recent disturbing claims, based on epidemiological data, which suggest that subjects with only modestly raised iron stores are at greater risk of developing malignancy[8] and ischaemic heart disease[9]. These current uncertainties raise a most important question and that is the degree to which the body's control mechanism can protect it from unwanted iron. The sources of the iron include the diet itself, fortification iron and extraneous iron. In this regard, special attention needs to be directed to those individuals who have a predisposition to absorb iron excessively.

Effects of dietary variations: Results of single-meal radioisotopic absorption studies have shown that the range of absorption of non-haem iron varies manyfold, depending on the presence of inhibitors, such as tea, and enhancers, such as meat and ascorbic acid[15,18]. These findings raise questions as to their long term effects in subjects consuming Western-type diets. In this regard, attempts at dietary manipulation over longer periods in normal volunteers have shown that bioavailability is affected by dietary variations but changes in the absorption rate have been less dramatic than would have been anticipated from single absorption studies. In one study a mean absorption figure of 6.4 per cent was obtained for subjects consuming their usual diet; comparable figures with strongly enhancing and inhibiting diets were 8.0 per cent and 3.2 per cent, respectively[53]. These results are not altogether surprising in the context of a varied Western-type diet, especially since the group tested included iron replete individuals. The point is underlined by a further study of the same type in which diets of high and medium bioavailability were compared. Bioavailability was significantly better in subjects with depleted iron stores but there were no differences in those with adequate stores[54]. These data suggest that both bioavailability and storage iron status are important and that at higher levels of iron stores, the body has the capacity to limit absorption in order to maintain iron balance.

The important role that dietary haem plays in ensuring adequate iron nutrition was discussed in a previous section. Of more relevance to the present discussion is the fact that its absorption is far less affected by the size of the body iron stores[55]. For example, in one study in which a standard meal containing meat was fed, the absorption of non-haem iron in iron replete and iron deficient subjects varied between 2.5 and 25 per cent, whereas that of haem iron ranged only between 25 and 47 per cent[40]. In addition, the percentage absorption of haem iron does not seem to vary much when differing amounts are fed. For example, when the haem iron content of a meal was increased from 0.3 to 4.5 mg in one study the percentage absorption remained relatively fixed at about 20 per cent[56]. These experimental findings suggest that stores above what have been regarded as the upper limit of normal way could accumulate in subjects consuming large amounts of meat. Recent epidemiological data from Australia, in which the meat consumption is high, suggest that this may, indeed, be so[5]. Studies in volunteers from a banking corporation and an insurance corporation, revealed median concentrations of serum ferritin in males at different ages that were more than double those previously reported. These figures translated to a body store of about 1900 mg and the difference remained high even when confounding variables, such as excessive ethanol consumption, were removed.

Effects of fortification iron and extraneous iron: Of most direct relevance to nutritional programmes are questions relating to the possible long term effects of iron fortification programmes on iron replete individuals, and especially adult males[52]. At present, evidence in this regard is inconclusive. A comparison of longitudinal survey data obtained in the NHANES II study (1976–1980) with pilot data from the NHANES III study (1987–1988) suggest that serum ferritin levels may have risen[57]. However, when the effects of iron fortification have been studied more directly, limited evidence has been obtained which suggests that control mechanisms may remain effective with small increments in dietary iron intake. In one study, an adult male with normal stores was given 10 mg iron daily as ferrous sulfate for 500 days without any significant change occurring in the serum ferritin level[58]. Similar results were noted in a fortification trial in an Indian population in which $NaFe^{III}EDTA$ was added to curry powder to provide approximately 7.5 mg extra dietary iron per day over a 2 year period[59]. Although the prevalence of anaemia in women dropped dramatically, there was no significant rise in serum ferritin levels in males who were over the age of 18 years at the beginning of the study.

The discussion thus far has focused on the possible deleterious effects of the relatively small amounts of fortification iron which are present in the diets of a number of countries throughout the world[60]. Further insight into this problem can be contained by examining what happens when much larger amounts of iron are ingested over extended periods. In this context, the dietary iron overload that is still prevalent in blacks living in rural parts of southern Africa merits special comment[1]. The extra iron is derived from the containers used for the preparation of brewed alcoholic beverages and is in a high bioavailable form. The dietary intake of iron in subjects consuming such drinks is often several times normal and iron overload of varying degrees has been found in a large proportion of males in affected populations[61]. It has been assumed until recently that this form of iron overload is solely due to environmental factors but this view has recently been challenged and it has been suggested that there is also a genetic component, different from the HLA-linked one responsible for hereditary haemochromatosis[62]. The evidence included the following points - a bimodal distribution of transferrin saturations in subjects exposed to increased dietary iron, the fact that only 17 per cent of subjects with an increased dietary intake are iron overloaded and, thirdly, the occurrence of the disorder in some young subjects. In addition, segregation analysis of iron overload pedigrees indicated that the effect was attributable to interaction with a single gene rather than being polygenic or due to environmental factors alone. This evidence can be regarded as suggestive but not conclusive. If confirmed, however, it will indicate that the absorbing mechanisms of normal subjects have the capacity to protect the body from very large quantities of iron in the diet.

Iron fortification and phenotypic expression in iron loading disorders: The two situations in which genetic factors have been definitely identified as being responsible for disordered iron balance leading to iron overload are hereditary haemochromatosis and iron- loading anaemias, such as thalassaemia major[7]. In the first, iron usually accumulates at a rate of about 2 mg daily, with clinical manifestations usually occurring between the 4th and 6th decades. The prevalence of the HLA-linked iron-loading gene responsible for the disorder varies in different Caucasoid populations, with between 0.3 and 4.0 per 1000 being homozygous. Phenotypic expression depends, not only on the severity of the metabolic defect and on the presence of sufficient quantities of absorbable iron in the diet, but also on physiological losses from the body. For example, menstruation in females and a smaller dietary intake diminish the positive balance so that full phenotypic expression occurs 10 times less often than in men[7]. Individuals heterozygote for the gene may exhibit modest increases in body iron but haemochromatosis does not develop[63]. With the widespread use of iron fortification which has occurred in industrialized countries over the past decades, it might have been anticipated that phenotypic expression might occur at younger ages and that more homozygotes would be presenting to hospitals with the fully developed disease[52]. This does not, however, seem to have occurred, at least in terms of hospital statistics. Between 1979 and 1987 the hospitalization rates of 4–13 per 100,000 persons in Medicaid (1984) and the National Health Discharge Survey (1979–1987) were similar to the estimates from 1955[64]. These results suggest that many subclinical cases are still being missed or that full phenotypic expression does not occur in many affected homozygous individuals or that the gene frequency is lower than previously calculated. The rate of iron accumulation in the iron-loading anaemias, such as thalassaemia major, is greater than in hereditary haemochromatosis (± 4–5 mg daily) and, as a result, clinical manifestations occur by the second decade. However, these conditions have less direct relevance to iron nutritional programmes, since affected individuals are identified clinically at an early age and, in any event, are usually maintained on blood transfusions which in themselves load the body with massive amounts of iron[65].

References

1. Bothwell, T.H., Charlton, R.W., Cook, J.D. & Finch, C.A. (1979): *Iron metabolism in man.* Oxford: Blackwell Scientific Publications.
2. Crichton, R.R. (1991): *Inorganic biochemistry of iron metabolism.* London: Ellis Horwood.
3. Baker, E. & Morgan, E.H. (1994): Iron transport. In: *Iron metabolism in health and disease*, eds. C.H. Brock, J.W. Halliday, M.J. Pippard & L.W. Powell, pp. 63–95. London: W.B. Saunders.
4. Cook, J.D., Finch, C.A. & Smith, N.J. (1976): Evaluation of the iron status of a population. *Blood* **48,** 449–455.

5. Leggett, B.A., Brown, N.N., Bryant, S.J., Duplock, L., Powell, L.W. & Halliday, J.W. (1990): Factors affecting the concentration of serum ferritin in a healthy Australian population. *Clin. Chem.* **36,** 1350–1355.

6. Ballot, D.E., MacPhail, A.P., Bothwell, T.H., Gillooly, M. & Mayet, F. (1989): Fortification of curry powder with NaFe(III)EDTA in an iron deficient population: initial survey of iron status. *Am. J. Clin. Nutr.* **49,** 156–161.

7. Bothwell, T.H., Charlton, R.W. & Motulsky, A.G. (1995): Haemochromatosis. In: *The metabolic and molecular basis of inherited disease*, eds. C.R. Scriver, A.L. Beaudet, W.S. Sly & D. Valle, pp. 2237–226. New York: McGraw Hill.

8. Stevens, R.G., Jones, D.Y., Micozzi, M.S. & Taylor, P.R. (1988): Body iron stores and the risk of cancer. *N. Engl. J. Med.* **319,** 1047–1052.

9. Salonen, J.T., Nyyssnen, K., Korpela, H., Tuomilehto, J., Seppänen, R. & Salonen, R. (1992): High stored iron levels are associated with excess risk of myocardial infarction in Eastern Finnish men. *Circulation* **86,** 803–811.

10. Green, R., Charlton, R., Seftel, H., Bothwell, T., Mayet, F., Adams, B., Finch, C. & Layrisse, M. (1968): Body iron excretion in man. A collaborative study. *Am. J. Med.* **45,** 336–353.

11. Dubach, R., Moore, C.V. & Callender, S. (1955): Studies in iron transport and metabolism. IX. The excretion of iron as measured by the isotope technique. *J. Lab. Clin. Med.* **45,** 599–615.

12. Hallberg, L. (1992): Iron requirements. Comments on methods and some crucial concepts in iron nutrition. *Biol. Trace. El. Res.* **35,** 25–45.

13. Nilsson, L. & Sölvell, L. (1967): Clinical studies on oral contraceptives - a randomized, double blind, cross over study of 4 different preparations. *Acta Obstet. Gynecol. Scand.* **46,** (Suppl 8), 1–39.

14. Layrisse, M. & Roche, M. (1964): The relationship between anaemia and hookworm infection. Results of surveys of a rural Venezuelan population. *Am. J. Hyg.* **79,** 279–301.

15. Hallberg, L. (1981): Bioavailability of dietary iron in man. *Ann. Rev. Med.* **1,** 123–147.

16. Derman, D.P., Bothwell, T.H., Torrance, J.D., MacPhail, A.P., Bezwoda, W.R., Charlton, R.W. & Mayet, F.G.H. (1981): *Scand. J. Haematol.* **29,** 18–24.

17. Charlton, R.W., Bothwell, T.H. & Seftel, H.C. (1973): Dietary iron overload. *Clin. Haematol.* **2,** 383–404.

18. Charlton, R.W. & Bothwell, T.H. (1983): Iron absorption. *Ann. Rev. Med.* **34,** 55–68.

19. Layrisse, M., Martinez-Torres, C., Méndez-Castellano, H., Taylor, P., Fossi, M., Lopes de Blanco, M. & Landaeta-Jimenez, M. (1990): Relationship between iron bioavailability from diets and the prevalence of iron deficiency. *Food Nutr. Bull.* **12,** 301–309.

20. Layrisse, M., Martinez-Torres, C., Cook, J.D., Walker, R. & Finch, C.A. (1973): Iron fortification of food: its measurement by the extrinsic tag method. *Blood* **41,** 333–352.

21. Hallberg, L., Brune, M. & Rossander, L. (1986): Effect of ascorbic acid on iron absorption from different types of meals. Studies with ascorbic acid given in different amounts with different meals. *Am. J. Appl. Nutr.* **40A,** 107–113.

22. Hallberg, L., Brune, M. & Rossander, L. (1989): Iron absorption in man: ascorbic acid and dose-dependent inhibition by phytate. *Am. J. Clin. Nutr.* **49,** 140–144.

23. Siegenberg, D., Baynes, R.D., Bothwell, T.H., Macfarlane, B.J., Lamparelli, R.D., MacPhail, A.P., Schmidt, U., Tal, A. & Mayet, F. (1991): Ascorbic acid prevents the dose-dependent inhibitory effect of phenols and phytates on non-heme iron absorption. *Am. J. Clin. Nutr.* **53,** 537–541.

24. Gillooly, M., Bothwell, T.H., Torrance, J.D., MacPhail, A.P., Derman, D.P., Bezwoda, W.R. & Mills, W. (1983): The effects of organic acids, phytates and polyphenols on the absorption of iron from vegetables. *Br. J. Nutr.* **49,** 331–347.

25. Hallberg, L., Brune, M., Erlandsson, M., Sandberg, A.S & Rossander-Hultén, L. (1991): Calcium effect of different amounts on non-heme and heme-iron absorption in humans. *Am. J. Clin. Nutr* **53,** 112–119.

26. Hurrell, R.F., Juillerat, M.A. & Reddy, M.B. (1992): Soy protein, phytate and iron absorption in humans. *Am. J. Clin. Nutr.* **56,** 573–578.

27. Lynch, S.R., Dassenko, S.A. & Cook, J.D. (1994): Inhibitory effect of a soybean-protein-related moiety on iron absorption in humans. *Am. J. Clin. Nutr.* **60,** 567–572.

28. Walters, G.O., Jacobs, A., Worwood, M., Trevett, D. & Thomson, W. (1975): Iron absorption in normal subjects and patients with idiopathic haemochromatosis: a relationship with serum ferritin concentration. *Gut* **16,** 188–192.

29. Bezwoda, W.R., Bothwell, T.H., Torrance, J.D., MacPhail, A.P., Charlton, R.W., Kay, G. & Levin, J. (1979): The relationship between marrow iron stores, plasma ferritin concentrations and iron absorption. *Scand. J. Haematol.* **22,** 113–120.

30. Baynes, R.D., Bothwell, T.H., Bezwoda, W.R., MacPhail, A.P. & Derman, D.P. (1987): Relationship between absorption of inorganic and food iron in field studies. *Ann. Nutr. Metab.* **31,** 109–116.

31. Finch, C.A. (1994): Regulation of iron balance in humans. *Blood* **84,** 1697–1702.

32. Hallberg, L., Hogdahl, A.M., Nilsson, L. & Rybo, G. (1966): Menstrual blood loss and iron deficiency. *Acta Med. Scand.* **180,** 639–650.

33. Bothwell, T.H., Pirzio-Biroli & G. & Finch, C.A. (1958): Iron absorption. I. Factors influencing absorption. *J. Lab. Clin. Med.* **51,** 24–36.

34. Skikne, B.S. & Cook, J.D. (1992): Effect of enhanced erythropoiesis on iron absorption. *J. Lab. Clin. Med.* **120,** 746–751.

35. Pootrakul, P., Kitcharoen, K., Pornpan, Y., Wasi, P., Fucharoen, S., Charoenlarp, P., Brittenham, G., Pippard, M.J. & Finch, C.A. (1988): The effect of erythroid hyperplasia on iron balance. *Blood* **71,** 1124–1129.

36. Cook, J.D. (1989): Adaptation in iron metabolism. *Am. J. Clin. Nutr.* **51,** 301–308.

37. Whittaker, P., Skikne, B.S., Covell, A.M., Flowers, C., Cooke, A. & Lynch SR (1991): Duodenal iron proteins in idiopathic haemochromatosis. *J. Clin. Invest.* **83,** 261–267.

38. Huebers, H., Huebers, E., Csiba, E., Rummel, W. & Finch, C.A. (1983): The significance of transferrin for intestinal iron absorption. *Blood* **61,** 283–290.

39. Baynes, R.D. (1994): Iron absorption. In: *Iron metabolism in health and disease*. eds. J.H. Brock, J.W. Halliday, M.J. Pippard & L.W. Powell, pp. 150–187. London: W.B. Saunders.

40. Conrad, M.E. & Umbreit, J.N. (1993); A concise review: iron absorption - the mucin-mobilferrin-integrin pathway. A competitive pathway for metal absorption. *Am. J. Hematol.* **42,** 67–73.

41. Teichmann, R. & Stremmel, W. (1990): Iron uptake by human upper small intestine microvillous membrane vesicles. Indication for a facilitated transport mechanism mediated by a membrane iron-binding protein. *J. Clin. Invest.* **86,** 2145–2153.

42. Rosenmund, A., Gerber, S., Huebers, H. & Finch, C. (1980): Regulation of iron absorption and storage iron turnover. *Blood* **56,** 30–37.

43. Cavill, I., Worwood, M. & Jacobs, A. (1975); Internal regulation of iron absorption. *Nature* **256,** 328–329.

44. Finch, C.A., Huebers, H., Eng, M. & Miller, L. (1982): Effect of transfused reticulocytes on iron exchange. *Blood* **59,** 364–369.

45. Cook, J.D., Dassenko, S. & Skikne, B.S. (1990): Serum transferrin receptor as an index of iron absorption. *Br. J. Haematol.* **75,** 603–610.

46. Yoshida, K., Furihata, K., Takeda, S., Nakamura, A., Yamamoto, K., Morita, H., Hiyamuta, S., Ikeda, S., Shimizu, N. & Yanagisiwa, N. (1995): A mutation of the ceruloplasmin gene in association with systemic haemosiderosis in humans. *Nature Genet.* **9,** 267–272.

47. Norrby, A. & Sölvell, L. (1974): Iron absorption and haemoglobin regeneration in posthaemorrhagic anaemia. Studies on the absorption pattern during oral iron therapy. *Scand. J. Haematol.* (Suppl 20) 15–32.

48. Finch, S., Haskins, D. & Finch, C.A. (1950): Iron metabolism. Hematopoiesis following phlebotomy. Iron as a limiting factor. *J. Clin. Invest.* **29,** 1078–1086.

49. Monsen, E.R., Hallberg, L., Layrisse, M., Hegsted, D.M., Cook, J.D., Mertz, W. & Finch, C.A. (1978): Estimation of available dietary iron. *Am. J. Clin. Nutr.* **31,** 134–141.

50. FAO/WHO Joint Expert Consultation Report. Requirements of vitamin A, iron, folate and vitamin B_{12} (1988): *Food Nutrit. Ser.* **23,** FAO.

51. DeMaeyer, E. & Adiels-Tegman, M. (1985): The prevalence of anaemia in the world. *World Health Stat. Q.* **38,** 302–316.

52. Bothwell, T.H. & Charlton, R.W. (1982): A general approach to the problem of iron deficiency and iron overload in the population at large. *Sem. Hematol.* **19,** 54–67.

53. Cook, J.D., Dassenko, S.A. & Lynch, S.R. (1991): Assessment of the role of nonheme-iron availability in iron balance. *Am. J. Clin. Nutr.* **54,** 717–722.

54. Hultén, L., Gramatkovski, E., Gleerup, A. & Hallberg, L. (1995): Iron absorption from the whole diet. Relation to meal composition, iron requirements and iron stores. *Eur. J. Clin. Nutr.* **49,** 794–808.

55. Carpenter, C.E. & Mahoney, A.W. (1992): Contributions of heme and nonheme iron to human nutrition. *Crit. Rev. Food Sci. Nutr.* **31,** 333–367.

56. Bezwoda, W.R., Bothwell, T.H., Charlton, R.W., Torrance, J.D., MacPhail, A.P., Derman, D.P. & Mayet, F.G. (1983): The relative dietary importance of haem and non-haem iron. *S. Afr. Med. J.* **64,** 552–556.

57. Looker, A.C., Gunter, E.W., Cook, J.D., Green, R. & Harris, J.W. (1991): Comparing serum ferritin values from different population study. National Center for Health Statistics. *Vital. Health Stat.* **2,** (III) 1–18.

58. Sayers, M.H., English, G. & Finch, C.A. (1994): The capacity of the store-regulator in maintaining iron balance. *Am. J. Hematol.* **47,** 194–197.

59. Ballot, D.E., MacPhail, A.P., Bothwell, T.H., Gillooly, M. & Mayet, F. (1989): Fortification of curry powder with NaFe(III)EDTA in an iron deficient population: report of a controlled iron-fortification trial. *Am. J. Clin. Nutr.* **49,** 162–169.

60. Bothwell, T.H. & MacPhail, A.P. (1992): Prevention of iron deficiency by food fortification. In: *Nutritional anemias*, eds. S.J. Forman & S. Zlotkin, pp.183–192. New York: Raven Press.

61. Bothwell, T.H. & Isaacson, C. (1962): Siderosis in the Bantu. A comparison of the incidence in males and females. *Brit. Med. J.* **1,** 522–524.

62. Gordeuk, V., Ndambire, S., Emmanual, J., Nakanza, N., Chapanduka, Z., Randall, M., Boone, P., Romano, P., Martell, R.W., Yamashita, T., Eller, P., Mukiibi, J., Hasstedt, S.J., Samowitz, W., Edwards, C.Q. & West, G. (1992): Iron overload in Africa. Interaction between a gene and dietary iron content. *N. Engl. J. Med.* **326,** 95–100.

63. Powell, L.W., Jazwinska, E. & Halliday, J.W. (1994): Primary iron overload. In: *Iron metabolism in health and disease*, eds. J.H. Brock, J.W. Halliday, M.J. Pippard, L.W. Powell pp. 227–270. London: W.B. Saunders.

64. Gable, C.B. (1992): Haemochromatosis and dietary iron supplementation: Implications from US mortality morbidity and health survey data. *J. AM. Diet. Ass.* **92,** 208–212.

65. Pippard, M.J. (1994): Secondary iron overload. In: *Iron metabolism in health and disease*, eds. J.H. Brock, J.W. Halliday, M.J. Pippard & L.W. Powell, pp. 271–309. London: W.B. Saunders.

Iron Nutrition in Health and Disease, edited by Leif Hallberg and Nils-Georg Asp

Chapter 2

Control of cellular iron transport and storage at the molecular level

Lukas C. Kühn

Swiss Institute for Experimental Cancer Research, CH- 1066 Epalinges Lausanne, Switzerland

Summary

Iron is both essential and potentially toxic for cells. It is generally assumed, therefore, that iron homeostasis should be carefully controlled. Indeed, in healthy individuals there is a constant balance between iron recycling and tissue consumption, as well as between small organismic losses and intestinal iron absorption. This steady state equilibrium is the result of mechanisms whereby individual cells control iron uptake, storage, utilization and release. Not only proliferating cells, but also cells involved in particular iron-related functions are capable of sensing intracellular 'free' iron and adjusting to specific physiological needs by regulating the key mediators for iron uptake and storage, transferrin receptor and ferritin, respectively. Recent research has elucidated the molecular nature of this feedback system. The control mechanisms involve changes in mRNA translation and stability. This is achieved by interaction of regulated mRNAs with cytoplasmic iron regulatory proteins (IRP-1 and IRP-2), whose RNA-binding activity is highly sensitive to changes in iron levels. IRPs are also modulated by substances such as nitric oxide, hydrogen peroxide and possibly phosphorylation. Thus, there exists a network of adaptive processes in response to both an unbalance in iron and natural stimuli. Further investigations should clarify their full significance to iron physiology in various tissues and possibly provide new insight into certain disorders of iron metabolism and the control of intestinal iron absorption.

Iron as an essential element in cellular metabolism

Iron plays a role of central importance in oxygen transport by haemoglobin and myoglobin. As a constituent of the active site in numerous enzymes, iron participates also in many key reactions of the cellular metabolism, notably in mitochondrial electron transport, the citric acid cycle, reactions of detoxification and the synthesis of deoxyribonucleotides (Table 1; for reviews see Refs 1 and 2.) The catalytic action of iron is often, but not exclusively, related to the redox properties of the element. Depending on the protein, iron is either incorporated into haem, associated with an Fe-S cluster or directly protein-bound. Since many iron-dependent functions are essential to cell survival, it is evident that iron has to reach the sites of protein assembly in the cytoplasm or organelles in adequate amount and appropriate form as di- or trivalent iron (whether complexed or not is unknown). This is particularly critical in proliferating cells which have to resynthesize the entire set of cellular enzymes. Therefore, a multicellular organism must have appropriate mechanisms of iron absorption from nutrition, distribution to tissues and transport across cell layers and membrane barriers.

In man about 70 per cent of the 3–5 g total body iron is present in haemoglobin, some 3–5 per

Table 1. Mammalian proteins containing iron

Proteins	Function	Location
Haem-containing proteins		
Haemoglobin	Transport of oxygen	Erythrocyte
Myoglobin	Binding of oxygen	Muscle
Cytochromes (b, c, c_1, a, a_3), cytochrome oxidase	Electron transfer in respiratory chain	Mitochondrion
Catalase, peroxidase	Enzymatic cleavage of peroxides	Peroxisome
Dioxygenases, mono-oxygenases (several, some without haem, cytochromes P450)	Hydroxylations detoxification steroid synthesis	Several tissues liver microsomes adrenal gland
Iron-Sulphur-containing proteins		
Dehydrogenases (several flavoproteins)	Electron transfer	Mitochondrion
Aconitase	Citric acid cycle	Mitochondrion
Iron-binding proteins		
Ribonucleotide-reductase	Deoxynucleotide synthesis	Cytoplasm
Transferrin	Carrier of iron	Serum
Lactoferrin	Carrier of iron	Mucosal secretions
Iron-storage proteins		
Ferritin	Iron deposits	Cytoplasm

cent in muscle myoglobin, and about 10 per cent in other cellular proteins. The remaining iron is stored in ferritin, which forms a hollow shell composed of 24 heavy and light subunits that can accommodate in its internal space up to 4500 Fe^{3+} ions in the form of ferrihydrite. Although transient storage of iron is a natural phenomenon of all cells, it has also been looked upon as a detoxification mechanism, since iron in its 'free', non-protein-bound form catalyses the formation of reactive oxygen species (see Chapter 21).

In order to maintain the supply of iron to all cells, and particularly those of the bone marrow involved in haemoglobin synthesis, there exists a dynamic exchange between tissues. This amounts to about 30 mg daily and derives predominantly from the degradation of senescent erythrocytes in reticuloendothelial cells. Comparatively, only a small fraction is absorbed from nutrition (1–3 mg), just enough to compensate the moderate losses from the organism. This daily recycling of close to 1 per cent of the body iron involves the major carrier of iron in serum, transferrin, which can bind two Fe^{3+} ions. The total amount of transferrin in serum (about 2 mg/ml) is such that on average every protein molecule will get loaded and deliver iron twice per day. Yet, under normal conditions only about 30–40 per cent of the transferrin-binding sites get saturated, and at any time no more than 0.15 per cent of the body iron circulates in serum. This underlines the highly dynamic removal of iron from circulation, too. Diferric transferrin is endocytosed and unloaded wherever it encounters cell surface receptors for transferrin. These receptors constitute the admission sites of iron to cells, and their expression limits its access. Iron-59 uptake is proportional to the endocytosis of transferrin in primary erythroid cells[3] and fibroblast cell lines with artificially over-expressed transferrin receptors[4]. This relationship holds true only as long as the iron-binding capacity of transferrin is not exceeded. Beyond this threshold, notably in iron overload, mechanisms of non-transferrin-bound iron uptake come into play[5].

Although transferrin receptor can be considered as the major gate for iron entry into cells, we should not think of it as the only iron uptake mechanism. Particularly in liver parenchymal cells, but also some other cell types additional ways to absorb iron were found: notably transport of non-protein-bound iron[5], ferritin receptors[6,7] and asialoglycoprotein receptors which may capture desialylated transferrin[8] contribute to iron uptake. Moreover, products of haemolysis, haem-haemopexin complexes [9] and haemoglobin-haptoglobin complexes[10,11] are specifically absorbed in the liver.

Cellular iron absorption at the molecular level, an only partially solved problem

In most cells the key molecule for iron uptake is the surface receptor for transferrin (reviewed in Refs 5 and 12). This receptor binds preferentially iron-loaded transferrin and mediates its endocytosis. The receptor is a glycosylated protein of 760 amino acids with a single transmembrane spanning region and a 65 amino acid NH_2-terminal domain that interacts with coated vesicle components during endocytosis[13–15]. The receptor forms disulfide-linked homodimers, and each subunit has one transferrin-binding site in its extracellular domain. Receptors are continuously internalized in coated vesicles, independently of their loading with transferrin[16,17], and reach the endosomal compartment from where they recycle to the cell surface within minutes. Under physiological conditions most surface receptors become saturated with transferrin, since the concentration of diferric transferrin is about 100-fold above the K_d for the ligand- receptor interaction ($K_d = 5 \times 10^{-9}$ M) and shows rapid association kinetics at neutral pH. These receptor- transferrin complexes remain stable in the low pH (about 5.5) of the endosome. However, iron dissociates from transferrin at low pH and is transported across the endosomal membrane. It is only after receptor recycling to a neutral pH at the cell surface that apotransferrin dissociates rapidly, making both the ligand and receptor available for further rounds of iron absorption[18–21]. This entire pathway takes about 15 min. The number of receptors, as well as their endocytosis and recycling rates are limiting to the accumulation of $^{59}Fe^{3+}$. However, since endocytosis serves many other nutritional purposes, the formation of coated vesicles is a rather constitutive process, and rates of receptor recycling vary within a range of no more than threefold in different cell types or physiological conditions (reviewed in Ref. 12). In contrast, transferrin receptor numbers can change much more, due both to transcriptional and post-transcriptional regulation of gene expression.

Transferrin receptors are readily detected on rapidly dividing cells where 10,000 to 100,000 molecules are commonly found on tumour cells or cell lines in culture. In contrast non-proliferating cells show much lower expression, and receptors are frequently undetectable. For example, stimulation of lymphocytes with mitogenic agents induces receptor mRNA from a virtually undetectable to a significant and at least 50-fold higher level within less than 4 h. This induction is the result of an early transcriptional activation and a subsequent stabilization of the mRNA in the cytoplasm[22,23]. Besides, in certain tissues with specific iron-related functions, such as reticulocytes synthesizing haemoglobin or placenta and brain endothelium that ensure iron transport across cell layers, transferrin receptors persist after differentiation even when cell growth has largely stopped. It seems likely that this is also due to transcriptional control mechanisms. Thus, at large, transferrin receptor expression seems to correlate with the genuine needs for cellular iron.

Unfortunately, besides the role of transferrin as the serum iron carrier and the surface transferrin receptors in its capturing and endocytosis, we remain astonishingly ignorant about many other aspects of iron absorption. An important gap in our knowledge concerns iron transport across membranes, be it at the intestinal microvillus membrane, the hepatocyte plasmamembrane, or the endosomal membrane. The description of iron release from reticuloendothelial cells remains similarly incomplete. It seems likely that transmembrane transport in vertebrate cells is mediated by one or more ion-transport systems. Recent progress was made on kinetic aspects of non-transferrin-bound iron transport in reticulocytes and hepatocytes from certain iron chelates, citrate, ascorbate or iron sulfate in isotonic sucrose (reviewed in Refs 5 and 24). A weak point of most studies remains, however, the lack of information about the membrane proteins involved. Two groups have come forward with iron-binding proteins on the microvillus surface that they consider as facilitators of iron transport[25–28]. One of them, a 56 kDa protein which binds iron (mobilferrin) was also found associated with integrins at the surface of K562 erythroleukaemia cells[29]. Since iron transport across membranes is thought to require reduction of iron and a protein with multiple transmembrane helices to form a channel, it is quite unlikely that these iron-binding proteins or integrins are sufficient to explain the transport mechanism. Whereas bacteria or plants use specific chelators and distinct, probably non-conserved mechanisms of iron uptake, it is possible that studies on the yeast *Saccharomyces cerevisiae* may bring new insights to iron transport in vertebrates. Iron transport in yeast requires at least a surface oxidoreductase, a multiple transmembrane spanning protein and a copper-containing oxidase that have been genetically identified and cloned[30–32].

Coordinate control of iron uptake, storage and utilization

Many key proteins in mammalian cell iron metabolism are controlled by intracellular iron availability. However, absolutely exceptional and unseen in any biological system is the type of coordinate control exerted by iron, which can be qualified as self-regulatory and which involves specific mRNA-protein interactions in the cytoplasm (for recent reviews see Refs 33–36). The discovery of these specific feedback mechanisms started with studies by Munro and co-workers who found that translation of ferritin was induced by iron and repressed after iron chelation[37]. They showed that a region in the 5^1 untranslated region of H and L ferritin mRNAs was both necessary and sufficient to permit this repression[38]. This region forms a specific RNA stem-loop structure, a so called 'iron responsive element' (IRE)[39] (Fig. 1) which interacts with a cellular protein known as 'iron regulatory protein' (IRP)[40]. Binding of IRP to the IRE of ferritin mRNAs prevents ribosome attachment and inhibition of translation[38,41–43]. As a result ferritin and iron storage decrease in iron deprived cells. *In vitro* this interaction can be measured by the incubation of ^{32}P-labelled RNA with cytoplasmic cell extracts[40,44]. Using this assay it was shown that IRP becomes active as an RNA-binding protein when cells are deprived of iron, i.e. in the presence of an iron chelator[44,45]. In contrast, the RNA-binding activity of IRP is inactivated by sufficient iron supply. The intermediate target most likely is a 'free' chelatable iron pool in the cytoplasm which then influences IRP.

By now six different mRNAs have been shown to contain one or more IREs (Fig. 1). In addition to those of H- and L-ferritin mRNA, a single IRE is present in the 5^1 untranslated regions of erythroid 5-aminolevulinate synthase[46,47], porcine mitochondrial aconitase mRNA[47] and *Drosophila melanogaster* succinate dehydrogenase subunit b mRNA[84]. Each of these proteins (except for mitochondrial aconitase which remains to be studied) is iron-dependently regulated in its translation by the same control mechanism as ferritins. In the case of 5-aminolevulinate synthase, it has been postulated that translational inhibition may slow protoporphyrin synthesis in erythroid cells when iron is limiting[48–50]. It remains less clear why certain enzymes that function in the citric acid cycle should be regulated by iron levels.

A very interesting mRNA with IREs is that of transferrin receptor mRNA as it contains five such RNA stem-loop structures clustered in the middle of an exceptionally long 3^1 untranslated region[39]. Under low iron conditions, each of these IREs can bind one cytoplasmic IRP[44,51]. Based on correlative studies and extensive mutational analysis, it has been concluded that the IRE-IRP interactions stabilize transferrin receptor mRNA, presumably by preventing endonucleolytic cleavage by an RNase in the vicinity of the IREs[44,52]. A potential site for cleavage within the regulatory region has been identified, but the putative endonuclease remains to be defined[53]. This iron-dependent regulation of transferrin receptor mRNA leads to a threefold induction of surface transferrin receptor in response to iron chelation[54]. As a consequence the cells internalize more iron[13].

Although transferrin receptor is regulated opposite to ferritin, the two mechanisms cooperate to restore the 'free' intracellular iron pool. Less iron storage and enhanced iron uptake will

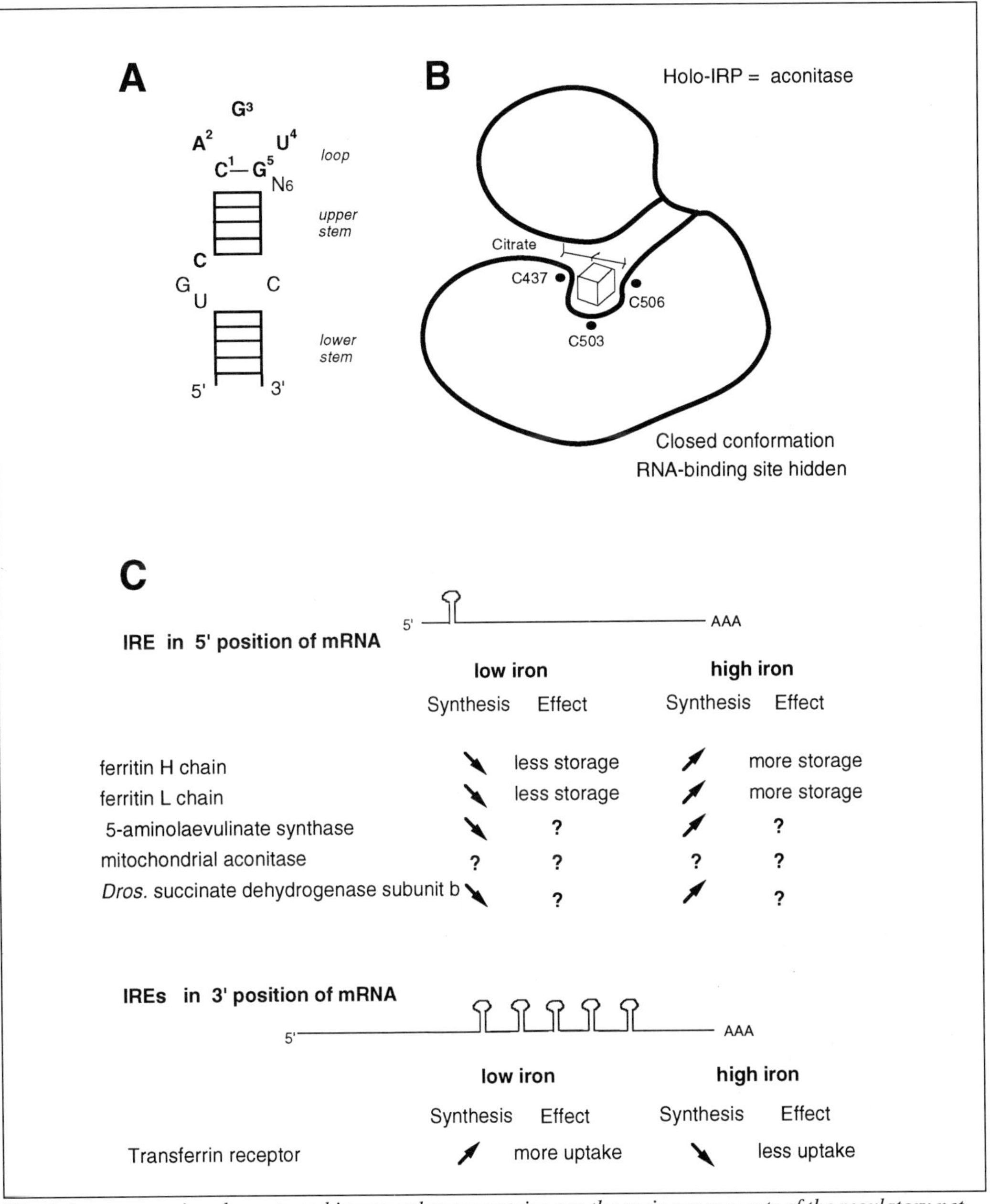

Fig. 1. Iron responsive elements and iron regulatory proteins are the main components of the regulatory network in iron metabolism. The typical wild-type IRE (A) is highly conserved in evolution and present in all mRNAs that are regulated. The IRE is an RNA stem-loop in which an upper stem with five paired nucleotides and a lower stem of variable length confer stability to the structure. 5′ to the upper stem is always an unpaired C, and a six-nucleotide loop comprises almost invariably the sequence CAGUGN. The schematic representation of IRP-1 (B) is based on the crystal structure of mitochondrial aconitase. IRP-1 is itself an aconitase when there is enough cytoplasmic iron to form a [4Fe–4S]-cluster. However, in iron deprived conditions, IRP-1 lacks the cluster and adopts a conformation that interacts strongly with IREs. Various mRNAs (C) are regulated by IRE-IRP interactions with physiological consequences as indicated.

make more iron available for the biosynthesis of iron-containing proteins. This is required when cells are confronted with an iron deprived situation due to insufficient iron supply or a physiological change like the onset of cell proliferation. Under high iron conditions, however, the regulatory balance will be inverted, and the increased iron storage along with lower iron uptake can protect the cells from iron overload and the production of damaging radicals.

Iron regulatory proteins, the sensory switch of iron homeostasis

Recent evidence shows that there exist two distinct IRPs (IRP-1 and IRP-2) with 79 per cent sequence similarity in mammals[55,56] (Table 2). IRP-1 is present in all tissues with a most prominent expression in liver, kidney and intestine[56–58]. IRP-1 was shown to be identical with a cytoplasmic aconitase and under conditions of normal iron supply it contains a [4Fe-4S]-cluster which is bound to three cysteine residues[59–61]. The mature enzyme converts citrate to isocitrate, but lacks entirely RNA-binding activity (Fig. 1). In contrast, under conditions of iron deprivation, the enzyme cannot mature to the holoprotein, and instead apoprotein without an iron-sulfur cluster accumulates[61,62]. This apoprotein binds IREs with high affinity, but lacks aconitase activity. It can therefore be concluded that the formation and insertion of the iron-sulfur cluster is a decisive event in the control of RNA binding. It seems likely that IRP undergoes a structural change when the iron-sulfur cluster is inserted such that the RNA-binding site gets hidden. By site-directed mutagenesis of cysteines which hold the cluster it was possible to modify IRP-1 such that it remained constitutively in its IRE-binding conformation, independent of cellular free iron levels[63,64]. Expression of such a mutated IRP in a cell line provokes permanent changes in the expression of ferritin and transferrin receptor[65].

Besides iron levels, several conditions can perturb the RNA-binding activity of IRP-1. *In vitro*, the apoprotein readily forms intramolecular disulfide bridges between the unoccupied cysteines of the cluster-binding site, and this inhibits binding to the IRE[63]. It is conceivable, therefore, that the reduction potential in an iron deprived cell may influence the IRE-IRP interaction. However, freshly isolated apo-IRP is usually found to be active, suggesting that the cytoplasmic environment is sufficiently reducing due to glutathione. IRP-1 is a rather stable protein, and full IRE-binding activity in cells is only obtained after about 12–15 h of iron deprivation[44]. This raises the question as to whether the active form derives from *de novo* synthesis of apoprotein and/or iron-sulfur cluster disassembly in the holoprotein. Translation inhibitors, cycloheximide or anisomycin, delay apoprotein accumulation, but do not entirely abolish it[66]. In other words, the apoprotein accumulates both by *de novo* synthesis or from the

Table 2. Distinctive features of iron regulatory proteins

Properties	IRP-1	IRP-2	References
Molecular mass	98 kDa	105 kDa	55, 56, 81–83
Tissue distribution	wide	more restricted	55, 57, 58
Induction by iron deprivation	yes	yes	44, 55, 66, 76
Inactivation in high iron by	Fe-S cluster	protease	55, 60, 61, 66, 76
Relative affinity for IRE	0.61 nM	0.63 nM	58
Migration of RNA in bandshift assay[1)]	slow	faster	40, 58, 74, 80
Elution from DEAE-Sephacel[1)]	25 mM KCl	150-200 mM KCl	58
Recognition by anti-IRP-1 peptide 1-13	yes	no	58
Activation by 2% β-mercaptoethanol	yes	no	58, 74

[1)] This difference has been reported for mouse and rat IRPs, whereas human IRP-1 and IRP-2 comigrate and have presumably a similar charge.

holoprotein by disassembly of the iron-sulfur cluster. Furthermore, IRP-1 is artificially activated to become IRE-binding by the presence of high concentrations of 2-mercaptoethanol. This does not involve the disassembly of the Fe-S cluster[63].

Recent evidence shows that natural cellular compounds NO and H_2O_2 also strongly activate IRP-1. Induction of NO synthase by interferon in macrophages leads to a response within about 12 h, similar to that seen with an iron chelator[67,68], and this affects ferritin and transferrin receptor levels[69]. It is accompanied by the loss of cytoplasmic aconitase activity[67]. The response can be mimicked *in vitro* with recombinant IRP-1 and NO gas in solution, but remains somewhat incomplete leaving doubts as to whether NO is capable of promoting the disassembly of Fe-S clusters or whether it acts only as an iron chelator[67]. In contrast, activation of IRP-1 by H_2O_2 is much more rapid and occurs within 30 min[70,71]. This effect seems sensitive to okadaic acid and was, therefore, postulated to involve a protein phosphatase[71]. Ascorbic acid known to reduce iron has an opposite effect when added to cells and tends to stimulate ferritin synthesis possibly by inactivating IRP[72]. Finally it was also reported that IRP-1 is a substrate for phosphorylation at serine residues, and that this may influence its RNA-binding activity[73]. The physiological implications of these compounds or modifications are still not entirely understood at present. The possible links between iron metabolism and natural stimulators of NO synthesis, H_2O_2 accumulation or protein phosphorylation need to be explored further. Since cytokines play a role in inflammation, it would not be surprising if changes in IRP activity occurred that might explain inflammation- related redistribution of iron.

The second IRE-binding protein, IRP-2, has only recently been characterized[55,56,58,74]. It shares numerous features with IRP-1, notably a high affinity for IRE-containing mRNAs (Table 2). At least *in vitro* IRP-2 was shown to inhibit ferritin translation[75]. IRP-2 is readily detected by IRE-protein bandshift assays in rodents, but IRE-IRP-2 complexes of human cell extracts comigrate with those of IRP-1 and cannot easily be distinguished, unless specific antibodies are used[58,74]. The activity of this IRP-2 is less abundant than that of IRP-1 in most cells[58]. In mouse tissue extracts IRP-2 is clearly visible in intestine and brain[55,58]. Unlike IRP-1, IRP-2 has no aconitase activity, and it remains uncertain that its RNA-binding activity is regulated by an Fe-S cluster[74]. It seems rather that IRP-2 decays rapidly in high iron conditions[55,76]. This may offer cells yet another way to regulate iron levels in response to specific stimuli. Interestingly, IRP-2 gets more strongly induced under certain experimental conditions than IRP-1[77,78].

We have recently analysed the possibility that IRP-1 and IRP-2 may have different target mRNAs and have determined by appropriate selection procedures the RNA-binding specificity of each protein[79] (submitted). They both show strongest affinity for the naturally occurring wild-type IRE (Fig. 1). However, certain mutations in the IRE are tolerated and induce only a moderate loss in affinity. IRP-1 and IRP-2 recognize a spectrum of suboptimal IRE-like sequences that are overlapping but not identical. For the time being all known IREs in mRNAs correspond to the highly conserved wild-type sequence, and it remains unknown whether there exist mRNAs with variant IRE sequences. At least none have been detected yet in computer searches of databases. Besides this issue, the present analysis has left us with specific IRE targets that are selectively recognized by either IRP-1 or IRP-2. These reagents should prove useful in distinguishing the RNA-binding activity of IRP-1 and IRP-2, particularly in human cells where complexes comigrate.

Possible role of IRP in intestinal iron absorption

The coordinate feedback regulation of iron at the level of mRNA is a central feature of iron metabolism of all vertebrates and probably conserved in non-vertebrate species[74,80]. As all cells express IRPs and are potentially sensing iron levels, they are likely to adjust ferritins and transferrin receptor accordingly. That the iron status of an individual is reflected in its ratio of circulating transferrin receptor and ferritin (see Chapter 4) is strong support for this premise. We have previously found that proliferating cells (for example lymphocytes) are very sensitive to variations in extracellular iron, presumably since their own iron stores get exhausted by the active process of iron-protein synthesis[22,23]. It would seem that intestinal cells should not make an exception. The dividing crypt cells are exposed to serum and receive iron from transferrin via the receptor which is exclusively on the basolateral surface of epithelial cells. Thus, they can sense the body iron status and should synthesize ferritin accordingly. This ferritin is thought to serve as the barrier for incoming iron from nutrition[24]. It seems possible, however, that a specific mRNA coding for a iron transporter itself contains an IRE and is accordingly regulated. This is obviously highly speculative. For the time being it is possible to assess how intestinal cells regulate IRP in response to circulating body iron: the tools for investigations about the physiological relevance of the IRE-IRP interactions are largely available now.

Acknowledgements

This work was supported by the Swiss National Science Foundation.

References

1. Cammack, R., Wrigglesworth, J.M. & Baum, H. (1990): Iron-dependent enzymes in mammalian Systems. In: *Iron transport and storage*, eds. P. Ponka, H.M., Schulman & R.C. Woodworth, pp. 17–39. Boca Raton: CRC Press.
2. Crichton, R.R. (1991): *Inorganic biochemistry of iron metabolism*, pp. 7–263. Chichester: Ellis Horwood.
3. Iacopetta, B.J., Morgan, E.H. & Yeoh, G.C.T. (1982): Transferrin receptors and iron uptake during erythroid cell development. *Biochim. Biophys. Acta* **687,** 204–210.
4. Rothenberger, S., Iacopetta, B.J. & Kühn, L.C. (1987): Endocytosis of the transferrin receptor requires the cytoplasmic domain but not its phosphorylation site. *Cell* **49,** 423–431.
5. Baker, E. & Morgan, E.H. (1994) Iron Transport. In: *Iron metabolism in health & disease*, eds. J.H. Brock, J.W. Halliday, M.J. Pippard & L.W. Powell, pp. 63–95. London: W.B. Saunders.
6. Mack, U., Powell, L.W. & Halliday, J.W. (1983): Detection and isolation of a hepatic membrane receptor for ferritin. *J. Biol. Chem.* **258,** 4672–4675.
7. Adams, P.C., Powell, L.W. & Halliday, J.W. (1988): Isolation of a human hepatic ferritin receptor. *Hepatology* **8,** 719–721.
8. Beguin, Y., Bergamaschi, G., Huebers, H.A. & Finch, C.A. (1988): The behavior of asialotransferrin-iron in the rat. *Am. J. Hematol.* **29,** 204–210.
9. Morgan, W.T., Muster, P., Tatum, F., Kao, S.M., Alam, J. & Smith, A. (1993): Identification of the histidine residues of haemopexin that coordinate with heme-iron and of a receptor-binding region. *J. Biol. Chem.* **268,** 6256–6262.
10. Kino, K., Tsunoo, H., Higa, Y., Takami, M., Hamaguchi, H. & Nakajima, H. (1980): Haemoglobin-haptoglobin receptor in rat liver plasma membrane. *J. Biol. Chem.* **255,** 9616–9620.
11. Okuda, M., Tokunaga, R. & Taketani, S. (1992): Expression of haptoglobin receptors in human hepatoma cells. *Biochim. Biophys. Acta* **1136,** 143–149.
12. Kühn, L.C, Schulman, H.M & Ponka, P. (1990): Iron- transferrin requirements and transferrin receptor expression in proliferating cells. In: *Iron transport and storage*, eds. P. Ponka, H.M. Schulman & R.C. Woodworth, pp. 149–191. Boca Raton, Florida: CRC. Press.
13. Iacopetta, B.J., Rothenberger, S. & Kühn, L.C. (1988): A role for the cytoplasmic domain in transferrin receptor sorting and coated pit formation during endocytosis. *Cell* **54,** 485–489.

14. Miller, K., Shipman, M., Trowbridge, I.S. & Hopkins, C.R. (1991): Transferrin receptors promote the formation of clathrin lattices. *Cell* **65,** 621–632.

15. Collawn, J.F., Stangel, M., Kuhn, L.A., Esekogwu, V., Jing, S., Trowbridge, I.S. & Tainer, J.A. (1990): Transferrin receptor internalization sequence YXRF implicates a tight turn as the structural recognition motif for endocytosis. *Cell* **63,** 1061–1072.

16. Watts, C. (1985): Rapid endocytosis of the transferrin receptor in the absence of bound transferrin. *J. Cell. Biol.* **100,** 633–637.

17. Ajioka, R.S. & Kaplan, J. (1986): Intracellular pools of transferrin receptors result from constitutive internalization of unoccupied receptors. *Proc. Natl. Acad. Sci. USA* **83,** 6445–6449.

18. Morgan, E.H. (1981): Transferrin: biochemistry, physiology and clinical significance. *Molec. Aspects. Med.* **4,** 1–123.

19. Klausner, R.D, Ashwell, G., van Renswoude, J., Harford, J.B. & Bridges, K.R. (1983): Binding of apotransferrin to K562 cells: explanation of the transferrin cycle. *Proc. Natl. Acad. Sci. USA* **80,** 2263–2266.

20. Dautry-Varsat, A., Ciechanover, A. & Lodish, H.F. (1983): pH and the recycling of transferrin during receptor-mediated endocytosis. *Proc. Natl. Acad. Sci. USA* **80,** 2258–2262.

21. Morgan, E.H. (1983): Effect of pH and iron content of transferrin on its binding to reticulocyte receptors. *Biochim. Biophys. Acta* **762,** 498–502.

22. Testa, U., Kühn, L.C., Petrini, M., Quaranta, M.T., Pelosi, E. & Peschle, C. (1991): Differential regulation of iron regulatory element-binding protein(s) in cell extracts of activated lymphocytes *vs* monocytes-macrophages. *J. Biol. Chem.* **266,** 13925–13930.

23. Seiser, C., Teixeira, S. & Kühn, L.C. (1993): Interleukin-2-dependent transcriptional and post-transcriptional regulation of transferrin receptor mRNA. *J. Biol. Chem.* **268,** 13074–13080.

24. Skikne, B. & Baynes, R.D. (1994): Iron absorption. In: *Iron metabolism in health & disease*, eds. J.H. Brock, J.W. Halliday, M.J. Pippard & L.W. Powell, pp. 151–187. London: W.B. Saunders.

25. Stremmel, W., Lotz, G., Niederau, C., Teschke, R. & Strohmeyer, G. (1987): Iron uptake by rat duodenal microvillous membrane vesicles: evidence for a carrier mediated transport system. *Eur. J. Clin. Invest.* **17,** 136–145.

26. Teichmann, R. & Stremmel, W. (1990): Iron uptake by human upper small intestine microvillous membrane vesicles. Indication for a facilitated transport mechanism mediated by a membrane iron-binding protein. *J. Clin. Invest.* **86,** 2145–2153.

27. Conrad, M.E., Umbreit, J.N., Moore, E.G., Peterson, R.D. & Jones, M.B. (1990): A newly identified iron binding protein in duodenal mucosa of rats. Purification and characterization of mobilferrin. *J. Biol. Chem.* **265,** 5273 5279.

28. Conrad, M.E., Umbreit, J.N., Moore, E.G. & Rodning, C.R. (1992): identified iron-binding protein in human duodenal mucosa. *Blood* **79,** 244–247.

29. Conrad, M.E., Umbreit, J.N., Moore, E.G., Uzel, C. & Berry, M.R. (1994): Alternate iron transport pathway. Mobilferrin and integrin in K562 cells. *J. Biol. Chem* **269,** 7169–7173.

30. Askwith, C., Eide, D., Van Ho, A., Bernard, P.S., Li, L., Davis-Kaplan, S., Sipe, D.M. & Kaplan, J. (1994): The FET3 gene of S. cerevisiae encodes a multicopper oxidase required for ferrous iron uptake. *Cell* **76,** 403–410.

31. Dancis, A., Yuan, D.S., Haile, D., Askwith, C., Elde, D., Moehle, C., Kaplan, J. & Klausner, R.D. (1994): Molecular characterization of a copper transport protein in *S. cerevisiae*: an unexpected role for copper in iron transport. *Cell* **76,** 393–402.

32. Klausner, R.D. & Dancis, A. (1994): A genetic approach to elucidating eukaryotic iron metabolism. *FEBS. Lett.* **355,** 109–113.

33. Melefors, O. & Hentze, M.W. (1993): Iron regulatory factor - the conductor of cellular iron regulation. *Blood Reviews* **7,** 251–258.

34. Klausner, R.D., Rouault, T.A. & Harford, J.B. (1993): Regulating the fate of mRNA: The control of cellular iron metabolism. *Cell* **72,** 19–28.

35. Theil, E.C. (1994): Iron regulatory elements (IREs): a family of mRNA non-coding sequences. *Biochem. J.* **304,** 1–11.

36. Kühn, L.C. (1994): Molecular regulation of iron proteins. *Baillière's Clinical Haematology* **7,** 763–785.

37. Zähringer, J., Baliga, B.S. & Munro, H.N. (1976): Novel mechanism for translational control in regulation of ferritin synthesis by iron. *Proc. Natl. Acad. Sci. USA* **73,** 857–861.

38. Aziz, N. & Munro, H.N. (1987): Iron regulates ferritin mRNA translation through a segment of its 5′ untranslated region. *Proc. Natl. Acad. Sci. USA* **84,** 8478–8482.

39. Casey, J.L., Hentze, M.W., Koeller, D.M., Caughman, S.W., Rouault, T.A., Klausner, R.D. & Harford, J.B. (1988): Iron-responsive elements: regulatory RNA sequences that control mRNA levels and translation. *Science* **240,** 924–928.

40. Leibold, E.A. & Munro, H.N. (1988): Cytoplasmic protein binds *in vitro* to a highly conserved sequence in the 5′ untranslated region of ferritin heavy- and light- subunit mRNAs. *Proc. Natl. Acad. Sci. USA* **85,** 2171–2175.

41. Walden, W.E., Patino, M.M. & Gaffield L. (1989): Purification of a specific repressor of ferritin mRNA translation from rabbit liver. *J. Biol. Chem.* **264,** 13765–13769.

42. Goossen, B., Caughman, S.W., Harford, J.B., Klausner, R.D. & Hentze, M.W. (1990): Translational repression by a complex between the iron-responsive element of ferritin mRNA and its specific cytoplasmic binding protein is position-dependent *in vivo*. *EMBO J.* **9,** 4127–4133.

43. Gray, N.K. & Hentze, M.W. (1994): Iron regulatory protein prevents binding of the 43S translation pre-initiation complex to ferritin and eALAS mRNAs. *EMBO J.* **13,** 3882–3891.

44. Müllner, E.W., Neupert, B. & Kühn, L.C. (1989): A specific mRNA-binding factor regulates the iron-dependent stability of cytoplasmic transferrin receptor mRNA. *Cell* **58,** 373–382.

45. Rouault, T.A., Hentze, M.W., Caughman, S.W., Harford, J.B. & Klausner, R.D. (1988): Binding of a cytosolic protein to the iron-responsive element of human ferritin messenger RNA. *Science* **241,** 1207–1210.

46. Cox, T.C., Bawden, M.J., Martin, A. & May, B.K. (1991): Human erythroid 5-aminolevulinate synthase: promoter analysis and identification of an iron-responsive element in the mRNA. *EMBO J.* **10,** 1891–1902.

47. Dandekar, T., Stripecke, R., Gray, N.K., Goossen, B., Constable, A., Johansson, H.E. & Hentze, M.W. (1991): Identification of a novel iron-responsive element in murine and human erythroid delta-aminolevulinic acid synthase mRNA. *EMBO J.* **10,** 1903–1909.

48. May, B.K., Bhasker, C.R., Bawden, M.J. & Cox, T.C. (1990): Molecular regulation of 5-aminolevulinate synthase. Diseases related to heme biosynthesis. *Mol. Biol. Med.* **7,** 405–421.

49. Bhasker, C.R., Burgiel, G., Neupert, B., Emery-Goodman, A., Kühn, L.C. & May, B.K. (1993): The putative iron-responsive element in the human erythroid 5-aminolevulinate synthase mRNA mediates translational control. *J. Biol. Chem.* **268,** 12699–12705.

50. Melefors, O., Goossen, B., Johansson, H.E., Stripecke, R., Gray, N.K. & Hentze, M.W. (1993): Translational control of 5-aminolevulinate synthase mRNA by iron-responsive elements in erythroid cells. *J. Biol. Chem.* **268,** 5974–5978.

51. Koeller, D.M., Casey, J.L., Hentze, M.W., Gerhardt, E.M., Chan, L.N., Klausner, R.D. & Harford J.B. (1989): A cytosolic protein binds to structural elements within the iron regulatory region of the transferrin receptor mRNA. *Proc. Natl. Acad. Sci. USA* **86,** 3574–3578.

52. Casey, J.L, Koeller, D.M., Ramin, V.C., Klausner, R.D & Harford, J.B. (1989): Iron regulation of transferrin receptor mRNA levels requires iron-responsive elements and a rapid turnover determinant in the 3′ untranslated region of the mRNA. *EMBO J.* **8,** 3693–3699.

53. Binder, R., Horowitz, J.A., Basilion, J.P., Koeller, D.M., Klausner, R.D. & Harford, J.B. (1994): Evidence that the pathway of transferrin receptor mRNA degradation involves an endonucleolytic cleavage within the 3′ UTR and does not involve poly(A) tail shortening. *EMBO J.* **13,** 1969–1980.

54. Müllner, E.W. & Kühn, L.C. (1988): A stem-loop in the 3′ untranslated region mediates iron-dependent regulation of transferrin receptor mRNA stability in the cytoplasm. *Cell* **53,** 815–825.

55. Samaniego, F., Chin, J., Iwai, K., Rouault, T.A. & Klausner, R.D. (1994): Molecular characterization of a second iron-responsive element binding protein, iron regulatory protein 2 - structure, function, and post-translational regulations. *J. Biol. Chem.* **269,** 30904–30910.

56. Guo, B., Brown, F.M., Phillips, J.D., Yu, Y. & Leibold, E.A. (1995): Characterization and expression of iron regulatory protein 2 (IRP2). Presence of multiple IRP2 transcripts regulated by intracellular iron levels. *J. Biol. Chem.* **270,** 16529–16535.

57. Müllner, E.W., Rothenberger, S., Müller, A.M. & Kühn, L.C. (1992): *In vivo* and *in vitro* modulation of the mRNA-binding activity of iron-regulatory factor. Tissue distribution and effects of cell proliferation, iron levels and redox state. *Eur. J. Biochem.* **208,** 597–605.

58. Henderson, B.R., Seiser, C. & Kühn, L.C. (1993): Characterization of a second RNA-binding protein in rodents with specificity for iron-responsive elements. *J. Biol. Chem.* **268,** 27327–27334.

59. Kaptain, S., Downey, W.E., Tang, C., Philpott, C.C., Haile, D., Orloff, D.G., Harford, J.B., Rouault, T.A. & Klausner, R.D. (1991): A regulated RNA binding protein also possesses aconitase activity. *Proc. Natl. Acad. Sci. USA* **88,** 10109–10113.

60. Haile, D.J., Rouault, T.A., Harford, J.B., Kennedy, M.C, Blondin, G.A, Beinert, H. & Klausner, R.D. (1992): Cellular regulation of the iron-responsive element binding protein: Disassembly of the cubane iron-sulfur cluster results in high-affinity RNA binding. *Proc. Natl. Acad. Sci. USA* **89,** 11735–11739.

61. Emery-Goodman, A., Hirling, H., Scarpellino, L., Henderson, B. & Kühn, L.C. (1993): Iron regulatory factor expressed from recombinant baculovirus: conversion between the RNA-binding apoprotein and Fe-S cluster containing aconitase. *Nucleic. Acids. Res.* **21,** 1457–1461.

62. Basilion, J.P., Kennedy, M.C., Beinert, H., Massinople, C.M., Klausner, R.D. & Rouault, T.A. (1994): Overexpression of iron-responsive element-binding protein and its analytical characterization as the RNA-binding form, devoid of an iron-sulfur cluster. *Arch. Biochem. Biophys.* **311,** 517–522.

63. Hirling, H., Henderson, B.R. & Kühn, L.C. (1994): Mutational analysis of the [4Fe-4S]-cluster converting iron regulatory factor from its RNA-binding form to cytoplasmic aconitase. *EMBO J.* **13,** 453–461.

64. Philpott, C.C., Haile, D., Rouault, T.A. & Klausner, R.D. (1993): Modification of a free Fe-S cluster cysteine residue in the active iron-responsive element-binding protein prevents RNA binding. *J. Biol. Chem.* **268,** 17655–17658.

65. DeRusso, P.A., Philpott, C.C., Iwai, K., Mostowski, H.S., Klausner, R.D. & Rouault, T.A. (1995): Expression of a constitutive mutant of iron regulatory protein 1 abolishes iron homeostasis in mammalian cells. *J. Biol. Chem.* **270,** 15451–15454.

66. Henderson, B.R. & Kühn, L.C. (1995): Differential modulation of the RNA-binding proteins IRP-1 and IRP-2 in response to iron. IRP-2 inactivation requires translation of another protein. *J. Biol. Chem.* **270,** 20509–20515.

67. Drapier, J.-C., Hirling, H., Wietzerbin, J., Kaldy, P. & Kühn, L.C. (1993): Biosynthesis of nitric oxide activates iron regulatory factor in macrophages. *EMBO J.* **12,** 3643–3649.

68. Weiss, G., Goossen, B., Doppler, W., Fuchs, D., Pantopoulos, K., Werner-Felmayer, G., Wachter, H. & Hentze, M.W. (1993): Translational regulation via iron-responsive elements by the nitric oxide/NO-synthase pathway. *EMBO J.* **12,** 3651–3657.

69. Pantopoulos, K. & Hentze, M.W. (1995): Nitric oxide signaling to iron-regulatory protein: direct control of ferritin mRNA translation and transferrin receptor mRNA stability in transfected fibroblasts. *Proc. Natl. Acad. Sci. USA* **92,** 1267–1271.

70. Martins, E.A.L., Robalinho, R.L. & Meneghini, R. (1995): Oxidative stress induces activation of a cytosolic protein responsible for control of iron uptake. *Arch. Biochem. Biophys.* **316,** 128–134.

71. Pantopoulos, K. & Hentze, M.W. (1995): Rapid responses to oxidative stress by iron regulatory protein. *EMBO J.* **14,** 2917–2924.

72. Toth, I., Rogers, J.T., McPhee, J.A., Elliott, S.M., Abramson, S.L. & Bridges, K.R. (1995): Ascorbic acid enhances iron- induced ferritin translation in human leukaemia and hepatoma cells. *J. Biol. Chem.* **270,** 2846–2852.

73. Eisenstein, R.S., Tuazon, P.T., Schalinske, K.L., Anderson, S.A. & Traugh, J.A. (1993): Iron-responsive element-binding protein. Phosphorylation by protein kinase C. *J. Biol. Chem.* **268,** 27363–27370.

74. Guo, B., Yu, Y. & Leibold, E.A. (1994): Iron regulates cytoplasmic levels of a novel iron-responsive element-binding protein without aconitase activity. *J. Biol. Chem.* **269,** 24252–24260.

75. Kim, H.Y., Klausner, R.D. & Rouault, T.A. (1995): Translational repressor activity is equivalent and is quantitatively predicted by in vitro RNA binding for two iron-responsive element- binding proteins, IRP1 and IRP2. *J. Biol. Chem.* **270,** 4983–4986.

76. Pantopoulos, K., Gray, N.K. & Hentze, M.W. (1995): Differential regulation of two related RNA-binding proteins, iron regulatory protein (IRP) and IRPB. *RNA* **1,** 155–163.

77. Cairo, G. & Pietrangelo, A. (1994): Transferrin receptor gene expression during rat liver regeneration. Evidence for post- transcriptional regulation by iron regulating factorB, a second iron- responsive element-binding protein. *J. Biol. Chem.* **269,** 1–5.

78. Chan, R.Y.Y., Seiser, C., Schulman, H.M., Kühn, L.C. & Ponka, P. (1994): Regulation of transferrin receptor mRNA expression. Distinct regulatory features in erythroid cells. *Eur. J. Biochem.* **220,** 683–692.

79. Henderson, B.R., Menotti, E., Bonnard, C. & Kühn, L.C. (1994): Optimal sequence and structure of iron-responsive elements. Selection of RNA stem–loops with high affinity for iron regulatory factor. *J. Biol. Chem.* **269,** 17481–17489.

80. Rothenberger, S., Müllner, E.W. & Kühn, L.C. (1990): The mRNA-binding protein which controls ferritin and transferrin receptor expression is conserved during evolution. *Nucleic Acids Res.* **18,** 1175–1179.

81. Hirling, H., Emery-Goodman, A., Thompson, N., Neupert, B., Seiser, C. & Kühn, L.C. (1992): Expression of active iron regulatory factor from a full-length human cDNA by in vitro transcription/translation. *Nucleic Acids Res.* **20,** 33–39.

82. Yu, Y., Radisky, E. & Leibold, E.A. (1992): The iron- responsive element binding protein. Purification, cloning, and regulation in rat liver. *J. Biol. Chem.* **267,** 19005–19010.

83. Patino, M.M. & Walden, W.E. (1992): Cloning of a functional cDNA for the rabbit ferritin mRNA repressor protein. Demonstration of a tissue-specific pattern of expression. *J. Biol. Chem.* **267,** 19011–19016.

84 Kohler, S., Henderson B.R., Kühn, L.C: Unpublished.

Iron Nutrition in Health and Disease, edited by Leif Hallberg and Nils-Georg Asp
©1996 John Libbey & Company Ltd., pp. 31–48

Chapter 3

Assessment of the prevalence and the nature of iron deficiency for populations: the utility of comparing haemoglobin distributions

Ray Yip[1], Rebecca J. Stoltzfus[2] and William K. Simmons[3]

[1]*Division of Nutrition, Centers for Disease Control and Prevention, Atlanta, GA, 30341, USA and United Nations Children's Fund (UNICEF), Jakarta, 10012 Indonesia ;* [2]*Division of Human Nutrition, School of Hygiene and Public Health, Johns Hopkins University, Baltimore, MD 21205, USA;* [3]*Caribbean Food and Nutrition Institute, Kingston, Jamaica*

Summary

Even though there are a number of well established haematoligic and biochemical tests to assess iron status, it is not always feasible to perform them under field conditions, especially in developing countries. Also, in such regions, factors other than poor iron intake, such as infections and hereditary disorders affecting red cell production, can interfere with the interpretation of iron-related tests. To overcome these limitations, we propose a simplified approach to asses iron status using only results form haemoglobin testing. The strategy of this approach is based on the observation that the most common reason for iron deficiency, poor dietary intake, has a differential impact on the iron status of children, women, and men. Whereas other factors affecting iron and haematological status lack such differential impact. This approach requires the comparison of haemoglobin distributions of children, women, and men froma specific population against their respective standard distributions (free from iron deficiency). Examples of populations with different factors contributing to iron deficiency from the Middle East, Africa, the Caribbean, and Alaska are used to illustrate this approach. The improved capacity of field testing for haemoglobin in recent years means more opportunity of assessing iron deficiency in countries when it is not always feasible to conduct the more comprehensive surveys using multiple iron tests.

Introduction

Several haematologic and biochemical tests are well established for screening or diagnosis of iron deficiency in individuals as well as for population-based assessment[1]. Even though the purpose of population-based assessment of iron deficiency differs from the purpose of screening individuals, the desirable features of the assessments overlap. The three common reasons for population-based or public health based application are: (1) characterization of the extent and nature of iron deficiency in communities; (2) planning and design for appropriate intervention programmes; and (3) monitoring and evaluation for the effects of programmes.

Issues related to the use of indicators for population-based assessment

As is true for all clinical tests, the most important features for a test designed to assess iron deficiency in an individual is adequate sensitivity, specificity and, the positive predictive value for this particular disorder. Although these are also desirable features for tests used in population-based assessment[2], the more important features are the feasibility of carrying out the assessment, and ability to compare with findings over time or across populations. One feature of using indicators for population-based assessment is that tests of limited value for individual-based assessment can still be useful in characterizing a population. One good example is the use of anaemia as a proxy of iron deficiency when anaemia may not be adequate for assessing iron status for an individual. This is because there are several conditions other than iron deficiency that can cause anaemia. Nevertheless, anaemia can serve as a useful indicator of iron deficiency in a population, because a population with overall high prevalence of anaemia is likely to have overall high prevalence of iron deficiency. Using an indicator for population-based assessment is analogous to estimating the size of an iceberg by measuring the tip of iceberg above the water. Anaemia can be viewed as the tip of the iceberg for iron deficiency.

In using an indicator to define the prevalence of the condition of interest, it is common to apply a cut-off point to the laboratory values for individual-based screening. For example, for haemoglobin <11.0 g/dl is a commonly used cutoff to define anaemia for young children who require further clinical evaluation, and it is also used for population-based assessment. One drawback of this approach is the tendency to regard only individuals with laboratory values below or above the cutoff as affected, and to focus intervention on those who meet the definition for the indicator, when in fact a much greater proportion of the population is affected. This is like using the tip of an iceberg to define the size of the iceberg without taking into account the larger portion underwater. One way to bypass this pitfall is to present the entire distribution of the laboratory findings against a reference or standard distribution which is free from iron deficiency. The proper application of the prevalence of an indicator based on a laboratory cut-off point is to view the prevalence as an index of severity; interpretation of this index requires knowledge from previous studies and the background of the populations.

Assessment of iron deficiency

Three options exist for assessing the status of iron nutrition in dietary iron intake assessment: use of single haematologic or biochemical test, and use of multiple biochemical tests. By far, anaemia as a single indicator is the most commonly used approach to assess iron status of a population. There are, however, limitations with this approach if not taken into account in the interpretation of the findings: (1) anaemia is not specific for iron deficiency in some parts of the world; (2) anaemia represents a more severe form of iron deficiency; and (3) anaemia may not have adequate predictor value for iron deficiency when iron deficiency is mild or when the prevalence for a population is low. To avoid some of these limitations and the common misapplication of the prevalence of anaemia as the proportion of the population affected by iron deficiency, we propose the use of the entire haemoglobin distribution.

Use of dietary intake of iron

Assessment of the dietary intake of iron is an indirect approach for estimating the status of iron nutrition. The main advantage of this approach is that, with proper training and procedures, it is not difficult to collect information on the quantity of food consumed and the frequency of consumption. Use of this method is highly feasible because it does not require laboratory procedures. Unfortunately, this technique has several limitations. Although study results indicate that the assessment of a relatively simple dietary pattern of infant feeding has a strong predictive value for the risk of iron deficiency in young children[3], studies in adults have shown a lack of correlation between estimated dietary iron intake and iron nutrition status. Assessment of dietary intake in infants is a useful approach because the majority of the diet is milk-based, so the iron content of the milk is the main determinant of iron status[4]. The poor correlation for adult dietary iron content and iron nutrition status is partly due to common use of a method that estimates the total dietary iron content, and which often fails to take into account the bioavailability of iron in food items and the fact that other dietary components can increase or decrease the absorption of iron[5]. Another reason that dietary iron assessment is of limited value, particularly in industrialized countries, is that, for women, menstrual blood loss that is higher than average is a major determinant of iron deficiency, a factor that appears to be more important than dietary iron intake.

Given the indirectness and limitations of dietary assessment for iron nutrition status, the most important role of dietary iron assessment is to complement the information on iron nutrition status that is based on laboratory assessment. This information can be helpful in defining the programme content of the food-based approaches that have potential to improve iron nutrition. Investigators can use dietary assessment as adjunct information in determining iron nutrition status. They can collect this information by using qualitative approaches as part of the effort to understand the nature of iron deficiency.

Use of single haematologic or biochemical test

A survey based on haemoglobin or haematocrit measurements to define the prevalence of anaemia in a population is the most common approach for assessing the extent of iron deficiency. There is good evidence to support the assumption that, in many parts of the world, iron deficiency is the predominant cause of anaemia. Operationally, because haemoglobin measurement is one of the most commonly performed laboratory tests worldwide, it is often feasible to obtain measurements of haemoglobin or haematocrit. The common approach of measuring the prevalence of anaemia for the maternal and child health population is useful for defining the severity of iron deficiency in a population. In a later section an expanded approach, comparing the entire haemoglobin distribution with reference distributions, will be described with several examples.

No single biochemical tests other than haemoglobin or haematocrit is commonly used to define iron nutrition status in a population. It is possible that serum ferritin levels could be used as an indicator of iron deficiency because low serum ferritin reflects low iron stores in the body is a more specific indicator for iron deficiency. High serum ferritin levels could also be used as an indicator for populations in which iron overload is a concern. In developed countries where iron deficiency anaemia is relatively uncommon, haemoglobin levels and/or anaemia are less sensitive in detecting variations in iron nutrition status among populations. Unlike serum ferritin which has no upper biological limit, the upper value of haemoglobin is regulated by tissue oxygen requirements which do not increase with increasing body iron load beyond what is sufficient for an optimal level.

Use of multiple biochemistry tests

Each of the well-known biochemical tests for iron reflects a different aspect of iron metabolism. Often, application of multiple tests for the same individual gives inconsistent results[6]. This problem has led to the development of a strategy to characterize nutrition iron status using multiple iron tests to define iron deficiency. This approach was developed for the assessment of iron status of the US population based on the National Health and Nutrition Examination Surveys (NHANES)[7,8].

The principle of applying multiple tests in parallel is that the certainty of iron deficiency increases with the increase of the number of abnormal tests. For the NHANES-based assessment, iron deficiency was defined as having abnormal results in two or more of three iron-related tests. Two models of multiple tests were used in the NHANES study: (1) the ferritin model, which uses the tests for serum ferritin, transferrin saturation, and erythrocyte protoporphyrin; and (2) the MCV model which uses the tests for mean corpuscular volume (MCV), transferrin saturation, and erythrocyte protoporphyrin[7]. There are two advantages of using multiple tests to define iron deficiency: (1) multiple indices allow differentiation of the severity of iron deficiency and; (2) this approach can be useful even when iron deficiency is not a common problem, as is the case in the USA.

However, the use of multiple tests has several disadvantages. The most obvious one is that the approach is relatively costly and operationally complex, and is thus not very feasible for a large-scale survey work in many parts of the world. It is also an approach mainly suited for use in more developed settings, where iron deficiency is often an isolated finding. In many less developed areas, high rates of infection or inflammatory conditions and other nutrient deficiencies impede the determination of iron deficiency in the population (because such conditions can interfere with biochemical tests for iron); the more recently developed transferrin receptor test is an exception[9,10]. The lack of agreement on cut-off points and standardized methods for some of the tests makes comparison of survey findings difficult. The use of multiple tests to assess iron nutrition status appears to be more suited for clinical studies based of well-defined population samples in limited locations than for large-scale population-based assessment.

Expanded use of the haemoglobin test

In addition to cost, feasibility and the appropriateness and limitations of different approaches with which to assess iron deficiency, several factors affect the choice of an assessment method. It is important to determine the cause(s) of anaemia and iron deficiency in a given population. Possible causes include decreased bioavailability of dietary iron, blood loss related to hookworm, infections that can interfere with iron metabolism, and nutritional deficiency other than iron such as vitamin A or folate deficiencies. Development of an assessment approach that would provide information and clues regarding cause(s) of anaemia and iron deficiency would be helpful. Because the risk of iron deficiency differs for children, women, and men in most populations, all these three groups need to be assessed. This method is based on the general knowledge of the causes of iron deficiency in relation to different stage of economic development and ecological conditions[11]. Table 1 summarizes the general risk for iron deficiency for subpopulations of children, women, and men for areas at different stages of economic development - less developed, intermediate and developed.

In recent years, there has been improvement in the feasibility of conducting haemoglobin testing for populations in remote field settings, related to the availability of a new-generation haemoglobin photometer, the HaemoCue (Angelholm, Sweden). The HaemoCue photometer is battery operated and uses a dry reagent (sodium azide) in a microcuvette for direct blood collection and measurement. The portability and stability of this system has made it more feasible to measure haemoglobin in

Table 1. Risk for iron deficiency and anaemia for subpopulations in areas with different stages of economic development

Stage of economic development	Children	Women	Men
Developed	**Low:** Iron fortified diet available **Moderate:** Lack of iron fortified diet	**Low:** Mainly for subset with excessive menstrual blood loss	**None**
Intermediate	**Moderate to high:** Lack of iron fortified diet	**Moderate:** Low iron bioavailability	**None to low**
Less developed	**High:** Lack of iron fortified diet and low iron bioavailability of supplementary food	**High:** Possibility that other factors in addition to iron deficiency contribute to anemia	**Low:** Not affected by hookworm **Moderate:** affected by hookworm

remote field settings without formal laboratory support. The accuracy and precision of haemoglobin values based on HaemoCue are comparable to those of the standard laboratory method[12]. All of the major case examples of haemoglobin distributions from different countries presented here were based on the HaemoCue system.

The extent and the nature of iron deficiency in different situations

Developed countries - adequate dietary iron intake and moderate iron deficiency

In industrialized societies, where dietary iron intake and bioavailability are relatively high, the modest level of iron deficiency anaemia is observed mainly in young children and women of childbearing age. A good example is a finding from the US national surveys (NHANES[7,8]). Young children are at greater risk of iron deficiency than older children and adults because rapid growth during infancy results in a relatively high requirement for iron[4]. In addition, the amount of iron in the infant diet is generally not adequate to meet iron requirements unless the diet is fortified with iron[3]. The relative lack of overlap in the dietary intake of infants and adults can put young children at risk for iron deficiency, even in countries where the adult diet is adequate in iron content and bioavailability. Data from studies conducted in Argentina, Canada and the United States support this proposition[13–15].

Women of childbearing age are at greater risk of iron deficiency than men because the average blood loss of 40–50 ml at each menstrual cycle increases their requirement for iron to an average 50 per cent higher than that for men[16]. For a small subset of women who have high menstrual blood loss exceeding 80 to 100 ml per cycle, it is difficult to meet their iron requirement with a diet that is otherwise adequate for most women. For this reason, in developed countries it is fair to assume that the primary cause of iron deficiency is menstrual blood rather than lack of iron content or lack of bioavailability of iron in the general diet. Studies have established that, in such a setting it is possible to observe a modest level of iron deficiency anaemia in young children and women of childbearing age but not in men[7,8].

Anaemia is not specific for iron deficiency in an individual especially when the prevalence is low. Also, because iron deficiency anaemia represents the more severe form of iron deficiency, not all individuals with iron deficiency have anaemia. Nevertheless, monitoring the prevalence of anaemia can still be a useful approach to determining iron deficiency in a population. The reduction of childhood anaemia in response to improved infant iron nutrition in the United States is an example of the usefulness of this approach[15,17]. (Fig. 1)

The NHANES are the few sources of broad population-based assessment in which multiple tests for iron were used. Consequently, we are able to use the NHANES data to characterize the optimal haemoglobin distribution to serve as a reference that can be helpful in assessing iron status for other populations. An optimal haemoglobin distribution can be defined after excluding the subset of the sample with biochemical evidence of iron deficiency (two or more of the three tests in the MCV model). Figure 2 illustrates the optimal haemoglobin levels for children under 5 years age, and for women and men 18–44 years of age in the USA. The distinct and generalized difference in haemoglobin distributions for children, women and men is the basis for applying age- and sex-specific criteria in defining anaemia.

Figure 3 shows the haemoglobin distribution for the 10 per cent in the women in the United States who had evidence of iron deficiency based on having two or more abnormal test for iron (the MCV model). This distribution is compared with that for the 90 per cent of the women who were regarded as non-iron deficient. The iron deficient group have a generalized downward shift if their haemoglobin distribution in contrast to the non-deficient group, but the overlap between the two distributions is substantial. This overlap suggests that the haemoglobin test has limited usefulness for detection of milder forms of iron deficiency because many subjects with iron deficiency have haemoglobin values above the standard cutoff point for anaemia of 12.0 g/dl for women.

From the perspective of population-based assessment, a modest downward shift of the entire haemoglobin distribution, as shown in Fig. 3, indicates that most if not all of the subjects had lower haemoglobin levels. This finding suggests that such a comparison of haemoglobin distribution can avoid the common pitfall of regarding only subjects with anaemia as iron deficient. Several examples are given later to further demonstrate the limitations of haemoglobin testing for detecting individuals with iron deficiency. However, this limitation does not negate the usefulness of haemoglobin testing for population- based assessment.

One major complication of using haemoglobin testing to assess iron deficiency is the need to apply appropriate criteria for reference. The haemoglobin distribution used for assessment of anaemia in a population is commonly adjusted for sex and age. Other non- pathological factors that can cause shifting of the haemoglobin distribution are altitude and pregnancy[18]. There is also increasing evidence that some races or ethnic groups may have distinct haemoglobin distributions that are independent of iron nutrition status[19]. Figure 4 shows a comparison of haemoglobin distributions for non-iron deficient black and white women based on the NHANES II data. If the same criteria for anaemia were used, the number of black women classified as anaemic would be three times the number of white women considered to be anaemic. For this reason, in using the haemoglobin test to define iron status, a reference haemoglobin distribution based on black subjects would be the appropriate reference for comparison with a population that was mainly of African extraction.

Areas with intermediate developments - low dietary iron intake or poor bioavailability as major cause of iron deficiency anaemia

In many parts of the world where economic development can be regarded as being at an intermediate stage, iron deficiency anaemia is quite common mainly among children and women. These areas include most of South and Central America, the Middle East, North Africa, and the northern part of Asia. In these regions anaemia is mainly due to poor bioavailability of dietary iron because of low intake of meat which contains the more bioavailable form of haem iron, and greater exposure to inhibitors of non-haem

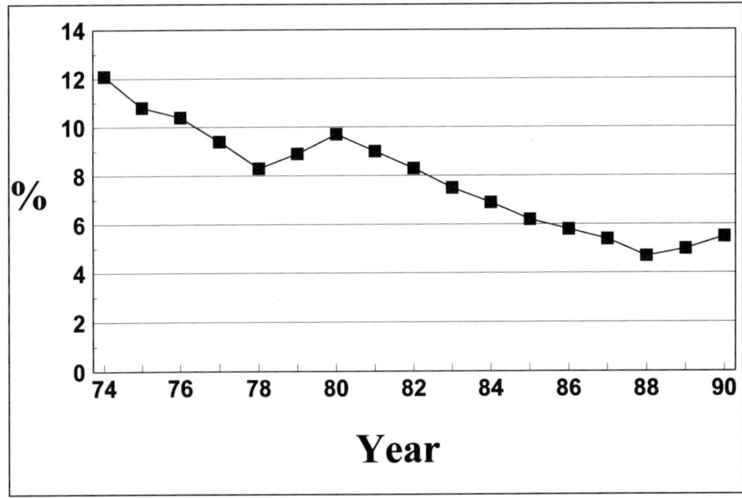

Fig. 1. This finding demonstrates that the prevalence of anaemia is a useful tool for the population-based monitoring of iron deficiency. Graph showing declining trend of anaemia in low income families in the United States. This trend reflects improved iron nutrition status. The improvement was related to a significant change in the iron content of the infant diet during the same time period[15].

Fig. 2. Graph showing distribution of haemoglobin levels for children aged 1 to 5 years and women and men aged 18 to 44 years. Data are from National Health and Nutritional Examination Surveys II, after exclusion of individuals with abnormal values for mean corpuscular volume (MCV), transferrin saturation and erythrocyte protoporphyrin. These distributions are used as a standard for comparison with haemoglobin distributions from other surveys.

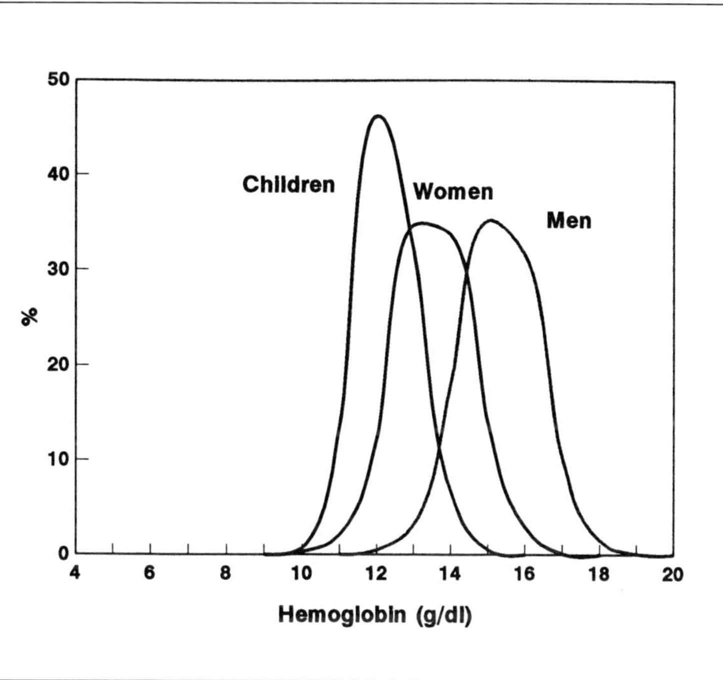

Fig. 3. Graph showing a comparison of the optimal haemoglobin distribution for women who were not iron deficient in NHANES II with the distribution for women who had abnormal results in two or more tests for iron nutrition. The women with iron deficiency made up approximately 10 per cent of the women in the USA. Haemoglobin values for women who had iron deficiency were lower than those for women who had no iron deficiency. Data are from the US National Health and Nutritional Examination Surveys (NHANES II).

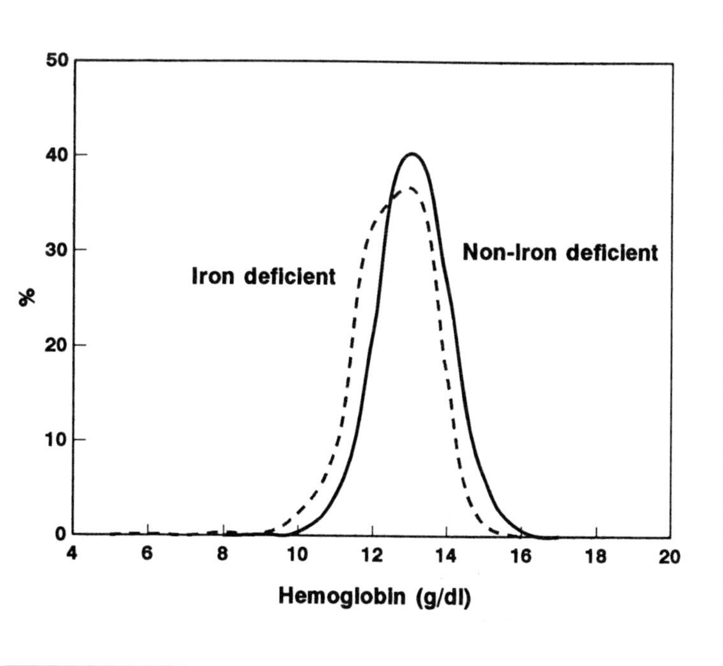

iron absorption, such as phytate in grain and tannic acid in tea. In these areas other major causes of anaemia, such as malaria or iron deficiency related to gastrointestinal blood loss due to hookworm, are rare or the condition is mild. Except for instances of greater severity or higher prevalence, the pattern of anaemia is similar to the pattern for developed countries in that it mainly affects young children and women. This finding indicates that when low dietary content or poor bioavailability of iron is the main reason for iron deficiency, the prevalence or severity of anaemia can be used as an index of iron nutrition status.

The Middle East is a region where, for the most part, poor iron intake is the major cause of anaemia. Figure 5 shows the haemoglobin distributions for children, women, and men of the Palestinian refugees residing in Syria, Jordan, Lebanon, the West Bank and Gaza, using the optimal or the non-iron deficient haemoglobin distribution based on the US sample (NHANES II) as a comparison[11]. The Palestinian refugees did not have an adequate source of iron in the infant diet; consumption of meat is relatively low because of low socioeconomic status; and tea consumption is common and starts in late infancy. Comparison of the distributions shown in Fig. 5 indicates that the prevalence of anaemia is relatively high for Palestinian children and women, as indicated by a substantial downward shift in haemoglobin distribution. The distribution for Palestinian men is not very different from that for men in the USA. This finding indicates that even when iron intake is grossly inadequate for children and women, men still do not suffer from significant iron deficiency. The marked shift of haemoglobin distribution for children and women indicates that most of them were affected by iron deficiency, not just those below the common anaemia cut-offs.

Another example is based on the national iron deficiency survey of Grenada for which, in addition to haemoglobin testing, serum ferritin level was also determined. Analysis of this survey confirms that a similar differential shift of haemoglobin distribution between women and men, as observed in the Middle East, is indeed the result of iron deficiency. In Grenada, where

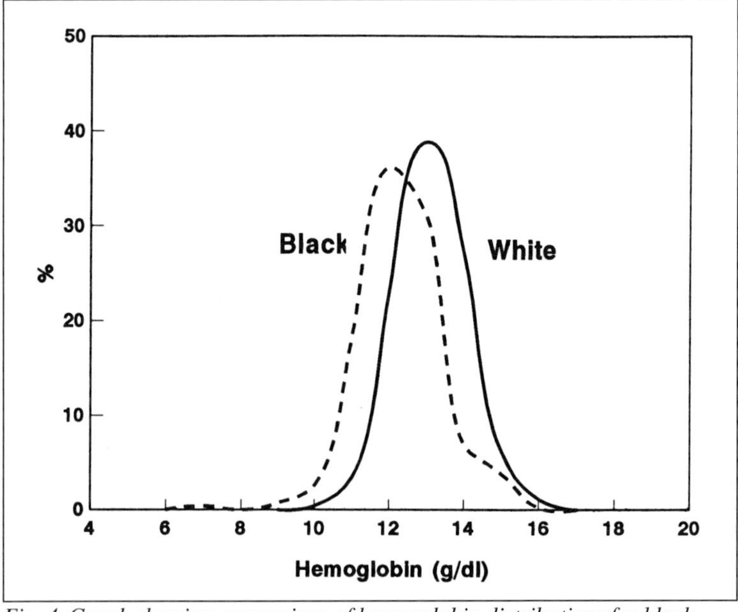

Fig. 4. Graph showing comparison of haemoglobin distributions for black women and white women who were not iron deficient. Haemoglobin values for black women were lower than those for white women. Data are from the US National Health and Nutritional Examination (NHANES II) .

there is little problem with hookworm infection or malaria, poor iron intake or low iron bioavailability is the only plausible explanation for iron deficiency anaemia observed. Their haemoglobin distribution for men is similar to that for non-iron deficient black men in the USA (Fig. 6a). Haemoglobin levels for Grenadian women were substantially lower than those for non-iron deficient US black women (Fig. 6b). This finding suggests high rates of iron deficiency in Grenadian women.

However, when only the small subset of non-iron deficient Grenadian women (serum ferritin levels ≥ 30 µg/l) was retained, their haemoglobin distribution was found to be similar to that for non-iron deficient US black women (Fig. 6c). This finding clearly indicates that the marked shift of haemoglobin distribution for the entire sample of Grenada women was mainly related to iron deficiency. That few Grenadian men had a low serum ferritin level confirms our impression that it is possible for men in a population to have little or no iron deficiency, even when women in the same population have substantial iron deficiency.

On the basis of these two examples, a case can be made that inclusion of adult men in an anaemia survey can yield information that will be useful in determining the nature of iron deficiency in women and children.

Less developed countries - causes of anaemia in addition to low dietary iron intake

From the point of view of economic development, by far the most challenging areas for assessing iron nutrition status are the less developed countries that comprise a substantial part of sub-Saharan Africa and South and Southeast Asia. In these regions, beyond poor dietary intake of iron contributes to the common and severe iron deficiency observed, hookworm infection often plays a major role by causing

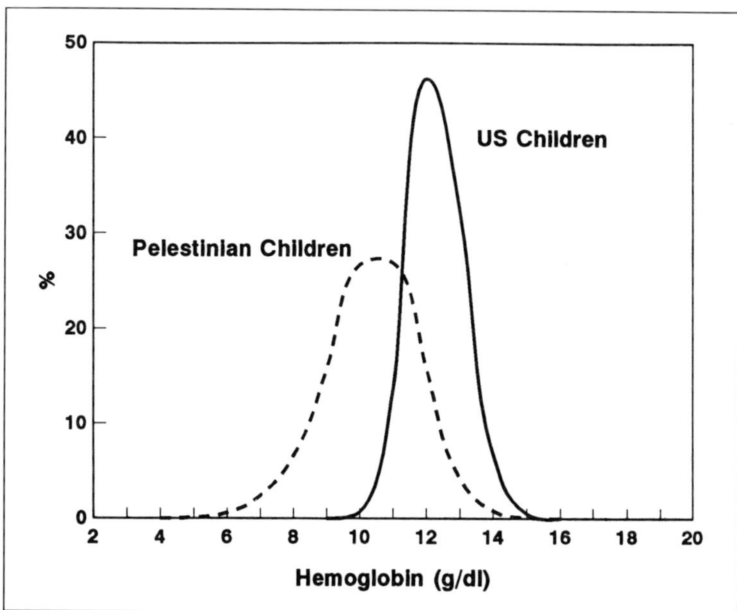

Fig. 5. Graphs showing lower haemoglobin levels for Palestinian children (Fig. 5a above), women (Fig. 5b), and men (Fig. 5c) than for children, women and men in the US population. The Palestinian refugees residing in five areas in the Middle East were surveyed in 1990. Haemoglobin levels in this population were mainly affected by low iron intake and poor bioavailability of dietary iron. There were no other major causes for anaemia or blood loss. Haemoglobin distributions indicated substantial iron deficiency in children and women but not men[11].

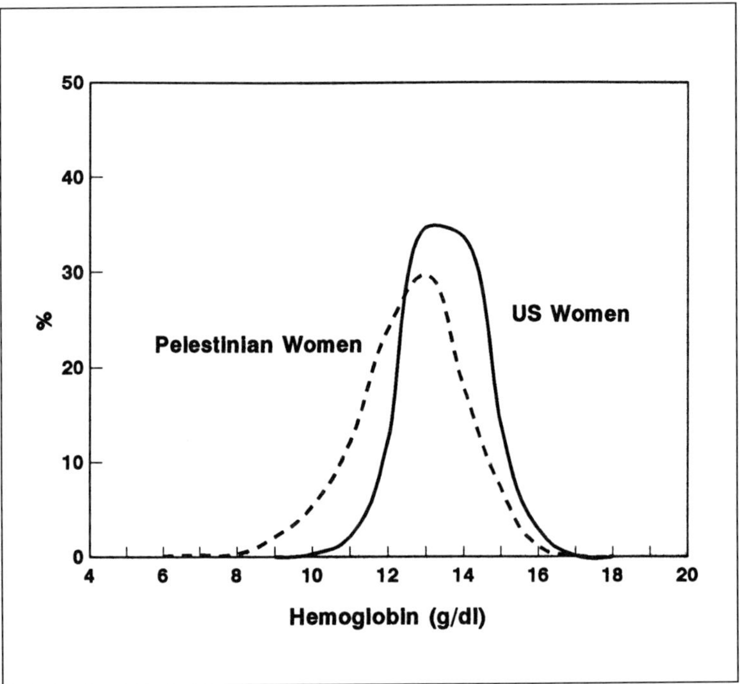
50
40
30
20
10
0
%
4
6
8
10
12
14
16
18
20
Hemoglobin (g/dl)
US Women
Pelestinian Women

Fig. 5b

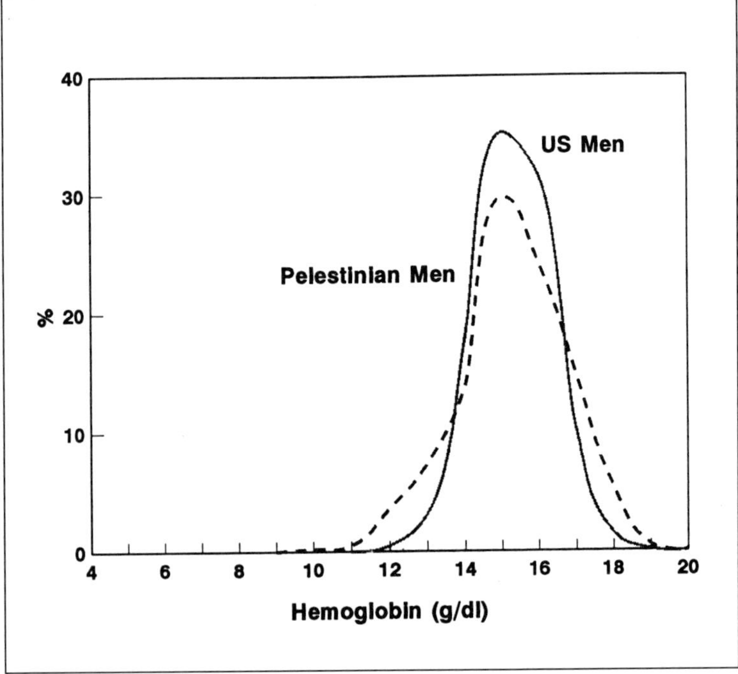
40
30
20
10
0
%
4
6
8
10
12
14
16
18
20
Hemoglobin (g/dl)
US Men
Pelestinian Men

Fig. 5c

clinically significant gastrointestinal (GI) blood loss[20]. Factors other than iron deficiency contributing to anaemia is also common: infections include malaria and hereditary haemoglobinopathies and defects in red blood cell production. All these conditions render the use of haemoglobin levels for assessing iron deficiency difficult. Unfortunately, the use of biochemical tests for iron is not an alternative because infections and inflammatory conditions can affect iron metabolism and make it difficult to interpret most tests for determining levels of iron. In less developed countries, it is also less feasible to implement biochemical tests for population-based or large-scale assessment. Despite its limitations, haemoglobin testing appears to be the most viable option for assessment of iron deficiency in the populations of the less developed countries.

The finding of a high prevalence of anaemia or low haemoglobin levels for children and women in less developed countries is to be expected. The finding that men also have anaemia requires other forms of evaluation in order to determine the likely cause of the anaemia. One major possibility is that men are iron deficient and hookworm infection is a likely cause in many tropical areas. The proper determination of the intensity of hookworm infection is to perform limited stool examination for hookworm egg counts. In the case of malaria or nutritional deficiency as possibilities for the high rates of anaemia among men, assessment of haemoglobin response during therapeutic trials for subjects with anaemia may be the best approach for defining the nature of the anaemia. In a recent study of combined vitamin A and iron supplementation for pregnant women with anaemia

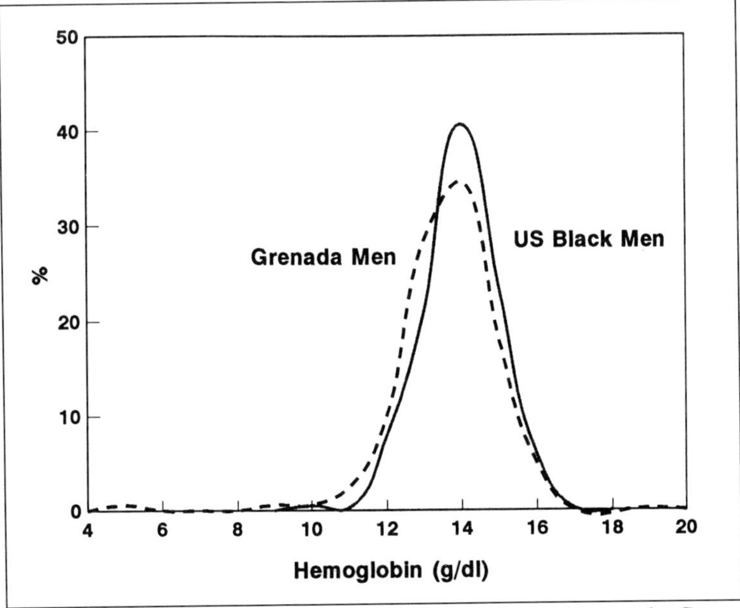

Fig. 6. Graphs showing comparisons for haemoglobin distributions for Grenadian men versus that for black men in the United States. (Fig. 6a, above), and for Grenadian women versus black women with no iron deficiency (Fig. 6b). Haemoglobin levels for Grenadian women were substantially lower than those for black women in the USA (Fig. 6b). This finding indicates high rates of iron deficiency for Grenadian women. For Grenadian women with serum ferritin levels ≥30 µg/ml, who made up less than half of the total sample of women, the haemoglobin distribution is similar to that for black women in the USA who were not iron deficient (Fig. 6c). This finding indicates that the shift of haemoglobin distribution for the entire sample of women was mainly related to iron deficiency.

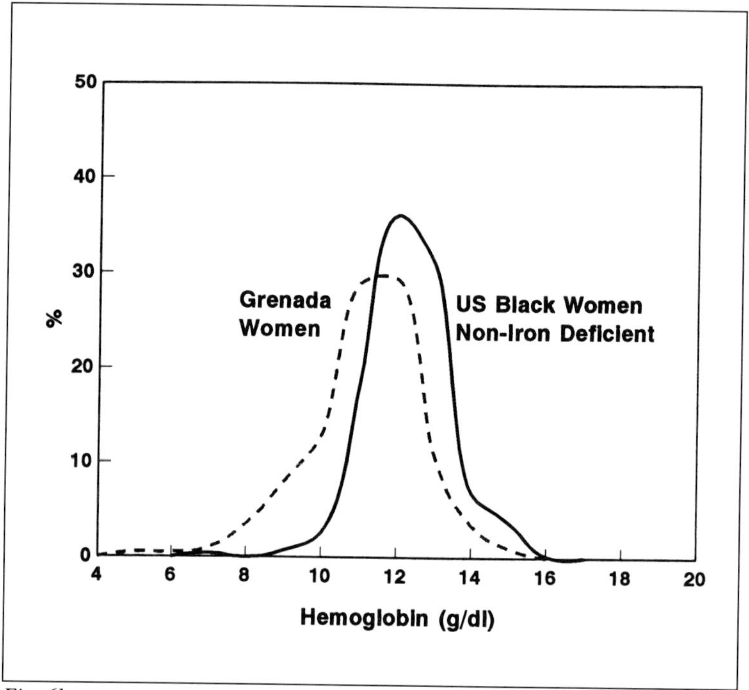
50
40
30
20
10
0
%
4
6
8
10
12
14
16
18
20
Hemoglobin (g/dl)
Grenada
Women
US Black Women
Non-Iron Deficient

Fig. 6b

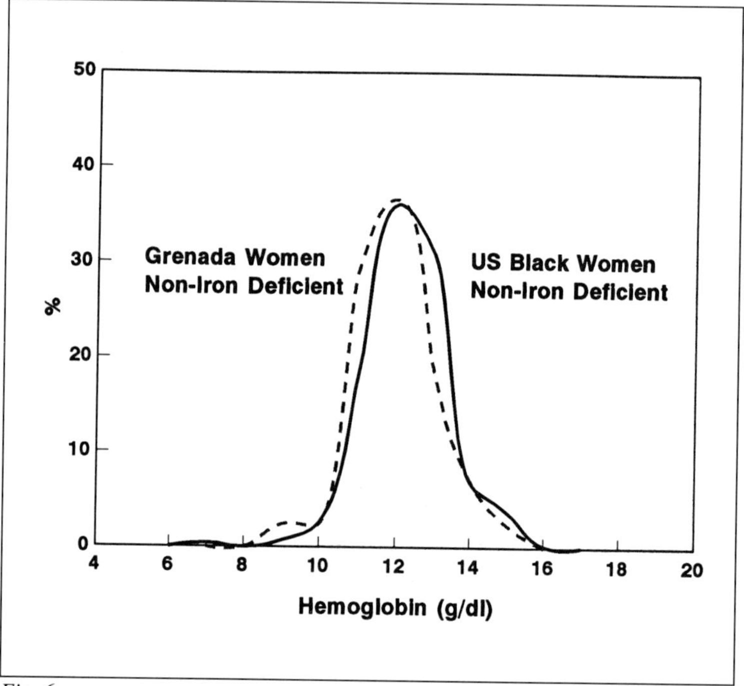
50
40
30
20
10
0
%
4
6
8
10
12
14
16
18
20
Hemoglobin (g/dl)
Grenada Women
Non-Iron Deficient
US Black Women
Non-Iron Deficient

Fig. 6c

Table 2. Proportion of pregnant women with anaemia responding to dietary supplements with increase in haemoglobin to ≥ 11.0 g/dl).*

Treatment	No of patients	Response (%)	95% Confidence interval
Placebo	62	16	7–29
Vitamin A only	63	35	22–48
Iron	63	60	54–79
Iron and vitamin A	63	97	88–99

* Data from Suharno *et al.*[20]

Table 3. Amount of blood loss estimated by quantitative stool haeme analysis and prevalence of anaemia for Zanzibar children with different hookworm loads[a]

Hookworm infection degree of disease hookworm load (eggs/per gram of faeces)	No. of children	Mean faecal haemoglobin (mg/g of stool)	(%) With anaemia[b]
None 0	45	1.24	49
Light 1–9999	83	1.46	57
Moderate 2000–3999	19	2.96	68
Heavy ≥ 4000	56	8.79	80

[a] Data from Stoltzfus *et al.* [22]

[b] Children were considered to have anaemia if haemoglobin levels were < 11.0 g/dl.

in Indonesia, investigators found that vitamin A deficiency together with iron deficiency contributed substantially to the high rates of anaemia observed[20] Table 2 details the response to vitamin A and iron supplementation for that study conducted by Suharno *et al.*

Example of areas with low dietary iron intake and common gastrointestinal blood loss

In the tropics hookworm infection with resulting iron deficiency is the most common epidemic form of blood loss anaemia; it affects mainly older children and adults[20,21]. In a recent study of school-age children in Zanzibar, Stoltzfus *et al.* found a remarkable correlation between iron deficiency anaemia and GI blood loss related to hookworm infection using a quantitative method in determining faecal blood content (HaemoQuant) (Table 3). For the heavily infected children, the estimated daily blood loss was more than 5 ml[22]. Rates of anaemia ranged from 49 per cent for children without hookworm infection to 80 per cent for those with heavy infection. The high rates of anaemia for those children without hookworm infections fit with the general impression of low iron intake in this population and were confirmed by serum ferritin testing.

Figure 7 shows comparisons of haemoglobin distributions for Zanzibar school-age children and adult men with those for black children and black men in the United States. The marked downward shift of haemoglobin distribution for men in Zanzibar suggests that they have substantial rates of anaemia due to GI blood loss related to hookworm infection. An unusual example of adequate dietary iron intake but increased gastrointestinal blood loss

Another example of common GI blood loss and iron deficiency affecting the haemoglobin distributions for both men and women is the recently discovered epidemic form of *Helicobactor pylori* gastritis in the Alaskan Eskimo natives in the Arctic region[23]. Unlike the population affected by hookworm in the tropics,

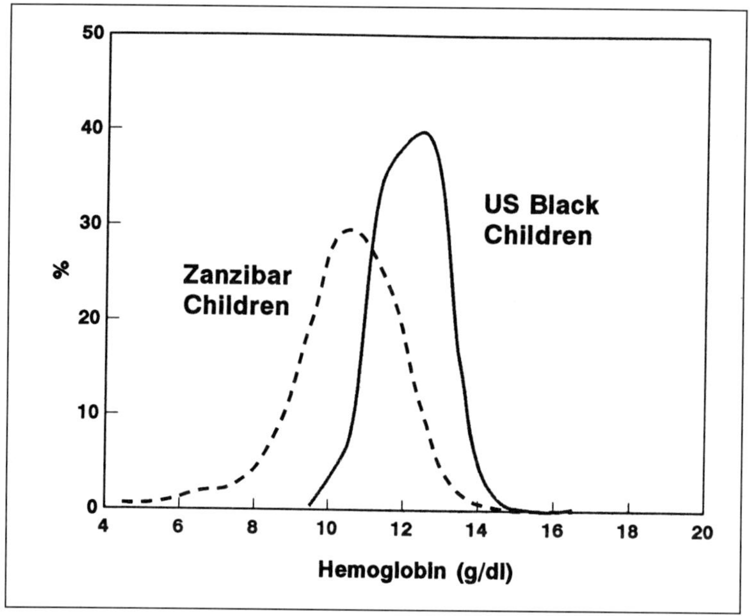

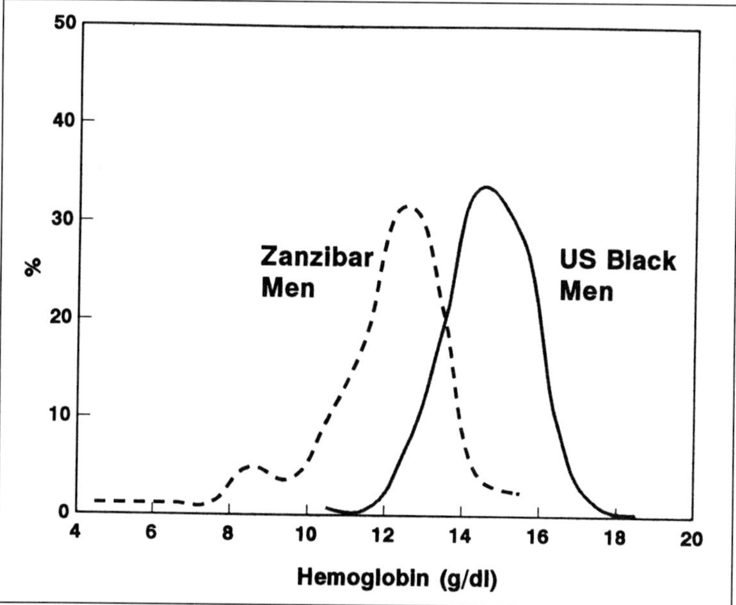

Fig. 7. Graphs showing comparisons of haemoglobin distributions for Zanzibar children (top), and Zanzibar men (bottom). Black children and black men with no iron deficiency, in the USA, are the reference. These comparisons indicate that hookworm infection and the resulting gastrointestinal blood loss is related to decreased haemoglobin levels. This finding suggests that the substantial rates of anaemia in the country are related to gastrointestinal blood loss due to infection with hookworm.

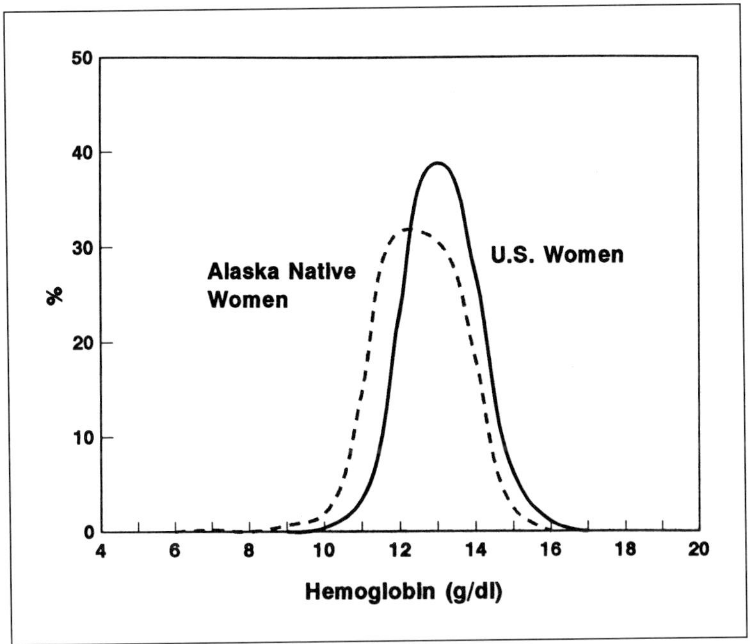

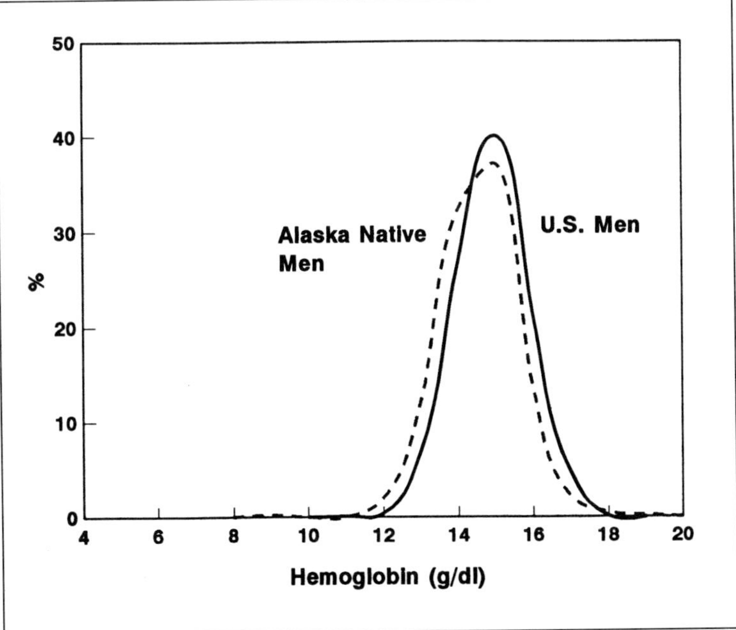

Fig. 8. Graphs showing comparisons of haemoglobin distribution for Alaskan Eskimo Native men (top) and women (bottom) versus those for men and women in the USA. These results show a modest trend toward lower haemoglobin levels for both Alaskan men and women, because of iron deficiency related to increased gastrointestinal blood loss due to an atypical presentation. Heliobactor pylori gastritis is common in the Arctic region. The iron deficiency is not severe because dietary iron intake is adequate in this population.

where iron intake is generally low, Alaskan Eskimos have adequate iron intake with rich sources of haem iron from fish and land and marine mammals[24]. The increased occult GI bleeding due to gastritis resulted in lower iron stores and thus prevalence of iron deficiency for both men and women that were higher than those for men, and women in the US general population[25].

Figure 8 shows comparisons between the haemoglobin distributions for Alaskan Eskimo men and women against the optimal distributions based on the US sample. In contrast to the optimal distribution, the Alaskan men had a slightly but generalized lower haemoglobin distribution suggesting many of them were affected by iron deficiency. This is confirmed by the fact that the Alaskan men had a median serum ferritin level of 31 g/ml in contrast to the value of 132 μg/ml for men in the USA. This finding indicates that when iron deficiency anaemia is relatively mild or the prevalence is not high, serum ferritin can better differentiate the iron nutrition status of populations. The main constraint against using serum ferritin level as an indicator of iron deficiency is the lack of a field test, which limits its use for large-scale surveys.

The two examples from Zanzibar and Alaska support the proposition that it is useful to examine the haemoglobin distribution or prevalence of anaemia for men. This approach can be helpful in differentiating iron deficiency that is mainly due to low iron intake or to excessive blood loss. For this reason, the addition of a sample of men should be considered for anaemia surveys which usually focus only on maternal and child populations.

Conclusions

The predictive value of haemoglobin testing is limited when screening individuals for iron deficiency in areas where prevalence of iron deficiency is low, but haemoglobin testing can be useful for population-based monitoring. The comparison between haemoglobin distributions for children, women, and men and respective standard distributions can provide valuable diagnostic information concerning the cause of iron deficiency in the population. In areas with multiple causes of anaemia, the use of treatment response may be the only alternative for determining the nature of anaemia other than iron deficiency. The proposed approach of comparing haemoglobin distributions or prevalence of anaemia against standard distributions for children, women and men has the potential for increasing the feasibility of iron deficiency assessment in countries where it is not always feasible to conduct comprehensive surveys by using multiple tests for iron. In developed countries where iron deficiency is mild and iron overload is a concern, the use of serum ferritin levels to monitor iron nutrition status should also be considered.

References

1. Dallman, P.R., Yip, R. & Oski, F.A. (1992): Iron deficiency and related nutritional anemia. In: *Hematology of infancy and childhood*, ed. O. Nathan, pp. 413–450. Philadelphia, PA: W.B. Saunders.
2. Centers for Disease Control. (1988) Guidelines for evaluating surveillance systems. *MMWR* **37,** (suppl. no. S–5): 1–18.
3. Pizarro, F., Yip, R., Dallman, P.R., Olivares, M., Hertrampf, E. & Walter, T. (1991): Iron status with different infant feeding regimens: relevance to screening and prevention of iron deficiency. *J. Pediatr.* **118,** 687–692.
4. Dallman, P.R., Siimes, M.A. & Stekel, A. (1980): Iron deficiency in infancy and childhood. *Am. J. Clin. Nutr.* **33,** 86–118.
5. Monsen, E.R., Hallberg, L., Layrisse, L. *et al.* (1978): Estimation of available dietary iron. *Am. J. Clin. Nutr.* **31,** 134–141.

6. Dallman, P.R., Reeves, J.D., Driggers, D.A. & Lo, E.Y.T. (1981): Diagnosis of iron deficiency: the limitation of laboratory tests in predicting response to iron treatment in 1-year-old infants. *J. Pedatr.* **98,** 376–381.

7. Expert Scientific Working Group (1985): Summary of a report on assessment of iron nutritional status of the United States population. *Am. J. Clin. Nutr.* **42,** 1318–1330.

8. Yip, R., Johnson, C. & Dallman, P.R. (1984): Age-related changes in laboratory values used in the diagnosis of anemia and iron deficiency. *Am. J. Clin. Nutr.* **39,** 427–436.

9. Yip, R. & Dallman, P.R. (1988): The role of inflammation and iron deficiency as causes of anemia. *Am. J. Clin. Nutr.* **48,** 1295–1300.

10. Skikne, B.S., Flowers, C.H. & Cook, J.D. (1990): Serum transferrin receptor: A quantitative measure of tissue iron deficiency. *Blood* **75,** 1870–1876.

11. Yip, R. (1994): Iron deficiency: Contemporary scientific issues and international programmatic approaches. *J. Nutr.* **124,** 1479S–1490S.

12. Van Schenck, H., Falkensson, M. & Lundberg, B. (1986): Evaluation of HaemoCue, a new device for determining hemoglobin. *Clin. Chem.* **32,** 526–529.

13. Calvo, E.B. & Ginazzo, N. (1990): Prevalence of iron deficiency in children aged 9–24 months from a large urban area of Argentina. *Am. J. Clin. Nutr.* **52,** 534–540.

14. Chan-Yip, A. & Gary-Donald, K. (1978): Prevalence of iron deficiency anemia Chinese children aged 6 to 36 months in Montreal. *Can. Med. Assc. J.* **136,** 373–378.

15. Yip, R., Binkin, N.J., Fleshood, L. & Trowbridge, F.L. (1987): Declining prevalence of anemia among low-income children in the United States. *JAMA* **258,** 1619–1623.

16. Hallberg, L., Högdahl, A., Nilsson, L. & Rybo, G. (1966): Menstrual blood loss - a population study. *Acta Obstet. Gynecol. Scand.* **45,** 320–351.

17. Ryan, A.S., Martinez, G.A. & Yip, R. (1990): Changing patterns of infant feeding in the United States: evidence to support improved iron nutrition status in childhood. Recent knowledge on iron and folate deficiencies in the world. Colloque *INSERM* Paris, **197,** 631–640.

18. Centers for Disease Control. CDC criteria for anemia in children and childbearing age women. (1989): *MMWR* **38,** 400–404.

19. Johnson-Spear, M. & Yip, R. (1994): Hemoglobin difference between black and white women with comparable iron status: justification for race-specific anemia criteria. *Am. J. Clin. Nutr.* **60,** 117–121.

20. Suharno, D., West, C.E., Karyadi, D. & Hautvast, G.A.J. (1993): Supplementation with vitamin A and iron for nutritional anemia in pregnant women in West Java, Indonesia. *Lancet* **1342,** 1325–1328.

21. Pawlowski, Z.S., Schad, G.A. & Stott, G.J. (1991): *Hookworm Infection and Anemia: An Approach to Prevention and Control.* Geneva, Switzerland: The World Health Organization.

22. Stoltzfus, R.J., Albnico, M., Chwaya, H.M. *et al.* (1995) The role of hookworm-related blood loss in iron deficiency anemia: A study of Zanibar children. *Abstr. Exp. Biol.*

23. Yip, R. Limburg, P. Ahlquist, D., O'Niell, A. & Kruse, D. An epidemic form of iron deficiency anemia due to gastrointestinal bleeding related to *Helicobactor pylori* gastritis among Alaska Natives (unpublished).

24. Nobmann, E.D., Byers, T., Lanier, A.P., Hankin, J.H., Jackson, M.Y. (1992): The diet of Alaska Native adults 1987–1988. *Am. J. Clin. Nutr.* **55,** 1024–1032.

25. Petersen, K.M., Parkinson, A.J., Nobmann, E.D., Bulkow, L. & Yip, R. (1996): High Prevalence of Iron Deficiency Anemia among Alaska Natives: Inadequate Intake or Unexpected Loss? *J. Nutr.* (in press).

Iron Nutrition in Health and Disease, edited by Leif Hallberg and Nils-Georg Asp
©1996 John Libbey & Company Ltd., pp. 49–58

Chapter 4

The use of the serum transferrin receptor for the assessment of iron status

James D. Cook, Barry Skikne and Roy Baynes

Division of Hematology, Department of Medicine, Kansas University Medical Center, Kansas City, KS 66160–7402, USA

Summary

The transferrin receptor is a key iron-related protein which regulates the influx of transferrin iron to all body cells. A soluble form of the transferrin receptor has been identified in human serum which reflects the total body mass of cellular transferrin receptor. Clinical measurements of the serum receptor are of value as a measure of total erythropoiesis and for the detection of iron deficiency. In over 90 per cent of patients with iron deficiency anaemia, there is a distinct elevation in serum receptor levels which averages about 3–5-fold. The major clinical utility of the serum transferrin receptor is in distinguishing patients with the anaemia of chronic disease from those with iron deficiency anaemia, a distinction that commonly requires a bone marrow examination for stainable iron. Preliminary studies also indicate that the serum transferrin receptor and/or the receptor:ferritin ratio can identify the development of iron deficiency in patients with ongoing inflammation or infection. In population studies, the receptor:ferritin ratio is a valuable index of iron status because it quantitatively reflects body iron over the entire spectrum of iron balance encountered in humans.

Introduction

The evolution of our understanding of the manner in which extracellular iron is transported to the interior of cells is an intriguing chapter in cell biology. It has long been known that iron is bound in the plasma and extracellular fluid to transferrin, a specific carrier protein for iron, but the mechanism for the cellular uptake of iron-loaded transferrin was obscure until a specific receptor for the carrier protein was identified. The biochemical nature of this cellular transferrin receptor and of the intracellular pathways it follows in the process of iron uptake and transport have been extensively characterized. A valuable byproduct of these investigations was the detection of the soluble form of the transferrin receptor in human serum. During the past decade, there has been a rapid accumulation of knowledge regarding the factors affecting the concentration of serum transferrin receptor. Its measurement has proved to be a valuable indicator of total erythroid activity and the degree of tissue iron deficiency. The focus of the present review is on the use of the serum transferrin receptor in identifying iron deficiency and assessing its severity.

Cellular transferrin receptor

Biochemistry

The biochemical composition of the cellular form of the transferrin receptor and its physicochemical properties has been the subject of several reviews[1–4]. The transferrin receptor is a dimeric protein, each monomer containing 760 amino acids with a molecular mass of 95 kDa. The transferrin receptor is anchored in the plasma membrane, having a small cytoplasmic tail containing 61 amino acids, an intramembrane portion containing 28 amino acids and a large carboxyterminal extracellular domain containing 671 amino acids. There are four glycosolation sites, at positions 104, 251, 317 and 272. The gene for transferrin receptor is located on chromosome 3.

Function

The primary function of cellular transferrin receptor is to sequester diferric transferrin and deliver it to the interior of the cell for the synthesis of iron-containing compounds. This is accomplished by receptor-mediated endocytosis, a process common to several receptors for which transferrin uptake serves as the prototype. The affinity of the transferrin receptor varies with the iron content of its ligand. At physiological pH, the affinity is highest for diferric, intermediate for monoferric, and negligible for apotransferrin. After transferrin binds to its receptor, the complexes are gathered together on the cell surface over clathrin-coated pits which then invaginate to form an endocytic vesicle within the cell. As the pH of the vesicle falls below 6.0 by protonation, the affinity of transferrin for iron is lost and the released iron is transported across the endocytic membrane to an unknown cytosolic carrier. Meanwhile, apotransferrin having high receptor affinity at the more acidic pH remains attached to its receptor within the endosome and is promptly returned to the surface of the cell where it is released to the extracellular fluid on return to physiological pH. The transit time through the intracellular pathway is between 3 and 12 min.

All body cells contain transferrin receptor on their surface at some point in their early development but the highest density occurs in tissues requiring a large continuous supply of iron. In humans, about 75 per cent of the body mass of cellular transferrin receptor is contained in the erythroid bone marrow compartment and this proportion increases further in clinical conditions associated with enhanced erythropoiesis. The highest density of transferrin receptor is on intermediate normoblasts with a decline of 80–90 per cent in late normoblasts and a virtual disappearance in mature circulating red blood cells. The two other major tissue sites containing transferrin receptor are the liver and placenta. The human placenta is especially rich in transferrin receptor which ensures an adequate supply of iron to the fetus. Consequently, human placenta is an ideal tissue for isolation and purification of the protein.

Synthesis

An intriguing aspect of intracellular iron metabolism is the manner in which the synthesis of transferrin receptor and the storage protein, ferritin, are regulated[5,6]. Their synthesis is precisely coordinated by a 28 base nucleic acid sequence which forms a stem-loop structure termed the iron response element (IRE). Five of these IREs are to be found in the 3′ untranslated region of transferrin receptor mRNA and a single one in the 5′ untranslated ferritin mRNA. A 95–100 kDa bifunctional cytosolic protein termed the IRE-binding protein (IRE-BP) interacts with these IRE segments to control ferritin and transferrin receptor synthesis in a reciprocal fashion. The affinity of the IRE-BP for the IRE varies with its iron content which is in turn related to the iron status of the cell. When the IRE-BP is saturated with iron, it has aconitase-like activity with reduced affinity for the IRE, whereas when iron is lacking in the cell, the IRE-BP loses its aconitase activity and a cleft develops in the molecule which facilitates its binding to the IRE. When the IRE-BP binds to the IRE on the transferrin receptor mRNA, it protects the mRNA from degradation and thereby enhances synthesis of the transferrin receptor. When the IRE-BP binds to the ferritin mRNA, it impairs the translation of the ferritin mRNA by inhibiting the formation of polysomes, thereby reducing ferritin synthesis. In this unique system of coordinately regulated synthesis, the cytosolic concentration of iron reciprocally controls the synthesis of two of the major iron proteins in the body.

Serum transferrin receptor

Early data on the degradation product of cellular transferrin receptor was based on *in vitro* studies of maturing sheep reticulocytes[7,8]. Evidence was obtained by these workers that at least a portion of the transferrin receptor is lost from the cell as small microvesicles called exosomes in which the transferrin receptor is positioned exteriorly. Based on evidence that the transferrin receptor is highly expressed in malignant tissue, a search for circulating transferrin receptors in human sera was made using commercially available monoclonal antibodies against the cell surface receptor[9,10]. Transferrin receptor was invariably detected in human serum. It was originally postulated that this immunoreactive material was derived from the exosomal pathway of degradation and was therefore in particulate form. Studies in human serum have subsequently shown that virtually all of the circulating transferrin receptor is in a fully soluble form and cannot be removed by high speed centrifugation[11]. The presence of a free or soluble form of transferrin receptor was confirmed by other laboratories using various immunological methods[12,13].

Biochemistry

It was initially suggested that the immunologically reactive material in human serum was intact transferrin receptor[9,13]. However, when a significant quantity of transferrin receptor protein was isolated from human serum using a monoclonal affinity column, electrophoretic and amino acid sequence studies demonstrated that the circulating protein was a monomeric fragment of intact receptor[14]. As compared with molecular masses of 190 kDa and 95 kDa for purified placental transferrin receptor under non-reducing and reducing conditions, respectively, electrophoretic analysis of the purified serum protein showed a molecular mass of 85 kDa under both conditions. When amino acid sequence analysis was performed on the material isolated from serum, it was demonstrated to consist of a truncated fragment of intact receptor with the cleavage site between arginine (100) and leucine (101). The finding of a truncated form is in keeping with soluble forms that have been demonstrated for a variety of surface receptors for protein hormones and growth factors. The precise biological function of these receptor fragments has not been determined and in many cases, they presumably represent the results of cellular degradation of the receptor. This is supported by studies using polyclonal antibodies to specific peptide sequences in the extracellular and cytoplasmic domains of the transferrin receptor, indicating that proteolytic cleavage is involved in the production of the serum transferrin receptor[15]. *In vitro* studies using various protease inhibitors have suggested that this proteolysis is mediated by a serine protease[16].

Because the concentration of serum transferrin is several orders of magnitude higher than the monomeric fragments of transferrin receptor in serum, it is assumed that the serum transferrin receptor circulates as a complex with serum transferrin. This is supported by studies showing that more than 95 per cent of the receptor immunoreactivity in serum can be removed by precipitating with antibodies against transferrin[13]. The exact composition of the circulating ligand- receptor complex is unknown. The receptor fragment presumably blocks the cellular uptake of complexed transferrin but the proportion of circulating transferrin which is complexed with the serum transferrin receptor is too low for this inhibition to have any physiological or pathological significance.

Assay methods

The first reported assay for the measurement of serum transferrin receptor was a two-site immunoradiometric assay (IRMA) using commercially available monoclonal antibodies, OKT9 and B 3–25, developed against the cell surface receptor[9,10]. Similar mean values of 251 and 256 µg/l were reported in healthy male and female subjects, respectively. Subsequent assays have used immunological reagents developed against transferrin receptor purified from human placenta. An enzyme-linked immunoassay (EIA) reported by Flowers *et al.* using monoclonal antibodies prepared against isolated transferrin receptor gave a 20-fold higher normal mean value of 5.6 mg/l with no appreciable difference between male and female subjects[12]. In studies undertaken to reconcile the discrepancy in values obtained with the IRMA and monoclonal EIA, the difference was shown to be related to whether free or complexed transferrin was used as the standard. The monoclonal EIA gave similar values with the two standards, whereas the monoclonal IRMA varied depending on whether the standard was free or bound. Another assay approach has been to use polyclonal antibodies developed against the transferrin-receptor complex and subsequently adsorbed with purified transferrin. Normal mean values with this polyclonal EIA have ranged between 5 and 8.3 mg/L[13,17,18].

It is apparent that there are major differences in reported values with different assay systems. Nevertheless, the relative decreases or increases in serum transferrin receptor values reported in different disease states are remarkably similar. The 20-fold difference in normal values between the monoclonal IRMA and monoclonal EIA is probably related to the fact that the monoclonals in the IRMA were developed against membrane-bound transferrin receptor which is mainly free rather than transferrin bound. The antibodies for both the monoclonal and polyclonal EIA were developed against complexed transferrin receptor which is the form of the transferrin receptor that presumably exists in serum. Relatively small differences in reported values with the monoclonal and polyclonal EIA are likely due to minor differences in the purified transferrin receptor standard rather than a systematic difference in the specificity of the immunological reagents.

Serum transferrin receptor and the assessment of iron status

Iron deficiency anaemia

A key finding in early studies of the serum transferrin receptor was a distinct elevation in patients with iron deficiency anaemia. In the initial report by Kohgo *et al.*, an increase in serum transferrin receptor of 2.8 times above normal was observed in 41 patients with iron deficiency anaemia[10]. A similar increase of 3.2-fold was reported later in 19 patients with iron deficiency anaemia using the monoclonal EIA[12]. In the latter study, the mean serum transferrin receptor concentration was 18.0 mg/l as compared to a mean of 5.6 mg/l in healthy men and women. With the polyclonal EIA, the average increase reported in 13 patients with iron deficiency anaemia was 4.1 times higher than normal[13]. In a more recent study employing a commercial assay, the mean serum transferrin receptor concentration in 19 patients with iron deficiency anaemia was 5.3 as compared to 1.7 mg/l in 19 controls giving a relative increase in iron deficiency anaemia of 3.1[19]. The small differences in the relative increase of serum transferrin receptor in patients with iron deficiency anaemia presumably reflect differences in the severity of the iron deficiency. Nevertheless, despite widely different assay systems, a consistent 3–5-fold increase in serum transferrin receptor occurs in patients with iron deficiency anaemia and there is little or no overlap with values in normal subjects.

Iron deficiency without anaemia

The earliest stage of iron deficiency is depleted iron stores which is best identified by a serum ferritin concentration ≤ 12 μg/l. A significant further decline in body iron must occur before the haemoglobin concentration falls below the cut-off levels for anaemia. Once anaemia has developed, any further reduction in haemoglobin concentration reliably reflects the severity of tissue iron deficiency. Milder deficiency occurring between the point of storage iron depletion and the development of anaemia is commonly referred to as either iron deficient erythropoiesis or iron deficiency without anaemia. The latter has been difficult to identify and quantify because most of the available laboratory measurements of iron status are neither sensitive nor specific for iron deficiency.

The serum transferrin receptor measurement has been shown to be a reliable quantitative measure of tissue iron deficiency prior to the development of anaemia. Varying degrees of mild iron deficiency were induced by performing repeated phlebotomies of 150–250 ml of blood weekly in six male and eight female volunteer subjects[20]. When the haemoglobin concentration in each volunteer subject was reduced by more than 20 g/l from baseline, phlebotomies were discontinued. The amount of iron remaining in stores or the deficit in tissue iron was calculated weekly with this protocol from the amount of haemoglobin iron removed. The average duration of the phlebotomy programme was 13 weeks, the average amount of iron removed was 792 mg and the median deficit in tissue iron produced by phlebotomy was 339 mg iron.

As anticipated, the decline in serum ferritin concentration was directly proportional to the reduction in body iron stores. There was little or no change in the serum transferrin receptor concentration until stores were fully depleted but, with continuing phlebotomy, there was a progressive rise in serum transferrin receptor concentration that was proportional to the deficit in tissue iron. The serum transferrin receptor concentration with the onset of anaemia was 8.8 mg/l as compared with the baseline mean of 5.3 mg/l. Thus, the degree of tissue iron deficiency was modest as compared with the threefold elevation in serum transferrin receptor observed in patients with iron deficiency anaemia. A key finding in this study was that between the point of storage iron depletion and the development of anaemia, the only laboratory parameter which accurately reflected the degree of tissue iron deficiency was the serum transferrin receptor concentration.

In this phlebotomy study, the serial changes in body iron were accurately portrayed by two laboratory measurements, the serum ferritin and serum transferrin receptor; the former declined with storage iron depletion, whereas the latter increased with progressive tissue iron deficiency. Because of the reciprocal relationship between these two parameters, the receptor:ferritin ratio was proportional to body iron throughout the entire range of iron status induced by serial phlebotomy. The mean receptor:ferritin ratio increased from below 100 at baseline to over 2000 at the conclusion of the phlebotomy programme. The median ratio was approximately 500 at the point that iron stores were fully depleted. There was a precise linear relationship between the logarithm of the receptor:ferritin ratio and body iron stores.

The receptor:ferritin ratio will have its major utility in the assessment of the iron status of different segments of a population. In preliminary epidemiologic studies of the receptor:ferritin ratio, mean values have ranged from 40 in healthy adult males to approximately 350 in teenage girls with intermediate values of 151 and 72 in pre- and post-menopausal women, respectively (Cook, unpublished observations). The receptor:ferritin ratio proved to be a valuable tool in assessing the effect of iron supplementation in pregnant Jamaican women[21]. The median value of the receptor:ferritin ratio in control women given no iron supplement was 1200, as compared to 470 in women given one of two forms of iron supplementation. Moreover, as in the phlebotomy study by Skikne *et al.*[20], the cumulative frequency distribution of the log receptor:ferritin ratio was linear in both the control and iron-treated women, suggesting that iron stores in a given segment of the population are normally distributed and that there are no separate populations of normal and iron deficient individuals. If confirmed in other studies, arbitrary cut-off points for laboratory measurements of iron status in an attempt to define iron deficiency or iron sufficiency in a population are misleading.

Iron deficiency in pregnancy

The assessment of iron status during pregnancy has been a perplexing problem. Although the haemoglobin concentration is often used as an index of iron deficiency, it is greatly influenced by the expansion in both red cell mass and plasma volume of the mother during gestation. Because the plasma volume usually increases disproportionately, a dilutional anaemia results which is difficult to distinguish from iron deficiency anaemia. The diagnostic utility of the serum ferritin as an index of iron status is also greatly diminished during pregnancy because of the dramatic fall in serum ferritin which accompanies the mobilization of iron stores for expansion of the red cell mass. Other laboratory measurements that are commonly used to identify iron deficient erythropoiesis, such as the erythrocyte protoporphyrin and mean corpuscular volume, are also of limited value during gestation because they do not become abnormal for several weeks after the onset of iron deficiency.

It was initially reported that the serum transferrin receptor is elevated during pregnancy[22]; the authors assumed that the increase in serum transferrin receptor was derived from the placenta which is a rich source of receptor protein. However, in a later study, the serum transferrin receptor concentration in 176 women in third trimester pregnancy was 5.96 ± 2.3 mg/l, similar to the values observed in nonpregnant control women[23]. The frequency distributions in pregnant and control women were also comparable. Using a combination of laboratory measurements of iron status, 13 of the 176 women fulfilled the criteria for iron deficiency anaemia. The serum transferrin-receptor concentration was significantly elevated above the cutoff of 8.5 mg/l in 11 out of these 13 women. Together with the receptor:ferritin ratio findings in pregnant Jamaican women, these results indicate that the serum transferrin receptor is a useful measure of iron deficiency during pregnancy and the receptor-ferritin ratio may be even more so.

Anaemia of chronic disease

The anaemia of chronic disease develops in a wide spectrum of clinical disorders associated with chronic infection, inflammation or neoplastic disease exclusive of marrow metastasis, blood loss or haemolysis. The anaemias associated with renal failure, hepatic insufficiency or endocrinopathies are not included with the anaemia of chronic disease which is largely a diagnosis of exclusion. The anaemia of chronic disease is undoubtedly the most common cause of anaemia encountered in clinical practice. In one recent series, 90 out of 172 patients with anaemia or 52 per cent met the diagnostic criteria of the anaemia of chronic disease[24]. The anaemia of chronic disease is particularly common in the elderly. In one study of anaemic patients over the age of 65 years who underwent extensive laboratory testing including a bone marrow examination, 113 (or 44 per cent) had the anaemia of chronic disease as compared to 94 (or 36 per cent) with iron deficiency anaemia. These two forms of anaemia therefore accounted for 80 per cent of the anaemias seen in this elderly population group[25].

Despite several decades of investigation, the exact mechanism for the anaemia of chronic disease remains obscure. One of the characteristic features is hypoferremia in the face of normal or increased amounts of storage iron. The transferrin saturation is usually reduced and the total iron-binding capacity is also lower rather than increased as in iron deficiency anaemia . With protracted inflammation or infection, laboratory evidence of iron deficient erythropoiesis eventually develops and is best identified by a fall in mean corpuscular volume below 80 fl or an increase in erythrocyte protoporphryin. The red cell distribution width was initially proposed as a means of distinguishing iron deficiency anaemia from the anaemia of chronic disease but subsequent clinical studies have not demonstrated it to be a reliable means of distinguishing these two major forms of iron deficient erythropoiesis[26,27]. The one unequivocal feature that distinguishes iron deficiency anaemia from the anaemia of chronic disease is the amount of stainable iron in macrophages evaluated by bone marrow examination; iron is invariably absent in iron deficiency anaemia, but present and often increased in the anaemia of chronic disease.

Because of the impaired haemoglobinization of red cell precursors due to a curtailment in their iron supply, defective release of iron from macrophages has long been considered the underlying defect in the anaemia of chronic disease. However, defective production of erythropoietin for any given degree of anaemia may be an even more important factor. For example, studies in patients with rheumatoid arthritis who are often considered the prototype for the anaemia of chronic disease have shown that the log of the serum erythropoietin concentration is inversely related to the haemoglobin concentration but the regression line is displaced downwards in comparison to patients without inflammation[28]. Nevertheless, serum erythropoietin levels are invariably higher than in individuals without anaemia. This indicates that the inflammatory process has impaired the bone marrow response to erythropoietic stimulation. In defining the pathogenesis of the anaemia of chronic disease, emphasis has recently been placed on the disturbance in cytokine elaboration[29]. The elaboration of several cytokines including tumour-necrosis factor, interferons and interleukin-1 with an inflammatory response is now believed to play a central role in the development of the anaemia of chronic disease. Collectively, these cytokines are apparently responsible for the block in iron release from stores, the impairment in erythropoietin production and the dampened response to erythropoietin by the erythroid marrow.

The challenge to the clinician presented with an anaemic patient and laboratory evidence of iron deficient erythropoiesis is to distinguish the anaemia of chronic disease from iron deficiency anaemia. This often requires a bone marrow examination that typically demonstrates stainable iron in the anaemia of chronic disease but absent iron in iron deficiency anaemia. A less invasive approach is to measure the serum ferritin concentration, which is characteristically below 18–20 µg/l in iron deficiency anaemia and normal or elevated in the anaemia of chronic disease. However, although a study in the elderly has shown that the serum ferritin concentration is the best predictor for distinguishing iron deficiency anaemia from the anaemia of chronic disease, values commonly fall in the non-diagnostic range between 18 and 100 µg/l[25,30]. Thus, 70 out of 235 patients with either iron deficiency anaemia or non-iron deficiency anaemia (or approximately 30 per cent) had serum ferritin values between these levels. Of these 70 patients, 30 had iron deficiency anaemia while 40 had some other form of anaemia. Because of the elevation in serum ferritin which occurs with even modest inflammation, it is not an entirely reliable method for identifying patients with iron deficiency anaemia.

Clinical studies have shown that the serum transferrin receptor concentration remains normal in most patients with the anaemia of chronic disease, in contrast to the elevation typically seen in patients with iron deficiency anaemia[31]. In an initial report, serum transferrin receptor measurements were performed in 41 patients with the anaemia of chronic disease and 17 patients with iron deficiency anaemia. All but one patient with iron deficiency anaemia had elevated serum transferrin receptor values, whereas only four out of the 41 patients with the anaemia of chronic disease had a serum transferrin receptor value above the upper cut-off level for normal. When patients with more severe anaemia as defined by a haemoglobin concentration more than 25 g/l below normal were compared, there was a complete separation between the anaemia of chronic disease and iron deficiency anaemia using serum transferrin receptor values.

These findings were confirmed in a more recent study in which serum transferrin receptor concentrations were compared in 19 patients with iron deficiency anaemia and 14 patients with the anaemia of chronic disease[19]. The serum transferrin receptor concentration was increased in all but one of the patients with iron deficiency anaemia, whereas it remained normal in all patients with the anaemia of chronic disease. When these two series are combined, there are 42 patients with iron deficiency anaemia and 58 patients with the anaemia of chronic disease. Thirty-nine out of 42 patients with iron deficiency anaemia had elevated serum transferrin receptor concentrations (sensitivity 93 per cent), whereas 54 out of 58 patients with the anaemia of chronic disease had normal serum transferrin receptor concentrations (specificity 93 per cent). The positive predictive value for the serum transferrin receptor which is the proportion of patients with an elevated level who had iron deficiency anaemia was 91 per cent, whereas the negative predictive value or the proportion of patients with the anaemia of chronic disease who had normal serum transferrin receptor concentrations was 54 out of 57 or (95 per cent). These data indicate that bone marrow examinations to detect stainable iron may not be necessary in the majority of patients presenting with hypoproliferative anaemia and signs of iron deficient erythropoiesis.

Concurrent anaemia of chronic disease and iron deficiency anaemia

Preliminary studies suggest that the serum transferrin receptor concentration can also detect iron deficiency in patients with the anaemia of chronic disease. Two groups of patients with chronic inflammation and the anaemia of chronic disease who are especially prone to the development of iron deficiency anaemia are patients with rheumatoid arthritis or inflammatory bowel disease. In both these patient groups, iron deficiency occurs commonly because of chronic gastrointestinal blood loss. In a recent study by Pettersson *et al.*, the serum transferrin receptor concentration was measured in 34 anaemic patients, 11 of whom had iron deficiency anaemia and 23 had concurrent chronic rheumatoid disease and the anaemia of chronic disease[32]. In the latter group, bone marrow examinations demonstrated concurrent iron deficiency anaemia in 13, whereas the remaining 10 had stainable iron. The receptor:ferritin ratio was of particular value in identifying the patients with the anaemia of chronic disease who had concurrent iron deficiency. Thus, the receptor:ferritin ratio was below 50 in all 10 patients with the anaemia of chronic disease, whereas higher ratios were observed in 11 out of 13 patients with rheumatoid disease and concurrent iron deficiency anaemia. In a more recent study, 14 patients with inflammatory bowel disease underwent bone marrow examinations to determine the presence or absence of iron deficiency[33]. An increase in the receptor:ferritin ratio was observed in nine out of 10 patients with concurrent iron deficiency anaemia but none of the patients with stainable iron in the bone marrow.

When the data in patients with rheumatoid disease and inflammatory bowel disease are combined, a total of 36 patients with the anaemia of chronic disease have been evaluated of whom 23 had concurrent iron deficiency anaemia based on bone marrow examinations. Twenty of these 23 patients had an elevated receptor:ferritin ratio giving a sensitivity of 87 per cent, whereas none of the patients with stainable iron had an elevated level giving a specificity of 100 per cent. The overall diagnostic accuracy of the receptor:ferritin ratio was 92 per cent. Thus, although more clinical information is needed, it appears that a subset of patients with the anaemia of chronic disease who are susceptible to iron deficiency can be identified in most cases by the serum transferrin receptor or, preferably, receptor:ferritin ratio values.

Specificity of the serum transferrin receptor

It should be noted that there are a variety of haematologic disorders in which the serum transferrin receptor concentration is elevated in the absence of iron deficiency. This occurs because the red cell precursors in the bone marrow account for at least two-thirds of the serum transferrin receptor concentration and any increase in the size of the erythroid marrow is therefore parallelled by an increase in serum transferrin receptor concentration.

The most widely used clinical classification of anaemia is one in which anaemia is divided into hypoproliferative, ineffective erythropoiesis and haemolysis. In the latter two categories, the serum transferrin receptor concentration is typically elevated in the absence of iron deficiency. Haemolytic anaemia can be readily identified by an elevation in reticulocyte count which in most cases parallels the rise in serum transferrin receptor concentration[34]. It is more difficult to identify patients with ineffective erythropoiesis because the expansion in erythroid marrow is not accompanied by an increase in reticulocyte count. However, the proportion of anaemic patients with ineffective erythropoiesis is limited. In patients with megaloblastic anaemia or a myelodysplastic syndrome, an elevation in mean corpuscular volume will exclude iron deficiency in most cases. In population studies, the major diagnostic problem will be in distinguishing iron deficiency anaemia from thalassaemia major in regions where this genetic defect is common. However, these patients can usually be identified by clinical examination. It is possible that the serum transferrin receptor concentration may be useful in screening infants for thalassemia major in these countries.

For identifying iron deficiency anaemia, it is therefore recommended to limit the use of the serum transferrin receptor measurement to the evaluation of patients with hypoproliferative anaemia as defined by a low or normal reticulocyte count and laboratory evidence of iron deficient erythropoiesis. Unfortunately, many anaemic patients have more than one pathophysiological mechanism for their anaemia, which may create diagnostic confusion. Despite these limitations, the serum transferrin receptor concentration is of major value in assessing body iron status in otherwise healthy individuals, in distinguishing patients with iron deficiency anaemia from those with the anaemia of chronic disease, and in identifying the development of iron deficiency in patients with the anaemia of chronic disease.

References

1. Huebers, H.A. & Finch, C.A. (1987): The physiology of transferrin and transferrin receptors. *Physiol. Rev.* **67,** 520–582.

2. Trowbridge, I.S. (1988): Transferrin receptor as a potential therapeutic target. *Prog. Allergy* **45,** 121–146.

3. Ward, J.H. (1987): The structure, function, and regulation of transferrin receptors. *Invest. Radiol.* **22,** 74–83.

4. Seligman, P.A. (1983): Structure and function of the transferrin receptor. *Prog. Hematol.* **13,** 131–147.

5. Klausner, R.D., Rouault, T.A. & Harford, J.B. (1993): Regulating the fate of mRNA: The control of cellular iron metabolism. *Cell* **72,** 19–28.

6. Brittenham, G.M. (1991): Disorders of Iron Metabolism: Iron Deficiency and Overload. In: *Hematology: Basic principles and practice*, eds. R. Hoffman, E. Benz, S.J. Shattil, B. Furie & H.J. Cohen, pp. 327–349. Edinburgh: Churchill Livingston.

7. Pan, B.T. & Johnstone, R.M. (1983): Fate of the transferrin receptor during maturation of sheep reticulocytes *in vitro*: selective externalization of the receptor. *Cell* **33,** 967–978.

8. Pan, B.T. & Johnstone, R. (1984): Selective externalization of the transferrin receptor by sheep reticulocytes *in vitro*. Response to ligands and inhibitors of endocytosis. *J. Biol. Chem.* **259,** 9776–9782.

9. Kohgo, Y., Nishisato, T., Kondo, H., Tsushima, N., Niitsu, Y. & Urushizaki, I. (1986): Circulating transferrin receptor in human serum. *Br. J. Haematol.* **64,** 277–281.

10. Kohgo, Y., Niitsu, Y., Kondo, H. *et al.* (1987): Serum transferrin receptor as a new index of erythropoiesis. *Blood* **70,** 1955–1958.

11. Baynes, R.D., Skikne, B.S. & Cook, J.D. (1994): Circulating transferrin receptors and assessment of iron status. *J. Nutr. Biochem.* **5,** 322–330.

12. Flowers, C.H., Skikne, B.S., Covell, A.M. & Cook, J.D. (1989): The clinical measurement of serum transferrin receptor. *J. Lab. Clin. Med.* **114,** 368–377.

13. Huebers, H.A., Beguin, Y., Pootrakul, P., Einspahr, D. & Finch, C.A. (1990): Intact transferrin receptors in human plasma and their relation to erythropoiesis. *Blood* **75,** 102–107.

14. Shih, Y.J., Baynes, R.D., Hudson, B.G. & Cook, J.D. (1993): Characterization and quantitation of the circulating forms of serum transferrin receptor using domain specific antibodies. *Blood* **81,** 234–238.

15. Baynes, R.D., Shih, Y.J., Hudson, B.G. & Cook, J.D. (1994): Identification of the membane remnants of transferrin receptor using domain specific antibodies. *J. Lab. Clin. Med.* **123,** 407–414.

16. Baynes, R.D., Shih, Y.J., Hudson, B.G. & Cook, J.D. (1993): Production of the serum form of the transferrin receptor by a cell membrane associated serine protease. *Proc. Soc. Exp. Biol. Med.* **204,** 65–69.

17. Beguin, Y., Lipscei, G., Thoumsin, H. & Fillet, G. (1991): Blunted erythropoietin production and decreased erythropoiesis in early pregnancy. *Blood* **78,** 89–93.

18. Beguin, Y., Loo, M., Zik, S.R., Sautois, B., Lejeune, F. & Rorive, G. (1995): Quantitative assessment of erythropoiesis in haemodialysis patients demonstrates gradual expansion of erythroblasts during constant treatment with recombinant human erythropoietin. *Br. J. Haematol.* **89,** 17–23.

19. Punnonen, K., Irjala, K. & Rajamaki, A. (1994): Iron- deficiency anemia is associated with high concentrations of transferrin receptor in serum. *Gen. Clin. Chem.* **40,** 774–776.

20. Skikne, B.S., Flowers, C.H. & Cook, J.D. (1990): Serum transferrin receptor: A quantitative measure of tissue iron deficiency. *Blood* **75,** 1870–1876.

21. Simmons, W.K., Cook, J.D., Bingham, K.C. *et al.* (1993): Evaluation of a gastric delivery system for iron supplementation in pregnancy. *Am. J. Clin. Nutr.* **58,** 622–626.

22. Kohgo, Y., Niitsu, Y., Nishisato, T., *et al.* (1988): Immunoreactive transferrin receptor in sera of pregnant women. *Placenta* **9,** 523–531.

23. Carriaga, M.T., Skikne, B.S., Finley, B., Cutler, B. & Cook, J.D. (1991): Serum transferrin receptor for the detection of iron deficiency in pregnancy. *Am. J. Clin. Nutr.* **54,** 1077–1081.

24. Cash, J.M. & Sears, D.A. (1989): The anemia of chronic disease: Spectrum of associated diseases in a series of unselected hospitalized patients. *Am. J. Med.* **87,** 638–644.

25. Guyatt, G.H., Patterson, C., Ali, M., *et al.* (1990): Diagnosis of iron-deficiency anemia in the elderly. *Am. J. Med.* **88,** 205–209.

26. Flynn, M.M., Reppun, T.S. & Bhagavan, N.V. (1986): Limitations of red blood cell distribution width (RDW) in evaluation of microcytosis. *Am. J. Clin. Pathol.* **85,** 445–449.

27. Baynes, R.D., Flax, H., Bothwell, T.H., Bezwoda, W.R., Atkinson & P., Mendelow, B. (1986): Red blood cell distribution width in the anemia secondary to tuberculosis. *Am. J. Clin. Pathol.* **85,** 226–229.

28. Baer, A.N., Dessypris, E.N., Goldwasser, E. & Krantz, S.B. (1987): Blunted erythropoietin response to anaemia in rheumatoid arthritis. *Br. J. Haematol.* **66,** 559–564.

29. Means, R.T. & Krantz, S.B. (1992): Progress in understanding the pathogenesis of the anemia of chronic disease. *Blood* **80,** 1639–1647.

30. Guyatt, G.H., Oxman, A.D., Ali, M., Willan, A., Mcilroy, W. & Patterson, C. (1992): Laboratory diagnosis of iron-deficiency anemia: An overview. *J. Gen. Intern. Med.* **7,** 145–153.

31. Ferguson, B.J., Skikne, B.S., Simpson, K.M., Baynes, R.D. & Cook, J.D. (1992): Serum transferrin receptor distinguishes the anemia of chronic disease from iron deficiency anemia. *J. Lab. Clin. Med.* **119,** 385–390.

32. Pettersson, T., Kivivuori, S.M. & Siimes, M.A. (1994): Is serum transferrin receptor useful for detecting iron-deficiency in anaemic patients with chronic inflammatory diseases? *Br. J. Rheumatol.* **33,** 740–744.

33. Colton, C., Geraci, K., Tahsildar, H. *et al.* (1995): Serum transferrin receptor/ferritin ratio is a reliable predictor of iron deficiency anemia in inflammatory bowel disease patients. *Gastroenterology* **108,** A800 (abstract).

34. Beguin, Y., Clemons, G.K., Pootrakul, P. & Fillet, G. (1993): Quantitative assessment of erythropoiesis and functional classification of anemia based on measurements of serum transferrin receptor and erythropoietin. *Blood* **81,** 1067–1076.

Iron Nutrition in Health and Disease, edited by Leif Hallberg and Nils-Georg Asp
©1996 John Libbey & Company Ltd., pp. 59–64

Chapter 5

Iron nutrition in pubertal boys

M.A. Siimes and R. Anttila

Division of Pediatric Hematology & Oncology, Children's Hospital, University of Helsinki, FIN-00290 Helsinki, Finland

Summary

Few studies have considered the development of iron status in healthy pubertal boys, although it is known that body weight, blood volume, muscle mass and haemoglobin increase during and after puberty in response to elevated iron needs. We monitored 60 healthy boys through their puberty. Body growth, pubertal status and laboratory studies of iron metabolism were followed up. We observed a close correlation between individual haemoglobin and testicular volumes or testosterone levels in boys at any given age but only after mid-puberty. We also observed an association between haemoglobin and IGF-I or IGFBP-3. These observations suggest that the mediators of growth hormone may play a role in the determination of the individual's haemoglobin level. We anticipated that the boys with the fastest growth, and accordingly with the largest iron needs, should show some evidence of inferior iron status. However, we observed no correlation between haemoglobin and growth rate. We speculate that the boys with large individual iron needs are able to stimulate their gastointestinal absorption of iron to meet the needs. Serum ferritin decreased along with pubertal development, particularly in individuals with fastest growth. This decrease started at early puberty. The decreasing iron stores may have an important stimulatory effect on iron absorption which probably accounts for the majority of the increased iron needs. Accordingly, the decreasing serum ferritin may be a part of physiological development in prevention of iron deficiency.

Iron needs are different in boys and girls during puberty. In addition to menstruation several factors may be identified which have an influence on the iron needs. The timing of puberty and body growth spurt are different in the girls and boys. In girls, the pubertal development and the period of maximal body growth begin simultaneously. In boys, the puberty starts at a later age than in the girls. Moreover, the pubertal development begins at a mean age of 12.3 years and the growth spurt later, at a mean age of 14.0 years. Testosterone secretion should have an effect on erythropoiesis, and consequent iron requirements for haemoglobin synthesis. The relative proportion between the blood volume and the body weight, which is usually around 0.064, is dependent on the intensity of physical activity. In general, adolescent boys indulge in more intensive training than do girls. In such boys, the relative blood volume may rise which further increases iron requirements. Further, in boys the average proportion of muscle to fat increases which is another factor that elevates iron needs.

The development of iron status is poorly studied in healthy pubertal boys. The average haemoglobin increases during and after puberty. The haemoglobin concentrations are about 155 (90 per cent range 140–170 g/l) in adult males and about 135 g/l (120–150 g/l) in adult females.

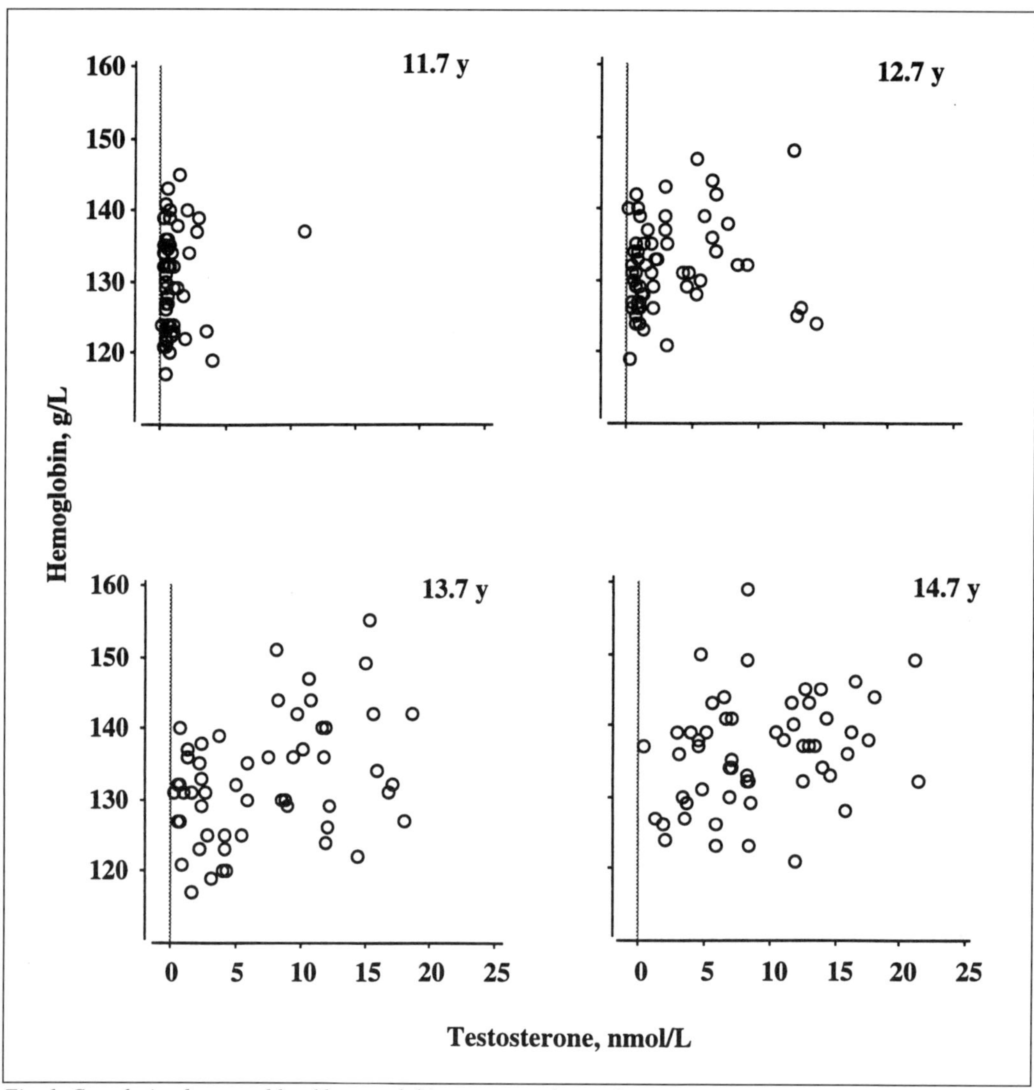

Fig. 1. Correlation between blood haemoglobin concentration and serum testosterone concentration at ages 11.7–14.7 years[2].

Some studies have shown that this difference develops surprisingly slowly, over a period of 4–5 years.

In a recent study we followed 60 healthy boys at 3 month intervals through puberty[1,2]. An opportunity to participate in the study was offered to 84 boys of the same secondary school level in three schools near the Children's Hospital in Helsinki. Most of the boys were from upper middle class families. The study was approved by the parents, the school authorities, and those responsible for school health, and by the Ethics Committee of the Children's Hospital. Written information about the study was sent to the families. Of the 84 boys, 62 agreed to participate. Two boys decided not to continue, leaving 60 boys for the study. Medical history and physical examination indicated that all the boys were healthy except three, who used seasonal medication for asthma. Epilepsy was diagnosed in one boy during the study and he was started on oxicarbamazepine medication. These boys were included in the study.

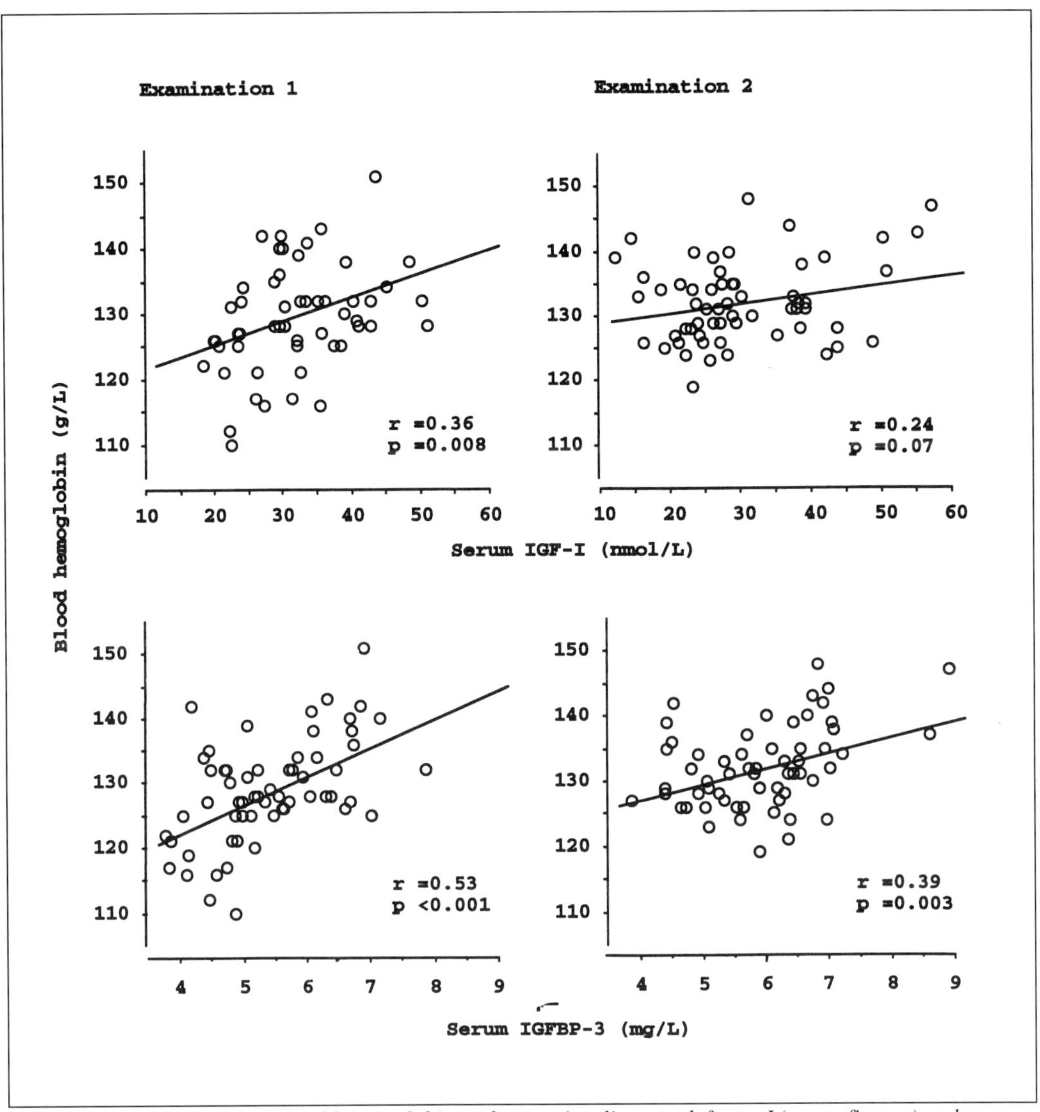

Fig. 2. Correlation between blood haemoglobin and serum insulin growth factor I (upper figures) and serum insulin-like growth factor binding protein-3 (lower figures) in 60 pubertal boys measured twice, with a 9-month interval[1].

At each examination, body weight was measured on the same platform scale, the boys wearing small shorts only. Height was measured on a Harpenden scale with 0.1 cm precision. Genital and pubic hair stages were assessed according to Tanner[3]. The length and width of the testicles were also measured with a ruler to the nearest mm in a lying position. Testicular volume was calculated from the formula 0.52 × longitudinal axis (in cm) × tranverse axis (in cm). Mean testicular volumes were used[1,2]. We estimated changes in muscle mass by determining the greatest diameter of the right quadriceps muscle by an ultrasound method[4].

Venous blood was drawn between 0830 and 1400 hrs. Haemoglobin concentration and heamatocrit value were measured with a Coulter Counter T 890. Serum ferritin concentrations were determined by a two-site chemiluminometric immunoassay with an automatic analyser

(Ciba Corning ACS:180, Switzerland). The red blood cell iron was calculated[5]. The serum testosterone concentration was measured by radioimmunoassay.

At the beginning of the study the mean age of the boys was 11.7 ± 0.05 years. Of the 60 boys, 35 had mean testicular volumes less than 2.0 ml and were considered prepubertal. The other 25 boys had testicular volumes ranging from 2.0 to 6.8 ml. At the end of the study, 3 years later, all boys were pubertal. Of the 60 boys, eight had reached genital stage 5 and were considered postpubertal.

We observed a close correlation between individual haemoglobin, and testicular volumes or testosterone levels in boys at any given age, but only after the average pubertal stage has advanced so that the median testicular volume has doubled (Fig. 1). Other studies indicate that mean haemoglobin continues to rise, by about 10 g/l, during the 2 year period after the age of 15 years when development is less likely to depend on testosterone[2].

An additional regulatory mechanism of haemoglobin level may occur via growth hormone and its mediators. Several pieces of *in vitro* data indicate that insulin-like growth factor system (IGF-I) is involved in the regulation of erythropoiesis[6,7]. Some findings *in vitro* indicate that one-third of the regulation is erythropoietin dependent and one-third is IGF-I dependent. We have also observed a close association between the haemoglobin level and the serum concentration of IGF-I or insulin like growth factors's binding protein (IGFBP-3) in healthy pubertal boys[1] (Fig. 2.). These observations suggest that testosterone may not be the direct stimulator of erythropoiesis, but mediators of growth hormone may play a role in the determination of the individual's haemoglobin level[1].

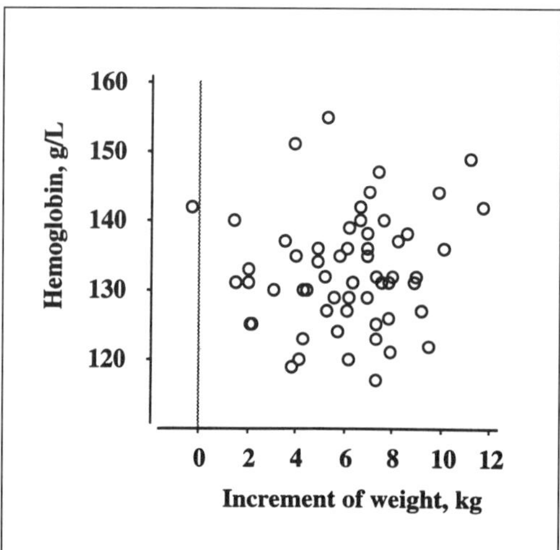

Fig. 3. Correlation between the haemoglobin concentration at age 13.7 years and the preceeding annual increment of body weight.

In our study the individual increments of body weight varied greatly; from –0.6 to +10.0 kg between ages 11.8 and 12.7 years, from –0.3 to +11.7 kg between ages 12.7 and 13.7 years and from –4.3 to +14.6 kg between ages 13.7 and 14.7 years. If one assumes that the ratio of blood volume to body weight remained similar and was 64 ml/kg, the annual balance in red blood cell iron varied in the individuals from negative to +319 mg, to +433 mg, and to +628 mg, respectively. However, it is more probable that the blood volume and muscle mass are more variable and dependent on the individual physical activity. These variations have an extra influence on the iron needs. If so, the differences in iron needs between the boys may be even larger than indicated by the above-mentioned increments in red blood cell iron.

Thus, we anticipated that individual growth rates would have an influence on the haemoglobin concentration during the period of the fastest growth. Accordingly, the boys with largest iron needs should have some evidence of marginal iron lack and those with the least iron needs should not have such evidence. However, our data indicate that there is no correlation between the haemoglobin and growth rate (Fig. 3.). This was a surprising observation. We speculate that it means that the boys with large iron needs are able to increase their gastrointestinal absorption of iron to meet these needs. The serum ferritin decreased along with pubertal development and particularly in individuals with fastest growth. This decrease started at early puberty, by genital stage 2. Thus, it is likely that the tissue iron stores are rapidly mobilized during male puberty, even before the period of most rapid growth. The decreasing iron stores may have an important stimulatory effect on iron absorption which probably accounts for the majority of the increased iron needs. Accordingly, the decreasing serum ferritin may be a part of physiological development rather than evidence of iron insufficency.

In contrast to the above-mentioned findings, we did find a correlation between the genital development and haemoglobin concentration (Table 1).

We have used five different criteria of iron deficiency, all of which have recently been used for pubertal maturation studies in Ireland, Canada, Sweden, USA and Australia[8–12]. The analysis showed that the incidence of iron deficiency was 2–3 per cent by any criteria in the beginning of our study. In later pubertal development it varied between 0 and 35 per cent (Table 2). These findings indicate that iron status has a continuous spectrum, making cut-off points for the diagnosis of iron deficiency highly arbitrary and misleading.

Conclusions

This is a first longitudinal study of haemoglobin concentration and iron status in healthy pubertal boys.

The haemoglobin concentration increases more slowly than the testosterone secretion as estimated by serum testosterone levels, testicular volumes or Tanner's pubertal or genital staging.

In contrast, the decrease in serum ferritin occurs early in pubertal development. It probably augments intestinal iron bioavailability,

Individual haemoglobin level depends on growth hormone status as estimated by insulin-like growth factor I or its binding-protein 3.

Table 1. Haemoglobin concentration in relation to age and individual genital status in a group of 60 healthy boys. Values are g/l ± SEM. Number of subjects is shown in parentheses[2].

	Age in years			
Genital Stage	**11.7**	**12.7**	**13.7**	**14.7**
G1	129 ± 1.0 (35)	129.7 ± 1.4 (6)		
G2	130.8 ± 1.5 (25)	130.1 ± 1.7 (10)	129.2 ± 2.4 (9)	130.5 ± 6.5 (2)
G3		132.4 ± 1.1 (29)	129.2 ± 1.4 (20)	134.3 ± 1.7
G4		135.7 ± 2.8 (9)	135.3 ± 1.3 (24)	135.3 ± 1.2 (35)
G5			141.8 ± 6.3 (5)	141.9 ± 3.4 (9)

Table 2. Incidence of iron deficiency by age in a group of 60 healthy pubertal boys in Helsinki as assessed by five different criteria (from Ireland, Canada, Sweden, United States and Australia [8–12] before and after iron medication[2].

Ferritin (μg/l) **Transferrin iron saturation (%)**	**< 10** **any** **Ref. 8**	< 15 any **Ref. 9**	**< 16** **any** **Ref. 10**	**< 10** **< 16** **Ref. 11**	**< 12** **< 16** **Ref. 12**
Mean age (years)					
11.7	2	3	3	2	3
12.2	0	5%	8	0	0
12.7	0	7	8	0	2
13.2	8	33	35	0	2
13.7	12	27	31	7	10
After iron medication					
13.9	2	9	12	0	0

The individual's rise in body weight is variable and determines iron needs. However, the lack of correlation between haemoglobin concentrations and body weight increments indicates that elevated iron needs are compensated for by stimulated iron absorption.

It is extremely difficult to estimate the prevalence of iron deficiency by any available criteria. However, the prevalence depends on genital stage. Most of the boys respond to iron medication regardless of their iron status.

References

1. Anttila, R., Koistinen, R., Seppala, M., Koistinen, H. & Siimes, M.A. (1994): Insulin-like growth factor I and insulin-like growth factor binding protein 3 as determinants of blood haemoglobin concentration in healthy subjects. *Pediatr. Res.* **36,** 754–8.

2. Anttila, R. & Siimes, M.A. (1995): Development of iron status and response to iron medication in pubertal boys. *J Paediatr. Gastroenterol Nutr.* **22**, 3127.

3. Tanner, J.M. (1962): *Growth at adolescence*, 2nd ed. Oxford: Blackwell Scientific.

4. Koskelo, E.K., Kivisaari, L.M., Saarinen, U.M. & Siimes, M.A. (1991): Quantitation of muscles and fat by ultrasonography: A useful methods in the assessment of malnutrition in children. *Acta Paediatr. Scand.* **80,** 682–687.

5. Green, R., Charton, R. & Seftel, H. *et al.* (1968): Body iron excretion in man. *Am. J. Med.* **4,** 336–353.

6. Kurtz, A., Hartl, W., Jelkmann, W., Zapf, J. & Bauer, C. (1985): Activity in fetal bovine serum that stimulates erythroid colony formation in fetal mouse livers is insulin-like growth factor I. *J. Clin. Invest.* **76,** 1643–1648.

7. Boyer, S.H., Bishop, T.R., Rogers, O.C., Noyes, A.N., Frelin, L.P. & Hobbs, S. (1992): Roles of erythropoietin, insulin-like growth factor I and unidentified serum factor in promoting maturation of purified murine erythroid colony-forming units. *Blood* **80,** 2503–2512.

8. Armstrong, P.L. (1989): Iron deficiency in adolescents. *Br. J. Med.* **289,** 499.

9. Valberg, L.S., Sorbie, J., Ludvig, J. & Pelletie, O. (1976): Serum ferritin and the iron status of Canadians. *Can. Med. Assoc. J.* **114,** 417–421.

10. Hallberg, L., Hulten, L., Lindstedt, G. *et al.* (1993): Prevalence of iron deficiency in Swedish adolescents. *Pediatr. Res.* **34,** 680–687.

11. Expert Scientific Working Group (1985): Summary of a report on assessment of the iron nutritional status of the United States population. *Am. J. Clin. Nutr.* **42,** 1318–1330.

12. English, R.M. & Bennett, S.A. (1990): Iron status of Australian children. *Med. J. Austr.* **152,** 582–586.

Iron Nutrition in Health and Disease, edited by Leif Hallberg and Nils-Georg Asp
©1996 John Libbey & Company Ltd., pp. 65–74

Chapter 6

Influence of age on laboratory criteria for the diagnosis of iron deficiency anaemia and iron deficiency in infants and children

Peter R. Dallman[1], Ann C. Looker[2], Clifford L. Johnson[2] and Margaret Carroll[2]

[1]*Department of Pediatrics, School of Medicine University of California - San Francisco, San Francisco, California 94143, USA,* [2]*Division of Health Examination Statistics, National Center for Health Statistics, Hyattsville, Maryland 20782, USA*

Summary

We present some of the results related to diagnosis of iron deficiency from the first half of the Third National Health and Nutrition Examination Survey (NHANES III), conducted in the United States between 1988 and 1994. For the diagnosis of anaemia, haemoglobin curves for the mean and 5th percentiles (mean −1.645 SD) were derived after excluding individuals with other laboratory evidence of iron deficiency. Prevalence of iron deficiency was defined on the basis of having at least 2 of 3 iron status measures abnormal (transferrin saturation, erythrocyte protoporphyrin and either MCV or serum ferritin) and iron deficiency anaemia as having, in addition, a haemoglobin value below the mean −1.645 SD. The prevalence of iron deficiency in infants 1 to 2 years of age was 5 to 10 per cent, and about half had iron deficiency anaemia. Between the ages of 3 and 11 years, there was a lower prevalence of iron deficiency and <2% had iron deficiency anaemia. In females, the prevalence of both conditions rose in adolescence and the childbearing years to about 8 to 13 per cent with iron deficiency and 2 to 4 per cent with iron deficiency anaemia. Among adolescent and young adult males, however, only <1% had iron deficiency anaemia.

Introduction

Reference standards and cut-off values according to age and sex for haemoglobin and other measures of iron status have gradually become more satisfactory over the past few decades[1]. Reference values are now derived from studies of specific healthy groups of individuals or from national nutrition survey data based on a representative sample of the population. In both cases, there is an effort to exclude persons with clinical or laboratory evidence of common causes of anaemia, such as iron deficiency and infection so that they do not bias the results for what should theoretically be a healthy reference population.

Studies that are specifically designed for the purpose of obtaining reference values have the advantage of concentrating on that objective and emphasizing the age groups of greatest interest. This type of study is still the major source of reference values for infants under the age of one year[2] and for pregnant women[3]. National nutrition surveys, however, have the advantage of being more broadly based, since they reflect a representative sample of the population. They also allow comparisons among different age, socioeconomic, and racial or ethnic groups[4].

In this report, we will review some of the results of the first half of the Third National Health and Nutrition Examination Survey (NHANES III) that was conducted in the United States between 1988 and 1994. This survey included a large collection of laboratory studies related to iron nutrition. The data provide a basis for deriving haemoglobin curves for infancy and childhood and for describing the relationship between pubertal stage and haemoglobin concentration for adolescent males. In addition, one can derive cut-off values for other laboratory tests of iron status and make some preliminary estimates of the prevalence of iron deficiency and iron deficiency anaemia.

Design of the Third National Health and Nutrition Examination Survey (NHANES III)

The recently completed NHANES III survey (1988–1994) included a total sample of about 40,000 persons, studied in 89 US locations. Children under the age of 5 years were substantially oversampled, comprising 23 per cent of the survey group, although only representing 9 per cent of the population. This degree of oversampling makes the survey particularly useful for iron status-related data in children.

The two largest minority groups in the USA, blacks and Mexican-Americans, were also oversampled. Each group accounted for about 30 per cent of the sample, although only 12 per cent of the US population is black and 5 per cent is Mexican-American. In the analysis of the data, the oversampling is corrected for by assigning each person a sample weight according to the number that he or she represents in the population. Consequently, the weighted analyses should provide information representative of the population as a whole.

In respect to childhood iron status, the survey incorporated several improvements over earlier ones. Venipunctures were obtained on a relatively high percentage of infants (about 69 per cent), the group in which this is most difficult. Ferritin was determined on all persons 1 year of age and over. Red cell distribution width (RDW) was obtained on a national US sample for the first time. The advantages of this test are its apparent high specificity and sensitivity in the diagnosis of iron deficiency[5] and the fact that, like the MCV, it is obtainable as a part of an automated blood count. The haemoglobin and iron status data from the first half of the survey (1988–1991) are now available and are the basis for the discussion that follows.

Haemoglobin curves for infants, children and adolescents

The haemoglobin reference population consisted of non-black individuals and excluded those who are most likely to have iron deficiency on the basis of having more than one abnormal value for other laboratory analyses by criteria to be discussed below (under the heading Laboratory tests for iron status). Since reference haemoglobin values of whites were almost exactly the same as those of Mexican-Americans, the groups were combined to yield larger sample sizes. Figure 1 shows the haemoglobin curves at the mean and the mean minus 1.645 standard deviations for reference populations of males and females aged 1–27 years. Since the reference haemoglobin values have a Gaussian distribution, the value corresponding to the mean minus 1.645 standard deviations is equivalent to the 5th percentile. However, the standard deviation approach is used because it is a statistically more reliable determination than the 5th percentile, especially for the smaller sample sizes, which average about 60 for each yearly interval among adolescent males or females. These relatively small sample sizes help to account for the fact that above the age of 11 years, where separate analyses by sex begin, values fluctuate more than at earlier ages. The haemoglobin curves were smoothed by the cubic spline method, the same statistical procedure that has been used to obtain growth curves for children[6,7].

The shapes of the haemoglobin curves for boys and girls are essentially the same as those published for whites 16 years ago[8]. The median

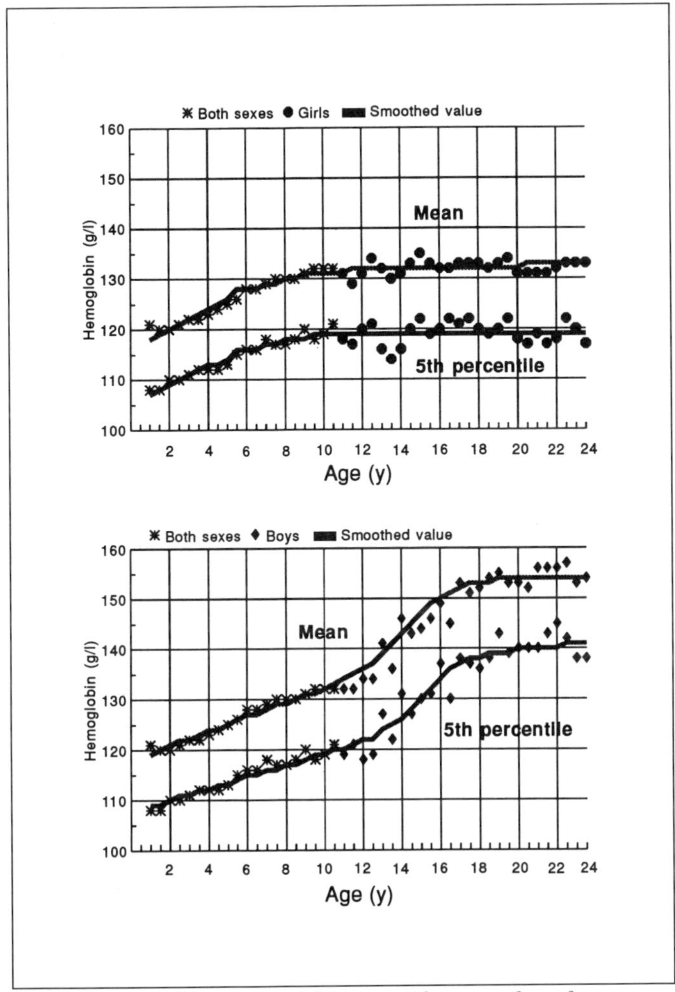

Fig. 1. Haemoglobin mean and 5th percentile curves for reference populations of females (upper panel) and males (lower panel) 1 – 25 years of age in NHANES III, phase 1, 1988–1991.

Table 1. Cut–off values for laboratory tests of iron status

Age (year)	Transferrin saturation (< %)	Serum ferritin (< ng/ml)	Erythrocyte protoporphyrin (> μg/dl RBC)	MCV (< fl)
1–2	9	10	70[a]	77
3–5	12	10	70	79
6–11	14	12	70	80
12–15	14	12	70	82
> 16	15	12	70	85

[a]1.24 mol/l RBC.

values reported in 1979 were slightly higher. The differences were greatest in infants 1–2 years of age, who had median and mean values of 125 g/l compared to 120 g/l in NHANES III. The diagnosis of anaemia in children on the basis of the haemoglobin curves offers the distinct advantage of reflecting the gradual nature of the changes in concentration with age.

The NHANES III haemoglobin reference values tabulated by age group are shown in Table 2. The mean and the mean minus 1.645 standard deviations (SD) correspond to the 50th and 5th percentiles. The mean minus 2 SD, equivalent to the 2.5th percentile, is also shown. The tabulated values (Table 2) represent age ranges of 2 or more years, and are least precise near ages at which haemoglobin values shift abruptly by 3–11 g/l. Consequently, use of the curves in the analysis of survey results should allow a more accurate estimate of the prevalence of anaemia. However, in many settings, the use of tabulated values is simpler and more convenient.

The NHANES III cut-off value for infants 1–2 years of age was 109 g/l at the 5th percentile. This figure rounds out to the commonly used cutoff value of 110 g/l. The use of a cut-off at the 5th percentile can be expected to identify 5 per cent of normal children as anaemic. This figure seems excessively high if haemoglobin screening is done in a population where iron deficiency is rare. Two standard deviations below the mean, equivalent to the 2.5th percentile, would yield a cutoff of 107 g/l and might be more appropriate in that situation. The 5th percentile as a cut-off is advantageous when using the analysis of haemoglobin in combination with other laboratory measures of iron status to estimate the prevalence of iron deficiency anaemia. When laboratory criteria are used in combination in this manner, it becomes more difficult to meet several stringent criteria. Consequently, cut- off values have to be relaxed to avoid missing the majority of individuals with iron deficiency.

After age 18 years, when values for adolescent males reach the adult platcau, the mean haemoglobin for non-blacks was 152 g/l, as it was for whites in NHANES II about 12 years earlier. These values are also quite close to the mean of 151 g/l recently reported for 3975 18-year- old men on enrollment into military service in Sweden[9]. Only 0.17 per cent of that large group was found to have iron deficiency anaemia. The mean minus 2 SD (the 2.5th percentile equivalent) was 135 g/l for the Swedish young men, identical to the value for the 16–19-year-old males in NHANES (Fig. 1, Table 2).

After the age of 12 years, haemoglobin values in females scarcely change. The mean remains at 133 g/l, the 5th percentile equivalent at 118–121 g/l, and the 2.5th percentile equivalent at 115–118 g/l.

Table 2. Haemoglobin reference values for non-blacks derived from NHANES III, part 1, 1988–1991. Individuals with more than one abnormal or missing value for ferritin, transferrin saturation, erythrocyte protoporphyrin, or mean corpuscular volume were excluded. The mean minus 1.645 SD is equivalent to the 5th and the mean minus 2 SD to the 2.5th percentile

			Haemoglobin (g/l)		
Sex	**Age (y)**	**N**	**Mean**	**Mean – 1.645 SD**	**Mean – 2 SD**
M, F	1–2	399	120	109	107
M, F	3–5	756	123	112	109
M, F	6–11	1055	130	118	115
F	12–15	218	133	118	115
F	16–19	200	133	121	118
F	20–49	1149	133	118	115
M	12–15	207	141	124	120
M	16–19	224	152	138	135
M	20–49	1469	152	137	133

Criteria for anaemia in adolescent males

The age of sexual maturation is highly variable[10] and is a strong influence on the haemoglobin concentration in males[11,12]. Boys who have matured early can be expected to have higher concentrations of haemoglobin than those of the same chronological age who will mature later. The higher haemoglobin values in sexually mature males compared to females is attributable to their high levels of testosterone[13]. The Tanner stages of sexual maturity were determined in NHANES III: stage 1 represents the immature, preadolescent state; stage 5, the mature, adult genitalia; and stages 2–4 are intermediate in development. The greatest variability in sexual maturation is from 12 to 13 years of age, when there are likely to be individuals at all five stages. At 13 years of age, the mean haemoglobin concentration was about 10 g/l higher in the more mature males at stages 4 and 5 than in less mature individuals at stages 1, 2 and 3. Differences of this magnitude make it useful to take the stage of maturation into account in interpreting borderline haemoglobin values.

Laboratory tests for iron status

Serum ferritin

Other than the haemoglobin and haematocrit, the serum ferritin is probably the most widely used laboratory test for iron status. A lower normal limit of of 12 mg/l is generally accepted for adults and one of 10 mg/l in children. These cut-off values are at the 5th percentile of the serum ferritin reference distribution for children and women in NHANES III (obtained after excluding those with more than one other laboratory abnormality of iron status by the criteria listed in Table 1).

Serum ferritin concentrations were substantially higher in NHANES III than in NHANES II. For example, the 50th percentile for the large reference population of non-black women 20–49 years of age was 43 mg/l in the more recent survey, as compared to 30 mg/l only 12 years earlier. Corresponding values were also much higher in men of the same age group, 135 mg/l versus 93 mg/l. Values in children have also risen. These results would seem to indicate increasing iron stores in the population as a whole. However, there is a possibility that changes in methodology might also play a role[14].

Erythrocyte protoporphyrin

Reference values for this laboratory test have decreased considerably since NHANES II, especially in young children. Among children 1–2 years of age, for example, the 95th percentile value for a reference population was 86 µg/dl RBC (1.53 µmol/l RBC) in NHANES II. The corresponding figure in NHANES III was 67 µg/dl RBC (1.19 µmol/l RBC), a decrease of 22 per cent. High erythrocyte protoporphyrin values are found not only in association with iron deficiency, but also with elevated blood lead concentrations. The decline in erythrocyte protoporphyrin values is paralleled by a dramatic decrease in blood lead levels over the same period[15]. In NHANES II (1976–1980), the median blood lead concentration of all persons was 13 µg/dl (0.63 µmol/l). The corresponding value for NHANES III, phase 1 (1989–1991) was 3.0 µg/dl (0.14 µmol/l). The decline for ages 1–5 was even greater. In NHANES II, the median blood level was 15 µg/dl (0.72 µmol/l) compared to 3.7 µg/dl (0.18 µmol/l) in NHANES III, phase 1. These changes can be attributed to the removal of 99.8 per cent of lead from gasoline and the removal of lead from soldered cans over the same period. Under the more recent circumstances, erythrocyte protoporphyrin should be a more specific test for iron deficiency.

In the analysis of NHANES II, erythrocyte protoporphyrin concentrations above 80 µg/dl RBC (1.42 µmol/l RBC) were considered abnormal for ages 1–2 years and a cut-off of 70 µg/dl RBC (1.24 µmol/l RBC) was used for ages 5 years and older. Current reference distributions make it possible to propose a single cutoff value of 70 µg/dl RBC (1.24 µmol/l RBC) (Table 1). This value is at or slightly above the 95th percentile for the reference populations of both women and young children. The mean reference erythrocyte protoporphyrin concentration in men was about 10 µg/dl RBC (0.18 µmol/l RBC) lower than in women.

Table 3. Reference red cell distribution width (RDW) values and prevalence of iron deficiency (Ferritin model) by RDW status in Blacks

Sample	Reference RDW (percentiles)		Per cent with iron deficiency	
	50th	95th	RDW ≤ 14.0	RDW > 14.0
Children, 1–2 years	12.7	14.3	2	30
Women, 20–49 years	12.6	13.7	6	65

Table 4. Prevalence of low haemoglobin (Hb) in non-Blacks by RDW status

Sample		Percentage with low Haemoglobin	
	Hb cut-off (g/l)	RDW ≤ 14.0	RDW > 14.0
Children, 1–2 years	< 109	6	28
Women, 20–49 years	< 119	5	36

Mean corpuscular volume (MCV)

In NHANES III, values for MCV in the reference populations of non-blacks were about 1–2 fl higher in all groups than corresponding values for for whites in NHANES II. The difference may be at least partly attributable to the manner in which the MCV has been derived. In NHANES II, the MCV was based on the haematocrit determined by centrifugation of the blood sample, whereas in NHANES III a Coulter-derived haematocrit was used. MCV, like haemoglobin, varies markedly with age, but male and female values are identical or nearly so. Blacks were excluded from the reference population for MCV because of lower values that are thought, like those for haemoglobin, to have a genetic basis.

The cut-off values for MCV that were used in NHANES II were close to the 2.5 percentile of the reference population. However, the resulting values, ranging from <73 fl at ages 1–2 years to > 80 fl in adults, were too low to identify many individuals with iron deficiency when used in combination with transferrin saturation and erythrocyte protoporphyrin. For this reason and because of the rise in MCV values probably due to changes in methodology, we used higher cut-off values than previously (Table 1). The tabulated cut-off values correspond to the 5th percentiles of the reference distributions in NHANES III, in accord with the setting of cut-off values for serum ferritin and erythrocyte protoporphyrin.

Transferrin saturation

In contrast to serum ferritin values which have risen, serum iron and transferrin saturation have declined compared to NHANES II. This can be attributed partly to a change in methodology that corrects for the interference of copper in the assay and that lowers serum iron values by about 9 µg/dl (1.6 µmol/l). This results in a much larger discrepancy at low iron concentrations than at higher ones. Another difference relates to the marked diurnal fluctuations in serum iron concentration. In NHANES III, more blood samples were drawn late in the day, when serum iron values are normally lower than in the morning.

The cut-off values listed in Table 1 were accordingly lowered from the familiar 16–15 per cent for adults and from the widely used 10–9 per cent for infants 1–2 years of age. These values approximate the 10th percentiles of the NHANES III reference populations for women 20–49 years and infants 1–2 years of age, respectively. Fifth percentile values, which would be more in line with cut-off values for other iron status measures, would result in still lower values: 11 per cent in women 20–49 and 7 per cent in infants 1–2 years of age.

Red cell distribution width (RDW)

The RDW measures variability in red cell size, which increases early in the course of iron deficiency. Initial studies of the RDW about 18 years ago indicated that it would reliably distinguish individuals with anaemia of infection, inflammatory disease, or β-thalassemia trait from those with iron deficiency anaemia[5]. Although it has been somewhat disappointing in this respect[16,17], the test still retains its major advantage of being provided as part of the routine blood count by many of the larger clinical laboratories. A disadvantage is that no generally applicable cut-off values can be recommended since results vary according to the instrument used in the analysis.

In NHANES III, RDW was measured on Coulter Electronics model S Plus Jr. Median values in the reference populations of children and young adults ranged between 12.4 and 12.8. The 95th percentile reference value was 14.3 in children 1–2 years of age, but was lower, ranging from 13.2 to 13.8 in all other age and sex groups to age 49.

Using a single RDW cutoff of 14.0 for the sake of simplicity, a remarkably high 65 per cent of women aged 20–49 years with an elevated RDW were also iron deficient by the ferritin model (Table 3) and 36 per cent were also anaemic (Table 4). The corresponding figures for women with a normal RDW of were 6 and 5 per cent, respectively. In children aged 1–2 years, the same cutoff did not yield as large a proportion of iron deficient and anaemic individuals. This may indicate a need for a slightly higher cutoff for this age group, reflecting their slightly higher value at the 95th percentile of the reference population.

Prevalence of iron deficiency, and iron deficiency anaemia

In the NHANES II survey (1976–1980), prevalence of iron deficiency (impaired iron status) was estimated by using combinations of three tests of iron status. The basis for the use of multiple tests was the earlier observation that populations with only one abnormal test out of three had scarcely more anaemia than one with all normal test results[18]. The prevalence of anaemia was substantially higher in those who had abnormal iron status by two or three tests.

By the so called MCV model, individuals were considered iron deficient if at least two out of

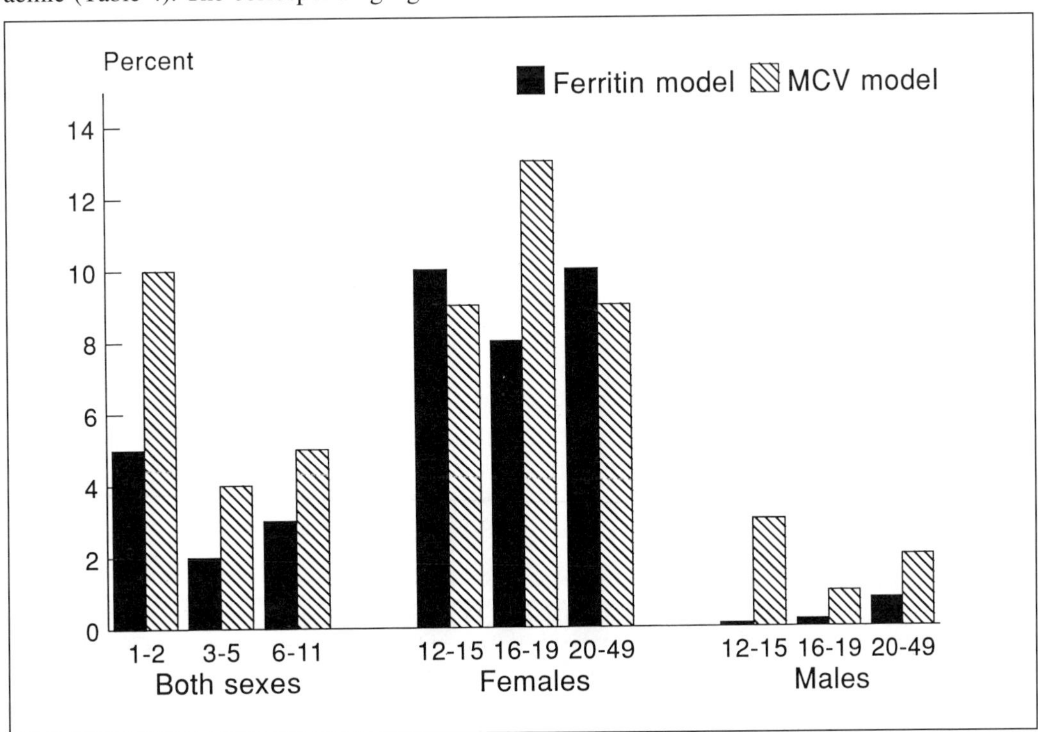

Fig. 2. Prevalence of iron deficiency in NHANES III, phase 1, 1988–1991.

three tests, MCV, transferrin saturation and erythrocyte protoporphyrin, were abnormal. By the ferritin model, the same approach, i.e. at least two out of three indicators, was taken, substituting serum ferritin for the MCV. This dual approach was taken largely because in NHANES II serum ferritin was only available for a subsample of individuals over the age of 3 years. However, it was decided to use the available serum ferritin data because of the advantages of this test in reflecting the abundance of storage iron and having abnormally low values only in response to a lack of iron. The MCV and ferritin models were used to determine the prevalence of iron deficiency in the analyses of the NHANES III, phase 1 data, but with the cut-off values shown in Table 1. Individuals who also had anaemia were considered to have iron deficiency anaemia.

From the Table 1 cutoffs, the prevalence of iron deficiency was higher by the MCV model than by the ferritin model for most groups (Fig. 2). For ages 1–2 years, the prevalences of iron deficiency were 10 and 5 per cent, respectively. Iron deficiency anaemia was found in 3 and 5 per cent, respectively (Fig. 3). For ages 3–5 and 6–11 years, the prevalence of iron deficiency declined and iron deficiency anaemia was found in 2 per cent or less by both models.

In contrast to the NHANES II findings, iron deficiency anaemia remained below 1 per cent in adolescent males. However, females between 12 and 15, and between 16 and 19 years of age had a higher prevalence of iron deficiency (8–13 per cent) and iron deficiency anaemia (2–4 per cent) in NHANES III than in NHANES II. Among women aged 20–49 years, the prevalences of both iron deficiency and iron deficiency anaemia remained essentially the same as in adolescence, 9–10 per cent and 3–4 per cent, respectively. Among males 20–49 years of age, as expected, fewer than 1 per cent had iron deficiency anaemia.

Among women 20–49 years of age, the largest group of individuals at risk, some idea of severity could be obtained by determining the degree of anaemia. Women with iron deficiency but without anaemia had mean haemoglobin

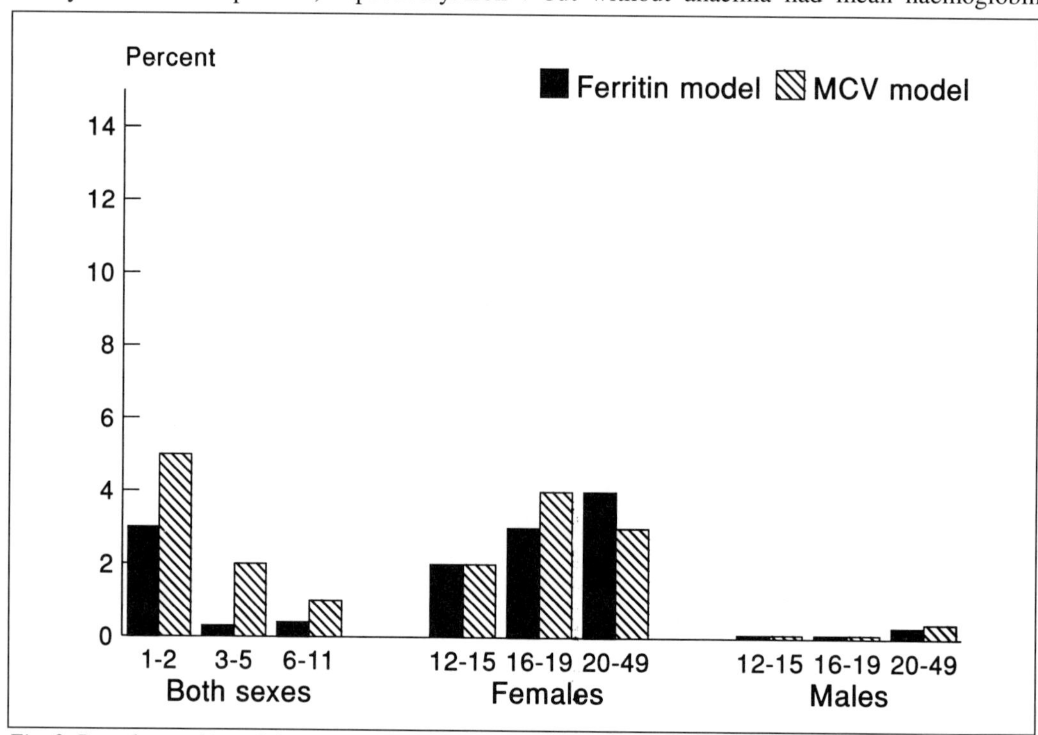

Fig. 3. Prevalence of iron deficiency anaemia in NHANES III, phase 1, 1988–1991.

concentrations of 128 g/l and 126 g/l, respectively, by the ferritin and MCV models, only 5 and 7 g/l lower than the mean of 133 g/l in the normal reference population. Women with iron deficiency anaemia had mean haemoglobin concentrations of 104 g/l and 106 g/l, respectively, by the ferritin and MCV models. These values are substantially below the normal mean and roughly 15 g/l below the commonly used cutoff of 120 g/l. This degree of anaemia seems great enough to warrant continued efforts to detect and prevent iron deficiency among the most vulnerable groups.

It is difficult to make comparisons between NHANES II and NHANES III, phase 1 for trends that might have taken place in iron status in the intervening 12 or so years. Some changes in methodology (transferrin saturation, MCV and possibly ferritin) and the effect of decreased blood lead levels on erythrocyte protoporphyrin have already been mentioned. When the Table 1 cutpoints are applied for all tests other than erythrocyte protoporphyrin, for which cutpoints specific to each survey were used, no major changes in prevalence are evident. For ages 1–2 years, 11 per cent were iron deficient by the MCV model in NHANES II, compared to 10 per cent in NHANES III phase 1. By the ferritin model, the prevalence of iron deficiency was only a relatively low 5 per cent in NHANES III phase 1. Other survey data have provided strong evidence of a substantial decline in prevalence of anaemia in infants and young children in the USA[19,20]. Such a decline would be in accord with the increased use of iron fortified formula and decreased consumption of cow's milk.

Among women 20–49 years of age, 9 per cent were iron deficient by the ferritin model in NHANES II and 10 per cent in NHANES III, phase 1. The results by the MCV model were also similar, with 8 per cent and 9 per cent, respectively. Neither showed any evidence of change between NHANES II and III. A lack of change was also noted in the prevalence of anaemia among low income pregnant women in the Centers of Disease Control pregnancy surveillance system[21].

Conclusions

The NHANES III survey provides an excellent opportunity to refine laboratory criteria for the diagnosis of anaemia and iron deficiency. The first phase of the survey has provided preliminary information for deriving haemoglobin curves and cut-off values for measures of iron status in children and adolescents, as well as estimates of prevalence of iron deficiency and iron deficiency anaemia. These results will become more valuable when they are based on the complete NHANES III survey in the near future.

References

1. Yip, R. (1994): Changes in iron metabolism with age. In: *Iron metabolism in health and disease*, eds. J. Brock, M. Pippard, J. Halliday & L. Powell, pp. 428–448. London: W.B. Saunders.
2. Saarinen, U.M. & Siimes, M.A. (1978): Developmental changes in red blood cell counts and indices of infants after exclusion of iron deficiency by laboratory criteria and continued iron supplementation. *J. Pediatr.* **92,** 412–416.
3. IOM (Institute of Medicine) (1990): Iron nutrition during pregnancy. In: *Nutrition during pregnancy. Report of the committee on nutritional during pregnancy and lactation*, Food and Nutrition Board. pp. 272–298. Washington, DC: National Academy Press.
4. Expert Scientific Working Group (1985): Summary of a report on assessment of the iron nutritional status of the United States population. *Am. J. Clin. Nutr.* **42,** 1318–1330.
5. Bessman, J.D., Gilmer, P.R. & Gardner, F.H. (1983): Improved classification of anemias by MCV and RDW. *Am. J. Clin. Pathol.* **80,** 322–326.
6. Smith, P.L. (1979): Splines as a useful and convenient statistical tool. *Am. Stat.* **33,** 57–62.

7. Stone, C.J. & Koo, C.Y. (1985): Additive splines in statistics. *Proc. Statistic. Comput. Sect. ASA* 45–48.

8. Dallman, P.R. & Siimes, M.A. (1979): Percentile curves for hemoglobin and red cell volume in infancy and childhood. *J. Pediatr.* **94,** 26–31.

9. Olsson, K.S., Marsell, R., Ritter, B., Olander, B., Åkerblom, Å., Östergård, H. & Larsson, O. (1995): Iron deficiency and iron overload in Swedish male adolescents. *J. Intern. Med.* **237,** 187–194.

10. Tanner, J.M. (1987): Issues and advances in adolescent growth and development. *J. Adolescent Health Care* **8,** 470–478.

11. Daniel, W.A. (1973): Hematocrit: maturity relationship in adolescence. *Pediatrics* **52,** 388–394.

12. Charache, S., Joffe, A. & Wong, H. (1987): Hematological changes during sexual maturation. *J. Adolescent. Health. Care.* **8,** 315–321.

13. Krabbe, S., Christensen, T., Worm, J., Christiansen, C. & Transbol, I. (1978): Relationship between haemoglobin and serum testosterone in normal children and adolescents and in boys with delayed puberty. *Acta Paediatr. Scand.* **67,** 655–658.

14. Pirkle, J.L., Brody, D.J., Gunter, E.W., Kramer, R.A., Paschal, D.C., Flegal, K.M. & Matte, T.D. (1994): The decline in blood lead levels in the United States. The National Health and Nutrition Examinations Surveys (NHANES). *JAMA* **272,** 284–291.

15. Looker, A.C., Gunther, E.W., Cook, J.D., Green, R. & Harris, J.W. (1991): Comparing serum ferritin values from different population surveys. National Center for Health Statistics. *Vital Health Stat.* **2,** 111.

16. Flynn, M.M., Reppun, T.S. & Bhagaavan, N.V. (1986): Limitations of red blood cell distribution Width (RDW) in evaluation of microcytosis. *Am. J. Clin. Pathol.* **85,** 445–449.

17. Baynes, R.D., Bothwell, T.H., Bezwoda, W.R., Gear, A.J. & Atkinson, P. (1987): Hematologic and iron-related measurements in rheumatoid arthritis. *Am. J. Clin. Pathol.* **87,** 196–200.

18. Cook, J.D., Skikne, B.S., Lynch, S.R. & Reusser, M.E. (1986): Estimates of iron sufficiency in the US population. *Blood* **68,** 726–731.

19. Yip, R., Walsh, K.M., Goldfarb, M.G. & Binkin, N.J. (1987): Declining prevalence of anemia in childhood in a middle-class setting: a pediatric success story? *Pediatrics* **80,** 330–334.

20. Yip, R., Binkin, N.J., Fleshood, L. & Trowbridge, F.L (1987): Declining prevalence of anemia among low-income children in the United States. *JAMA* **258,** 1619–1623.

21. Kim, I., Hungerford, D.W., Yip, R., Kuester, S.A., Zyrkowski, C. & Trowbridge, F.L. (1992): Pregnancy nutrition surveillance system – United States, 1979–1990. CDC Surveillance Summaries. *MMWR* **41,** 726–742.

Iron Nutrition in Health and Disease, edited by Leif Hallberg and Nils-Georg Asp
©1996 John Libbey & Company Ltd., pp. 75–79

Chapter 7

The importance of standardization of methodology for determination of iron status

Mark Worwood

Department of Haematology, University of Wales College of Medicine, Heath Park, Cardiff CF4 4XN, UK

Summary

The development of international reference standards and methods for the determination of blood haemoglobin concentration, serum iron concentration and total iron-binding capacity and serum ferritin concentration is reviewed. The impact of standardization on practice is discussed along with the problems which remain in carrying out longitudinal studies of the iron status of populations and comparing population surveys.

Introduction

Monitoring of the iron status of a population in terms of the prevalence of iron deficiency anaemia and the levels of storage iron (ferritin and haemosiderin iron in the tissues) is an important task because changes in overall food consumption, in the composition of the diet, the introduction of fortification or an increase in the consumption of tonics and supplements may lead to changes in iron status which have significant consequences for the health of the population.

Until 1972 the primary measurements were the haemoglobin concentration as an indicator of anaemia and measurements of serum iron concentration and transferrin saturation as an index of iron deficiency (the absence of storage iron). Since then the serum ferritin concentration has largely replaced serum iron determination as an index of storage iron and other measurements such as erythrocyte protoporphyrin and serum transferrin receptor have been introduced to detect iron deficient erythropoiesis. In normal subjects serum ferritin concentrations are related to levels of storage iron from absence to excess and are less labile than serum iron concentrations. However, both serum ferritin and serum iron concentrations are influenced by infection, inflammation and liver disease and their use in epidemiological studies require careful evaluation[1].

If haemoglobin iron or ferritin concentrations are to be compared in a longitudinal study or if different surveys are to be compared, then it is essential to eliminate methodological variability which causes differences in accuracy and precision between different parts of the survey or different studies.

Reference standards and methods

Comparibility of assays is best achieved by obtaining international agreement on defining both

Table 1. International standards and methods

Determination	Standard	Method
Haemoglobin	WHO[15]	Yes[15]
Serum iron	See Ref. [16]	ICSH[16, 17]
TIBC	No	ICSH 'best' method[18]
Ferritin	WHO[19]	No

The current WHO standards are haemoglobincyanide, 5th Standard, 1985 distributed by Rijksinstitut voor de Volksgezondheid, Postbus 1, 3720 BA Bilthoven, Netherlands, and ferritin human spleen, 2nd International Standard (80/578) distributed by NIBSC Hertfordshire, EN6 3QG, UK

reference standards and methods and by using these in surveys along with appropriate quality control procedures to demonstrate the consistency of the measurement.

This aim has not yet been achieved for all assays. For haemoglobin there is both a WHO International Standard and a reference method (Table 1). For serum iron there is a reference method accepted by the International Committee for Standardization in Haematology (ICSH) and revised in 1990. This describes the preparation of a reference standard, although the standard is not available either from a WHO laboratory or commercially. It has not proved possible to define a universally acceptable method for determining the total iron-binding capacity (TIBC) of transferrin in serum. This is a measure of transferrin concentration and is required for the calculation of the transferrin saturation ((serum iron concentration/TIBC) × 100). The ICSH (Expert Panel on Iron) has recommended a method in which the excess iron added to saturate the transferrin is removed by the addition of magnesium carbonate. An intrinsically better approach is the direct, immunological determination of transferrin concentration but although such methods are in widespread use international standards and reference methods have not been agreed.

Serum ferritin concentrations are determined immunologically and there are many varieties of assay using radioactive, enzymic or fluorescent labels. There is a WHO reference standard but no internationally accepted reference method.

Methodological and biological variability of assays

The blood assays vary greatly in both methodological and biological stability (Table 2).

Table 2. Overall variability of assays for iron status (within subject, day-to-day CV for healthy subjects)

Reference	Haemoglobin	Serum ferritin	Serum iron	TIBC	EP
Dawkins *et al.*[2]	–	15(MF)	–	–	–
Gallagher *et al.*[20]	1.6(F)	15(F)	–	–	–
Statland and Winkel[21]	–	–	29(F)	–	–
Statland *et al.*[22]	–	–	27(M)	–	–
Statland *et al.*[23]	3(MF)	–	–	–	–
Pilon *et al.*[24]	–	15(MF)	29(MF)	–	–
Romslo and Talstad[25]	–	13(MF)	33(MF)	11(MF)	12(MF)
Borel *et al.*[4]	4(MF)	14(M)	27(M)	–	–
Borel *et al.*[4]	4(F)	26(F)	29(F)	–	–

Haemoglobin concentrations are stable and the simple and well-standardized method of determination ensures relatively low day-to-day variation in individuals. The more complicated procedures involved in immunoassays mean higher methodological variation for ferritin assays (coefficient of variation (CV) of at least 5 per cent) and this, coupled with some physiological variation, gives an overall CV for serum ferritin for an individual over a period of weeks of the order of 15 per cent. There is little evidence of any significant diurnal variation in serum ferritin concentration[2]. The serum iron determination is an example of extremes with reasonably low methodological variation coupled with high physiological variation, giving an overall 'within subject' CV of approximately 30 per cent when venous samples are taken at the same time of day. A diurnal rhythm has been reported with higher values in the morning than in late afternoon, when concentrations may fall to 50 per cent of the morning value[3]. The circadian fluctuation is due largely to variation in the release of iron from the reticuloendothelial system to the plasma. Results from a number of studies of overall variability are given in Table 2 but is should be noted that the type of blood sample, length of study period and the statistical analysis vary from study to study. The somewhat higher variability for haemoglobin and ferritin reported by Borel *et al.*[4] may be due to their use of capillary blood and plasma. Pootrakul *et al.*[5] have demonstrated that mean plasma ferritin concentration is slightly higher in capillary specimens than venous specimens and that within and between sample variation was approximately three times greater. Variability was less in capillary serum but still greater than in venous serum.

These results have clear implications for the use of these assays in population studies[6,7] and in the assessment of individual patients[4]. With increasing coefficient of variation the predictive value of the test is reduced. For accurate diagnosis, either a multiparameter analysis is required or the assay of several samples.

Impact of standardization on practice

Haemoglobin determinations are now accurate and reproducible with automated blood counters using the cyanmet haemoglobin method and the WHO reference standard for primary calibration. Direct comparisons between surveys is possible[8].

For serum iron and TIBC measurements the situation is unsatisfactory. Serum iron is determined in many clinical laboratories using automatic analysers but Tietz *et al.*[9] have demonstrated significant differences between iron concentrations when samples are assayed with automatic, clinical chemistry analysers and the ICSH method. These differences are particularly marked at the lower end of the range where diagnosis of iron deficiency is the principle diagnostic application. No comparable comparisons of TIBC methods are available and the agreement between transferrin determinations and determination of TIBC by the ICSH recommended method was not good[10].

The provision of a reference standard improved the accuracy of serum ferritin determination[11] but differences between assays remain and 'normal ranges' show significant variations[12].

Meta-analysis and longitudinal studies

At present it is possible to compare results of haemoglobin determinations between surveys. This is not the case for serum iron or ferritin assays. The difficulties involved in comparing surveys which have taken place decades apart with the use of different assay procedures and standards can be illustrated with two reports. Hallberg *et al.*[13] wished to compare ferritin concentrations on samples collected in 1968–69 and assayed in 1974 with results obtained with assays in use in 1992. They were able to do this by correcting assay results from the first survey according to the known differences in potency between the original standard and the first international standard for ferritin. However, this cannot provide absolute assurance and the effects of storage are difficult to assess. The recent attempts to monitor changes in iron status in the US population by comparing results from NHANES series have shown that without common assays and standards such comparison is not feasible[14].

For future surveys it remains essential to ensure that an international standard is used as the reference and that the methodology remains available for later studies or that samples are properly stored to allow retrospective comparison.

References

1. Worwood, M. (1994): Laboratory Determination of iron Status. In: *Iron Metabolism in Health and Disease*, eds. J.H. Brock, J.W. Halliday, M.J. Pippard & L.R. Powell. pp. 449–476. London: W.B. Saunders.

2. Dawkins, S.J., Cavill, I., Ricketts, C. & Worwood, M. (1979): Variability of serum ferritin concentration in normal subjects. *Clin. Lab. Haematol.* **1,** 41–46.

3. Bothwell, R.H., Charlton, R.W., Cook, J.D. & Finch, C.A. (1977): Iron metabolism in man. Oxford: Blackwell Scientific.

4. Borel, M.J., Smith, S.M., Derr, J. & Beard, J.L. (1991): Day-to-day variation in iron status indices in healthy men and women. *Am. J. Clin. Nutr.* **54,** 729–735.

5. Pootrakul, P., Skikne, B.S. & Cook, J.D. (1983): The use of capillary blood for measurements of circulating ferritin. *Am. J. Clin. Nutr.* **82,** 289–293.

6. Looker, A.C., Sempos, C.T., Liu, K., Johnson, C.L. & Gunter, E.W. (1990): Within-person variance in biochemical indicators of iron status: effects on prevalence estimates. *Am. J. Clin. Nutr.* **52,** 541–547.

7. Wiggers, P., Dalhoj, J., Hyltoft Peterson, P., Blaabjerg, O. & Horder, M. (1991): Screening for haemochromatosis: influence of analytical imprevision diagnostic limit and prevalence on test validity. *Scand. J. Clin. Lab. Invest.* **51,** 143–148.

8. De Maeyer, E. & Adiels-Tegman, M. (1985): The prevalence of anaemia in the world. *World Health Stat. Quart.* **38,** 302–216.

9. Tietz, N.W., Rinker, A.D. & Morrison, S.R. (1994): When is a serum iron really a serum iron? The status of serum iron measurements. *Clin. Chem.* **40,** 546–551.

10. Huebers, H.A., Eng, M.J., Josephson, B.M., Ekpoom, N., Rettmer, R.L., Labbe, R.F., Pootrakul, P. & Finch, C.A. (1987): Plasma iron and transferrin iron-binding capacity evaluated by colorimetric and immunoprecipitation methods. *Clin. Chem.* **33,** 273–277.

11. ICSH (Expert Panel on Iron) (1994): Preparation, characterization and storage of human ferritin for use as a standard for the assay of serum ferritin. *Clin. Lab. Haemat.* **6,** 177–191.

12. Dawson, D.W., Fish, D.I. & Shackleton, P. (1992): The accuracy and clinical interpretation of serum ferritin assays. *Clin. Lab. Haemat.* **14,** 47–52.

13. Hallberg, L., Bengtsson, C., Lapidus, L., Lindstedt, G., Lundberg, P.A. & Hulten, L. (1993): Screening for iron deficiency: an analysis based on bone-marrow examination and serum ferritin determination of a population sample of women. *Brit. J. Haematol.* **85,** 787–798.

14. Looker, A., Gunter, E., Cook, J., Green, R. & Harris, J. (1991): Problems in comparing serum ferritin values from population surveys. Vital and Health Statistics Series 2 *Data Evaluation and Methods Research*. (111), 1–19.

15. ICSH (1978): Recommendations for reference method for haemoglobinometry in human blood and specifications for international haemoglobincyanide reference preparation. *J. Clin. Pathol* **31,** 139–143.

16. ICSH (1978): Recommendations for measurement of serum iron in human blood. *Brit. J. Haematol.* **38,** 291–294.

17. ICSH (1990): Revised recommendations for the measurements of the serum iron in human blood. *Brit. J. Haematol.* **75,** 615–616.
18. ICSH (1978): The measurement of total and unsaturated iron-binding capacity in serum. *Brit. J. Haematol.* **38,** 281–290.
19. ICSH (1985): Proposed international standard of human ferritin for the serum ferritin assay. *Brit. J. Haematol* **61,** 61–63.
20. Gallagher, S.A., Johnson, L.K. & Milne, D.H. (1989): Short-term and long-term variability of indices related to nutritional status 1: Ca, Cu, Fe, Mg, and Zn. *Clin. Chem.* **35,** 369–373.
21. Statland, B.E. & Winkel, P. (1977): Relationship of day- to-day variation of serum iron concentrations to iron-binding capacity in healthy young women. *Am. J. Clin. Pathol.* **67,** 84–90.
22. Statland, B.E., Winkel, P. & Bokieland, H. (1976): Variation of serum iron concentration in healthy young men: within day and day-to-day changes. *Clin. Biochem.* **9,** 26–29.
23. Statland, B.E., Winkel, P., Harris, S.C (1977): Evaluation of biologic sources of variation of leucocyte counts and other hematologic quantities using very precise automated analyzers. *Am. J. Clin. Pathol.* **69,** 48–54.
24. Pilon, V.A., Howantitz, P.J., Howanitz, J.H. & Domres, N. (1981): Day-to-day variation in serum ferritin concentration in healthy subjects. *Clin. Chem.* **27,** 78–82.
25. Romslo, I. & Talstad, I. (1988): Day-to-day variations in serum iron, serum iron binding capacity, serum ferritin and erythrocyte protoporphyrin concentrations in anaemic subjects. *Eur. J. Haematol.* **40,** 79–82.

Iron Nutrition in Health and Disease, edited by Leif Hallberg and Nils-Georg Asp
©1996 John Libbey & Company Ltd., pp. 81–95

Chapter 8

Methods to study dietary iron absorption in man - an overview

Leif Hallberg and Lena Hultén

Department of Internal Medicine, Section of Clinical Nutrition, University of Göteborg, Annedalsklinikerna, Sahlgrens Hospital, S-413 45 Göteborg, Sweden

Summary

Several methods are available to measure the absorption of iron from the diet. Each method has its limitations and advantages which are important considerations in the choice of method to study specific problems and in the interpretation of results.

The first method used in the 1930s and 1940s was the chemical balance method. Absorption was calculated as the difference between amounts of iron ingested and amounts excreted in the faeces. This difference is usually small and difficult to measure with precision. It is also difficult to identify the start and end of the faecal sampling period, a fact requiring long balance periods, in turn leading to increased risk of systematic losses. In patients with gastrointestinal disorders there is also a risk of subclinical blood loss. Using patients with ileostomy to study iron absorption the sampling problems are greatly reduced but other sources of systematic errors remain. Applied with great care the chemical balance method provided early information about the magnitude of the absorption of dietary iron.

When radioiron was introduced to measure iron absorption, inorganic radioiron was first given as a drink during ingestion of various 'standard' meals. The purpose was mainly to study iron absorption in different clinical disorders. Absorption was measured as a radioiron balance or based on incorporation of radioiron into red cells. The accuracy of this method was never established. Radioiron was also used to label single food items biosynthetically. Absorption was measured as above. Absorption varied considerably both between foods and between subjects.

The extrinsic tag method, adding a radioiron tracer to single foods or composite meals, was a 'byproduct' of studies to validate the 'standard' meal method. Several studies were made to validate the extrinsic tag method, to develop optimal experimental designs and to express results in a way that took into consideration the effect of differences in individual iron status on iron absorption. The extrinsic tag method can be used, for example, to measure non-haem iron absorption from different meals, to search for and study various factors that may inhibit or promote non-haem iron absorption, and to study the bioavailability of iron in compounds used for iron fortification and to estimate the effect expected.

Comparative studies on the bioavailability of iron in different foods or meals should preferably be made in iron deficient subjects or in subjects who are iron replete but with low or moderate iron stores. The reason is that with increasing iron stores true differences in bioavailability will become successively less and thus more difficult to demonstrate. Recent findings show that differences in bioavailability may even disappear in subjects with high physiological iron stores as an effect of the efficient down- regulation of iron absorption with increasing iron stores.

Haem iron absorption can also be measured using an extrinsic tag. The tag, however, must be biosynthetically labelled with radioiron - usually haemoglobin produced in iron deficient animals. In most situations haem iron absorption can be well predicted from knowledge of individual iron status and haem iron intake.

Several methods are available to measure iron absorption from the whole diet. It may be measured with the chemical balance method, mentioned above. The rate of haemoglobin regeneration in subjects with iron deficiency anaemia can be also used to estimate the average iron absorption from the diet during the period of regeneration, provided that further blood loss can be excluded. A change in serum ferritin, as a measure of a change in iron stores, has also been used to estimate total iron absorption. A valid estimation, however, requires that a number of conditions are fullfilled, such as an initially optimal haemoglobin level, no infection or inflammation, initial serum ferritin preferably above 20 and below 50 µg/l. These facts limit its usefulness.

Recently a method was developed based on uniformly labelling all dietary non-haem iron to the same specific activity in all meals for periods of 1–4 weeks. This method was validated in two groups of menstruating women by comparing in each woman total iron absorption and total iron requirements based on body weights and measurements of menstrual blood losses.

Introduction

In 1937 a fundamental discovery was made by McCance and Widdowson who found that the body has very little capacity to excrete iron and that faecal iron represented almost entirely ingested iron that had not been absorbed[1]. Very small amounts of faecal iron originated from desquamated cells and considerable amounts of iron could only be lost by haemorrhage. Since then several methods have been devised to measure iron absorption, and especially dietary iron absorption which is to be discussed in the present paper. Each method has its limitations and advantages which are important considerations in the choice of method to study specific problems and in the interpretation of results.

Balance studies

The first iron absorption studies were made using the classical chemical balance technique[2,3]. A main problem with this method, measuring absorption as the difference between oral intake and faecal loss, is the fact that this difference is small - in normal men about 5–10 per cent of the intake - and technically difficult to measure with accuracy. It is also difficult to establish the start and end of the faecal sampling period. Long balance periods were thus required which in turn increases the risk for loss of faecal material. Losses of iron in the analytical procedures were reported in earlier reviews. Double-portion techniques with high-precision chemical analyses of food and faeces, long periods of a constant diet known in detail, meticulous care in planning the diet and collecting faeces made these balance studies very laborious and costly. The studies were also difficult for the subjects since metabolic ward conditions had to be applied. The main advantage of the method is that it measures iron absorption from the whole diet over a considerable time period. Some very careful studies were made in the 1940s with balance periods usually extended over several weeks[4,5]. These studies gave information about the magnitude of the total absorption of iron from the diet. Of course no information could be obtained about the absorption from individual meals. These early studies have been reviewed in detail[2,3]. Recently, very careful balance studies were reported using a controlled metabolic ward unit and a 5.5 week balance period[6].

Balance experiments have also been made using patients with ileostomy after proctocolectomy for ulcerative colitis[7]. The sampling of faeces was then very much facilitated. The method has many advantages and has been extensively used in several absorption studies. In studies on iron absorption the chemical analytical problems for iron remain, however. Moreover, a special problem in iron absorption studies is the possibility of minor blood losses from a sometimes diseased intestine and from the fistula when collecting the stools leading to even positive balance figures. With available methods minor blood losses in the collected stools are hard to exclude in balance studies on meat- containing diets, a fact that will greatly reduce the usefulness of this method for studies on iron absorption. By and large, chemical balance methods have been abandoned for the technical reasons given and because new, more exact methods are now available.

Radioiron labelled standard meals

When radioiron was introduced to measure iron absorption in man it was first used to study the absorption of iron salts in balance studies in patients with various disorders[8]. A few years later the first attempts were made to study food iron absorption by adding a tracer dose of radioiron labelled ferric chloride to a so-called standard meal[9,10]. The assumption was that the radioiron would admix with the food iron sufficiently well to provide an index of food iron absorption under different clinical conditions. Different investigators were using different 'standard' meals and the main purpose of the studies was to compare iron absorption in subjects with different iron status and different clinical conditions.

The absorption of the radioiron tracer added to the meal was measured either by collecting faeces (balance technique) or by measuring the incorporation of radioiron into red cells by estimating the blood volume from body weight and assuming that a certain fraction of the absorbed radioiron was incorporated into red cells. Later on the distribution of the absorbed iron was also calculated using another radioiron isotope given intravenously[11].

The extent of labelling of the food iron in the standard meals was unknown at this time. Only single administrations of labelled meals were given and the results were thus influenced by the day-to-day variation in absorption. No method was available to quantitatively express iron status in the individual subject and results were thus simply given as mean values within groups of normal and iron deficient subjects. Wide ranges of absorption were seen both within iron replete and iron deficient groups. At that time it also became evident that patients with achlorhydria or with partial gastrectomy absorbed non- haem iron less well but that haem iron was well absorbed[10,12–17].

Iron absorption from biosynthetically radioiron labelled foods

This method was introduced in 1951 by growing plants in solutions containing radioiron to get radioiron labelled vegetables and cereals or by injecting radioiron into animals to get labelled eggs, meat, haemoglobin and liver[18]. The measurements of iron absorption from the labelled foods were based on faecal sampling or incorporation of radioiron into red cells. This pioneering work led to the observations that different foods varied considerably in bioavailability and that haem iron was absorbed differently[2]. At that time the absorption of iron from a meal was assumed to be a simple sum of the absorption of iron from different foods with different bioavailabilities contained in a meal. This simple concept, however, was not quite compatible with early observations by Roche and Layrisse[2] that addition of maize or black beans seemed to modestly reduce the absorption of iron from labelled beef and that the addition of beef to labelled black beans significantly increased the absorption from the beans. The positive effect of ascorbic acid on non-haem iron absorption was also observed in these early studies.

This was by and large the situation in 1967 when Carl Moore summarized the available knowledge about iron absorption from foods by saying that data were inadequate to provide any satisfactory conclusion about the amounts of iron absorbed from the diet, that a good guess would be that healthy subjects absorb 5–10 per cent, and iron deficient patients 10–20 per cent of the dietary iron[2].

Extrinsic tag method

Introduction

In 1969 a joint IEAA-WHO project was started to examine the systematic errors of the standard meal technic in order to develop a simple method that might be used in field studies mainly in developing countries. Different biosynthetically radioiron labelled foods (e.g. maize, wheat and soybeens) were prepared by Dr R Walker in the Department of Botany at the University of Washington in Seattle, USA. These labelled foods were then sent to the four cooperating laboratories in Seattle, Caracas, Johannesburg and Göteborg. In the first studies we prepared and served the labelled foods together with a solution taken as a drink and containing an iron salt labelled with another radioiron isotope.

These first studies showed that considerably more iron was absorbed from the iron solution than from the biosynthetically labelled foods. The extrinsic label thus markedly and to a varying extent overestimated the absorption of the biosynthetically labelled foods. However, by mixing the extrinsic tracer into the food, instead of taking it as a drink, the unexpected observation was made that the extrinsic, added tracer and the intrinsic, biosynthetic tracer were absorbed to the same extent[19–21]. This was true for all foods studied. It was true for labelled bread made of well absorbed white wheat, and it was also true for bread containing the poorly absorbed bran fraction. A series of studies were then made by the groups cooperating in the project to develop and validate the technique[21–26]. By giving foods labelled with both an extrinsic and an intrinsic tracer the plasma activity curves of the two tracers were identical[27]. Adding extra iron, extra ascorbic acid or an inhibitor such as desferrioxamine did not change the finding that the two tracers were absorbed to the same extent. Mixing biosynthetically radioiron-labelled eggs, having a low iron absorption when given alone, with biosynthetically radioiron labelled white wheat, having a very high absorption when given alone, showed that when the two foods were used to make an omelet the two tracers were absorbed to the same extent[27]. This observation also strongly supported the hypothesis that there is a rapid and complete isotopic exchange between native food iron and an added inorganic radioiron tracer and the pool concept was developed[28]. A rapid isotopic exchange also took place in patients with gastric achlorhydria and in patients who had had a partial gastric resection. Labelling only one component of a meal gave the same result as uniformly labelling all iron-containing components in a meal[29]. Early on it was suggested that a similar isotopic exchange should occur with tracers added to other minerals, such as zinc, manganese and calcium.

These early observations implied that it became possible to homogenously label all non-haem iron in meals and thus, for the first time, to measure iron absorption from composite meals, to study the interaction of different foods on iron absorption, to measure effects of meal preparation on iron absorption. Methods were also devised to measure the bioavailability of iron from compounds used for iron fortification. Several studies were also made by different groups to identify factors enhancing or inhibiting the absorption, especially of non-haem iron and to quantitate the effects of such factors under different conditions. Among factors studied were meat and other proteins, ascorbic acid and other organic acids, phytate and other inositol phosphates, various polyphenols and various drinks including tea, coffee, legumes, fruits and spices. All these studies are presented in another paper. Several studies were also made of the absorption of iron from different meals - typical breakfast meals[30], lunch and dinner meals[31], Western meals[32] and meals typical for different developing countries[33]. The groups working in this field all used two radioiron isotopes simultaneously, which greatly facilitated such studies by making each subject his own control.

There are a few exceptions to the uniform labelling of foods with the extrinsic tracer. An example is ferritin and haemosiderin[34,35]. Another is unpolished unmilled rice where the aleuron layer probably forms a barrier that delays the rate of isotopic exchange[27]. Many foods, especially in developing countries, contain a considerable amount of iron originating from contaminating dust and soil. This contamination iron may constitute the main part of the iron in many meals. To calculate the absolute amount of iron absorbed it is thus necessary to get a measure of the total amount of non-haem iron in the meal that exchanges with the added tracer. The bioavailability of the contamination iron cannot be directly determined. An *in vitro* method has been devised, however, to measure the extent of isotopic exchange between the added tracer and the iron present in the meal under simulated gastrointestinal luminal conditions[36,37]. Since some soil iron exchanges quite well *in vitro* with an added tracer, the nutritional importance of soil iron should not be disregared. Soil iron probably plays a key role in the iron nutrition of many animals, such as the pig and the elephant. Soil iron might well have had an important role for iron nutrition in man in primitive societies, especially to cover the high iron requirements in weaning infants and toddlers. Most iron compounds used for iron fortification of foods, for example various forms of reduced iron, do not completely exchange with an added tracer. To measure iron absorption from such compounds it is necessary to label them during their synthesis or by irradiation[38,39]. Labelled iron in sodium-iron EDTA presents another problem since its iron only partially exchanges with the food iron. This is especially marked for foods where the iron is poorly available, such as in maize. There are also data suggesting that some of the iron compounds present in milk do not fully exchange with an extrinsic tracer. This fact makes it difficult to translate iron absorption from a tracer added to milk into milk-iron absorption.

Experimental design

The extrinsic tag method has greatly facilitated measurements of food iron absorption. The principal problems remaining in such measurements are the day-to-day variation in iron absorption within the same subject and the marked variation between different subjects. These problems can be partly solved by choosing a suitable experimental design. The effect of the day-to-day variation in absorption can be reduced by administering multiple servings of tagged foods over several days. Usually two radioiron isotopes are used. If two meals A and B are to be compared the meals are given in a fasting state on consecutive days. To reduce the day-to-day variation in iron absorption two or more administrations of labelled meals can be given, for example, giving the meals on four consecutive days in the order ABBA. If more comparisons are to be made in the same subjects, A and B meals are first compared and the absorption measured two weeks later and then followed by the serving of meals C and D and measuring iron absorption again 2 weeks later. If reference doses (R) are given the design can be ABBA followed 2 weeks later by RR, preferably given on two consecutive mornings to reduce the effect of the day-to-day variation in absorption. If three meals are compared an alternative design is ABCR. The choice of design depends on the accuracy and precision required, availability of equipment, number of volunteers available for study and so on. The choice of experimental design has been discussed in previous papers[40,41].

The absorption is measured by analysing the content of ^{59}Fe and ^{55}Fe in a blood sample drawn two weeks after the administration of the last test meal. Whole body counting of ^{59}Fe can also be made to get the absolute content of ^{59}Fe retained, and to calculate the total amount of ^{55}Fe absorbed from the ratio of the tracers in the blood sample and the whole body count of ^{59}Fe. The low energy in ^{55}Fe makes it not measurable in the whole body counter.

In patients where the fraction of absorbed iron taken up by red cells is unknown or known to be incomplete (for example in patients with ineffective erythropoiesis or with haemochromatosis) it is necessary to use a whole body counter with a good geometry to calculate the total amount of iron retained. It is also possible to label the food with one radioiron isotope and to give an other radioiron isotope intravenously to calculate the fraction of absorbed iron that is taken up by red cells.

Selection of volunteers and experimental meals

The selection of volunteers for absorption studies is very important. In studies on the effect of different factors on food iron absorption and in comparative studies on the bioavailability of iron in different meals, it is essential to choose subjects who are not fully iron replete such as adult men. We have not been fully aware of the importance of this fact until recently.

It is well established that there is a close relationship between iron absorption and iron status. This fact will be more discussed later. For the present discussion consider the results from two recent studies where we measured the total amounts of iron absorbed over periods of 5–10 days. We studied four diets with different bioavailability in two groups of subjects[42,43] by homogenously labelling all meals with an extrinsic radioiron tracer to the same specific activity. Haem iron absorption from the meals was calculated as described later[42,43].

Each diet was thus represented by a regression line (Fig. 1). The slopes of the four regression lines converged to a point at about 40–60 on the

SF scale. The results show the marked effect of iron status on iron absorption and the marked effect of differences in bioavailability.

Our findings imply that true effects of a factor on iron absorption or true differences in bioavailability between meals will be difficult or impossible to observe in subjects with serum ferritin above the range 50–60 µg/l.

This means that the higher the serum ferritin, which usually means the more stored iron, the smaller is the difference between iron absorption from meals with different bioavailability.

Often the purpose of absorption studies is to measure the effect of certain factors on iron absorption or the absorption from different meals in borderline iron deficient/iron replete subjects, to be able to compare the nutititive value of different diets for iron, and to recommend diets that will reduce the prevalence of iron deficiency. Therefore, studies should mainly be made in iron deficient subjects or in subjects who are not wholly iron replete. Suitable subjects are thus, for example, menstruating women, blood donors and young men with serum ferritin below 40 µg/l.

In studies on the effect of single dietary factors on non-haem iron absorption the choice of basal diet to which the factor is added is also important. In studies on factors expected to enhance iron absorption it is preferable to select a basal diet with a rather low bioavailability. Similarily, to study the effect of adding a factor expected to inhibit iron absorption the basal meal should have a rather good bioavailability. These principles reduce the risk that falsely negative effects are obtained and imply that statistically significant effects of a magnitude that is nutritionally important may be detected using fewer subjects.

Analysing food iron absorption data

There is a considerable variation in iron absorption from meals and the diet between different subjects mainly related to differences in iron status. This is true both for iron deficient and iron replete subjects. To facilitate comparisons of iron absorption from different meals obtained in different subjects, measurement of iron ab-

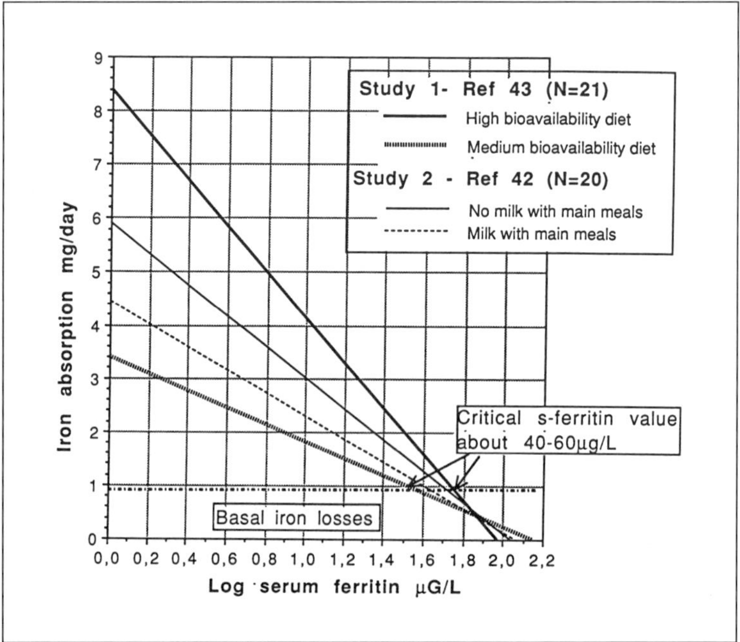

Fig. 1. Regression lines for the relationship between total amounts of iron absorbed and log serum ferritin in two studies[42,43]. The regression lines are statistically significantly different (P < 0.001).

sorption from a reference dose was early introduced. The dose recommended contains 3 mg elemental iron given as a ferrous salt in a solution containing ascorbic acid and administered in a fasting state in the morning[44]. This radioiron labelled dose is usually given 2 weeks after the measurement of food iron absorption is completed and the measurement of the absorption of the reference dose is then made after a further 2 weeks, by whole body counting or by measuring the radioiron content in a blood sample. Since this procedure prolongs the study by about 2 weeks, serum ferritin concentration or rather log serum ferritin was introduced as a measure of iron status and as an alternative basis for comparisons. Several studies have shown that there is a high correlation both between iron absorption and serum ferritin and between iron absorption from test meals and reference dose absorption[40,45,46].

Use of the reference dose has the disadvantage that it prolongs the study and that in order to give reliable results it must be taken in a strict fasting state which may be difficult to fully control. Use of serum ferritin has the disadvantage that it is influenced by external factors, such as a preceding simple infection, for example a common cold, and that this effect remains for a long time. The safest procedure is to use both methods, to carefully control the intake of the reference doses, and to take a medical history especially about preceding infection.

Iron absorption from 'single meals' versus absorption from whole diet

A very careful and extensive study was recently made comparing iron absorption from two types of single meals with markedly different bioavailability and from two kinds of diets with multiply labelled main meals served for 2 weeks[47]. These diets were also designed to have different bioavailability. They found that the difference between the two kinds of single meals (2.3 and 13.5 per cent) was greater than the difference between the two diets (3.2 and 8 per cent). Several reasonable explanations were given by the authors for these observations. Some readers of this comprehensive paper, however, seem to have misinterpreted these findings so far as to suggest that 'single meal' studies, in some unknown way, should give systematically incorrect results.

Studies on different factors influencing iron absorption are usually designed, for example, to study qualitatively whether a certain factor influences iron absorption or not, and to obtain some information about the relative quantitative importance of different single factors such as the dose-response relationship. The purpose may also be to study if there is a positive or negative interaction between different factors. The single meal studies are thus designed to specifically measure the effect of a certain factor under controlled experimental conditions.

There appears to be a general agreement that the absolute nutritional effect of a certain factor on iron absorption from the whole diet may be hard to predict from a few so-called single meal studies. In nutritional evaluation, consideration must include the levels of factors present in different meals, and also the frequency of consumption of different meals containing enhancing or inhibiting factors. It is important to emphasize that there is no evidence that the iron absorption measured from a single meal should in any way be systematically incorrect - the problem is to translate the measurements of iron absorption from single meals to iron absorption from the whole diet. Such translations can be made, however, using methods which will be discussed later.

Methods to measure iron absorption from the whole diet

Iron absorption from the whole diet can be estimated in different ways but there is hardly any simple method available for such direct measurements. Results obtained in studies using different methods are important, however, to get information about the magnitude of the absorption of iron from a certain diet and to estimate the effect expected of dietary modifications.

Chemical balance technique

As mentioned above it is possible to get information about the amounts of iron absorbed from the whole diet over a certain time period. The complexity of the method makes it difficult to use in comparative studies on iron absorption from different diets. When carefully applied, however, it can give very important results[6].

Rate of haemoglobin regeneration

The principle of this method is to measure the rate of haemoglobin regeneration in subjects with uncomplicated iron deficiency anaemia, who have no continued blood loss and who are served a diet with a known composition for a longer time period. The most extensive such study was the following[48,49]. A group of 10 healthy men, aged 20–29 years, were phlebotomized to a haemoglobin level of about 100 g/l over an average period of 3 months. One of the purposes of the study was to measure the amounts of stored iron by repeated phlebotomies. After the phlebotomy period haemoglobin regeneration was followed for an average period of 128 days. In each subject there was a linear increase in haemoglobin concentration, which was converted into red cell iron from measurements of blood volume both at the beginning and the end of the study. The average daily increase in red cell mass iron was 3.8 mg/day. By adding the estimated basal iron losses of 1 mg/day the total iron absorption from the diet was 4.8 mg/day. There was no stainable iron in the bone marrow smears at the beginning or at the end of the regeneration period and there was no available stored iron as shown by a new phlebotomy period. Seven-day dietary records were taken before and monthly during the regeneration period. The mean dietary iron intake was 18 mg/day (range 12.9–23.4 mg). As analysed in a previous paper[50] part of this iron was unavailable fortification iron and it could be calculated that there was on average 16 mg of available iron in the diet. This means that 30 per cent (4.8/16 = 30 per cent) was absorbed from the whole diet in these 10 subjects with iron deficiency anaemia. Iron absorption was also measured from a small radioiron-labelled inorganic iron dose both at the beginning and at the end of the study. The average absorptions were 82 and 83 per cent, respectively. At a reference dose absorption of 40 per cent the total amounts of iron absorbed from this diet would thus be 15 per cent. This figure is close to other calculations of the average absorption from the same diet in borderline iron replete/iron deficient subjects. The results of this study based on haemoglobin regeneration provide independent support for the validity of other methods used to measure iron absorption from the same type of diet.

Estimating iron absorption from an increase in serum ferritin

The principle for this method, that has been used in recent years, is that there is a relationship between serum ferritin and amount of stored iron and that iron stores are expected to increase when a subject is in a positive iron balance. The rate of change in serum ferritin would thus give a measure of the rate of absorption from the diet.

The use of this method requires that several conditions are fulfilled:

- A change in serum ferritin is expected only in subjects who have their individual optimal haemoglobin level. Otherwise the absorbed iron is first used to restitute the haemoglobin level.
- In subjects who have an intial SF in the range 50–60 µg/l, no further increase in iron stores is expected as we recently found. (This SF value is for women, the upper SF level in men remains unknown.)
- An important condition is that the subjects do not have or have not had any recent infections, inflammatory conditions, liver disease or other conditions that influence the SF level.
- Finally, it is hard to translate a change in SF into a change in amounts of stored iron. The correlation between iron stores measured by phlebotomy and serum ferritin is rather poor.

There are two main studies published on the relationship between SF and amount of mobilizable iron stores in 24 and 14 normal subjects, respectively[51,52]. There are also two minor studies each containing three subjects[53,54]. In total there are thus results available from 42 normal subjects (Fig. 2). SF ranged from almost zero to about 250 and amounts of mobilizable iron up to about 1700 mg iron. Statistical regression analyses showed a squared regression coefficient of only 0.447. Since most normal subjects have lower SF than 250, the relationship was also analysed in those 31 who had SF ≤ 100 g/l. This range has the greatest interest in attempts to predict iron stores from SF concentrations in epidemiological studies. The squared correlation coefficient was still only 0.506. If log SF is used instead of SF the squared correlation coefficient was lower, 0.386. These results imply that only half of the variation in SF can be ascribed to a variation in iron stores, and that predictions of iron stores from SF in single individuals and small groups have a low accuracy. A considerable part of the total variation in SF seen must be due to experimental errors in calculating iron stores and determining SF. Some of the variation may be due to a day-to-day variation in SF. Another part of the variation is probably due to individual differences in the relationship between iron stores and SF - a fact that was noted early on[53]. An important part of the variation in SF seems to be related to preceding or existing effects of different disorders, including a mild infection such as the common cold or alcohol consumption. There are thus good reasons to be very careful both when interpreting SF changes and when translating SF into iron stores. Another important conclusion of the present analyses is that rather large groups are needed to make meaningful comparisons of iron status between populations or the same population analysed at different times based on the distribution of SF and that various confounding factors must be carefully recorded and considered.

Labelling the whole diet using the extrinsic tag principle

In an early study we measured iron absorption from breakfast, lunch and dinner meals which were served as different puddings in which the relative amounts of provisions were close to the average amounts calculated from a 6 week master menu and from detailed supply records for the corresponing meals served at a military unit[55]. The non-haem iron in the puddings were extrinsically labelled with an inorganic tracer and haem iron with biosynthetically labelled haemoglobin. The total amounts of iron absorbed were measured from blood samples and whole body counting. The average absorption obtained corresponded well with the average iron requirements calculated in the 32 young enlisted men. This method is very laborious and we never tested the validity of using 'puddings'. With this experimental design the marked variation in bioavailability of non-haem iron between different meals was disregarded at that time.

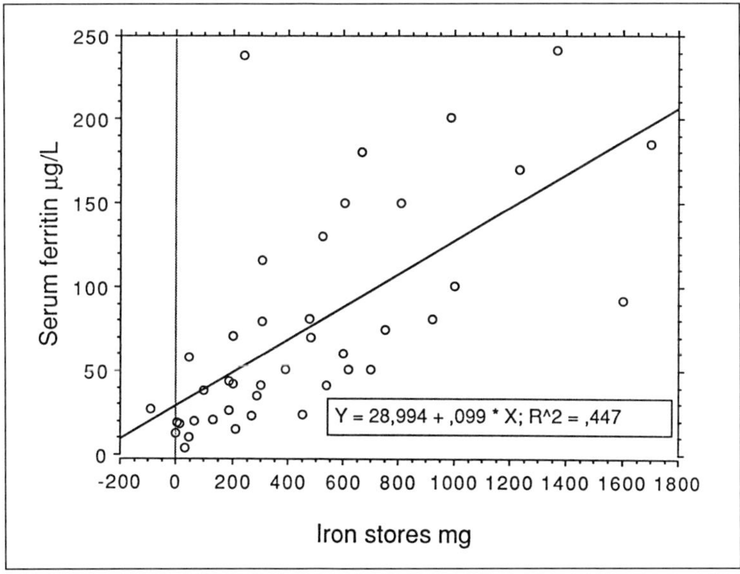

Fig. 2. The relationship between mobilizable iron stores by phlebotomy and initial serum ferritin in four studies.

Another attempt to calculate iron absorption from the whole diet was making a weighed mean values of iron absorption from a spectrum of meals to obtain absorption figures for the whole diet[50]. In these calculations differences in iron content and differences in frequency of consumption of different meals were considered. The average bioavailability of the potentially available iron in this pooled composite diet was 14.5 per cent in borderline iron deficient subjects. This method is less valid than direct measurements but give an approximation that is not far from results obtained with other methods. It shows, however, that data obtained in single meal studies on typical meals have no major systematic errors.

Recently, we developed a method where we measured non-haem iron absorption from all meals for time periods of 5 or 10 days by uniformly labelling all meals with an extrinsic inorganic radioiron tracer in amounts to obtain the same specific activity of the non-haem iron in all meals during all days[42,43]. In the studies made so far, however, haem iron absorption has been calculated from a known relationship between iron absorption from an inorganic reference dose and haem iron absorption[43]. In ongoing studies on men, we also label all haem iron with an extrinsic biosynthetically labelled haemoglobin tracer.

Some results from these studies were mentioned above when discussing the selection of subjects for iron absorption studies. The results from the four diets studied will be further discussed both in the present paper and in a later paper. Most meals were precooked and kept frozen until labelled and served in the laboratory. Iron-free foods were allowed to balance differences in energy requirements between the women.

To validate the method the absorption in each woman was related to her individual iron requirement, based on measurements of menstrual iron losses and estimations of basal iron losses calculated from body weight. As shown in Fig. 3 the agreements between absorption and requirements in the two studies are remarkably good. The agreement cannot be perfect since different diets were studied, and since the diets were not identical with the diets usually consumed by these women. The magnitude of iron

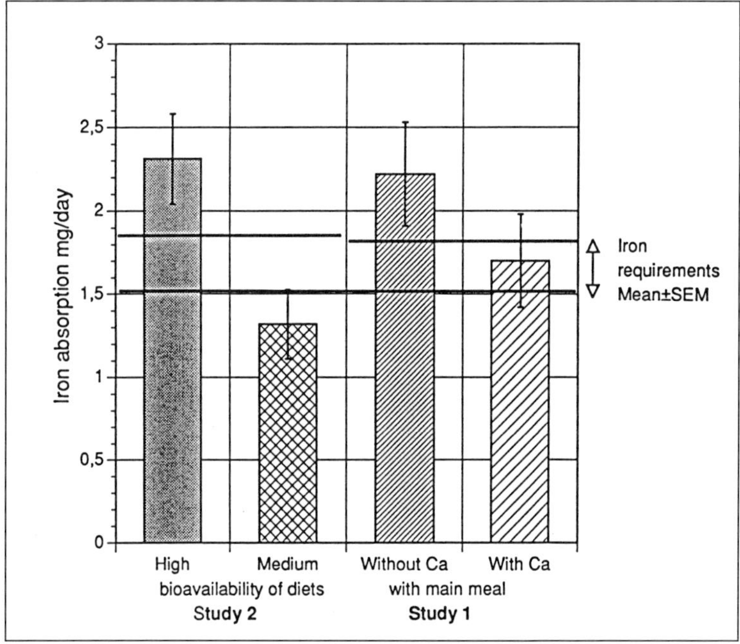

Fig. 3. Iron absorption from four diets in relation to iron requirements in two studies[42,43]. Mean and SEM values are plotted.

absorption and the magnitude of iron requirements, however, were the same.

In a discussion on single meals, the study by Cook *et al.*[47] is of relevance. The absorption of non-haem iron was measured from 28 main meals served during 2 weeks by serving with each of the main meals a wheat roll containing an inorganic radioiron tracer. Three different groups of subjects were served diets with different properties. One group of 15 subjects was instructed to consume a diet that was expected to have a high bioavalability by eating meat and ascorbic acid-rich foods. Another group was instructed to eat a low bioavailability diet with no meat and more inhibitors of iron absorption. A third group was instructed to eat as they usually did. The absorption from the 28 main meals served during 2 weeks by Cook *et al.* aimed at having a high and low bioavailability. It agreed very well with the results obtained from whole diets in our studies, which also aimed at having high and low bioavailability (Fig. 4). To be able to compare the results, all data were adjusted to the same iron status (SF 40 µg/l) by the method used by Cook *et al.* in their study.

The main conclusions of this comparison are:

- it is possible to measure iron absorption from the whole diet using extrinsic labelling;
- results obtained in the different studies agree very well;
- as expected, iron absorption agrees with iron requirements;
- differences in bioavailability of iron in realistic Western-type diets show marked differences.

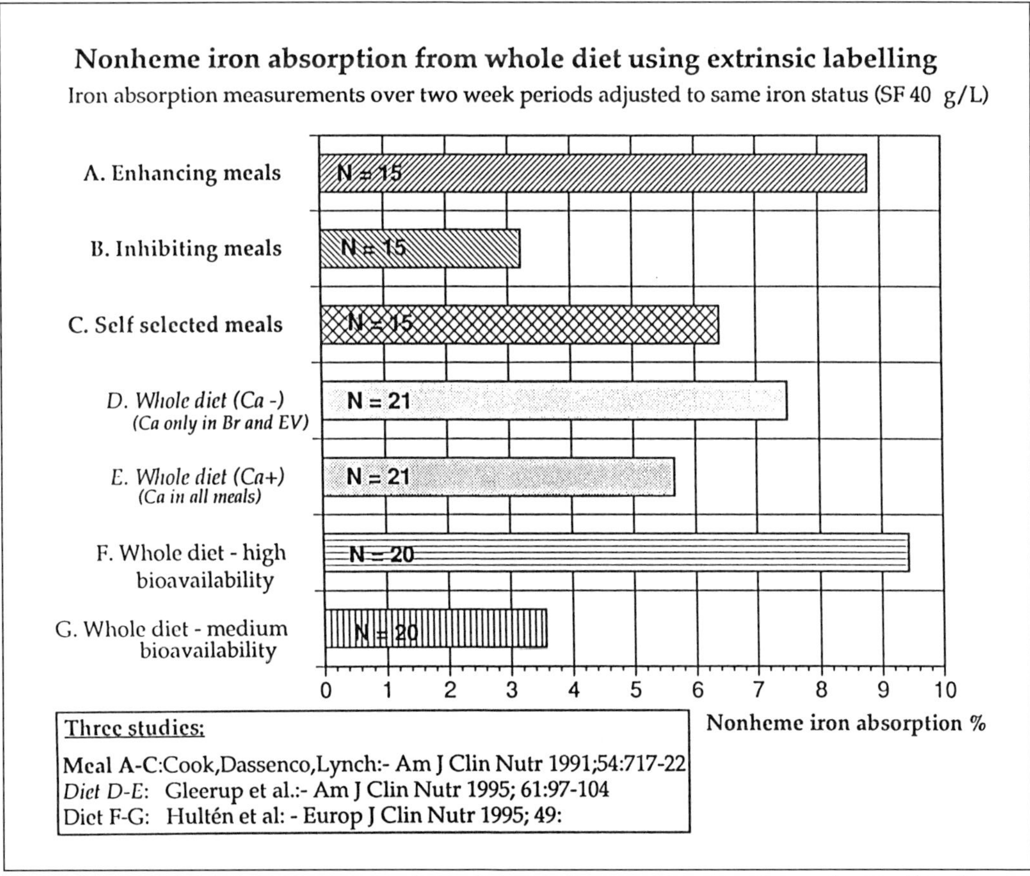

Fig. 4. Non-haem iron absorption from six diets adjusted to the same iron status (serum ferritin 40 µg/l).

Concluding remarks

Several methods are available with which to measure iron absorption from single foods, single meals and the whole diet. The choice of method depends on the problem to be studied and the resources available - the latter refers both to technical facilities and methodological experience. The access to motivated volunteers is an important limiting factor in basic experimental studies.

Over the years more and more has constantly been learned about systematic errors and methodological pitfals. This knowledge has been important both for the development of optimal experimental designs and for the interpretaion of results. The close cooperation between groups in different parts of the world working in the iron field for almost 40 years has been characterized not only by a natural competition but also by a friendly supportive attitude which has developed during much cooperative work and writing in most parts of the world.

Acknowledgements

This work was supported by Swedish Medical Research Council Project B95-19X-04721-20B, and by Swedish Council for Forestry and Agriculture Research Project 50.0267–93.

References

1. McCance, R.A. & Widdowson, E.M. (1937): Absorption and excretion of iron. *Lancet* **2,** 680–684.
2. Moore, C.V. (1968): The absorption of iron from foods. In: *Occurrence, causes and prevention of nutritional anaemias*, ed. G. Blix, pp. 92–102. Uppsala: Almquist Wiksells.
3. Josephs, H.W. (1958): Absorption of iron as a problem in human physiology. A critical review. *Blood* **13,** 1–54.
4. Johnstone, F.A., Frenchman, R. & Burroughs, E.D. (1948): The iron metabolism of young women on two levels of iron intake. *J. Nutr.* **35,** 453–465.
5. McMillan, T.S. & Johnstone, F.A. (1951): The absorption of iron from spinach and the effect of beef upon the absorption. *J. Nutr.* **44,** 383–398.
6. Hunt, J.R., Mullen, L.M., Lykken, G.I., Gallagher, S.K. & Nielsen, F.H. (1990): Ascorbic acid: effect on ongoing iron absorption and status in iron depleted young women. *Am. J. Clin. Nutr.* **51,** 649–655.
7. Andersson, H. (1992): The ileostomy model for the study of carbohydrate and sterol digestion in man. *Europ. J. Clin. Nutr.* **46,** S69–S76.
8. Dubach, R., Callender, S. & Moore, C.V. (1948): Studies in transportation and metabolism. VI. Absorption of radioactive iron in patients with fever and with anemia of varied etiology. *Blood* **3,** 526–540.
9. Sharpe, L.M., Peacock, W.C., Cooke, R. & Harris, R.S. (1950): The effect of phytate and other food factors on iron absorption. *J. Nutr.* **41,** 433–446.
10. Pirzio-Biroli, G., Bothwell, T.H. & Finch, C.A. (1958): Iron absorption II. The absorption of radioiron administered with a standard meal in man. *J. Lab. Clin. Med.* **51,** 37–48.
11. Saylor, L. & Finch, C.A. (1953): Determination of iron absorption using two isotopes of iron. *Amer. J. Physiol.* **170,** 372–376.
12. Cook, J.D., Brown, G.M. & Valberg, L.S. (1964): The effect of achylia gastrica on iron absorption. *J. Clin. Invest.* **43,** 1185–1191.

13. Stevens, A.R.J., Pirzio-Biroli, G., Harkins, H.N., Nyhus, L.M. & Finch, C.A. (1959): Iron metabolism in patients after partial gastrectomy. *Ann. Surg.* **149,** 534–538.

14. Baird, I.M. & Wilson, G.M. (1959): The pathogenesis of anaemia after partial gastrectomy. II. Iron absorption after partial gastrectomy. *Quart. J. Med.* **28,** 35–41.

15. Turnbull, A.L. (1965): The absorption of radioiron given with a standard meal after Polya partial gastrectomy. *Clin. Sci.* **28,** 499–509.

16. Hallberg, L., Sölvell, L. & Zederfeldt, B. (1966): Iron absorption after partial gastrectomy. A comparative study on the absorption from ferrous sulfate and haemoglobin. *Acta Med. Scand.* **Suppl. 445,** 269–275.

17. Goldberg, A., Lochhead, A.C. & Dagg, J.H. (1963): Histamine-fast achlorhydria and iron absorption. *Lancet* **1,** 848–850.

18. Moore, C.V. & Dubach, R. (1951): Observations on the absorption of iron from foods tagged with radioiron. *Trans. Ass. Amer. Physicians* **64,** 245–246.

19. Hallberg, L. & Björn-Rasmussen, E. (1972): Determination of iron absorption from whole diet. A new two-pool model using two radioiron isotopes given as haem and non-haem iron. *Scand. J. Haematol.* **9,** 193–197.

20. Cook, J.D., Layrisse, M., Martinez-Torres, C., Walker, R., Monsen, E. & Finch, C.A. (1972): Food iron absorption measured by an extrinsic tag. *J. Clin. Invest.* **51,** 805–815.

21. Björn-Rasmussen, E., Hallberg, L. & Walker, R.B. (1972): Food iron absorption in man. I. Isotopic exchange between food iron and inorganic iron salt added to food: studies on maize, wheat, and eggs. *Am. J. Clin. Nutr.* **25,** 317–323.

22. Björn-Rasmussen, E. (1973): Food iron absorption in man - III. Effect of iron salt, ascorbic acid and desferrioxamine on the isotopic exchange between native food iron and an extrinsic inorganic iron tracer. *Scand. J. Haematol.* **11,** 391–397.

23. Björn-Rasmussen, E. (1973): Food iron absorption in man. IV. Validity of the extrinsic tag two-pool method for measurement of dietary non-heme iron absorption in patients with various clinical disorders. *Scand. J. Gastroent.* **8,** 645–650.

24. Björn-Rasmussen, E. & Hallberg, L. (1974): Effect of ascorbic acid on iron absoirption from maize supplemented with ferrous sulfate. *Nutr. Metabol.* **19,** 94–100.

25. Disler, P.B., Lynch, S.R., Charlton, R.W., Bothwell, T.H., Walker, R.B. & Mayet, F. (1975): Studies on the fortification of cane sugar with iron and ascorbic acid. *Br. J. Nutr.* **34,** 141–152.

26. Sayers, M.H., Lynch, S.R, Jacobs, P., Charlton, R.W., Bothwell, T.H., *et al.* (1973): The effects of ascorbic acid supplementation on the absorption of iron in maize, wheat and soya. *Br. J. Haematol.* **24,** 209–218.

27. Björn-Rasmussen, E.J., Hallberg, L. & Walker, R.B. (1973): Food iron absorption in man. II. Isotopic exchange of iron between labelled foods and between a food and an iron salt. *Am. J. Clin. Nutr.* **26,** 1311–1319.

28. Hallberg, L. (1974): The pool concept in food iron absorption and some of ita implications. *Proc. Nutr. Soc.* **33,** 285–291.

29. Björn-Rasmussen, E., Hallberg, L., Magnusson, B., Rossander, L., Svanberg, B. & Arvidsson, B. (1976): Measurement of iron absorption from composite meals. *Am. J. Clin. Nutr.* **29,** 772–778.

30. Rossander, L., Hallberg, L., Björn-Rasmussen, E. (1979): Absorption of iron from breakfast meals. *Am. J. Clin. Nutr.* **32,** 2484–2489.

31. Hallberg, L. & Rossander, L. (1982): Absorption of iron from Western-type lunch and dinner meals. *Am. J. Clin. Nutr.* **35,** 502–509.

32. Hallberg, L. & Rossander, L. (1982): Bioavailability of iron from Western-type whole meals. *Scand. J. Gastroenterol.* **17,** 151–160.

33. Hallberg, L. & Rossander, L. (1984): Improvment of iron nutrition in developing countries: comparison of adding meat, soy protein, ascorbic acid, citric acid, and ferrous sulphate on iron absorption from a simple Latin American-type of meal. *Am. J. Clin. Nutr.* **39,** 577–583.

34. Layrisse, M., Martinez-Torres, C., Lenzi, M. & Leets, I. (1975): Ferritin iron absorption in man. *Blood* **45,** 688–698.

35. Martinez-Torres, C., Renzi, M. & Layrisse, M. (1976): Iron absorption by humans from haemosiderin and ferritin. Further studies. *J. Nutr.* **106,** 128–135.

36. Hallberg, L. & Björn-Rasmussen, E. (1981): Measurement of iron absorption from meals contaminated with iron. *Am. J. Clin. Nutr.* **34,** 2808–2815.

37. Hallberg, L., Björn-Rasmussen, E., Rossander, L., Suwanik, R., Pleehachinda, R. & Tuntawiroon, M. (1983): Iron absorption from some Asian meals containing contamination iron. *Am. J. Clin. Nutr.* **37,** 272–277.

38. Hallberg, L., Brune, M. & Rossander, L. (1986): Low bioavailability of carbonyl iron in man: studies on iron fortification of wheat flour. *Am. J. Clin. Nutr.* **43,** 59–67.

39. Forbes, A.L., Adams, C.E., Arnaud, M.J, *et al.* (1989): Comparison of *in vitro*, animal, and clinical determinations of iron bioavailability:International Nutritional Anemia Consultative Group Task Force report on iron bioavailability. *Am. J. Clin. Nutr.* **49,** 225–238.

40. Hallberg, L. (1980): Food iron absorption. In: *Methods in hematology*, eds. J.D. Cook, pp. 116–133. London: Churchill.

41. Magnusson, B., Björn-Rasmussen, E. & Rossander, L. (1981): Iron absorption in relation to iron status. Model proposed to express results of food iron absorption measurements. *Scand. J. Haematol.* **27,** 201–208.

42. Gleerup, A., Rossander-Hultén, L., Gramatkowski, E. & Hallberg, L. (1995): Iron absorption from the whole diet: Comparison of the effect of two different distributions of daily calcium intake. *Am. J. Clin. Nutr.* **61,** 97–104.

43. Hultén, L., Gramatkovski, E., Gleerup, A. & Hallberg, L. (1995): Iron absorption from whole diet. Relation to meal composition, iron requirements and iron status. *Europ. J. Clin. Nutr.* 49.

44. Layrisse, M., Cook, J.D., Martinez-Torres, C., Roche, M., Kuhn, I.N. & Walker, R.B. (1969): Food iron absorption: A comparison of vegetable and animal foods. *Blood* **33,** 430–443.

45. Bezwoda, W., Bothwell, T.H., Torrance, J.D., *et al.* (1979): The relationship between marrow iron stores, plasma ferritin concentrations and iron absorption. *Scand. J. Haematol.* **22,** 113–120.

46. Cook, J.D., Lipschitz, D.A., Miles, L.E.M. & Finch, C.A. (1974): Serum ferritin as a measure of iron stores in normal subjects. *Am. J. Clin. Nutr.* **27,** 681–687.

47. Cook, J.D., Dassenko, S.A. & Lynch, S.R. (1991): Assessment of the role of non heme-iron availability in iron balance. *Am. J. Clin. Nutr.* **54,** 717–722.

48. Norrby, A. (1974): Iron absorption studies in iron deficiency. *Scand. J. Haematol.* (Suppl 20) **20**, 5–125.

49. Olzon, E., Isaksson, B., Norrby, A. & Sölvell, L. (1978): Food iron absorption in iron deficiency. *Am. J. Clin. Nutr.* **31,** 106–111.

50. Hallberg, L. & Rossander-Hultén, L. (1991): Iron requirements in menstruating women. *Am. J. Clin. Nutr.* **54,** 1047–1058.

51. Walters, G.O., Miller, F.M. & Worwood, M. (1973): Serum ferritin concentration and iron stores in normal subjects. *J. Clin. Path.* **26,** 770–772.

52. Skikne, B.S., Flowers, C.H. & Cook, J.D. (1990): Serum transferrin receptor: A quantitative measure of tissue iron deficiency. *Blood* **75,** 1870–1876.

53. Birgegård, G., Högman, C., Killander, A., Levander, H., Simonsson, B. & Wide, L. (1977): Serum ferritin and 2,3-DPG during quantitative phlebotomy and iron treatment. *Scand. J. Haematol.* **19,** 327–333.

54. Charlton, R.W., Derman, D., Skikne, B. *et al.* (1977): Iron stores, serum ferritin and iron absorption. In: *Proteins of iron metabolism*, ed. E.D. Brown, pp. 387. Philadelphia, PA: Grune & Stratton.

55. Björn-Rasmussen, E., Hallberg, L., Isaksson, B. & Arvidsson, B. (1974): Food iron absorption in man. Application of the two-pool extrinsic tag method to measure heme and nonheme iron absorption from the whole diet. *J. Clin. Invest.* **53,** 247–255.

Iron Nutrition in Health and Disease, edited by Leif Hallberg and Nils-Georg Asp
©1996 John Libbey & Company Ltd., pp. 97–104

Chapter 9

Comparison of methods to estimate iron absorption

Göran Hallmans and Per Tidehag

Department of Nutritional Research, Umeå University, S–901 87 Umeå, Sweden

Summary

Based on our results in humans, we find it likely that the amount of iron available for absorption by the body and the resulting iron status will be only marginally affected if variations in the calcium content of the diet or meals within a diet are within normal physiological limits. We believe that the differences between the results of the small intestinal balance study and those of radioisotope studies, which have shown pronounced effects of high calcium levels, are the results of differences in experimental design and measurement method including the fact that the most dramatic differences in iron absorption have been seen in studies using very low diet calcium levels as controls.

On the basis of the results of the methodological study in humans we recommend that radioiron-labelled test diets should be given at all meals during test days and not as single meals in the morning after an overnight fast as the values obtained with the single meal technique may be inflated.

Although the mechanisms involved in the absorption process of iron are still obscure, it is very important to have methods available which mirror the various aspects of the absorption process. Combined isotope studies, small intestinal balance studies, and long-term studies related to iron status may be useful in this respect.

Introduction

The absorption of iron from food is dependent on the iron requirements of the individual and on the amount and bioavailability of dietary iron, which in turn is affected by various dietary factors. It is therefore important to have accurate and reliable methods for measuring iron absorption from both individual foodstuffs and whole meals.

Data are inconclusive as to whether animals and in particular rats represent a suitable model. The results from similar studies in rats and humans have often been inconclusive[1]. The use of humans in iron absorption studies is definitely to be preferred as no species translation will be necessary to interpret the results. Prior to the use of radioisotopes, the methods used in humans were time-consuming and sometimes inaccurate. The development of new radioiron techniques has altered this situation[2]. The use of well-established, conventional ileostomy subjects for balance studies (the small intestinal balance technique) has greatly increased the reliability of the balance method due to the short intestinal transit time[3].

The aims of our studies have been to evaluate different methods of measuring iron absorption in humans. The results presented are a summary of studies which have been published or will be submitted for publication.

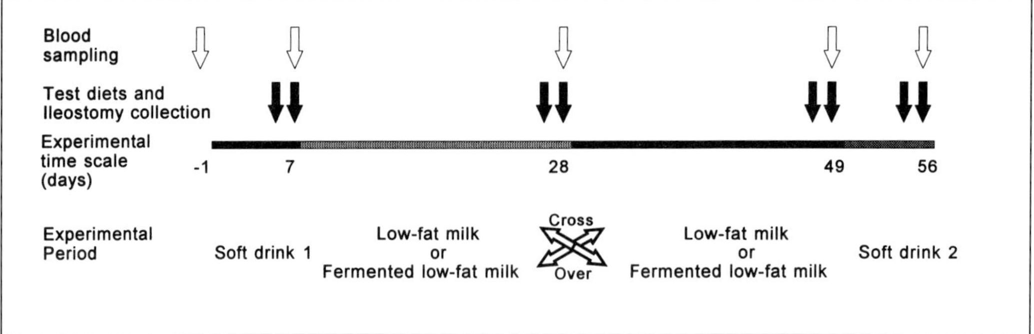

Fig. 1. The expiremental design in study I.

Materials and methods

The purpose of study I was to investigate the effect of dietary calcium on the absorption of iron, measured as the small intestinal balance of a complete diet in nine ileostomy subjects. The experiment lasted for 8 weeks, divided into four periods of 1, 3, 3 and 1 week, respectively[4] (Fig. 1). The beverage, 1000 ml/day, was distributed evenly among the three main meals and an evening snack. The subjects were instructed to keep their ordinary diets, with some restrictions to limit the intake of calcium and dietary fiber. The 95 per cent confidence intervals regarding the difference in iron absorption figures obtained from the balance experiments were calculated. From this result the difference in absorption to reach statistical significance, expressed as a percentage, was calculated for the combined calcium groups.

The purpose of study II (in preparation) was to evaluate the effect of a high-fibre diet (HFD) of oat bran versus a low-fibre diet (LFD) on iron metabolism in ileostomy subjects using three different methods: (1) iron status measured as changes in the concentration of ferritin over three weeks; (2) a small intestinal balance of an ordinary day at the beginning (day 3) and at the end (day 17) of the 3 week experiment; (3) single meal isotope retention experiments compared with a small intestinal balance study with four nutritionally identical meals with a high content of dairy products on day 18 (Fig. 2).

Two experimental groups followed one diet for 3 weeks and then the other diet for 3 weeks in a cross-over design. The subjects were studied for a total of 6 consecutive weeks on an outpatient basis except for days 3, 17 and 18 in each dietary period, for which the subjects were admitted to the research ward. When the patients stayed in their homes they were instructed

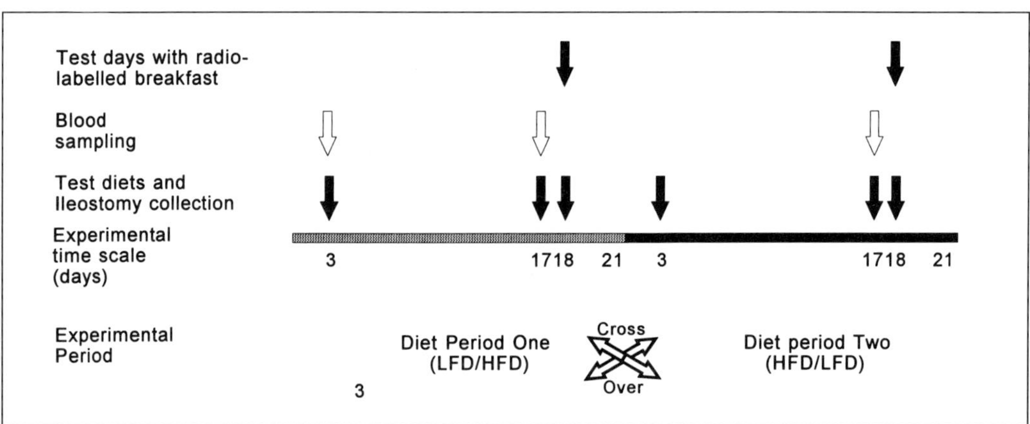

Fig. 2. The expiremental design in study II: LFD = low fibre diet; HFD = high fibre diet.

orally and in writing to eat premade experimental bread and their own home diet, which was modified to be low in dietary fibre. During both periods the subjects were given the same diet during days 3 and 17 with the exception of the bread. Endosperm wheat bread was given in the LFD and oat bran bread was given in the HFD. On day 18 they were given either a low-fibre porridge diet with the same low-fibre bread as on the LFD days or a high-fibre porridge diet with a high-fibre oat bran bread. Four identical meals were freshly prepared and served at 4 h intervals, and ^{59}Fe was added to the first meal.

The purpose of study III was to compare iron balances measured with the small intestinal balance method and iron absorption measured with isotope retention from one meal or several meals of both low- and high-fibre diets[5]. Two study periods of 5 successive days each were used. The same diet was consumed at each meal served during the 5 experimental days in both periods. The breakfast consisted of one-seventh, lunch of two-sevenths, and dinner of four-sevenths of the total intake during the day. The proportions of nutrients as well as stimulators and inhibitors of iron absorption were identical in all meals. During both day 4 and day 5 of each period the subjects were given breakfast meals labelled with ^{55}Fe and ^{59}Fe and lunch and dinner meals labelled with ^{59}Fe. The same specific activity was used in all meals.

Results

The effect of milk and fermented milk on small intestinal iron absorption (study I)

The apparent iron absorption (mg or per cent) measured as the small intestinal balance did not differ significantly between low and high calcium diets (Fig. 3). The 95 per cent confidence limit was ± 28 per cent, which means that an inhibition amounting to 29 per cent or more would have been required to obtain a statistically significant difference. There was a negative correlation between the apparent absorption (mean value day 1 and day 2) and the plasma ferritin concentration of the various periods (soft drink period 1, $r = -0.92$, $P < 0.001$; low-fat milk, $r = -0.77$, $P = 0.01$; fermented low-fat milk, $r = -0.94$, $P < 0.001$; soft drink period 2, $r = -0.74$, $P = 0.052$).

Effects of oat bran on the small intestinal balance and isotope retention (study II)

The plasma ferritin concentration decreased significantly during the LFD but not during the HFD. The content of phytic acid was high in the oat bran diet (inositol-6-phosphate on day 3 and

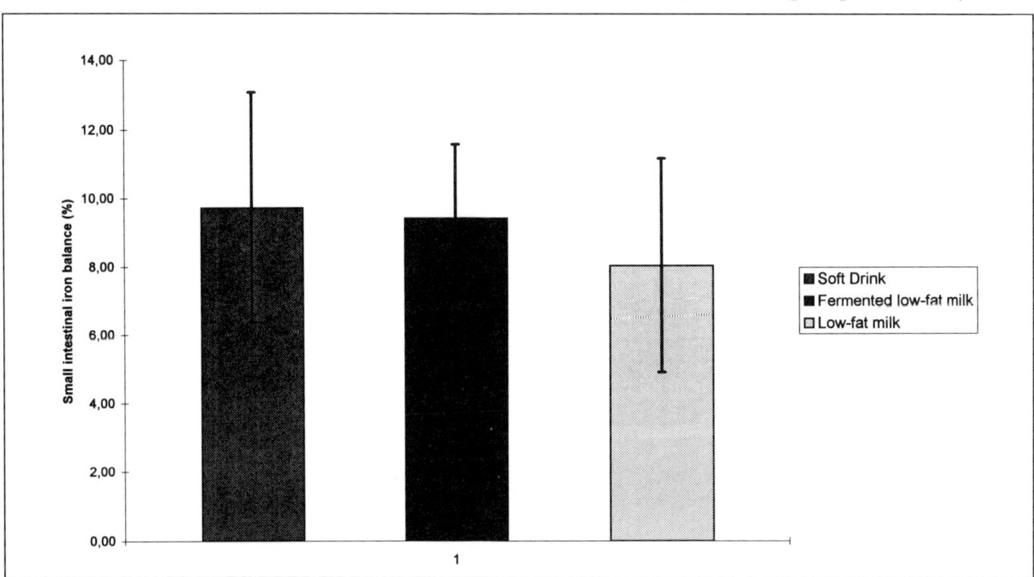

Fig 3. The mean small intestinal iron balance (study I). The bars represent one SEM.

day 17, 3.4 mmol; day 18, 5.5 mmol). A good mean recovery of phytic acid and fibre were seen in the ileostomy contents during both the HFD (day 18: phytic acid 100 per cent, fibre 101 per cent) and the LFD (day 18: phytic acid 93 per cent, fibre 105 per cent). No significant differences were found in fractional or absolute small intestinal iron balance in days 3 and 17. In day 18 a higher absolute small intestinal iron balance was seen in the HFD compared to the LFD.

During day 18 the fractional small intestinal balance of calcium from the HFD decreased compared with day 17, while the absorption of iron, magnesium and zinc increased (Fig. 4). Corresponding changes were also found on the LFD days for calcium, magnesium, and zinc.

A single-meal isotope retention experiment was performed in day 18 by labelling the breakfast meal. A low fractional isotope uptake (LFD = 1.87 ± 0.59 per cent, HFD = 0.64 ± 0.22 per cent) was observed in both groups. The fractional uptake was highest from the LFD.

Comparison of iron absorption from single meals or all meals using radioiron (study III)

The mean retention of radioiron from the low-fibre single meal given in the morning on two consecutive days was 2.87 ± 0.44 per cent, which is approximately 80 per cent higher than the retention of radioiron from the same diet served at every meal on both days. During the high fibre period the retention from the single morning meal was 3.45 ± 0.48 per cent and almost 50 per cent higher (not significant, P = 0.08) than that from the diet served as every meal during two days.

Discussion

The quantitative recovery of ileostomy effluents is supported by the nearly 100 per cent recovery of dietary phytic acid and/or dietary fibre in the ileostomy contents in our studies. When there is

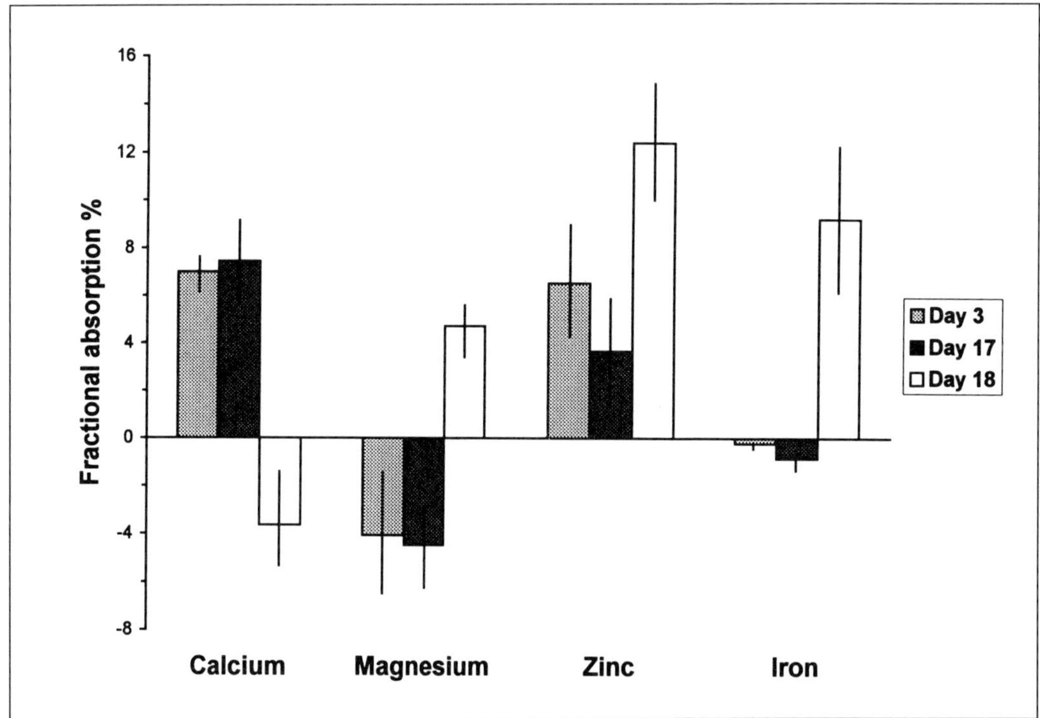

Fig 4. The mean small intestinal iron balance during the high fibre diet at days 3, 17 and 18 (study II). The bars represent one SEM.

a small difference between ingested iron and absorbed iron, the method is sensitive to errors, and contamination or measurement errors may affect the results. Further methodological studies are also needed to exclude the theoretically possible influence of bleeding from the stoma.

In study I no effect of the milk diet on iron absorption was seen. With the variations found in the material, a 29 per cent decrease in absorption from the combined calcium groups compared to the combined control groups was calculated to be required to reach the 0.05 significance level. In a long-term study on 109 free-living healthy, premenopausal women eating ordinary diets, ingestion of 1000 mg Ca, as the carbonate, daily with meals also did not appear to significantly influence their iron status over a 12 week period[6].

In the studies in which the most prominent and significant effects of calcium on iron absorption have been demonstrated, the initial calcium content has been considerably lower than in our study, i.e. lower than 40 mg/meal[7,8]. One interpretation would then be that rather than demonstrating an inhibition of iron absorption by high calcium concentrations in the diet, those studies may have demonstrated increased iron absorption in the control groups due to extremely low diet calcium concentrations.

One principal difference between studies in which calcium has been shown to markedly impair iron absorption and study I, is the different methods used to measure iron absorption. In our study, iron absorption was measured as small intestinal iron balance from a test diet over a 2 day period after at least 1 week of adaptation to the imposed calcium intake level, whereas most earlier studies used radioiron- labelled single meals. Thus there is a possibility that differences in the methods for measuring iron absorption may explain the differences in the results. It is well known that there is a marked variation in absorption of iron not only between different, apparently healthy, individuals but also in the same individual on different days, and that absorption measurements made over a period of time show compensation for low iron absorption from one meal by higher absorption from others[9]. In a recent study by Gleerup *et al.*[10], non-haem iron in all meals over a period of 10 days were labelled with radioisotopes of iron. The inhibitory effect of calcium was studied by distributing the same amount of calcium in two ways, either mainly with breakfast and evening meals or more evenly with all meals. About 30–50 per cent more iron was absorbed when calcium- rich products were avoided at the main meals, which was also less than the reduction of 50–60 per cent demonstrated in single-meal studies. Thus, studies of iron absorption from diets appear to give a lower effect of calcium on iron absorption than is seen in studies on meals.

One disadvantage with the ileostomy model is the difficulty in recruiting a sufficient number of subjects in good health who are willing to participate. It is thus very difficult to perform this kind of study in a strictly controlled manner using a large number of subjects. However, there is reason to believe that using the subjects as their own controls at least partially compensates for the low number of subjects. Although there is a large interindividual variation in both iron status and iron absorption, the two are well

Table 1. Pearson's product-moment correlations in study I between iron balance iron during different diet periods, tested using t-test (p)

	Soft drink period 1	**Low-fat milk**	**Fermented low-fat milk**	**Soft drink period 2**
Soft drink 1				
Low-fat milk	0.90 (p=0.001)			
Fermented low-fat milk	0.93 (p<0.001)	0.82 (p=0.007)		
Soft-drink period 2	0.90 (p=0.001)	0.77 (p=0.014)	0.89 (p=0.001)	

correlated (study I) and the four repeated measures of balance in each individual were also well correlated (Table 1). Thus the intraindividual variation is low and the interindividual variation in iron status should not confound the effects of diet (calcium) on iron absorption.

In the oat experiment (study II) we investigated the differences between single-meal measurements of iron absorption using isotope retention and conventional balance measurements in the same ileostomy subjects. In order to compare the two methods with each other, a diet corresponding to the composition of an ordinary Swedish breakfast was studied the whole day, i.e. identical meals were given four times during test day 18. The first meal was labelled with ^{59}Fe. A significantly higher fractional absorption of ^{59}Fe was observed from the LFD compared to the HFD. The results are in accordance with findings of Rossander–Hulthén *et al.*[11] who showed that oat bran and oat porridge markedly inhibited the absorption of non-haem iron. During the HFD the mean absorption of iron measured as ^{59}Fe was only 0.25 mg, compared with 2.7 mg when measured with the small intestinal balance technique. No correlation was found between the two methods of measuring iron absorption. The changes in mineral balances (Fe, Ca, Mg, Zn) during test day 18 on the HFD compared to test day 17 (Fig. 4) may indicate that the high concentrations of both calcium and phytate from the breakfast meal, which was almost exclusively based on cereal and dairy products, produced a calcium-phytate complex or other complex which decreased the absorption of calcium, while iron, magnesium and zinc were available for absorption. Our observations that high amounts of calcium and phytate increase iron absorption is supported by the results of Hallberg *et al.*[8], which suggested that phytate may reduce the inhibiting effect of calcium on iron absorption when using the single meal technique. The formation of a calcium–phytate complex is dependent on the molar ratios of calcium to phytate in the diets. The molar ratio of calcium to phytate was approximately 10 in the HFD. At molar ratios > 6 calcium phytate is considered to precipitate at pH conditions occurring in the intestine[12]. It is therefore possible that the inhibiting effect of phytate and calcium on iron absorption was reduced on day 18.

How can the differences in results between the single meal method and the intestinal balance method (study II) be explained in relation to isotope transfer and/or exchange in the intestinal mucosa? One hypothesis is that the isotopes do not always measure and/or represent what we believe them to measure and/or represent. The present results of study II might be an illustrative example of this. Although no common isotope pool exists in the small intestine, and the formation of complexes within the intestinal lumen might interfere with isotope transfer in an uncontrolled manner, the presence of complexes and/or other factors may cause a variation in the release pattern of isotopes over the whole length of the intestine, followed by differences in isotope exchange in the intestinal mucosa. As a consequence the isotope uptake may in some fractions be different from the 'true' iron absorption. The methodological problems with the balance method have been mentioned previously.

There may be several explanations which separately or combined may explain the differences observed between the results of the single meal design and the daily diet design (study III)[5]. One of them may be that the single meal was given after a 12 h period of fasting (overnight) compared to a 4 h period of fasting before the lunch and dinner meals. This difference in fasting period length may account for the greater absorption from the breakfast meal than the average for the same diet throughout the whole day.

A second factor which may explain the differences in results is that the single meal given in the morning represented only one-seventh of the total daily intake and, therefore, only one-seventh of the total iron intake as well as the intake of stimulators and inhibitors of iron absorption. As the intake of iron in the morning was comparatively low, this may have given rise to a higher fractional iron absorption from the morning meal. The ratios of iron, calcium, phytic acid and fibre to each nother were equal in all the meals, to avoid the possibility that differences in absorption between the single meal and daily diet design could be caused by differences in the relative proportions of enhancers and inhibitors from meal to meal as was the case in the studies of Gleerup *et al.*[10] and Cook *et al.*[13]. If the total amount of enhancers and/or inhibitors is important (e.g. calcium), obvious differences were present between the meals and the concentration of calcium was high also in the morning meal (≈ 200 mg).

A third explanation of the results might be related to the sequencing of the differences in accumulation and transfer of iron within/through the intestinal mucosa. Not all the iron taken from the lumen into the intestinal cells is necessarily transferred into plasma. A variable proportion may be stored within the mucosal cells and later discarded when the cells exfoliate[14,15]. In addition, about 30 per cent of the cells in the intestine will be renewed during the night's fasting, and consequently some of the iron within the cells will be lost. This means that more ^{59}Fe from the dinner will be lost than ^{55}Fe from breakfast before it gets a chance to be absorbed.

Conclusions

Based on our results in humans, we find it likely that the amount of iron available for absorption by the body and the resulting iron status will be only marginally affected if variations in the calcium content of the diet or meals within a diet are within normal physiological limits. We believe that the differences between the results of the small intestinal balance study and those of radioisotope studies, which have shown pronounced effects of high calcium levels, are the results of differences in experimental design and measurement method including the fact that the most dramatic differences in iron absorption have been seen in studies using very low diet calcium levels as controls.

On the basis of the results of the methodological study in humans we recommend that radioiron-labelled test diets should be given at all meals during test days and not as single meals in the morning after an overnight fast as the values obtained with the single meal technique may be inflated. In some situations the single meal technique may exaggerate the effects of dietary factors on iron absorption as suggested by Cook *et al.*[13]. We therefore recommend that the results of single meal studies as a measure of iron absorption should be interpreted with caution.

The different methods used (isotope retention versus small intestinal balance) to measure fractional iron absorption in two experiments gave significantly different results. We found no inhibitory effect of oat on iron absorption measured as net absorption using the chemical balance technique. In contrast the fractional absorption of ^{59}Fe was inhibited by oat bran. Some of the results (day 18) may be explained by the formation of calcium-phytate complexes within a diet with a very high content of cereals and dairy products.

Although the mechanisms involved in the absorption process of iron are still obscure, it is very important to have methods available which mirror the various aspects of the absorption process. Combined isotope studies, small intestinal balance studies, and long-term studies related to iron status may be useful in this respect.

References

1. Reddy, M.B. & Cook, J.D. (1991): Assessment of dietary determinants of nonheme-iron absorption in humans and rats. *Am. J. Clin. Nutr.* **54,** 723–728.

2. Hallberg, L. & Björn-Rasmussen, E. (1972): Determination of iron absorption from whole diet. A new two-pool model using two radioiron isotopes given as haem and non-haem iron. *Scand. J. Haematol.* **9,** 193–197.

3. Sandberg, A.S, Andersson, H., Hallgren, B., Hasselblad, K. & Isaksson, B. (1981): Experimental model for *in vivo* determination of dietary fibre and its effect on the absorption of nutrients in the small intestine. *Br. J. Nutr.* **45,** 283–294.

4. Tidehag, P., Sandberg, A. S., Hallmans, G., Wing, K., Türk, M., Holm, S. & Grahn, E. (1995): The effect of milk and fermented milk on iron absorption and iron status in ileostomy subjects. *Am. J. Clin. Nutr.* **62,** 1216–1220.

5. Tidehag, P., Hallmans, G., Wing, K., Sjöström, R., Ågren, G., Lundin, E. & Zhang, J.X. (1996): A comparison of iron absorption from single meals and daily diets using radioiron (Fe-55/Fe-59). *Br. J. Nutr.* **75**, 281–289

6. Sokoll, L.J. & Dawson-Hughes, B. (1992): Calcium supplementation and plasma ferritin concentrations in premenopausal women. *Am. J. Clin. Nutr.* **56,** 1045–1048.

7. Hallberg, L., Brune, M., Erlandsson, M., Sandberg, A.S. & Rossander-Hulten, L. (1991): Calcium: effect of different amounts on nonheme- and heme-iron absorption in humans. *Am. J. Clin. Nutr.* **53,** 112–119.

8. Hallberg, L., Rossander-Hulthén, L., Brune, M. & Gleerup, A. (1992): Calcium and iron absorption: mechanism of action and nutritional importance. *Eur. J. Clin. Nutr.* **46,** 317–327.

9. Sandberg A.-S, Hasselblad, C. & Hasselblad, K. (1982): The effect of wheat bran on the absorption of minerals in the small intestine. *Br. J. Nutr.* **48,** 185–191.

10. Gleerup, A., Rossander-Hulthén, L., Gramatkovski, E. & Hallberg, L. (1995): Iron absorption from the whole diet: comparison of the effect of two different distributions of daily calcium intake. *Am. J. Clin. Nutr.* **61,** 97–104.

11. Rossander-Hulthén, L., Gleerup, A. & Hallberg, L. (1990): Inhibitory effect of oat products on non-haem iron absorption in man. *Eur. J. Clin. Nutr.* **44,** 783–791.

12. Wise, A. (1983): Dietary factors determining the biological activities of phytate. *Nutr. Abstr. Rev.* **53,** 791–806.

13. Cook, J.D., Dassenko, S.A. & Lynch, S.R. (1991): Assessment of the role of nonheme-iron availability in iron balance. *Am. J. Clin. Nutr.* **54,** 717–722.

14. Charlton, R.W., Jacobs, P., Torrance, J.D., Bothwell, T.H. (1965): The role of the intestinal mucosa in iron absorption. *J. Clin. Invest.* **44,** 543–554.

15. Conrad, M.E.J. & Crosby, W.H. (1963): Intestinal mucosal mechanisms controlling iron absorption. *Blood* **22,** 406–415.

Iron Nutrition in Health and Disease, edited by Leif Hallberg and Nils-Georg Asp
©1996 John Libbey & Company Ltd., pp. 105–115

Chapter 10

Dietary factors influencing iron absorption – an overview

Lena Rossander-Hulthén and Leif Hallberg

Institute of Internal Medicine, Department of Clinical Nutrition, Göteborg University, Annedalsklinikerna, Sahlgrenska University Hospital, Göteborg, Sweden

Summary

There are two kinds of iron in the diet with respect to the mechanism for absorption - haem and non-haem iron. Haem iron is derived mainly from meat and forms only a small fraction of the dietary iron, 5–10 per cent in Western countries. Non-haem iron is thus the major part of dietary iron.

These two kinds of iron probably utilize two different receptors on the mucosal cells for their absorption. Their absorption is differently affected by the iron status of the subjects.

Various dietary factors markedly affect the absorption of non-haem iron, whereas the absorption of haem iron is much less affected by external factors.

Three main factors influence the absorption of non-haem iron: iron status, the amount of potentially available non-haem iron and the balance between dietary factors influencing the bioavailability. Non-haem iron can be considered as a pool and the chemical properties of the non-haem iron pool are a resultant of all ligands present in the gastrointestinal lumen. Foods may contain ligands which strongly bind iron ions, inhibiting absorption. Other dietary factors may enhance iron absorption.

The major enhancers of non-haem iron absorption from the common pool are meat and ascorbic acid. Meat has a double promoting effect on iron absorption. It provides the usually well-absorbed haem iron and it has an independent absorption-promoting effect on iron absorption.

Other less powerful promoters have been identified that may, under certain conditions, play a promoting role. These include organic acids such as citric acid, malic acid, tartaric acid and lactic acid, and alcohol.

Various soy products, such as miso and certain soy sauces are associated with enhanced iron absorption.

Dietary factors inhibiting non-haem iron absorption include phytates, iron-binding polyphenols and calcium. Phytates strongly inhibit iron absorption in a dose-dependent relationship and even small amounts have a marked effect.

It is probably only certain structures (galloyl and catechol groups) in the phenolic molecules which have the ability to react with iron. Only a few groups bind iron so strongly that absorption is influenced. Galloyl groups are the main structure interfering with iron absorption. The amount and choice of drinks taken with meals are important but also certain spices, vegetables and cereals may markedly reduce absorption.

Earlier studies in humans show less consistent results on the effect of calcium on iron absorption. In recent research in humans a strong dose-related inhibition of the absorption of iron by calcium was found with a maximal inhibiting effect of 50–60 per cent over the range 150–300 mg Ca. The inhibiting effect was the same when calcium was given as calcium chloride, milk or cheese. Studies on single composite meals showed that calcium, given as milk or cheese, strongly inhibited absorption of non-haem iron.

Calcium also inhibited the absorption of haem iron to the same extent as non-haem iron, suggesting that the interaction is probably located in the mucosal cell in a transport step which is common for both haem and non-haem iron.

A recently developed method, based on uniformly labelling all dietary non-haem iron to the same specific activity in all meals, has made it possible to measure iron absorption from the whole diet over periods of 1–4 weeks. This method made it possible to measure the amount of iron absorbed from different diets, in relation to the composition of the different diets and to individual iron requirement.The method has been used to quantify the overall effect on iron absorption of different calcium intakes (milk, cheese) at the main meals.

Introduction

There are two kinds of iron in the diet with respect to mechanisms of absorption: haem and non-haem iron.

The amounts of iron absorbed are determined by the amounts of these two kinds of iron and the balance between different factors enhancing or inhibiting the absorption.

Haem and non-haem iron absorption

Haem iron is absorbed as a porphyrin iron complex and is therefore not exposed to the inhibitory ligands in the diet which affect the bioavailability of non-haem iron[1]. Haem iron is absorbed by a special receptor on the mucosal cell[2]. Within the mucosal cell, the iron is released from the porphyrin molecule by a specific enzyme, haem-oxygenase[3,4]. The iron released then leaves the mucosal cell in the same chemical form as non-haem iron, using a final common pathway for haem and non-haem iron[5]. Non-haem iron competes with many complexing ligands in the intestinal lumen. There is convincing evidence that absorption of ferrous iron is superior to ferric iron in man since ferric iron forms stronger complexes with various ions, such as hydroxyl groups[6]. It is probable that iron can only be absorbed into the cells and pass the mucosal membrane in its ferrous form[7]. Reducing substances in the mucin layer of the mucosal cells are probably required for iron to be absorbed.

Haem iron in the diet

Haem iron in haemoglobin and myoglobin in meat usually constitute only 10 per cent or less (1–2 mg), of the total iron intake in Western mixed diets. Both haem and non-haem iron are markedly influenced by iron status of the subjects, but haem iron to a lower degree. The average absorption of haem iron in meat is usually around 25 per cent but may vary from about 10 to 40 per cent[8–11]. Haem iron absorption is markedly improved by the presence of meat. Haem iron can be degraded and converted to non-haem iron if foods are cooked at a high temperature for too long[12,13]. Calcium is the only known dietary factor that inhibits haem iron absorption[14].

Non-haem iron in the diet

Non-haem iron in cereals, vegetables, fruits, roots, pulses and beans forms the main part of dietary iron. The absorption is very much influenced by the individual iron status[15,16]. Moreover, a number of dietary factors have been shown to influence the bioavailability of non-haem iron (Table 1). The bioavailability may vary more than 20-fold, depending on the composition of the meal[17].

The great number of known and unknown factors influencing iron absorption has stimulated research to find alternative methods with which to assess iron absorption, e.g. animal and *in vitro* models.

In vitro studies

Several attempts have been made to design *in vitro* systems that will accurately predict absorption in humans. Even if some studies on some foods suggest a rather good relationship with results obtained in man, there are considerable exceptions. This may be due to effects of gastrointestinal motility, transit time, pH, enzyme concentrations and diffusion barriers, all affecting the proportion of ingested iron that is absorbed. *In vitro* systems determining ioinizable, soluble or dialysable iron after enzymatic digestion under physiological conditions have been developed[18,19]. Their major use is in pre-

Table 1. Factors influencing dietary iron absorption

- **Haem iron absorption**
  - Amount of heme iron, especially as meat
  - Content of calcium in meal
  - Food preperation (time, temperature)
- **Non-Haem iron absorption**
  - Iron status of subjects
  - Amount of potentially available non-haem iron (adjustment for fortification iron and contamination iron)
  - Balance between plus and minus factors

Plus factors	Minus factors
• Abscorbic acid	• Phytate
• Meat/Fish	• Iron-binding polyphenols
• The "Sauerkraut factor" (fermented foods)	• Calcium
	• Soy protein

dicting trends rather than absolute levels of iron absorption[20,21].

Animal models

There are two main differences in iron absorption between rat and man. First, considerable higher fractions of iron are absorbed by the rat. Second, the marked effects in man of factors such as bran, ascorbic acid and meat are not seen in the rat[22]. These facts make this model unsuitable for predicting dietary iron absorption in man.

Studies in man

The use of two radioiron isotopes has greatly facilitated the study of factors influencing iron absorption by making each person his own control consuming meals with/without the factor. Some points are specially important to emphasize in studies on the effect of different factors on iron absorption and in comparative studies on the bioavailability. It is important to choose subjects who are not fully replete. Recent sudies have shown that in female iron replete subjects with iron stores amounting to about 500 mg (serum ferritin about 50–60 μg/l), the absorption is more or less the same from several diets with widely different bioavailability[23]. This implies that it is hard, if not impossible, to observe the effect of inhibiting and enhancing factors in such subjects. Another important point in studies on the effect of single factors on non-haem iron absorption is the choice of basal diet to which the factor is added. In a study of the effect of adding a factor expected to inhibit iron absorption the basal meal should have a rather high bioavailability in order to detect true effects in a reasonable number of subjects. Similarly, in studies on factors expected to enhance iron absorption it is preferable to select a basal diet with a rather low bioavailability.

These recommendations reduce the risk of obtaining falsely negative effects. Morover, statistically significant effects of a magnitude that is nutrionally important may be detected using fewer subjects. Much knowledge has been obtained so far by several groups about the effects of different factors.

This paper, however, does not allow a review of all work in this field by different groups. The purpose is mainly to review the main results obtained in human studies.

Factors enhancing non-haem iron absorption

Ascorbic acid

It has been observed that ascorbic acid is a very powerful enhancer of non-haem iron. Native ascorbic acid in fruits, vegetables and juices increases iron absorption to the same extent as synthetic vitamin C. There is a clear dose-effect relationship. In a comprehensive study on infant cereals it was found that there was a threefold increase in iron absorption when the ascorbate: iron ratio was 1.5:1. When the ratio was to 3:1 there was a sixfold increase in iron absorption[24]. In another study Lynch and Cook found a two-phase dose-response curve[25]. In studies on the effect of ascorbic acid on iron absorption from different meals we found a strong exponential dose-related effect of ascorbic acid on non-haem iron absorption. The relationship was much affected by the composition of the meals[26]. The main effect on iron absorption was achieved by the first 25–100 mg of ascorbic acid in a meal and the increase in absorption by a further addition is relatively less marked. More ascorbic acid is needed to achieve a certain absolute increase in iron absorption if more inhibitors are present in a meal[27–29].

Cooking may completely or partially destroy the ascorbic acid. The extent of destruction depends on the time and method of food preparation. Even prolonged warming of food may destroy the ascorbic acid and therefore have a deleterious effect on the bioavailability of dietary iron[30].

The main mechanism for the action of ascorbic acid appears to be a reduction of ferric to ferrous iron[7]. Iron can probably only pass the mucosal membrane in its ferrous form, which implies that ascorbic acid also seems to play a role in the mucin layer. Ascorbic acid could also have a role in reducing the formation of poorly soluble and poorly available ferric complexes with, for example, hydroxyl ions, certain phosphate ions, phytates and iron polyphenol complexes. The effect of ascorbic acid on iron absorption is so marked and essential that its effect on iron absorption should be considered as one of the physiological roles of ascorbic acid in the body.

In a comprehensive study by Cook *et al.*[31] the effect of large doses of ascorbic acid supplementation had a very small effect on serum ferritin as an indicator of iron stores. The exception was one male iron-deficient blood donor who showed a significant response. Some factors need to be considered in the interpretion of this rather negative results. One is that most subjects were iron replete and possibly therefore did not further increase their stores.

Another comprehensive study on the effect of ascorbic acid was made by Hunt *et al.*[32]. These studies were made in iron deficient volunteers and iron absorption was measured in very careful 5,5 weeks chemical balances. This finding thus supports the previous conclusion that ascorbic acid may have a rather small effect in fully replete subjects.

Meat, poultry, fish and seafood

An enhancing effect of meat and fish was first reported by Layrisse *et al.* in 1968[33]. This observation has since been confirmed in many other studies[34,35].

Meat has two roles in iron nutrition. It provides haem iron, on average about 50 per cent of iron in meat (beef, pork and lamb) with a variation from 10 to 70 per cent. Meat also contains an unknown factor that markedly enhances the absorption of both haem and non-haem iron. This enhancing factor is also present in poultry, fish and other seafood[36]. The nature of this factor is still unknown. The enhancing effect of meat on non-haem iron absorption seems to relate specifically to muscle protein, and not to animal protein in general. The mechanism whereby meat facilitates non-haem iron absorption is not clear.

Iron from haem or haemoglobin given alone is poorly absorbed but, given with meat[10], it is well absorbed. It has been suggested that the presence of these proteins maintains haem in the monomeric state, thus preventing the formation of poorly absorbed macromolecular haem polymers.

Many attempts to isolate the potentiating meat factor of animal tissue proteins have been made, since understanding the nature of this factor and its isolation could be of potential value in enhancing iron absorption from less bioavailable foods. Several canditates have been identified as contributing to the meat factor. Cysteine is one of the suggested amino acids enhancing non-haem iron absorption[37]. Another group has identified cysteine-containing residues as contributing to the meat effect[38].

Further work is clearly required to finally identify the meat factor.

Fermented products and organic acids

Recently it was found that fermented cabbage (sauerkraut) had a marked enhancing effect on iron absorption. In further studies on this factor it was noted that during fermentation there is a production of lactic acid and other organic acids, pH is lowered and the phytase activated. Other lactic acid-fermented vegetables added to a meal were found to increase iron absorption (Rossander-Hulthén *et al.* unpublished data).

The fresh vegetables (carrots, turnips, onions) contained small amounts of phytate, which was hydrolysed during the fermentation. The amount of iron absorbed was increased when the fermented vegetables were added to a white wheat roll (the fractional absorption increased from 13.6 to 23.6) and also when added to phytate-rich meals with wholemeal rye and wheat rolls, the fractional absorption increased from 5.2 to 10.4. This indicates the formation of iron-promoting factors in lactic acid-fermented vegetables.

Lactic acid has been identified as the factor that enhances iron absorption from sorghum- and maize-derived beers[39,40]. In some studies citric acid has been found to increase non-haem iron absorption[40,41], Our studies have seen only a moderate effect when adding lactic acid but no effect with citric acid[42]. Addition of malic acid to a basal rice meal improved iron absorption[40,41] Tartaric acid found in white vines has been found to enhance iron absorption.

A very interesting new observation is that fermented soy products, such as miso and soy sauce, act as enhancers of non-haem absorption. Low-molecular-weight peptides and amino acids could be associated with enhanced iron absorption[43,44]. Since such soy sauces are widely used by many populations, especially in Asia, these observations may have very marked importance.

Inhibitors of non-haem iron absorption

A number of factors have been identified which inhibit non-haem iron absorption from the common pool such as phytates, polyphenols and calcium.

Phytate

Phytate is a salt of inositol hexaphosphates, acting as a storage of phosphates and minerals in grains, seeds, nuts, vegetables and fruits. In Western-type diets about 90 per cent of phytates originate from cereals. It was originally suggested by McCance and Widdowson[45], that phytate had a negative effect on iron absorption. Phytate strongly inhibits iron absorption in a dose-dependent fashion. Even rather small amounts of phytate have a marked effect[27]. These amounts were so small that they were not detectable by previously used methods. This fact has caused considerable confusion about its inhibiting effect.

Bran has a very high content of phytate. High-extraction flour thus has a much higher content of phytates than white wheat flour. In bread, part of the phytate in bran is degraded to phosphate and inositol phosphates with lower phosphate groups during the fermentation of the dough by the phytase present in flour. These inositol phosphates also inhibit iron absorption. There is a strong support for the opinion that phytate and not fibre in cereals is the main iron absorption inhibitory factor. This opinion is supported by the observations that sour dough fermentation of wholemeal rye bread to a very low phytate level gave the same high iron absorption as control rolls with a low fibre content and the same low phytate level[46].

Removal of phytate from bran using endogenous phytase or dilute hydrochloric acid results in significantly improved absorption. The absorption was not only improved, it was even better than white wheat rolls with the same low phytate content[47]. This could be explained by the additional removal of manganese. In later studies we found that manganese interferes with iron absorption, related to similar physiochemical properties and shared absorption pathway[48]. The inhibitory effect of bran on iron absorption is mainly due to its content of phytate. If a lot of bran is consumed with a meal low in iron, part of the observed inhibition may be related to the manganese content in bran.

The inhibitory effects present in beans, rice and a number of other cereals including sorghum, oat products, and in certain vegetables are mainly related to theis phytate content. The phytate content of rice may vary from region to region based on differences in soil nutrients and also on differences in milling practice[28]. Wet milling of wheat reduces phytate content[29].

The exact mechanism by the inhibition of phytate is unknown. The formation of diferric and tetraferric phytate complexes makes the iron unavailable for absorption by the mucosal cell.

In strict vegetarians, with a chronic intake of a high phytate diet, there is poor iron absorption from phytate-cotaining meals[49]. This finding suggests that populations eating a diet with a high phytate content are unable to improve iron absorption from this type of diet by adaptation of the intestinal mucosal cell.

Ascorbic acid counteracts the inhibition of phytate. The more phytate present in a meal, however, the more ascorbic acid is needed to balance this inhibition[27,29]. Unfortunately, however, in most diets in the world the ascorbic acid content usually is too low to effectively counteract the inhibition of iron absorption by phytate.

Iron-binding phenolic compounds

It is well known that that tea is a strong inhibitor of iron absorption. Some vegetables and cereals have also been reported to to have such properties. The effect has been mainly related to the content of tannin, belonging to the huge family of polyphenols. The structure of thousands of phenolic compounds have been described. These phenolic compounds are widespread in nature. Recently, we found that the inhibiting effect can mainly be ascribed to the content of galloyl groups in different foods and spices. A spectrophotometric method has been developed to quantifying the amount of catechol and galloyl groups present in phenolic compounds[50]. We have found a strong relationship between the content of galloyl groups in different foods and the inhibition of iron absorption[51,52]. Such groups are common in tea, coffee, in some red wines, some spices and certain vegetables[40]. Other structures, such as chlorogenic acid, may also bind iron, e.g. in coffee, but the effect is small[52].

As with the phytates, addition of ascorbic acid to the meal can more or less counteract the inhibition, depending on the relationship between amounts of iron-binding phenolic compounds and ascorbic acid[29,51]

Soy protein

The addition of soy protein to a meal reduces the fraction of iron absorbed. This inhibition is mainly explained by its high content of phytates[53–57]. It has been suggested that some higher-molecular-weight protein might bind iron in the duodenum and contribute to the inhibition by soy. Some support for this hypothesis comes from recent studies demonstrating improved iron bioavailability from traditional fermented soy products that have a reduced proportion of the higher-molecular-weight protein fraction as a result of processing[43]. In another recent study a protein-related moiety contained in the conglycinin fraction was postulated as an inhibitor of non-haem iron absorption, the effect of which is relatively independent of the presence of phytate[58]. Replacement of meat with soy flour has been shown to lower the total amount of iron absorbed, including haem iron[57]. In infant foods containing soy products, the inhibiting effect can be overcome by the addition of ascorbic acid[55].

Calcium

Studies in animals suggest that calcium interferes with the absorption of iron[59]. The earlier results in man were less consistent than in animals[60]. Recently, several studies have shown that there is a true inhibitory effect of calcium on iron absorption[61].

It was also found that calcium inhibited the absorption of haem iron.

The mechanism is unknown, but the balance of evidence strongly suggests that the inhibition is not localized to the gastrointestinal lumen but to the mucosal cell itself and to the common final transfer step for haem and non-haem iron. A condition for inhibition is that iron and calcium are in the same meal. When the intake of calcium and iron was separeted in time (2 h and 4 h) no inhibition was seen[62]. Giving the same amount of calcium (about 900 mg in the daily menu) but avoiding dairy calcium in the two main meals (lunch and dinner), increased total iron absorption by 40 per cent[63].

These results are based on a recently developed method in which comparisons were made of non-haem iron absorption from two 10-day periods with an identical meal menu, including a wide variation, but with different distribution of the dairy calcium. All meals in the two periods were labelled with radioiron to a uniform specific activity and using two differnt radioiron isotopes.

Studies are now underway to examine the overall effects of other dietary factors (e.g. ascorbic acid, meat and phytate) with the same new method.

Iron absorption data in relation to iron nutrition – some pitfalls

Absorption studies in iron replete subjects

Using the method of extrinsic labelling of the whole diet for periods of 5–10 days the total amount of iron absorbed from four diets so far been studied. The data were analysed by relating absorption to iron status expressed as seum ferritin in all subjects. Several investigators have reported that there is a straight line relationship between log serum ferritin and absorption of iron from iron salts and meals. Two new observations were made in our recent studies when iron absorption was expressed as total amount of iron absorbed from the diet over several days. One finding was that with increasing serum ferritin, iron absorption decreased to levels below the basal iron losses, implying that no further accumulation of iron could take place beyond this point. The other finding was that diets with markedly different bioavailabilities showed no difference in the amount of iron absorbed when serum ferritin had reached a certain high level. This implies that meaningful comparisons of iron absorption from meals or diets should not be made in fully iron replete subjects. This is also valid for analyses of the effect of different factors on iron absorption.

Statistical analyses of relationships between dietary factors and iron status

Several dietary factors have been shown to influence the absorption of especially non-haem iron. Some of these factors have shown a rather marked effect (e.g. meat, ascorbic acid, tea, calcium). Therefore, it may seem to be a simple procedure to establish the true nutritional importance of such factors in a population by statistical analyses of relationships between the content of such factors in the diet and measures of iron status, for example, serum ferritin. As a matter of fact several studies have shown such statistically significant relationships. In an extensive study in Finland it was found that a low meat intake and a high milk intake were associated with iron deficiency[64]. In a study in France it was found that the intake of meat, dairy products and coffee was significantly associated with serum ferritin[65]. In a study in the USA a high red meat intake was associated with high serum ferritin[66], and in Australia it was demonstrated that the meat intake accounted for a significant part of the variation in serum ferritin.

In some studies no relationship was found, for example, between the intake of ascorbic acid or ascorbic acid-rich foods and serum ferritin. At first sight this may seem strange, as the absorption-promoting effect of ascorbic acid is well documented. There are different explanations and it is necessary to critically examine the conditions for this kind of statistical analysis. Iron status is determined by the balance between iron absorption and iron requirements. If, for example, the variation of iron requirements is much greater than the variation in bioavailability of the dietary iron, then it would be hard to observe a relationship between the intake of a certain dietary factor and iron status. If one were to examine the effect of tea on iron absorption or, rather, its nutritional importance for iron status in a population where the intake is both high and rather uniform, then one would not find such a relationship even if the tea had reduced iron absorption by, say, one-third or more in most subjects. Similarily, if one were to examine the relationship between intake of milk and iron status in young children, no effect is expected if almost all children have a high milk intake. The examples illustrate a classical statistical trap that must be avoided. There must be a certain variation in the intake of the factor to be studied and also a certain variation in requirements to justify such statistical analyses. Absence of a statistically significant relationship between the intake of a certain food or a certain component and its relationship with iron status must therefore be interpreted with caution.

Conclusion

Recent studies show that several common variables in the composition of the diet, such as the amounts of meat and fish, the choice of ascorbic acid-rich vegetables and fruits eaten with the meals, the kind of bread and other cereal products consumed, the selection of spices, and the selection of drinks with the meal, all strongly influence the bioavailability of the dietary iron. Increased knowledge and increased information about these factors may be important tools in the prevention of iron deficiency in both industrialized and developing countries.

Acknowlegements

This work was supported by Swedish Council for Forestry and Agriculture Research Project 50.0267–93 and Project 50.0120–95

References

1. Turnball, A., Cleton, F. & Finch, C.A. (1962): Iron absorption. IV. The absorption of hemoglobin iron. *J. Clin. Invest.* **41,** 1897–907.

2. Gräsbäck, R., Kouvonen, I., Lundberg, M. & Tenhunen, R. (1979): An intestinal receptor for heme. *Scand. J. Haematol.* **23,** 5–9.

3. Weintraub, L., Weinstein, M., Huser, H.-J. & Rafal, S. (1968): Absorption of hemoglobin iron. The role of heme-splitting substance in intestinal mucosa. *J. Clin. Invest.* **47,** 531–539.

4. Raffin, S., Woo, C., Roost, K., Price, D. & Schmid, R. (1974): Intestinal absorption of hemoglobin iron-heme cleavage by mucosal heme oxygenase. *J. Clin. Invest.* **54,** 1344–1352.

5. Hallberg, L. & Sölvell, L. (1967): Absorption of hemoglobin iron in man. *Acta Med. Scand.* **181,** 335–354.

6. Brise, H. & Hallberg, L. (1962): Absorbability of different iron compounds. *Acta Med. Scand.* (Suppl) **17,** 23–37.

7. Wollenberg, P. & Rummel, W. (1987): Dependence of intestinal iron absorption on the valency state of iron. *Arch. Pharmacol.* **336,** 578–582.

8. Martinez-Torres, C. & Layrisse, M. (1971): Iron absorption from veal muscle. *Am. J. Clin. Nutr.* **24,** 531–540.

9. Heinrich, H., Gabbe, E. & Kugler, G. (1987): $^{59}Fe^{2+}$ and hemoglobin-^{59}Fe absorption in human beings do not require gastric juice or intrinsic factor. *Biochem. Med.* **5,** 472–482.

10. Hallberg, L., Björn-Rasmussen, E., Howard, L. & Rossander, L. (1979): Dietary heme iron absorption. A discussion of possible mechanisms for the absorption-promoting effect of meat and for the regulation of iron absorption. *Scand. J. Gastroenterol.* **14,** 769–779.

11. Bezwoda, W.R., Bothwell, T.H., Charlton, W., Torrance, J., MacPhail, A.P., Derman, D.P. & Mayet, F. (1983): The relative dietary importance of haem and non-haem iron. *S. Afr. Med. J.* **64,** 552–526.

12. Schricker, B.R. & Miller, D.D. (1983): Effects of cooking and chemical treatment on heme and non-heme iron in meat. *J. Food. Sci.* **48,** 1340–1349.

13. Martinez-Torres, C., Leeb, I., Taylor, P., Ramirez, J., del Valle Camacho, M. & Layrisse, M. (1986): Heme, ferritin and vegetable iron absorption in humans from meals denatured of heme iron during the cooking of beef. *J. Nutr.* **116,** 1720–1725.

14. Hallberg, L., Rossander-Hulthén, L., Brune, M. & Gleerup, A. (1993): Inhibition of haem-iron absorption in man by calcium. *Brit. J. Nutr.* **69,** 533–540.

15. Magnusson, B., Björn-Rasmussen, E., Hallberg, L., & Rossander, L. (1981): Iron absorption in relation to iron status. Model proposed to express results of food iron absorption measurements. *Scand. J. Haematol.* **27,** 201–8.

16. Baynes, R., Bothwell, T.H., Bezwoda, W.R., MacPhail, A.P. & Derman, D.P. (1987): Relationship between absorption of inorganic and food iron in field studies. *Ann. Nutr. Metab.* **31,** 109–16.

17. Hallberg, L. & Rossander, L. (1982): Absorption of iron from Western-type lunch and dinner meals. *Am. J. Clin. Nutr.* **35,** 502–9.

18. Schricker, B.R., Miller, D.D., Rasmussen, R.R. & Van Campen, D. (1981): A comparison of *in vivo* and *in vitro* methods for determining availability of iron from meals. *Am. J. Clin. Nutr.* **34,** 2257–63.

19. Forbes, A.L., Adams, C.E., Arnaud, M.J. *et al.* (1989): Comparison of *in vitro*, animal, and clinical determinations of iron bioavailability: International Nutritional Anemia Consultative Group Task Force report on iron bioavailability. *Am. J. Clin. Nutr.* **49,** 225–238.

20. Hurrell, R.F., Lynch, S.R., Trinidad, T.P., Dassenko, S.A. & Cook, J.D. (1988): Iron absorption in humans: bovine serum albumin compared with beef muscle and egg white. *Am. J. Clin. Nutr.* **47,** 102–107.

21. Hurrell, R.F., Lynch, S.R., Trinidad, T.P., Dassenko, S.A. & Cook, J.D. (1989): Iron absorption in humans as influenced by bovine milk proteins, *Am. J. Clin. Nutr.* **49** 546–552.

22. Reddy, M.B. & Cook, J.D. (1991): Assessment of dietary determinants of nonheme-iron absorption in humans and rats. *Am. J. Clin. Nutr.* **54,** 723–728.

23. Hulthén, L., Gramatkovski, E., Gleerup, A. & Hallberg, L. (1995): Iron absorption from the whole diet. Relation to meal composition, iron requirements and iron stores. *Eur. J. Clin. Nutr.* **49,** 794–808.

24. Derman, D.P., Bothwell, T.H. & MacPhail, A.P. (1980): Importance of ascorbic acid in the absorption of iron from infant foods, *Scand. J. Haematol.* **25,** 193–201.

25. Lynch, S.R. & Cook, J.D. (1980): Interaction of vitamin C and iron, *Ann. NY. Acad. Sci.* **335,** 32–44.

26. Hallberg, L., Brune, M. & Rossander, L. (1986): Effect of ascorbic acid on iron absorption from different types of meals, *Ann. Nutr. Appl. Nutr.* **40A,** 97–113.

27. Hallberg, L., Brune, M. & Rossander, L. (1989): Iron absorption in man: ascorbic acid and dose-dependent inhibition by phytate, *Am. J. Clin. Nutr.* **49,** 140–144.

28. Tuntawiroon, M., Sritongkul, N., Rossander-Hulthén, L., Hallberg, L. & Brune, M. (1990): Rice and iron absorption in man. *Eur. J. Clin. Nutr.* **44,** 489–497.

29. Siegenberg, D., Baynes, R.D. & Bothwell, T.H. (1991): Ascorbic acid prevents the dose-depedent inhibitory effects of polyphenols and phytates on nonheme-iron absorption. *Am. J. Clin. Nutr.* **53,** 537–541.

30. Hallberg, L., Rossander, L., Persson, H. & Svahn, E. (1984): Deleterious effects of prolonged warming of meals on ascorbic acid content and iron absorption. *Am. J. Clin. Nutr.* **39,** 577–581.

31. Cook, J.D., Watson, S.S., Simpson, K.M., Lipschitz, D.A. & Skikne, B.S. (1984): The effect of high ascorbic acid supplementation on body iron stores. *Blood* **64,** 721–726.

32. Hunt, J.R., Mullen, L.M., Lykken, G.I., Gallagher, S.K. & Nielsen, F.H. (1990): Ascorbic acid: Effect on ongoing iron absorption and status in iron-depleted young women, *Am. J. Clin. Nutr.* **51,** 649–655.

33. Layrisse, M., Martinez-Torres, C. & Roche, M. (1968): The effect of interaction of various foods on iron absorption. *Am. J. Clin. Nutr.* **21,** 1175–83.

34. Layrisse, M., Martinez-Torres, C., Cook, J.D., Walker, R. & Finch, C.A. (1973): Iron fortification of food: its measurement by the extrinsic tag method. *Blood* **41,** 333–352.

35. Björn-Rasmussen, E. & Hallberg, L. (1979): Effect of animal proteins on the absorption of food iron in man. *Nutr. Metab.* **23,** 192–202.

36. Cook, J.D. & Monsen, E.R. (1976): Food iron absorption in human subjects. III. Comparison of the effect of animal proteins on nonheme iron absorption. *Am. J. Clin. Nutr.* **29,** 859–867.

37. Martinez-Torres, C., Romano, E. & Layrisse, M. (1981): Effect of cysteine on iron absorption in man. *Am. J. Clin. Nutr.* **34,** 322–327.

38. Taylor, P.G., Martinez-Torres, C., Romano, E.L. & Layrisse, M. (1986): The effect of cysteine-containing peptides released during meat digestion on iron absorption in humans, *Am. J. Clin. Nutr.* **43,** 68–71.

39. Derman, D.P., Bothwell, T.H., Torrance, J.D. *et al.* (1980): Iron absorption from maize (Zea mays) and sorghum (Sorghum vulgare) beer. *Brit. Med. J.* **43,** 271–279.

40. Gillooly, M., Bothwell, T.H., Torrance, J.D. *et al.* (1983): The effects of organic acids, phytates and polyphenol absorption of iron from vegetables. *Br. J. Nutr.* **49,** 331–42.

41. Ballot, D., Baynes, R.D., Bothwell, T.H. *et al.* (1987): The effects of fruit juices and fruits on the absorption of iron from a rice meal. *Br. J. Nutr.* **57,** 331–343.

42. Hallberg, L. & Rossander, L. (1984): Improvement of iron nutrition in developing countries: comparisons of adding meat, soy protein, ascorbic acid, citric acid, and ferrous sulphate on iron absorption from a simple Latin American-type of meal. *Am. J. Clin. Nutr.* **39,** 577–583.

43. MacFarlane, B.J., van der Riet, W.B., Bothwell, T.H. *et al.* (1990): Effect of traditional soy products on iron absorption. *Am. J. Clin. Nutr.* **51,** 873–880.

44. Baynes, R.D., MacFarlane, B.J., Bothwell, T.H. *et al.* (1990): The promotive effect of of soy sauce on iron absorption in human subjects. *Eur. J. Clin. Nutr.* **44,** 419–424.

45. McCance, R.A. & Widdowson, E.M. (1942): Mineral metabolism of healthy adults on white and brown bread dietaries. *J. Physiol.* **101,** 44–85.

46. Brune, M., Hallberg, L., Rossander-Hulthén, Gleerup, A. & Sandberg, A-S. (1992): Iron absorption from bread. Inhibiting effects of cereal fiber, phytate and inositol phosphates with different numbers of phosphate groups. *J. Nutr.* **122,** 442–449.

47. Hallberg, L., Rossander, L. & Skånberg, A.-B. (1987): Phytates and the inhibitory effect of bran on iron absorption in man. *Am. J. Clin. Nutr.* **45,** 988–996.

48. Rossander-Hulthén, L., Brune, M., Sandström, B., Lönnerdal, B. & Hallberg, L. (1991): Competitive inhibition of iron absorption by manganese and zinc in humans. *Am. J. Clin. Nutr.* **54,** 152–156.

49. Brune, M., Rossander, L. & Hallberg, L. (1989): Iron absorption: no intestinal adaptation to a high-phytate diet. *Am. J. Clin. Nutr.* **49,** 542–545.

50. Brune, M., Hallberg, L. & Skånberg, A-B. (1991): Determination of iron-binding phenolic groups in foods. *J. Food. Sci.* **56,** 128–132.

51. Tuntawiroon, M., Sritongkul, N., Brune, M., Rossander–Hulthén, L. & Hallberg, L. (1991): Dose-dependent inhibitory effect of phenolic compounds in food on nonheme-iron absorption in man. *Am. J. Clin. Nutr.* **53,** 554–557.

52. Brune, M., Rossander, L. & Hallberg, L. (1989): Iron absorption and phenolic compounds: importance of different phenolic structures. *Eur. J. Clin. Nutr.* **43,** 547–558.

53. Cook, J.D., Morck, T.A. & Lynch, S.R. (1981): The inhibitory effect of soy products on nonheme iron absorption in man. *Am. J. Clin. Nutr.* **34,** 2622–2629.

54. Morck, T.A., Lynch, S.R. & Cook, J.D. (1982): Reduction of the soy-induced inhibition of nonheme iron absorption. *Am. J. Clin. Nutr.* **36,** 219–228.

55. Gillooly, M., Torrance, J.D., Bothwell, T.H. *et al.* (1984): The relative effect of ascorbic acid on iron absorption from soy-based and milk-based infant formulas. *Am. J. Clin. Nutr.* **40,** 522–527.

56. Derman, D.P., Ballot, D., Bothwell, T.H. *et al.* (1987): Factors influencing the absorption of iron from soya-bean protein products. *Br J Nutr,* **57,** 345–353.

57. Hallberg, L. & Rossander, L. (1982): Effect of soy protein on nonheme iron absorption in man. *Am. J. Clin. Nutr.* **36,** 514–520.

58. Lynch, S.R., Dassenko, S.A., Cook, J.D., Juillerat, M.-A. & Hurrell, R.F. (1994): Inhibitory effect of a soybean-protein-related moiety on iron absorption in humans. *Am. J. Clin. Nutr.* **60,** 567–572.

59. Barton, J.C., Conrad, M.E. & Parmeley, R.T. (1983): Calcium inhibition of inorganic iron absorption in rats. *Gastroenterology* **84,** 90–101.

60. Monsen, E.R. & Cook, J.D. (1976): Food iron absorption in human subjects. IV. The effect of calcium and phosphate salts on the absorption of non-heme iron. *Am. J. Clin. Nutr.* **29,** 1142–1148.

61. Hallberg, L., Brune, M., Erlandsson, M., Sandberg, A.-S. & Rossander-Hulthén, L. (1991): Calcium: effects of different amounts on nonheme- and heme-iron absorption in humans. *Am. J. Clin. Nutr.* **53,** 112–119.

62. Gleerup, A., Rossander-Hulthén, L. & Hallberg, L. (1993): Duration of the inhibitory effect of calciumon non-haem iron absorption in man. *Eur. J. Clin. Nutr.* **47,** 875–879.

63. Gleerup, A., Rossander-Hulthén, L., Gramatkovski, E. & Hallberg, L. (1995): *Am. J. Clin. Nutr.* **61,** 97–104.

64. Takkunen, H. & Seppänem, R. (1975): Iron deficiency and dietary factors in Finland. *Am. J. Clin. Nutr.* **28,** 1141–1147.

65. Galan, P., Hercberg, S., Soustre, Y., Dop, M.C. & Dupin, S. (1985): Factors affecting iron stores in french female students. *Human Nutr. Clin. Nutr.* **39,** C: 279–287.

66. Worthington-Roberts, B., Beskin, M. & Monsen, E. (1988): Iron status of premenopausal women in a university community and its relationship to habitual dietary sources of protein. *Am. J. Clin. Nutr.* **47,** 275–279.

Iron Nutrition in Health and Disease, edited by Leif Hallberg and Nils-Georg Asp
©1996 John Libbey & Company Ltd., pp. 117–121

Chapter 11

Validity of databases on dietary iron - some examples

W. Becker

Nutrition Division National Food Administration, P.O. Box 622, S-751 26 Uppsala, Sweden

Summary

Data on iron in foods are available in most food composition databases and are used for calculation of iron intake in dietary surveys. The validity of the iron data in the food databases has been studied using duplicate diets, analyses of selected foods or market baskets, and food intake data based on dietary surveys or food availability.

Studies carried out in Europe and the USA have shown that analysed values for daily intakes deviated from calculated values by –10 to +30 per cent. Even larger differences are seen when the iron intakes are expressed on an energy basis. Reasons for these differences could be variations in the iron content of foods, contamination in connection with analysis and food preparation, dietary methodology and inadequacies in databases. It can be concluded that there is a need for high quality analytical data on the iron content of foods and diets and that food database compilers should validate the iron data included.

Introduction

Data on iron in foods are available in most food composition tables and databases and are used for calculation of iron intakes in dietary surveys. The data are generally based on a mixture of analytical and calculated values of domestic and foreign origin. A common view has been that the variation in iron content of foods is low and that iron data are internationally similar. Is this true and how valid are the included data? In this short review, data from studies comparing analysed and calculated intakes of iron published during the last decade are discussed.

Validity of iron in databases

As for most nutrients there are relatively few published studies that have compared calculated with analysed iron intake data. The methods used include analyses of duplicate diets, analyses of a selection of foods or market baskets, and food intake data based on dietary surveys or food availability.

Studies carried out in Europe and the USA have shown that analysed values on daily iron intakes deviated from calculated values by –10 per cent to +30 per cent (Table 1). In a market basket study covering the 60 most consumed foods in Sweden, the analysed iron content was 16 mg/day, whereas the calculated content was 18 mg/day, a difference of about –10 per cent[1]. The selection of foods was based on food availability data. The foods were analysed raw after preparation of the edible part. Interestingly, there were virtually no regional differences, indicating that major foods sold in the relail outlets are similar over the country. An earlier

Swedish study with a similar design showed a similar result[2].

In the US total diet study 1982–1987, comprising 234 foods, the difference between the analysed and calculated (USDA food composition database) iron content was on average only +3 per cent, with a variation from –6 per cent to +20 per cent depending on age and sex group[3]. In a total diet study carried out the UK[4] the analysed dietary content was 8 per cent higher than the calculated content.

In a study of 40 Finnish men, duplicate diets were prepared on the basis of 24 h recalls. Individual dishes were prepared before analysis. The analysed daily iron intake was found to be similar (+5 per cent) to the calculated value[5]. In a survey of 22 pregnant US women[6] duplicate portions of what was eaten by each subject during one day was collected under supervision of a nutritionist. The nutrient content of the daily diets were analysed and calculated. The analysed daily iron intake was found to be about 30 per cent higher than the calculated value. In a survey of 30 British civil servants[7], different dietary methods were used to calculate the nutrient intake and the subjects also collected duplicates of all foods consumed during one week. The analysed daily intake deviated from the calculated intakes by –2 per cent to +28 per cent. In another British study 61 13–14 year old boys and girls kept a written, weighed record of all food and drink consumed every 6th day for 7 weeks[8]. Duplicate portions of the food were also collected on each day and analysed for iron and other nutrients. The iron content of the analysed food did not differ from that of the calculated for girls but for boys it was 11 per cent lower. When the iron intakes found in the above studies are expressed on an energy basis differences up to 40 per cent are seen (Table 1). The table also indicate that iron intake can vary between and within countries.

It is obvious that one could expect differences in iron content when direct analyses of individ-

Table 1. Analysed and calculated dietary iron content of diets in different studies

Study	Iron content (mg/d)					
	Analysed	Calculated	% diff[1] A-C	% diff mg/MJ	Dietary method[2]	Reference
Swedish Weekly Diet 1980	14	15.5	–10	–10	FBS	2
Swedish Market Baskets 1987	16	18	–11	–11	FBS	1
US Total Diet 1982–87	8.7–16	8.2–16.9	+3	–	24 h	3
UK Total Diet study 1991	10.9	10.1	+8	–	HBS	5
Finnish men 1981	19.0	18.1	+5	+5	24 h	4
US pregnant women	14.4	11.0	+31	+42	24 h	6
British adults 1980s	18.5	14.4	+28	+34	24 h	7
		17.2	+8	+34	7 d wr	
		18.9	-2	+37	FFI	
		17.9	+3	+35	Fd purch	
British 13–14 yr boys	13.2	14.9	–11	–15	7d wr	8
British 14–14 yr girls	9.8	9.7	+1	–1	7d wr	8

[1] (analysed–calculated) × 100/calculated.
[2] FBS = Food balance sheets, 24 h = 24 hour recall, 7 d wr = 7 days weighed record, FFI = food frequency interview, Fd purch = 28 day purchase record, HBS = household budget survey (British National Food Survey).

Table 2. Variation in iron content of selected foods in some food composition tables

Food	*N*	Mean	Range	Country
Pork, lean	15	1.61	0.9–4.35	Sweden[a]
	8	0.62	0.52–0.75	Finland[b]
	6	0.89	0.64–1.15	Denmark[c]
	–	1.8	0.9–2.5	Germany[d]
Potatoes	21	0.59	0.41–1.58	Sweden
	20	0.67	0.56–0.84	Finland
	9	0.6	0.35–1.2	Denmark
	–	0.4	0.34–1.5	Germany
Chicken	15	1.14	0.43–2.45	Sweden
	4	0.67	0.43–0.84	Finland
	26	0.6	0.42–1.06	Denmark
Wheat flour, whole	7	5.0	3.4–8.1	Sweden
	7	5.2	4.1–5.9	Finland
	–	3.31	2.4–5.3	Germany
Cod	15	0.25	0.13–0.74	Sweden
	3	0.16	0.13–0.18	Finland
	4	0.2	0.12–0.22	Denmark
	–	0.44	0.4–0.52	Germany
Cabbage	16	0.38	0.16–1.18	Sweden
	5	0.38	0.35–0.41	Finland
	7	0.38	0.16–0.33	Denmark
Carrot	17	0.25	0.17–0.39	Sweden
	5	0.48	0.34–0.74	Finland
	10	0.4	0.19–1.03	Denmark
	–	2.1	0.4–4.8	Germany

[a]From Ref. 8. [b]From Ref. 9. [c]From Ref. 10. [d]From Ref. 11.

ual foods or diets are compared with data obtained from food composition databases, because the data are not based on the same food samples. As for other nutrients, the iron content of foods can vary substantially. Studies on Swedish foods have shown a considerable variation in the iron content of several foods ranging from meat to potatoes. Examples of the variation in iron content of some foods, taken from a selection of food tables, are shown in Table 2. In iron analysis the problem of contamination is not negligible and could be one reason for some of the high values reported, in addition to variations due to feeding, crop variety and soil.

Food preparation can affect the iron content. Losses of iron are generally small while cooking food in cast iron utensils can markedly increase the iron content of dishes, especially when pH is low. Such data are probably not frequently included in food databases. Studies in our own laboratory have shown that the iron content of certain meat dishes cooked in cast iron utensils increased 2–3-fold. The contribution of this extra iron to the overall iron intake is difficult to estimate. During the collection of duplicate food samples fruit and vegetables contaminated with small amounts of soil might be included by the individual and thus increase the iron content of the diet.

Other factors that might affect the reliability of iron intake data are dietary methodology and missing or inadequate values in databases. In the study of 30 British adults the iron intake was calculated from 24 h recalls, 7 day weighed food records, food frequency interviews, and 28 day food purchase records[7]. The analysed (duplicate diet) intake was from 2 per cent lower to 28 per cent higher than the intakes calculated from the dietary data (Table 1). -2When adjusted for energy intake, however, the magnitude of the deviations for the calculated dietary data were similar for all methods (Table 1).

Inadequacies in the databases can account for differences between analysed and calculated iron intakes. Iron is a particularly good example since fortification of foods with iron is common and practicies vary between countries and with time. In a duplicate diet study of 100 Danish men the anlalysed intakes of the 25 men that had the lowest and highest intakes was found to be 46 per cent and 14 per cent lower, respectively, than the calculated intakes (B. Sandström, personal communication). The main reason for the lower analysed intakes was that the fortification of flour had ceased about 1 year before the study and that the official database had not yet been fully updated.

Other mineral elements

In the studies reviewed, other mineral elements were also included in the analyses. In Table 3 results for some elements are compared with the iron data. No definitive conclusions can be made from these few studies with respect to the quality of the iron data, but the differences seen

Table 3. Percentage difference[a] between analysed and calculated intakes of certain minerals

Survey	Fe	Ca	Mg	Zn	Se	Mn	Dietary method	Reference
Swedish market baskets 1987	–11	–2	–8	< 1	+16	–	FBS	1
US total diet 1982–87	+3	-8	–7	< 1	–	<1	24 h	3
Finnish men 1981	+5	+5	+9	+3	+20	+16	24 h	5
US pregnant women 1980s	+31	+20	–2	–3	–	–	24 h	6
British 13–14 yr boys	–11	–	–	+1	–	–	wr	8
British 13–14 yr girls	+	–	–	–4	–	–	wr	8

[1] (analysed–calculated) × 100/calculated.
[2] FBS = Food balance sheets, 24 h = 24 hour recall, 7 d wr = 7 days weighed record, FFI = food frequency interview, Fd purch = 28 day purchase record, HBS = household budget survey (British National Food Survey).
[a](analysed–calculated) × 100/calculated.

for the iron data appear, with one exception, to be in the same range as for other elements.

Conclusions

An evaluation of the results of the reviewed studies show that the agreement between the analysed and calculated iron intakes in many cases is relatively good, taking into account the apparent sources of variation. However, analysed dietary data can deviate substantially from calculated data and each database compiler should validate the iron data included.

Although iron bioavailability may be even more important than the total amount ingested, it can be concluded that there is a need for high quality analytical data on the iron content of foods and diets.

References

1. Becker, W. & Kumpulainen, J. (1991): Contents of essential and toxic mineral elements in Swedish market-basket diets in 1987. *Br. J. Nutr.* **66,** 151–160.
2. Slorach, S., Gustafsson, I.-B., Jorhem, L. & Mattsson, P. (1983): Intake of lead, cadmium and certain other metals via a typical Swedish weekly diet. *Vår Föda* **35,** (suppl. 1) 1–16.
3. Pennington, J.A.T. & Wilson, D.B. (1990): Daily intakes of nine nutritional elements: Analysed vs. calculated values. *J. Am. Diet. Assoc.* **90,** 375–381.
4. Buss, D. (1994): Iron: The situation in the UK. In: *Report of Third Annual Meeting, FLAIR Eurofoods-Enfant Project*, Vilamoura, Portugal, 10–12 November 1993, pp. 51–54. Wageningen, the Netherlands:
5. Kumpulainen, J., Mutanen, M., Paakki, M. & Lehto, J. (1987): Validity of calculation method in estimating mineral element content of a pooled total daily diet as tested by chemical analysis. *Vår Föda.* **39,** (suppl. 1) 75–82.
6. Brennan, R.E., Kohrs, M.B., Nordstrom, J.W., Sauvage, J.P. & Shank, R.E. (1983): Composition of diets of low-income pregnant women: Comparison of analyzed with calculated values. *J. Am. Diet. Assoc.* **83,** 538–545.
7. Bull, N.L. & Wheeler, E.F. (1986): A study of different dietary survey methods among 30 civil servants. *Human Nutr. Appl. Nutr.* **40A,** 60–66.

8. Southon, S., Wright, A.J.A., Finglas, P.M., Bailey, A.L. & Belsten, J.L. (1992): Micronutrient intake and psychological performance of schoolchildren: consideration of the value of calculated nutrient intakes for the assessment of micronutrient status in children. *Proc. Nutr. Soc.* **51,** 315–324.

9. Livsmedelstabeller (1986): *Food composition tables*, 2nd edn. Uppsala: Swedish National Food Admistration.

10. Møller, A. (1989): *Food composition tables 1989*. Søborg: National Food Agency.

11. Souci, S.W., Fachmann, W. & Kraut, H. (1994): Food composition and nutrition tables. 5th revised and completed edition. Stuttgart: Medpharm Scientific Publishers.

12. Koivistonen, P. (ed.) (1980): Mineral element composition of Finnish foods: N, K, Ca, Mg, P, S, Fe, Cu, Mn, Zn, Mo, Co, Ni, Cr, F, Se, Si, Rb, Al, B, Br, Hg, As, Cd, Pb and ash. *Acta Agric. Scand.* Suppl. 22.

Iron Nutrition in Health and Disease, edited by Leif Hallberg and Nils-Georg Asp
©1996 John Libbey & Company Ltd., pp. 123–128

Chapter 12

Iron requirements and iron deficiency: Studies in premature infants

M.A. Siimes and S.M. Kivivuori

Division of Pediatric Hematology & Oncology, Children's Hospital, University of Helsinki, FIN-00290 Helsinki, Finland

Summary

Preterm infants are at risk of developing protein and iron deficiency. Concentration of transferrin is low. In contrast, serum iron is similarly elevated, resulting in highly elevated transferrin iron saturation. This is of concern in relation to oxidative metabolism. Iron stores of prematures may be mobilised at a slower rate than the requirements for haemoglobin synthesis. Thus, iron deficiency and progressive decrease in haemoglobin may occur even though tissue iron stores are present. The maintenance of normal haemoglobin concentration may be by far the best criterion of adequate iron nutrition under these conditions. The prematures with birth weight from 0.5 to 1 kg form a special group requiring further studies. Medicinal doses of iron may increase haemolysis in vitamin E deficient prematures. Prevention of vitamin E deficiency is important since preterm infants are born with relatively low vitamin E stores and suboptimal tocopherol concentrations. "Anaemia of prematurity" is associated with a low rate of erythropoiesis and low serum concentrations of erythropoietin. Most studies indicate that erythropoietin is safe and effective in treatment of anaemia and in prevention of red blood cell transfusions. Extra iron has been used to compensate the elevated iron requirements for haemoglobin synthesis. We have observed that serum ferritin was lower and serum transferrin receptor highly elevated in erythropoietin-treated infants, indicating that stimulated erythropoiesis results in evidence of iron deficiency which cannot be compensated by iron medication.

Iron nutrition is complicated in preterm-born infants. At birth their haemoglobin concentration is lower than in fullterm newborns. The concentrations of serum ferritin in cord blood are also low. Thus, the relative iron reserves in red blood cells and tissue stores per unit of body weight may also be lower than in full-term newborns.

There are five specific reasons for anaemia in premature infants:

1. Small premature infants usually require intensive care and multiple red blood cell transfusions to compensate for the blood drawn for laboratory tests soon after birth. These requirements are difficult to control in any clinical study dealing with haemoglobin concentration or iron nutrition. The volumes transfused and the consequent haemoglobin concentration depend on the criteria used[1].

2. Soon after birth the preterm infants are at risk of developing protein deficiency. This may im-

pair eythropoiesis. Further, the serum protein levels are low including the main iron-binding protein, transferrin. Because the serum iron concentration is similarly elevated as for full-term infants, the serum transferrin iron saturation may be highly elevated. The oversaturation of transferrin has been of some concern in oxidative metabolism[2].

3. Vitamin E is also needed in excess. Prevention of vitamin E deficiency is important as preterm infants are born with relatively low vitamin E stores and suboptimal tocopherol concentrations. However, medicinal doses of iron may increase haemolysis in vitamin E-deficient prematures and result in anaemia[3]. Today, this potential risk may exist primarily soon after birth in preterm patients who are not receiving enteral feeding or intravenous multivitamins.

4. 'Anaemia of prematurity' is associated with a low rate of erythropoiesis and low serum concentrations of erythropoietin[4]. The haemoglobin concentration decreases and reaches its lowest level at 6–9 weeks after birth in the prematures[5].

5. Iron deficiency may develop 6–8 weeks after birth. All preterm infants are also at risk of developing iron deficiency after this age unless given iron treatment or adequate formula to compensate the extremely large needs of body growth during the first year of life[6]. It is not uncommon that an infant may increase his body weight 8- or 10-fold during the first year. An even higher proportional increase may be needed in the iron requirement for red blood cells since the the haemoglobin mass rises faster than the body weight. The required dose of oral iron may depend on the birth weight and vary between 2 and 4 mg/kg/day. In Norwegian studies a dose of 18 mg pcr infant has been recommended[5]. Accordingly, the latter dose is high soon after birth and decreases per kilogram through the infancy. Nevertheless, infants with the lowest birth weight require iron treatment or a special formula since the required iron may not be obtained from the regular infant diet. The efficiency of iron deficiency prevention, however, depends on the criteria of iron deficiency selected. If similar cut-off points for red blood cell indices, serum ferritin, transferrin iron satu-

Table 1. Studies of recombinant human erythropoietin (rHuEpo) treatment in premature infants (birth weight < 2,000 gm).

Reference	rHuEpo IU/kg/wk	Administrion	Number of subjects patients + controls
Halperin *et al*[12]	75–300	s.c.	7 + 0
Halperin *et al*[11]	75–600	s.c.	18 + 0
Beck *et al*[13]	10–200	i.v.	16 + 0
Obladen *et al*[14]	70	s.c.	43 + 50
Ohls *et al*[15]	700	s.c.	10 + 9
Shannon *et al*[16]	200	i.v.	10 + 10
Shannon *et al*[17]	500–1,000	s.c.	4 + 4
Carnielli *et al*[18]	1,200	both	11 + 11
Bechensteen *et a*[5]	300	s.c.	14 + 15
Emmerson *et al*[19]	100–300	s.c.	16 + 8
Messer *et al*[20]	300–900	s.c.	31 + 20
Soubasi *et al*[21]	300	s.c.	3 + 0
Maier *et al*[22]	750	s.c.	120 + 121
Meyer *et al*[23]	600	s.c.	40 + 40
Kivivouri *et al*[24]	900	s.c.	21 + 34
Shannon *et al*[1]	500	s.c.	77 + 80

ration and other available tests are used, as for older children, a large population of preterm infants are iron deficient[7,8]. However, such cut-off points for the diagnosis of iron deficiency may prove to be arbitrary and misleading, and the maintanence of normal haemoglobin concentration may be by far the best criterion.

Some evidence indicates that very low birth weight infants who receive a large volume of packed red cells during hospitalization may accumulate iron stores sufficient for red cell production during the first 6 months of life. However, the iron stores may be mobilized at a rate that is slower than the requirements for haemoglobin synthesis[6]. If this happens, laboratory evidence of iron deficiency and progressive decrease in haemoglobin concentration may occur even though tissue iron stores are present.

With adequate nutrition and supplementation, prematures with birth weights above 1 kg generally catch up with the haemoglobin concentration of full term infants by age 4–6 months, even though haemoglobin concentration is also rapidly rising in the full-term infants. Thus, the haemoglobin concentration and cell blood counts should be within the limits of full-term infants after age 6 months[9].

Those prematures with a birth weight below 1 kg form a special subgroup, and further studies are required to establish their optimal treatment, including prevention of iron deficiency.

Use of human milk is of benefit in maintanance of optimal iron status in healthy full-term infants. This beneficial effect may occur through improved gastrointestinal function, resulting in a better bioavailability of nutrients including that of iron. However, the amount of human protein in the diet may be a rate-limiting factor of erythropoiesis in exclusively human milk-fed preterm infants. Accordingly, fortification of human milk with human milk protein may prevent most 'anaemia of prematurity'[10].

The use of erythropoietin has become popular in clinical practices. Most studies have indicated that treatment with recombinant human erythropoietin (rHuEpo) is safe and effective in the treament of anaemia and in the prevention of red blood cell transfusions (Table 1). The opti-

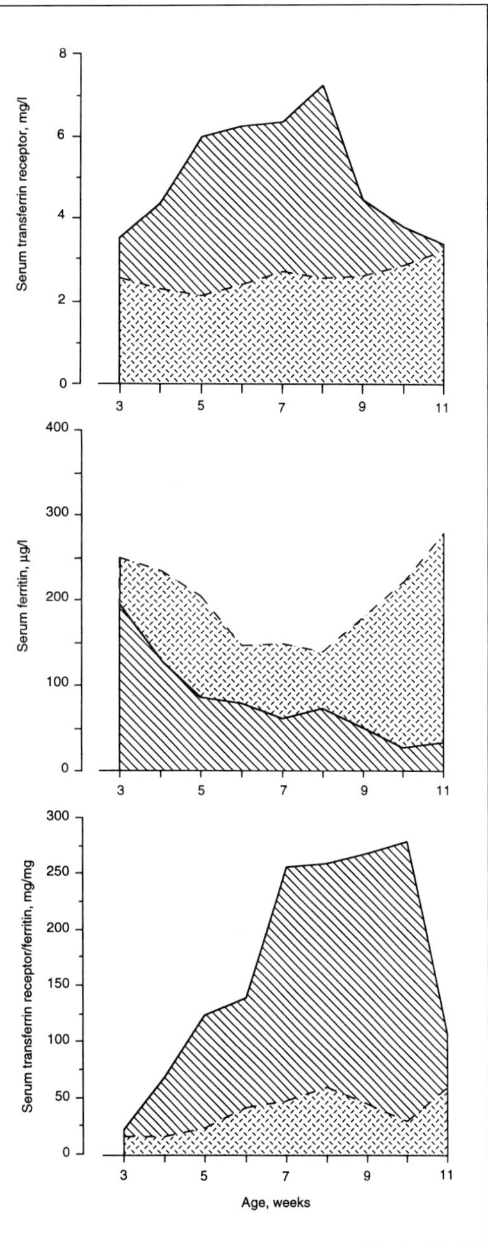

Fig. 1. Influence of rHuEpo treatment (dotted line) on the mean serum concentrations of transferrin receptor (upper figure) and ferritin (middle figure), and on the serum transferrin receptor/ferritin ratio (lower figure) compared to untreated infants (broken line). The rHuEpo treatment was started on the third week of life and continued for 3 weeks[24].

mal dose of rHuEpo has not been determined. Thus, a wide range of doses is used, usually from 300 to 1200 IU/kg/week. In the 15 studies the dosing and timing have varied greatly[1,5,11–23], Table 2. Prophylactic rHuEpo has been given in three such studies. Simultaneous iron supplementation has been used in every reported investigation. Both oral iron (from 2 to about 30 mg/kg/day) or intravenously administered iron (20 mg/kg/day) has been used to compensate the elevated iron requirements for haemoglobin synthesis.

Thus, the present data indicate that treatment with rHuEpo stimulates erythropoiesis and, consequently, the iron requirements for haemoglobin production even during the first weeks after the preterm birth are artificially and highly elevated. The infants are also left without the iron in the transfused red cells required without the rHuEpo treatment. A recent study with small prematures has shown that serum ferritin concentrations are lower, serum transferrin receptor concentrations higher and transferrin receptor:ferritin ratios highly elevated in the rHuEpo-treated infants, compared to similar infants without the treatment (Fig. 1)[24]. These findings may indicate that iron is marginally available under these conditions, even when given at 6 mg/kg/day which is one of the higher doses reported (Table 2). These findings may also indicate that the stimulated erythropoiesis results in evidence of iron deficiency which cannot be compensated for by iron medication. However, additional studies are needed for firm conclusions because the rise in serum tranferrin receptor may also be a secondary phenomenon of elevated erythropoiesis[25,26].

Conclusions

Preterm infants are at risk of developing iron deficiency after 2 months of age unless given iron fortified formula or supplementary iron.

The risk is larger in prematures with birth weights below 1000 g.

Table 2. Studies of rHuEpo treatment in premature infants (BW<2,000 gm): rHuEpo treatment in relation to iron medication

Reference	Age started (days)	**Duration of erythropoietin (weeks)**	**Dose of iron (mg/kg/day) peroral**
Halperin *et al*[12]	21-33	4	2
Halperin *et al*[11]	21-35	4	2–8
Beck *et al*[13]	25-59	4	3
Obladen *et al*[14]	4	3	2
Ohls *et al*[15]	41	3	2
Shannon *et al*[16]	10-35	6	3
Shannon *et al*[17]	8-28	6	6
Carnielli *et al*[18]	2	7	20[a]
Bechensteen *et a*[5]	21	4	18–36[b]
Emmerson *et al*[19]	9	5	6
Messer *et al*[20]	10	6	3-15
Soubasi *et al*[21]	7	6	3
Maier *et al*[22]	3	6	2
Meyer *et al*[23]	27	6	2–10
Kivivouri *et al*[24]	14-21	3	6
Shannon *et al*[1]	7-42	6	3-6

[a] intravenously
[b] mg of iron per infant

Treatment with rHuEpo stimulates erythropoiesis and is associated with a reduction in red blood cell transfusions.

Thus, the requirements of iron for stimulated haemoglobin synthesis are elevated.

This may lead to marginal iron deficiency. Elevated values for serum transferrin receptor and decreased values for serum ferritin during rHuEpo treatment support this possibility.

References

1. Shannon, K.M., Keith, J.F., Mentzer, W.C., Ehrenkranz, R.A., Brown, M.S., Widness, J.A., Gleason, C.A., Bifino, E.M., Millard, D.D., Davis, C.B., Stevenson, D.K., Alverson, D.C., Simmons, C.F., Brim, M., Abels, R.I. & Phibbs, R.H. (1995): Recombinant human erythropoietin stimulates erythropoiesis and reduces erythrocyte transfusions in very low birth weight preterm infants. *Pediatrics* **95,** 1–8.

2. Sullivan, J.L. (1977): Iron, plasma antioxidant, and the 'oxygenradical disease of prematurity'. *Am. J. Dis. Child* **142,** 1341–1344.

3. Williams, M.L., Shott, R.J., O'Neal, P.L. & Oski, F.A. (1975): Role of dietary iron and fat on vitamin E deficiency anemia of infancy. *N. Engl. J. Med.* **292,** 887–890.

4. Shannon, K.M. (1990): Anemia of prematurity: progress and prospects. *Am. J. Pediatr. Hematol. Oncol.* **12,** 14–20.

5. Bechensteen, A.G., Haga, P., Halvorsen, S., Whitelaw, A., Liestol, K., Lindemann, R., Grogaard, J., Hellebostad, M., Saugstad, O., Gronn, M., Daae, L., Refsum, H. & Sundal, E. (1993): Erythropoietin, protein, and iron supplementation and the prevention of anaemia of prematurity. *Arch. Dis. Child.* **69,** 19–23.

6. Lundstrom, U., Siimes, M.A. & Dallman, P.R. (1977): At what age does iron supplementation become necessary in low-birth-weight infants? *J. Pediatr.* **91,** 878–883.

7. Friel, J.K., Andrews, W.L., Matthew, J.D. *et al.* (1990): Iron status of verylow-birth-weight infants during the first 15 months of infancy. *Can. Med. Assoc. J.* **143,** 733–737.

8. Iwai, Y., Takanashi, T., Nakao, Y. & Mikawa, H. (1986): Iron status in low birth weight infants on breast and formula feeding. *Eur. J. Pediatr.* **145,** 63–65.

9. Lundstrom, U. & Siimes, M.A. (1980): Red blood cell values in low-birthweight infants: Ages at which values become equivalent to those of term infants . *J. Pediatr.* **96,** 1040–1042.

10. Ronnholm, K.A.R. & Siimes, M.A. (1985): Haemoglobin concentration depends on protein intake in small preterm infants fed human milk. *Arch. Dis. Child.* **60,** 99–104.

11. Halperin, D.S, Wacker, P., Lacourt, G., Felix, M., Babel, J.-F. & Wyss, M. (1992): Recombinant human erythropoietin in the treatment of infants with anaemia of prematurity. *J. Pediatr.* **121,** 661–667.

12. Halperin, D.S., Wacker, P., Lacourt, G., Felix, M., Babel, J.-F., Aapro, M. & Wyss, M. (1990): Effects of recombinant human erythropoietin in infants with the anemia of prematurity: A pilot study. *J. Pediatr.* **116,** 779–786.

13. Beck, D., Massarey, E., Meyer, M. & Calame, A. (1991): Weekly intravenous administration of recombinant human erythropoietin in infants with the anaemia of prematurity. *Eur. J. Pediatr.* **150,** 767–772.

14. Obladen, M., Maier, R., Segerer, H., Graul, E.L., Holland, D.M., Stewart, G., Jorch, G., Rabe, H., Linderkmap, O., Hoffmann, H.G, Houghton, F., Herrmann, Z., Scigalla, P. & Wardrop, C. (1991): Efficacy and safety of recombinant human erythropoietin to prevent the anemias of prematurity. In: *Erythropoietin in renal and non-renal anemias*, eds. H.J. Gurland, J. Moran, W. Samtleben, P. Scigalla & L. Wieczorek, pp. 314–326. Karger: Bastle.

15. Ohls, R.K. & Christensen, R.D. (1991): Recombinant erythropoietin compared with erythrocyte transfusion in the treatment of anemia of prematurity. *J. Pediatr.* **119,** 781–788.

16. Shannon, K.M., Mentzer, W.C., Abels, R.I., Freeman, P., Newton, N., Thompson, D., Sniderman, S., Ballard, R. & Rhibbs, R. (1991): Recombinant human erythropoietin in the anemia of prematurity: Results of a placebo-controlled pilot study. *J. Pediatr.* **118,** 949–955.

17. Shannon, K.M., Mentzer, W.C., Abels, R.I., Wertz, M., Thayer-Moriyama, J., Yi Li, W., Thompson, D., Decelle, S. & Rhibbs, R. (1992): Enhancement of erythropoiesis by recombinant human erythropoietin in low birth weight infants: A pilot study. *J. Pediatr.* **120,** 586–592.

18. Carnielli, V., Montini, G., Da Riol, R., Dall'Amico, R. & Cantarutti, F. (1992): Effect of high doses of human recombinant erythropoietin on the need for blood transfusions in preterm infants. *J. Pediatr.* **121,** 98–102.

19. Emmerson, A.J.B., Coles, H.J., Stern, C.M.M. & Pearson, T.C. (1993): Double blind trial of recombinant human erythropoietin in preterm infants. *Arch. Dis. Child.* **68,** 291–296.

20. Messer, J., Haddad, J., Donato, L., Astruc, D. & Matis, J. (1993): Early treatment of premature infants with recombinant human erythropoietin. *Pediatrics* **92,** 519–523.

21. Soubasi, V., Kremenopoulos, G., Diamandi, E., Tsantali, C. & Tsakiris, D. (1993): In which neonates does early recombinant human erythropoietin treatment prevent anemia of prematurity? Results of a randomized, controlled study. *Pediatr. Res.* **34,** 675–679.

22. Maier, R.F., Obladen, M., Scigalla, P., Linderkamp, O., Duc, G., Hieronimi, G., Halliday, H.L., Versmold, H.T., Moriette, G., Jorch, G., Verellen, G., Semmekrot, B.A, Grauel, E.L., Holland, B.M. & Wardrop, C.A.J. (1994): Effect of epoetin beta (recombinant human erythropoietin) on the need for transfusion in very-low-birth-weight infants. *N. Engl. J. Med.* **330,** 1173–1178.

23. Meyer, M.P., Meyer, J.H., Commerford, A., Hann, F.M., Sive, A.A., Moller, G., Jacobs, P. & Malan, A.F. (1994): Recombinant human erythropoietin in the treatment of the anemia of prematurity: Results of a doubleblind, placebo-controlled study. *Pediatrics* **93,** 918–923.

24. Kivivuori, S.M., Heikiheimo, M., Siimes, M.A. (1994): Early rise in serum concentration of transferrin receptor is induced by recombinant human erythropoietin in very low-birth-weight infants. *Pediatr. Res.* **36,** 85–89.

25. Kohgo, Y., Niitsu, Y., Kondo, H., Kato, J., Tsushima, N., Sasaki, K., Hirayama, M., Numata, T., Nishisato, T. & Urushizaki, I. (1987): Serum transferrin receptor as a new index of erythropoiesis. *Blood* **70,** 1955–1958.

26. Skikne, B.S., Flowers, C.H. & Cook, J.D. (1990): Serum transferrin receptor: a quantitative measure of tissue iron deficiency. *Blood* **75,** 1870–1876.

Iron Nutrition in Health and Disease, edited by Leif Hallberg and Nils-Georg Asp
©1996 John Libbey & Company Ltd., pp. 129–136

Chapter 13

Iron requirements and prevalence of iron deficiency in term infants during the first 6 months of life

Olle Hernell and Bo Lönnerdal

Department of Pediatrics, Umeå University, S-901 85 Umeå, Sweden and Department of Nutrition, University of California, Davis CA 95616, USA

Summary

The appropriate level of iron supplementation of infant formulas is still under discussion. In Europe, formulas generally contain 7 mg of iron/l (1 mg/100 kCal), whereas a more generous level of 12 mg/l (1.8 mg/100 kCal) is used in the USA. Both these levels of iron fortification prevent iron deficiency and anaemia during the first 6 months of life. Breast milk, however, only contains 0.2–0.4 mg of iron/l and iron deficiency is rarely seen in term breast fed infants at 6 months of age. In the present paper we summarize the results from two studies exploring the effect of formulas containing target levels of 4 and 2 mg of iron/l, respectively, on iron status of formula-fed term infants during the first 6 months of life. Term infants were either exclusively breast fed or fed experimental formulas containing 4 or 2 mg iron/l from 6 ± 2 (4 mg study) or 4 ± 2 (2 mg study) weeks to 6 months of age. In one formula in each of the studies part of the iron was provided as bovine lactoferrin rather than as $FeSO_4$. With respect to the 4 mg study there were no differences in haematological indices between groups at 6 months of age. All infants had satisfactory iron status, i.e. none of the infants was iron deficient as judged by conventional multiple criteria. In the 2 mg study, using the same design, there were no differences with respect to anthropometric measurements at any time point (1, 4 and 6 months of age), nor were there significant differences between the groups with respect to haematological parameters or iron status, including serum transferrin receptor levels, at 4 or 6 months of age. A single child was considered iron deficient by use of multiple criteria at 6 months of age. Based on these studies an iron fortification level of 2 mg of iron/l should be adequate for term infants up to 6 months of age.

Introduction

Iron deficiency is one of the most common nutrition disorders worldwide. In addition to affecting a large proportion of infants, children and women in the developing world, iron deficiency is the only nutrient deficiency of significant prevalence in virtually all developed nations as well[1]. Thus, iron deficiency, with or without anaemia, is still considered a major nutritional problem in infancy and childhood. In fact, infants fed formulas which have not been fortified with iron are at risk of developing iron deficiency anaemia as early as 4–6 months of age[2,3]. Consequently, most infant formulas in Europe contain 7–8 mg iron/l (1 mg/100 kCal), whereas most formulas in the USA contain 12–13 mg/l (1.8 mg/100 kCal). Although both these levels of iron fortification have been shown to prevent iron deficiency and anaemia during the first 6 months of life they should be compared to the average iron concentration of only 0.2–0.4 mg/l in human milk. Exclusively breast-fed infants rarely show any signs of iron deficiency at 6 months of age[4–6]. The considerably higher levels of iron in formulas has been used to compensate for a higher bioavailability of iron from human milk than from formula[7]. However, even if the bioavailability were only 1/10 that of human milk, which is probably an underestimation for modern formulas, a formula containing 4 mg iron/l should be sufficient to prevent iron deficiency at least during the first 6 months of life. If so, it would seem reasonable to lower the iron content of formulas because an excess of iron may have adverse effects, such as that due to prooxidative capacity of ferrous iron. In fact, it was recently shown that iron bioavailibility from modern whey-predominant infant formulas is higher than previously believed, and may in fact not be substantially lower than that from breast milk[8]. With this background, our objective was to study the effect of a lower level of iron fortification of infant formulas on iron status and haematological indices during the first 6 months of life in healthy term infants. We here summarize two studies conducted to explore the effects of using iron concentrations of 2 mg/l and 4 mg/l, on the iron status of exclusively formula-fed infants[6], (Hernell and Lonnerdal, submitted).

Iron is commonly added to infant formulas as iron sulfate, a soluble form of iron with high bioavalability. The small intestinal mucosa of infants has specific receptors that can bind lactoferrin[9], the major iron-binding protein in human milk, which, theoretically, may in turn facilitate iron absorption[10]. Since bovine lactoferrin can be obtained in large quantities commercially, we also evaluated the effects of iron provided in the form of lactoferrin on infant iron status. Lactoferrin-bound iron may have a high bioavailibility, will be in the ferric state (which is less prone to free radical-mediated reactions), and may also be less likely to interfere with the absorption of other trace elements[11]. We also evaluated the effect of nucleotide fortification of formula as this has been suggested to affect iron status[12].

Methods

Subjects

Healthy term infants in the first, 4 mg study were recruited at 6 ± 2 weeks of age, and in the second, 2 mg study at 4 ± 2 weeks of age at three well baby clinics in Umea, Sweden.

Study design

The infants were exclusively breast-fed (BF groups) or fed experimental formula until 6 months of age when the respective study was discontinued. Only limited amounts of selected fruit purées (containing no iron) were allowed at 4–6 months of age. Anthropometric measurements were taken monthly and venous blood samples on entry into the studies and then at 6 months of age (4 mg study) or at 4 and 6 months of age (2 mg study). All samples were drawn in the infant's home by the same research nurse and generally prior to a meal, i.e. 3–4 h after the previous meal. Haematological indices were determined on the day of collection. Serum was separated within a few hours and stored at –20 °C until analysed at the end of each study. Individual health records were kept for all infants and parents were contacted at least monthly by phone or visit. Both studies were approved by the Ethical Committee at Umea University.

Formula composition

The study formula was a milk-based whey-predominant (60/40) infant formula containing 13 g of protein, 4 mg of zinc and 460 mg of calcium per litre. In the 4 mg study[6] the target value for all experimental formulas was 4 mg of iron/l. In three of them the source of iron was ferrous sulfate ($FeSO_4$) and in one (4 mg, Lf + Se) one-third of the iron (1.4 mg) was provided as bovine lactoferrin and two-thirds (2.6 mg) as $FeSO_4$. Two of the formulas (4 mg, Lf + Se, and 4 mg + Se) were fortified with selenium as sodium selenite (Na_2SeO_3, 10 µg/l) and one (4 mg + Cu) with copper sulfate ($CuSO_4$, 0.4 mg/l). The last group (7 mg Fe) was the unmodified standard formula containing 7 mg iron, which served as the control formula. These levels were target values; the analysed values in the final products were slightly different as illustrated in Table 1. The standard formula in the 2 mg study was fortified with selenium (to a level of 15 μg/l) and copper (0.45 mg/l) as a consequence of the results of the 4 mg study, and contained 4 mg of iron as $FeSO_4$ (4 mg). The three experimental formulas all contained a target level of 2 mg of iron/l. In one of these (2 mg, Lf), bovine lactoferrin provided the major part of iron. Again, these were target levels, the analysed levels were slightly different. Notably, one of the 2 mg formulas (2 mg) contained only 1.6 mg iron/l (Table 1).

One of the experimental formulas (2 mg + N) was also fortified with nucleotides to levels resembling those of human milk (5′-AMP, 5′-CMP, 5′-GMP, 5′-IMP and 5′-UMP to a total level of 40 mg/l).

Analytical methods

Haematological indices and trace element status

Haemoglobin was analysed by the cyanomethaemoglobin method, MCV by Coulter counter, serum iron and transferrin by commercial kits (Boehringer Mannheim, Indianapolis, IN), and serum ferritin and serum transferrin receptor by ELISA-methods (R & D Systems; Minneapolis, MN). Serum zinc and copper were determined by atomic absorption spectrophotometry[13].

Table 1. Iron concentration of formulas used

Formula	Analysed value (mg/l)	Iron source
4 mg study		
7 mg	6.9	FeSO4
4 mg	4.3	FeSO4
4 mg + Se	4.4	FeSO4
4 mf, Lf + Se	3.8	FeSO4 2.5 mg, Lf-Fe 1.3 mg
2 mg study		
4 mg	4.0	FeSO4
2 mg	1.6 mg	FeSO4
2 mg, Lf	1.8	FeSO4 0.5 mg, Lf-Fe 1.3 mg
2 mg + N	2.2	FeSO4

Statistical analyses

Statistical analyses were performed using ANOVA. Data were tested for residuals and no skewness was found. Where the ANOVA indicated significant group differences ($P < 0.05$), multiple comparisons were performed using Tukey's method to identify which group differed ($P < 0.05$). Values in tables and figures are given as means ± SD.

Results

At the end of the 4 mg study there were no statistically significant differences between groups with respect to anthropometry or haematological indices. A single child had a serum-ferritin level < 12 μg/l. None was iron deficient using the combined criteria serum ferritin < 12 μg/l, serum Fe < 10 Mmol/L and MCV < 70 fl as recommended by the International Nutritional Anemia Consultation Group[14].

Figure 1a. shows the mean and standard deviations in haemoglobin concentration at 6 months of age and illustrates that there was no significant difference between groups. Within the groups, there was a large variation in serum ferritin levels, but the only significant difference was that the group fed a formula fortified with 4 mg $FeSO_4$ and selenium (4 mg + Se) had a significantly higher mean value than the 4 mg group also fortified with copper (4 mg + Cu). However, the important observation was that the 4 mg groups did not have significantly lower haematological values and iron status than the 7 mg group, or the breast-fed group (Fig. 2a).

Based on these results a reasonable question was whether a formula containing less iron, i.e. 2 mg of iron/l also would result in satisfactory iron status during the first 6 months of age. Analyses from this study has yet to be completed and the results should therefore be considered preliminary. However, again there were no significant differences at any age (1, 4 or 6 months of age) with respect to anthropometric measurements, nor were there any differences between groups with respect to haemoglobin concentrations (Fig. 1b). At 6 months of age, a single child had an MCV value below 70 fl which would be compatible with iron defi-

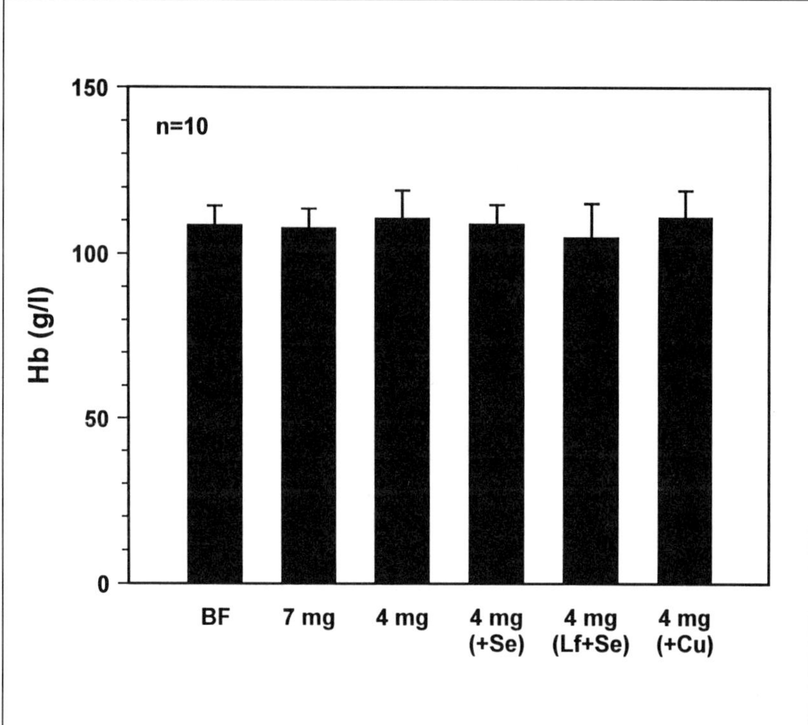

Fig. 1. Haemoglobin concentrations at 6 months of age (means ± SD).
a – 4 mg study
b – 2 mg study

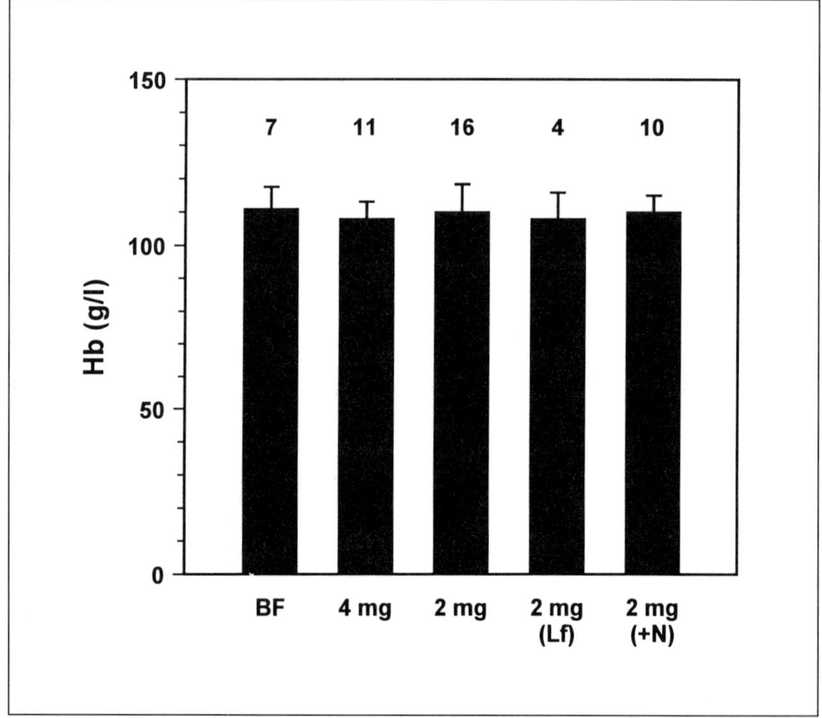

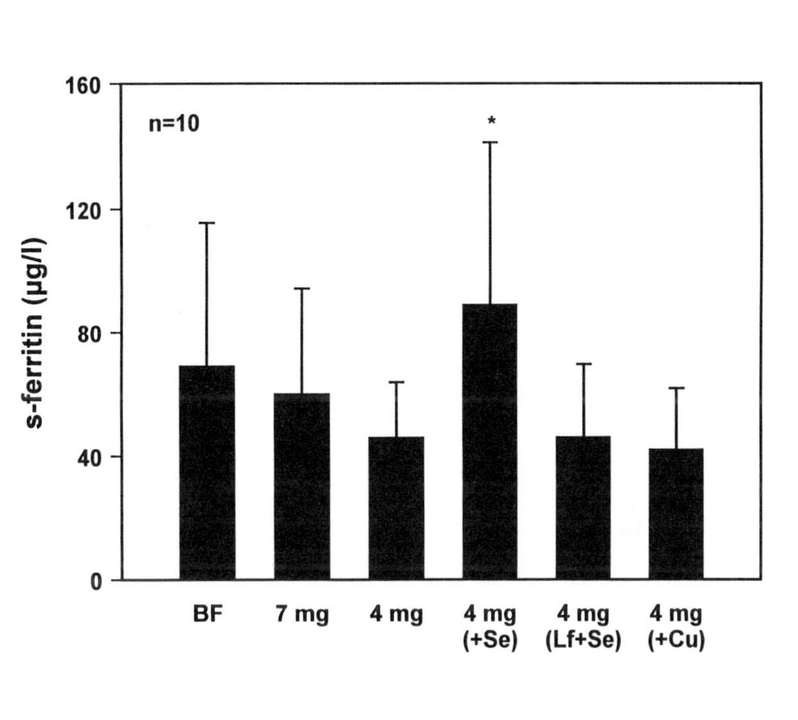

Fig. 2. Serum ferritin concentrations at 6 months of age (means ± SD).
a – 4 mg study
b – 2 mg study

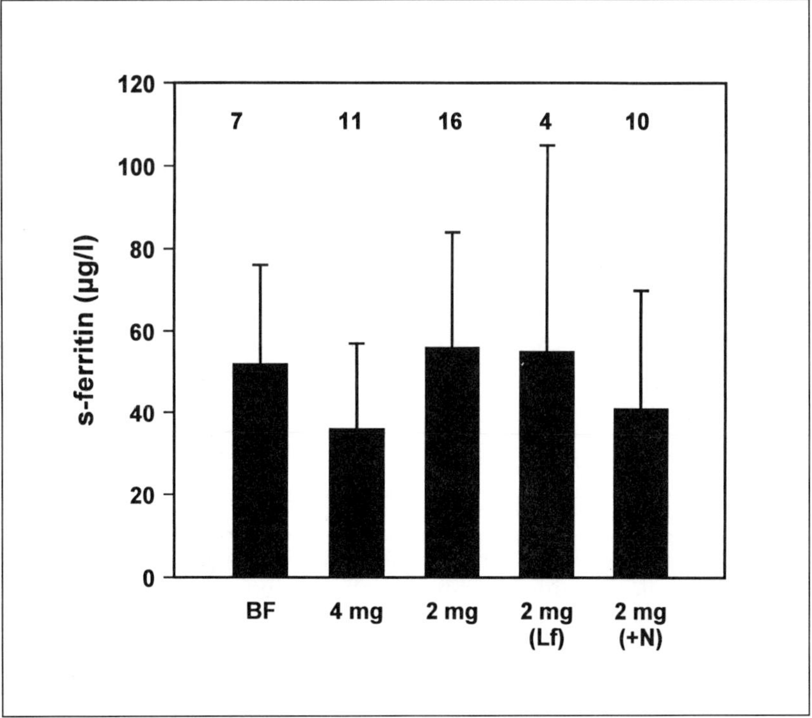

ciency. The corresponding haemoglobin value was 93 g/l but the serum ferritin value was 52 µg/l which makes iron deficiency less likely. There were no significant differences in MCV between groups at any point in time.

In the 2 mg study there was also a large variation in serum ferritin values within the groups, but at 6 months (or at the earlier time points) there were no significant differences between the groups (Fig. 2b). Three infants had serum ferritin < 12 ug/l, none of these was anaemic (Hb < 105 g/l), two had low iron saturation and one, belonging to the 2 mg/l group, also had an elevated TIBC value and was most probably iron deficient.

Serum transferrin receptor is a novel indicator of iron status which has been shown to reflect cellular iron needs[15,16] and, hence, is a potentially more sensitive indicator of iron deficiency than serum ferritin. The serum receptor levels increase when the cells become depleted of iron. The mean values of the 2 mg groups were not significantly higher than that of the 4 mg group, or the breast-fed infants, supporting the conclusion that none of the groups had become iron deficient at 6 months of age.

Discussion

It is generally agreed that infant formulas should be fortified with iron[17,18]; however, the appropriate level of iron to use is still under discussion. In the first study we found that, judged by haematological indices, all six groups of infants had satisfactory iron status at 6 months of age when the study was discontinued[6]. In fact, none of the infants had values that were lower than the commonly used cut-off levels, i.e. serum ferritin < 12 µg/l, serum Fe < 10 µM and MCV < 70 fl[14]. This was not unexpected since it has previously been shown in exclusively breast-fed infants that iron supplied from breast milk (0.2–0.4 mg/l) is adequate up to at least this age.

Even if iron may be absorbed more efficiently from breast milk than from milk-based infant formula[7], it seems unlikely that it would be more than 10 times better absorbed. Milk formulas contain both casein and whey proteins, which have been shown to affect iron absorption negatively[19], but also generous quantities of ascorbic acid and citrate which both have an enhancing effect on iron absorption[20].

A level of iron fortification of 4 mg/l may in fact provide ample safety margin to protect against iron deficiency. In the 2 mg study, the mean serum ferritin level of the infants fed 2 mg of iron/l was not significantly different than that of infants fed 4 mg of iron/l or breast-fed infants. The observation that out of 20 infants fed 2 mg iron/l we found only one with iron deficiency is probably due to a random effect, rather than as a consequence of inadequate provision of iron. Since infants fed unfortified formula receive approximately 0.7–1.0 mg iron/l and have unsatisfactory iron status[1,2], whereas infants that received formula with 1.6–2 mg iron/l had satisfactory iron status at 6 months of age, it appears that iron absorption from breast milk is at most five times higher than from modern whey-predominant milk-based formulas. This is in agreement with a study on infants fed radiolabelled breast milk or formula[7].

The effect of using bovine lactoferrin as an iron source in infant formula is difficult to assess[10]. We found no advantage with regard to iron status in these two studies, which is in agreement with others[21–23]. It is possible that only human lactoferrin will facilitate iron absorption in infants; however, it is also possible that formulas with 2 or 4 mg of iron/l both provide more iron than infants at this age require and that any beneficial effect of bovine lactoferrin would be difficult to observe in this situation. The potential advantage of providing iron in a biologically less harmful form, i.e. ferric iron, was not evaluated in this study and may require long-term studies in a large number of infants. However, the lower the iron concentration of the formula the lower the likelyhood of a potential harmful effect.

Some infant formulas are fortified with nucleotides to levels mimicking those of human milk. The reason for adding nucleotides have primarily been to stimulate the immune function of formula-fed infants[24], and possibly, affect mucosal growth[25] and/or differentiation[26]. In addition, one study has suggested an effect of nucleotides on iron status[12]. We found no significant effect of nucleotide fortification on iron status in our study; however, as mentioned above, all groups had satisfactory iron status which makes evaluation of any enhancer difficult.

In conclusion, breast feeding or feeding an adapted, whey-predominant, milk-based infant formula containing 2 mg of iron/l both result in satisfactory iron status up to 6 months of age. We found no beneficial effect of providing iron as bovine lactoferrin as compared to the currently used ferrous sulfate, and found no effect on iron status of fortification with nucleotides to levels typical of human milk. Hence, the results presented do not argue against the view that it would be safe to reduce the fortification level of whey-predominant, milk-based infant formulas to 2 mg iron/l.

Acknowledgements

We are grateful to research nurse Margaretha Henriksson for her excellent handling of all the practical aspects of the studies, and for taking care of participating infants and parents in a most professional and yet personal way. We are also grateful to Shannon Kelleher for expert assistance with the chemical analyses. Financial support from the Swedish Medical Research Council (grant No. 19X-0507) and Semper AB, Stockholm, Sweden are also gratefully acknowledged.

References

1. Yip, R. (1994): Iron deficiency: contemporary scientific issues and international programmatic approaches. *J. Nutr.* **124,** 1479S–1490S.

2. American Academy of Pediatrics, Committee on Nutrition (1969): Iron balance and requirements in infancy. *Pediatrics* **43,** 34–42.

3. Dallman, P.R., Siimes, M.A. & Stekel, A. (1980): Iron deficiency in infancy and childhood. *Am. J. Clin. Nutr.* **33,** 86–118.

4. Siimes, M.A., Salmenpera, L. & Perheentupa, J. (1984): Exclusive breast-feeding for 9 months: risk of iron deficiency. *J. Pediatr.* **104,** 196–199.

5. Duncan, B., Schifman, R.B., Corrigan, J.J. & Schaefer, C. (1985): Iron and the exclusively breastfed infant from birth to six months. *J. Pediatr. Gastroenterol. Nutr.* **4,** 21–25.

6. Lonnerdal, B. & Hernell, O. (1994): Iron, zinc, copper and selenium status of breast-fed infants and infants fed trace element fortified milk-based infant formula. *Acta Paediatr.* **83,** 367–373.

7. Saarinen, U.M., Siimes, M.A. & Dallman, P.R. (1977): Iron absorption in infants: high bioavailability of breast milk iron as indicated by the intrinsic tag method of iron absorption and by the concentration of serum ferritin. *J. Pediatr.* **91,** 36–39.

8. Davidsson, L., Kastenmayer, P., Yuen, M., Lonnerdal, B. & Hurrell, R.F. (1994): Influence of lactoferrin on iron absorption from human milk in infants. *Pediatr. Res.* **35,** 117–124.

9. Kawakami, H. & Lonnerdal, B. (1991): Isolation and function of a receptor for human lactoferrin in human fetal intestinal brush border membranes. *Am. J. Physiol.* **261,** G841–G846.

10. Lonnerdal, B. & Iyer, S. (1995): Lactoferrin: molecular structure and biological function. *Ann. Rev. Nutr.* **15,** 93–110.

11. Solomons, N.W. & Jacob, R.A. (1981): Studies on the bioavailability of zinc in humans. Effect on heme and nonheme iron on the absorption of zinc. *Am. J. Clin. Nutr.* **34,** 475–482.

12. Faelli, A. & Esposito, G. (1970): Effect of inosine and its metabolites on intestinal iron absorption in the rat. *Biochem. Pharmacol.* **19,** 2551–2554.

13. Clegg, M.S., Keen, C.L., Lonnerdal, B. & Hurley, L.S. (1981): Influence of ashing techniques on the analysis of trace elements in animal tissue. *Biol. Trace. Elem. Res.* **3,** 107–115.

14. International Nutritional Anemia Consultative Group (1979): Iron deficiency in infancy and childhood. New York: The Nutrition Foundation.

15. Kohgo, U., Niitsu, Y., Kondo, H., Kato, J., Tsushima, N., Sasahi, K., Hiayama, M., Numata, T., Nishisato, T. & Urushizaji, I. (1987): Serum transferrin receptor as a new index of erythropoiesis. *Blood* **70,** 1955–1961.

16. Skikne, B.S., Flowers, C.H. & Cook, J.D. (1990): Serum transferrin receptor: a quantitative measure of tissue iron deficiency. *Blood* **75,** 1870–1876.

17. European Society for Pediatric Gastroenterology and Nutrition (ESPGAN), Committee on Nutrition (1977): Committee report. 1. Recommendation for the composition of adapted formula. *Acta Paediatr. Scand.* **Suppl. 262,** 2–20.

18. American Academy of Pediatrics, Committee on Nutrition (1976): Iron supplementation for infants. *Pediatrics* **58,** 765–768.

19. Hurrell, R.F., Lynch, S.R., Trinidad, T.P., Dassenko, S.A. & Cook, J.D. (1989): Iron absorption in humans as influenced by bovine milk proteins. *Am. J. Clin. Nutr.* **49,** 546–552.

20. Gillooly, M., Bothwell, T.H., Torrance, J.D., MacPhail, A.P., Derman, D.P., Bezwoda, W.R., Mills, W., Charlton, R.W. & Mayet, F. (1983): The effects of organic acids, phytates and polyphenols on the absorption of iron from vegetables. *Br. J. Nutr.* **49,** 331–342.

21. Fairweather-Tait, S.J., Balmer, S.E., Scott, P.H. & Ninski, M.J. (1987): Lactoferrin and iron absorption in newborn infants. *Pediatr. Res.* **22,** 651–654.

22. Schulz-Lell, G., Dörner, K., Oldigs, H.D., Sievers, E. & Schaub, J. (1991): Iron availability from an infant formula supplemented with bovine lactoferrin. *Acta Paediatr. Scand.* **80,** 155–158.

23. Chierici, R., Sawatzki, G., Tamisari, L., Volpato, S. & Vigi, V. (1992): Supplementation of an adapted formula with bovine lactoferrin. 2. Effects on serum iron, ferritin and zinc levels. *Acta Paediatr.* **81,** 475–479.

24. Carver, J.D., Pimentel, B., Cox, W.I. & Bamess, L.A. (1991): Dietary nucleotide effects upon immune functions in infants. *Pediatrics* **88,** 359–363.

25. Uauy, R. (1994): Nonimmune systems responses to dietary nucleotides. *J. Nutr.* **124,** 157S–159S.

26. He, Y., Chu, S.W. & Walker, W.A.: (1992): Nucleotide supplements alter proliferation and differentiation of cultured human (Caco-2) and rat (IEC-6) intestinal epithelial cells. *J. Nutr.* **123,** 1017–1027.

Iron Nutrition in Health and Disease, edited by Leif Hallberg and Nils-Georg Asp
©1996 John Libbey & Company Ltd., pp. 137–148

Chapter 14

Iron requirements and prevalence of iron deficiency in adolescents. An overview

Susan J. Fairweather-Tait

Institute of Food Research, Norwich Laboratory, Norwich Research Park, Colney, Norwich NR4 7UA, UK

Summary

Adolescence is the period between childhood and adulthood, i.e. from puberty, the period at which the generative organs become capable of exercising the function of reproduction, to maturity. Some girls may enter puberty in their 10th year and attain maximum height by the age of 15, whereas boys generally begin their pubertal growth spurt later and only reach maximum growth rate in their 15th year.

Adolescence is a time of rapid growth and physical and psychological development. The post-pubertal growth spurt results in an increased requirement for iron. Rapid skeletal muscle development, together with expanding blood volume, create additional requirements for iron in both adolescent boys and girls. The timing of these extra demands is different for each sex, with maturational age being more important than chronological age. Adolescent females also have an additional demand created by the onset of menses. An allowance must also be made to allow the build up of iron stores as a reserve for future physiological demands, notably pregnancy. The overall daily iron requirements for adolescents are estimated to be 1.45–2.03 mg in boys and 1.22–1.46 mg in pre-pubertal girls, and 1.39–2.54 mg after menstruation has started.

Several fairly recent publications report data for iron status in adolescents. Mean Hb concentrations ranges are 129–151 g/l in boys and 128–134 g/l in girls, and serum ferritin ranges are 17.3–52.8 µg/l in boys and 14.2–43.0 µg/l in girls. In comparison, the values for UK adults for Hb are 148 g/l (men) and 132 g/l (women), and for serum ferritin are 106.9 µg/l (men) and 46.8 µg/l (women). It appears, therefore, that adolescents have lower body iron levels than adults. The reported prevalence of low iron stores (< 10/12 µg ferritin per litre of serum) in individual studies ranges from 1 to 43 per cent and iron deficiency anaemia (Hb < 120 g/l in girls, g/l in boys) ranges from 4 to 20 per cent, which suggests that adolescents are a vulnerable group with respect to iron nutrition.

There has been a gradual decline in iron intakes in the UK population, which is the result of changes in life-style (reduced energy expenditure, and hence a lower intake of food) and diet (composition of meals and dietary patterns). Correlations between haem iron intake (+) and calcium (–) with iron stores, but not total iron, coffee, tea or vitamin C, are reported in a large study on French subjects aged 6 months to 97 years. The lack of correlation between total iron intake and body iron is not surprising, since the key determinant is dietary iron bioavailability. However, other studies on adolescents report no clear-cut relationships between iron status and dietary measurements. This is probably due to the fact that indices of iron status reflect the balance between previous dietary supply and physiological requirements, thus simultaneous measures of intake and status may not be the appropriate way to examine any interdependency.

Furthermore, adolescents are a rather unstable group in that they undergo several stages of rapid growth (affecting iron stores), and may have erratic eating patterns.

Some adolescents have special needs for iron. It is obvious that girls with large menstrual losses have a high requirement for iron, but the need for iron by boys to achieve an increased red cell mass and the higher Hb concentration found in adult men must not be overlooked. Other 'at-risk' individuals include vegetarians, especially new vegetarians from non-vegetarian households, since meat is not only a good source of absorbable iron but also enhances the absorption of non-haem iron from the rest of a meal. Children consuming an unbalanced diet, who for example follow 'food fads' or try to lose weight by eating low-energy diets, are unlikely to receive adequate iron. Decreased iron stores have been reported in female runners, thus adolescent girls who perform sustained physical exercise are highly susceptible to iron deficiency. Pregnant adolescent girls are at particular risk, and usually require iron therapy.

Introduction

Adolescence is the period between childhood and adulthood, from puberty, the period at which the generative organs become capable of exercising the function of reproduction, to maturity. The age of puberty differs between individuals. Some girls may enter puberty in their 10th year, and attain their maximum height by the age of 15, whereas boys generally begin their pubertal growth spurt later and only reach maximum growth rate in their 15th year[1]. Puberty is delayed in the presence of chronic undernutrition[2], and delayed entry into puberty for girls and a prolonged puberty for boys was observed in a rural community in The Gambia, although this was not specifically related to the child's nutritional status[3]. In industrialized countries adolescence generally spans the ages of 10–15 years in girls, and 11–18 years in boys.

Recent data for the weights and heights of children at different ages were produced by the Panel on Dietary Reference Values[4]. The 50th centile values are given in Table 1, together with the calculated mean increase in bodyweight over the period of adolescence, where it can be seen that boys almost double their weight between the age of 10.5 and 19 years.

Iron requirements

Iron is needed to replace daily endogenous losses[4]; the figures for adults include haemolysed red blood cells (0.38 mg), bile (0.24 mg), desquamated gastrointestinal cells (0.14 mg), and urine (0.1 mg). This amounts to a mean total daily loss of 0.9 mg. In adolescents basal iron losses have been calculated as 0.62–0.90 and 0.65–0.79 mg/day for males and females, respectively[5]. In menstruating females iron is required to replace blood lost in menses, and in adolescence there is also an additional requirement for growth.

From 11.5 to 15.5 years of age boys gain 20.6 kg and girls gain 15.8 kg bodyweight. Using approximate estimates of blood volume in adults based on body mass[6] of 75 and 66 ml/kg bodyweight in males and females respectively, the 4 year growth increment is associated with an increase in the volume of blood of 1545 and 1043 ml respectively. Estimates of the quantity of iron needed for the extra blood (assuming blood Hb concentrations of 149 and 135 g/l in boys and girls, respectively[7], and an iron concentration of 3.47 mg/g Hb[4] are 0.55 mg/day in boys and 0.33 mg/day in girls.

The increase in lean body mass also requires iron, primarily for muscle myoglobin and also non-haem iron. The iron content of skeletal muscle is approximately 0.026 mg/g wet weight[8]. If half the increase in bodyweight is associated with greater muscle mass this will

Table 1. Weights (kg) of adolescents in the UK population

Age (y)	50th Centile	
	Boys	**Girls**
10.5	32.7	33.0
11.5	35.9	36.7
12.5	39.0	41.0
13.5	45.5	47.0
14.5	52.0	50.5
15.5	56.5	52.5
16-19	64.5	55.5
Weight increment		
10.5-19	31.8	22.5
11.5-15.5	20.6	15.8

require 0.18 and 0.14 mg iron per day in boys and girls, respectively.

In girls who have reached puberty, there is an additional requirement for iron to replace blood loss, and this will differ greatly between individuals. Hallberg *et al.*[9] measured menstrual blood loss and found that the mean blood loss per period in 15-year-old girls was 33.8 (SEM 2.4) ml in 95 individuals. Values for the 10th and 90th percentile were 10.4 and 65.1 ml respectively. Assuming a Hb value of 134 g/l[10], a blood loss of 33.8 ml results in a loss of 15.7 mg iron per period, equivalent to 0.56 mg iron per day. The range (10th to 90th percentile) is 0.17 to 1.08 mg iron per day.

Apart from iron that is utilized for tissue growth and replacement, and red blood cell production, it is considered prudent to build up iron stores as a reserve for future physiological demands, notably pregnancy[5,11]. The prevalence of low iron stores, assessed by serum ferritin concentrations, is fairly high in adolescents (see below). If stores are assumed to be depleted by the end of the adolescent growth spurt and the target iron storage level is 300 mg by the age of 20–25[11], the amount of absorbed iron required is in the range of 0.1–0.4 mg/day in boys and 0.1–0.2 mg/day in girls.

From the above calculations, the overall daily iron requirements for adolescent boys and girls (before menses starts) are estimated to be 1.45–2.03 mg/day and 1.22–1.46 mg/day, respectively. Once menstruation has begun, the requirements for girls (replacing blood losses incurred from the 10th to the 90th percentile) increases to 1.39–2.54 mg/day. These are, however, minimum values because the estimation of menstrual blood loss will always be an underestimate rather than an overestimate. The large range reflects the wide intersubject variation in blood loss, although intrasubject variations are much less marked[9].

Table 2(a). Mean (± SD) iron status (Hb, transferrin saturation (TfS), serum ferritin (SF), and transferrin receptor (TfR)) for groups of adolescent boys

n	**Age (y)**	**Hb (g/l)**	**TfS (%)**	**SF (Mg/l)**	**TfR (mg/l)**	**Reference**
322	9		22.2			17
254				41.3		
107	10–12	132 ± 7		14.6		18
62	11.7 ± 0.3	130 ± 7	21.6 ± 7.1	35.7 ± 17.2	3.8 ± 1.1	13
293	12		21.4			17
204				44.7		
24	12–13			27 ± 18		38
202	12–14	143 ± 11				22
140	13–14		31.4 ± 1.5			
19	13–14	129 ± 9		24 ± 9		39
118	13–15	141 ± 10			13.1	18
201	14		24.1 ± 10.8	27.3 ± 17.6	2.96 ± 0.93	15
266	15		23.8			17
176				45.7		
207	15–16	147 ± 8	32.7 ± 10.3	26.4 ± 1.7		10
86	16–18	150 ± 8		20.0		18
271	17		22.9 ± 10.9	52.8 ± 34.8	2.35 ± 0.53	15
86	14–18	143 (103–166)		173 (2.1–87.3)		40
~4000	18	151 ± 8	30.7 ± 12.4	36.8 ± 1.6		16

Body iron levels

The most useful biochemical indices of body iron levels are Hb, transferrin saturation, serum or plasma ferritin, and erythrocyte (or zinc) protoporphyrin[12]. These give an estimate of functional iron status as well as iron stores. Commonly used cut-off points for Hb concentration are 120 g/l for boys aged 11–14/15 years and 115–120 g/l for girls aged 11– 14/15[12]. The measurement of serum or plasma transferrin receptor concentration has been reported to be of little additional value when assessing the iron status of adolescent subjects[12].

Iron deficiency in infants, children and adults living in developing countries is very widespread. For example, Agha *et al.*[14] examined 13–20 year old children in Pakistan and found that 30 per cent of boys and 54 per cent of girls were iron depleted, and 17 per cent of boys and 18 per cent of girls were anaemic. In socially advanced countries the problem is less severe, but still exists, particularly amongst adolescents. A summary of results of studies investigating the iron status of adolescents in developed countries is given in Table 2. In the UK the mean reported values for Hb concentration (129–147 g/l in boys and 128–134 g/l in girls) and serum ferritin (17.3–52.8 μg/l in boys and 18.2–30.4 μg/l in girls) are lower than those reported for UK adults (Hb 148 g/l in men and 132 g/l in women, and serum ferritin 106.9 μg/l in men and 46.8 μg/l in women). It appears, therefore, that adolescents in general have lower body iron levels than adults.

Three studies examining iron stores in Swedish adolescents have recently been published. In 523 adolescents, aged 14–17 years, living in the city, suburb or countryside, Bergstrom *et al.*[15] reported serum ferritin values of less than 12

Table 2(b). Mean (± SD) iron status (Hb, transferrin saturation (TfS), serum ferritin (SF), transferrin receptor (TfR)) of groups of adolescent girls

n	Age (y)	Hb (g/l)	TfS (%)	SF (μg/l)	TfR (mg/l)	Reference
302	9		23.5			17
248				43.0		
83	10–12	133 ± 8		16.7		18
114	11–14	130 ± 11				21
267	12		22.6			17
195				37.9		
26	12–13			20 ± 16		38
197	12–14	133 ± 10				22
156	12–14		30.4 ± 1.6			22
35	13–14	128 ± 6		21 ± 12		39
102	13–15	134 ± 8		14.2		18
197	14		22.3 ± 10.8	27.3 ± 17.6	2.74 ± 1.01	15
230	15		22.3			17
143				31.7		
[a]40	14–17	134	32	35		41
220	15–16	134 ± 8	29.9 ± 10.7	18.2 ± 18.2		10
222	16–17	134 ± 7	21.3 ± 9.1	26.9 ± 18.9		42
78	16–18	132 ± 7		16.7		18
198	17		18.8 ± 9.9	29.5 ± 20.9	2.27 ± 0.67	15
148	14–18	133		15.3		40

[a]Cross-country runners.

μg/l in 5 per cent of boys and 15 per cent of girls, suggesting that the Swedish children have a higher iron stores than UK children as assessed from the limited number of small studies. Serum ferritin values increased with pubertal stage in boys but not in girls. Menstruating girls had a lower mean serum ferritin value (27.5 μg/l) than non-menstruating girls (40.4 μg/l), and girls taking oral contraceptives had a higher mean serum ferritin value (37.9 μg/l) than the other girls (27.9 μg/l). Olsson *et al.*[16] examined approximately 4000 teenage boys (aged 18 years) from three counties in Central Sweden, awaiting enrolment for military service, and found that only 0.4 per cent had low iron stores (serum ferritin < 12 μg/l). Amongst all the published values of measures of iron status in adolescents, this group had the highest iron status, which may be a characteristic of the subjects selected, or possibly the result of the widespread food iron fortification policy followed in Sweden. In contrast, Hallberg *et al.*[10] found in a sample of 427 children that 15 per cent of boys and 40 per cent of girls (aged 15–16 years, living in Göteborg) had low iron stores (serum ferritin below 16 μg/l). Since the authors found that haematological parameters started to decrease at serum ferritin values above 16 μg/l, they argued for a higher cut-off value for serum ferritin so as not to miss any individuals who were iron compromised. The conflicting results from these Swedish studies may be explained by the age difference of the subjects; the 2–3 year difference between 15/16 and 18 years of age may be sufficient time to replenish iron stores depleted as a result of pre- and post-pubertal growth.

Australian children aged 9–15 years, had a generally satisfactory iron status (based upon measurements of transferrin saturation and plasma ferritin concentration) except for the 15-year-old girls where plasma ferritin showed a marked decrease with age[17]. The prevalence of iron deficiency (low values of both plasma ferritin (< 12 g/l) and transferrin saturation (< 16 per cent)) was 9.2 per cent in these girls. In Canada, however, low iron stores (serum ferritin < 12 g/l) were found in 39 per cent of 10–18-year-old children studied, with no major differences relating to sex or age[18]. Low levels of serum ferritin were most frequent in boys aged 13–15 years (44 per cent), despite a high number with dietary iron intake above the recommended level[19], thus emphasizing the importance of dietary iron bioavailability rather than total iron intake.

According to the results of the second National Health and Nutrition Examination Survey, 1976–1980, the prevalence of iron deficiency in the US population was described as 'fairly low, with the exception of children aged 1–2 years, males aged 11–14 years, and females aged 15–44 years'[20]. This lends further support to the

Table 3. Prevalence of iron-eficiency anaemia and low iron stores in adolescents from the UK and Ireland

Study (ref)	Sex	Age (y)	*n*	Prevalence of iron deficiency
Ireland [40]	M	14.5–18.4	86	13%: Hb < 130 g/l 32%: serum ferritin <10 μg/l
	F		148	7%: Hb < 120g/L 43%: serum ferritin < 10 μg/l
London[38]	M	12–13	34	8%: serum ferritin < 10 μg/l
	F		32	28%: serum ferritin < 10μg/l
London[22]	M	12–14	202	4%: Hb < 122/126 g/l 1%: serum ferritin < 12 μg/l
	F		197	11%: Hb < 120 g/l 4%: serum ferritin < 12 μg/l
London21	F	11–14	114	20%: Hb < 120 g/l
Norwich[23]	M	13–14	19	11%: serum ferritin < 10 μg/l
	F		35	21%: serum ferritin < 10 μg/l

conclusion that adolescents are a high risk group with respect to iron deficiency.

As shown in Table 3, iron deficiency anaemia in different studies in the UK and Ireland ranges in boys from 4 per cent (Hb < 122/126 g/l) to 13 per cent (Hb < 130 g/l), and in girls from 7 to 20 per cent (Hb <120 g/l). From these relatively small studies it would appear that iron deficiency anaemia is fairly common in UK adolescents, particularly amongst girls. Ethnic background also appears to have an effect on iron status. Nelson *et al.*[21] found that 20 per cent of 11–14-year-old girls had a Hb < 120 g/l, but when examined according to mother's ethnic origin anaemia was found in 11 per cent of white, 22 per cent of Indian, 25 per cent of Pakistani and 50 per cent of Afro-Caribbean children.

The prevalence of low iron stores (< 10–12 μg ferritin per litre serum) found in different studies in the UK and Ireland ranges from 1 to 35 per cent in boys and from 4 to 43 per cent in girls. However, the prevalence of low ferritin values (1 per cent in boys and 4 per cent in girls) reported by Nelson *et al.*[22] should be viewed with caution because the same study reported a higher incidence of iron deficiency anaemia (from Hb measurements) than low iron stores. This indicates that the ferritin values were not an accurate reflection of body iron stores in some of the children. Although there is a close relationship between serum ferritin concentration and storage iron in healthy individuals, with infection, inflammation and certain disease states there is an increased rate of ferritin synthesis in the reticuloendothelial system, which is reflected by an elevated concentration of ferritin in serum.

Iron intake

There are a number of published reports on the iron intake of adolescents. The results are summarized in Table 4. Most studies determine iron intake by measuring food intake over a number of days, using one of a variety of techniques, such as weighed intake or questionnaire. Mean daily iron intake is then calculated from published values for the nutritional content of foods. Southon *et al.*[23] found good agreement between calculated and analysed (duplicate diet) values for iron ($r = 0.84$, $P < 0.001$), but the analysed values were slightly lower than the calculated values in the boys. The mean daily iron intakes of boys and girls were 14.9 and 9.7 mg, respectively, when analysed from duplicate diet collections, and 13.2 and 9.8 mg, respectively, when estimated from food table values.

Daily iron intakes increase with age, presumably in line with increasing energy requirements. In 10–11-year-old boys the mean daily iron intake is approximately 10 mg, and this increases to 12–20 mg in 14–18 year olds. Girls have a lower intake; at the age of 10–11, the mean daily intake is 8–10 mg, rising to 13 mg at the age of 17. The UK and France appear to have similar levels of intake, whereas higher

Table 4. Iron intake (mean ± SD, or median[a]) of adolescents

Age (y)	n	Daily intake (mg)	Country	Reference
Boys				
10-11	902	10.0 ± 2.3	UK	1
10-14	27	12.5[a]	France	29
11-12	184	11.7 ± 3.3	UK	24
12-13	35	10.9 ± 2.8	UK	38
12-14	202	12.3 ± 4.8	UK	22
13-14	19	13.2 ± 4.4	UK	23
14	147	17.5 ± 4.4	Sweden	15
14-15	513	12.2 ± 3.3	UK	1
14-18	28	14.4[a]	France	29
17	190	20.9 ± 6.2	Sweden	15
Girls				
10-11	821	8.6 ± 1.9	UK	1
10-14	28	10.1[a]	France	29
11-13	195	11.2 ± 3.8	UK	24
12-13	30	9.7 ± 2.9	UK	38
12-14	197	9.6 ± 3.5	UK	22
13-14	35	9.8 ± 3.0	UK	23
14	176	13.4 ± 3.8	Sweden	15
14-15	461	9.3 ± 2.5	UK	1
14-18	25	10.4[a]	France	29
17	158	13.4 ± 4.4	Sweden	15

intakes of iron are reported in Sweden, particularly in boys.

Moynihan *et al.*[24] examined the sources of dietary iron in 11–12 year old UK adolescents. The four most important sources of iron were meat and meat products (19 per cent), breakfast cereals (15 per cent), bread (12 per cent) and potatoes (including chips and crisps, 11 per cent). Chocolate contributed 4 per cent, and ranked more highly than vegetables (3 per cent); half of the vegetable contribution came from baked beans.

Intake–status relationship and bioavailability

Haematological parameters reflect body iron levels in the long term, whereas dietary intake data are generally collected over a short period of time. Thus, unless the intake data are truly representative of habitual diet, it is unlikely that the two measures will be significantly correlated. Furthermore, adaptive mechanisms operate to maintain homeostasis (Fig. 1). When dietary supply is limiting, the efficiency of absorption of iron increases, and when the supply is well in excess of requirements it falls.

Kerr *et al.*[25] made a detailed study of the relationship between dietary (24 h dietary recall) intake and biochemical measures of nutritional status in HANES I data. When adjusted for sociodemographic factors, regression analysis revealed a significant negative relationship ($P < 0.01$) between dietary iron intake and both serum iron ($R^2 = 0.156$) and transferrin saturation ($R^2 = 0.096$), i.e. serum values decreased with increasing consumption of iron. No relationship between iron intake and Hb or haematocrit was observed. The low R^2 values (which represent the percentage of variation in the dependent variable (iron status) accounted for by the regression equation) strongly suggest that iron intake data obtained from a 24 h recall is a poor predictor of an individual's iron status.

Other studies using more accurate methods of assessing iron intake have also reached the conclusion that intake is not a good predictor of iron status. Miles *et al.*[26] found no direct correlation between serum ferritin levels and iron intake in men and women. Similarly in adolescents, Southon *et al.*[23] demonstrated that serum ferritin values were not related to iron intake. Thus, because of the time needed to attain different planes of iron nutritional status, simultaneous measures of total iron intake and biochemical indices of status are not a useful way of investigating the effect of diet on body iron levels. The other very important reason why there is no association between iron intake and status is that total iron intake is not a good measure of absorbed iron, as this will depend on a number of dietary and host-related variables.

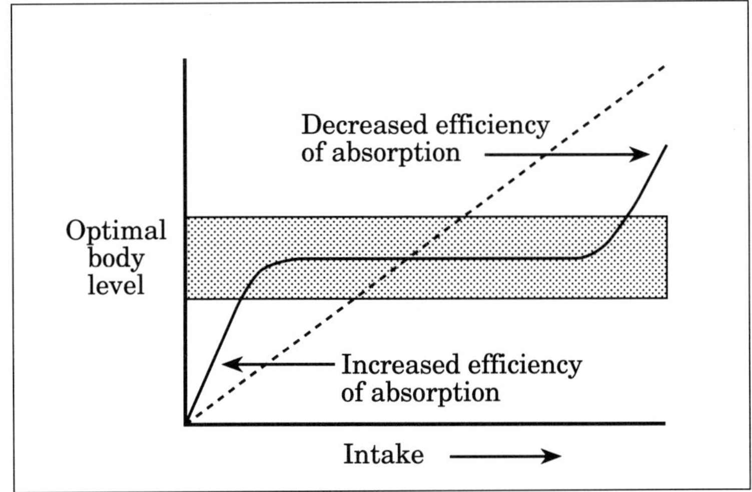

Fig. 1. Adaptive mechanisms involved in the maintenance of iron homeostasis

Thus the question of bioavailability must be considered.

Key dietary determinants of iron bioavailability include the enhancers ascorbic acid and animal protein, and the inhibitors phytate and polyphenols[27]. There is, as yet, no reliable way of predicting the amount of absorbable iron in a meal from knowledge of the food constituents, but a few attempts have been made to evaluate the effect of different levels of intake of modifiers of iron absorption on iron status. When Soustre *et al.*[28] examined the relationship between intake (g) of certain foods and serum ferritin in a group of 127 menstruating women, they found significant correlations ($P < 0.05$) with meat (positive), dairy products (negative), and coffee (negative), but not with fish, eggs, cereals, pulses, fruits and vegetables, or tea. More recently the same group analysed dietary intake and iron status data collected from a larger study of 1108 subjects, aged 6 months to 97 years old[29]. Multiple linear regression showed positive correlations between serum ferritin and haem ($P < 0.05$) and non-haem iron ($P < 0.01$) intake, a negative correlation with calcium intake ($P < 0.001$), but none with coffee, tea or ascorbic acid intake. In contrast Nelson *et al*[22]. observed that 12–14-year-old children with low iron and ascorbic acid intakes were more likely to be anaemic than those with high iron and ascorbic acid intakes (14.5 versus 2.3 per cent). Anaemia was more common in vegetarians than omnivores (25 versus 9 per cent). When examining the inter-relationships between dietary intake data and iron status, in addition to the time displacement already discussed, there are two other important factors to be taken into consideration. First, the dietary modifiers, such as ascorbic acid, will only exert an effect if they are present with the main meals and in sufficient quantity. For example, it is quite possible to have a high daily ascorbic acid intake, but if it is not associated with meals, there would be no enhancing effect on iron absorption. The second confounder is the use of serum ferritin as an index of iron stores. If some of the subjects have an elevated serum ferritin as a result of infection, then this will confound the statistical analyses.

Dietary recommendations

Dietary recommendations for iron intake in adolescents are, in general, derived from estimated physiological requirements multiplied by a 'bioavailability factor'. Values for some countries are given in Table 5. The UK and European recommendations are calculated assuming a dietary iron bioavailability of 15 per cent, and the US recommended dietary allowances (RDA) assume that 10–15 per cent of dietary iron is absorbed. The higher figures for girls living in the European Community[5] are based upon an absorbed iron requirement of 3.1 mg/day to meet the needs of 95 per cent of this subgroup of the population. For girls aged 11–14 years the daily iron requirements are estimated to be 0.65 mg for basal losses, 0.55 mg for growth, and 1.9 mg for menstrual losses (95th percentile). Basal losses are assumed to be lower than adults (0.9 mg), growth is similar to the figure derived earlier (0.33 mg for increased blood volume plus 0.14 mg for increased lean body mass), but the requirement for menstrual

Table 5. Dietary recommendations for iron (mg/day) in adolescents

		(2)LRNI	(3)EAR	(4)RNI
(1) UK				
Boys	11–18 y	6.1	8.7	11.3
Girls	11–18 y	8.0	11.4	14.8
(5) USA				(6)RDA
Boys	11–18 y			12
Girls	11–18 y			15
(7) Europe				(8)PRI
Boys	11–14 y			10
	15–17 y			13
Girls	11–14 y			†22
				‡18
	15–17 y			†21
				‡17

(1) Department of Health,[4]
(2) Lower Reference Nutrient Intake
(3) Estimated Average Requirement
(4) Reference Nutrient Intake
(5) National Research Council,[11]
(6) Recommended Dietary Allowances
(7) Reports of the Scientific Committee for Food,[5]
(8) Population Reference Intake

† Covers needs of 95% of population
‡ Covers needs of 90% of population

blood loss is higher. Published values from a large study in Sweden, before the introduction of oral contraceptives, showed that 1.08 mg iron per day replaced losses in 90 per cent of girls[9]. However, this group have recently argued that their findings are an underestimate, and suggest that losses are the same as in adult women[30]. In view of the fact that oral contraceptives reduce menstrual losses, it is likely that mean iron requirements to replace blood losses have decreased since the study carried out in the 1960s, not increased. Therefore there is still some uncertainty as to the exact requirements for iron to replace menstrual losses.

When iron intake data (Table 4) are compared with recommended dietary intakes, it is clear that, with the possible exception of Sweden, the diet of adolescents in industrialized countries is not adequate with respect to iron. The prevalence data for iron deficiency supports this finding, assuming that the cut-off values used to define iron deficiency are appropriate.

Vulnerable groups

Various subgroups of adolescents are more likely to become iron deficient, due to increased requirements for growth or pregnancy, or high menstrual losses, coupled with an inadequate diet. Adolescent pregnancies are prone to complications, such as an increased frequency of low birth weight, early delivery and perinatal mortality[31]. Infants with low birth weight will have reduced iron stores, which may well have future consequences. The assessment of body iron levels in pregnancy is not easy, hence the prevalence of iron deficiency in female adolescents is difficult to quantify[32]. However, the estimated high frequency of iron deficiency in female adolescents suggests that pregnant girls are at particular risk and require careful monitoring, and in many cases iron therapy.

Many adolescents, especially females, experiment with brief periods of food restriction ('dieting'), and a few develop anorexia nervosa. Low-energy diets, consumed by adolescents trying to lose weight or by children leading a sedentary lifestyle, are unlikely to provide adequate levels of iron unless the mixture of foods consumed is carefully selected. Nelson *et al.*[22] observed that anaemia was 3 times more likely in girls who had tried to lose weight during the preceding 12 months compared with those who had not (23 versus 7 per cent).

In the UK the number of adolescents who are vegetarian appears to be steadily increasing, particularly girls[33]. There are different types of vegetarian diet, including vegan (no food of animal origin), lacto- ovovegetarian (eggs and milk allowed), and 'semi' vegetarian diets in which some fish and/or white meat is consumed. In adolescents, avoiding meat may increase the likelihood of iron deficiency[22]. Compared to omnivores, vegetarians often have lower iron stores and are more likely to have iron deficiency anaemia[34]. Adolescents who become vegetarian in a household that already contains longstanding, well-informed vegetarians, will generally consume a balanced diet, since there will be a greater awareness of good vegetarian practices. 'New' vegetarians, however, are more vulnerable to iron deficiency[35] because simply eliminating meat from the diet is unlikely to result in an adequate diet. However, the greater variety of well-balanced vegetarian meals available in shops and restaurants, and increasing awareness of vegetarianism (e.g. popular articles and recipes) should make nutritional imbalances less likely.

Adolescents who are athletes or sportsmen/women must have sufficient iron in the body to ensure maximum oxygen capacity and to avoid adverse effects of impaired iron status on enzyme systems associated with energy production in muscles. Failure to maintain an adequate iron status may compromise performance levels and possibly make individuals more prone to injuries. Decreased iron stores have been reported in female adolescent runners[36]. The early weeks of intense aerobic training are associated with a moderate decrease in body iron reserves, and this is probably the result of mobilization of storage iron for an expanding red blood cell and muscle mass. In the highly-trained athlete, iron deficiency may be explained by an accelerated blood loss from the gastro-intestinal tract. Adolescent girls who perform intense physical exercise are highly susceptible to iron deficiency[37].

Acknowledgements

Parts of this paper are published with assistance from Tony Wright and Sue Southon in the Report of the British Nutrition Iron Task Force (British Nutrition foundation, in press). The author thanks Wendy Doyle and Sanna-Maria Kivivuori for access to raw data.

References

1. Department of Health (1989): *The Diets of British Schoolchildren*. Report on Health and Social Subjects No 36. London: HMSO.
2. Eveleth, P.B. & Tanner, J.M. (1976): World-wide variation in human growth. Cambridge: Cambridge University Press.
3. Lo, C., Jarjou, L., Poppitt, S., Cole, T.J. & Prentice, A. (1990): Delayed development of peak bone mass in West African adolescents. In: *Osteoporosis 1990*, Vol. 1, eds. C. Christiansen & K. Overgaard, pp. 73–77. Aalborg, Denmark: Handelstrykkeriet Aalborg Aps.
4. Department of Health (1991): *Dietary Reference Values for Food Energy and Nutrients for the United Kingdom*. Report on Health and Social Subjects No 41. London: HMSO.
5. Reports of the Scientific Committee for Food (1993): *Nutrient and Energy Intakes for the European Community*. Luxembourg: Office for the Official Publications of the European Communities.
6. Nadler, S.B., Hidalgo, J.U. & Block, T. (1962): Prediction of blood volume in normal human adults. *Surgery* **51,** 224–232.
7. Lentner, C. (1984): *Geigy Scientific Tables*, Vol. 3, Basle: Ciba-Geigy.
8. Torrance, J.D., Charlton, R.W., Schmaman, A., Lynch, S.R. & Bothwell, T.H. (1968): Storage iron in 'muscle'. *J. Clin. Path.* **21,** 495–500.
9. Hallberg, L., Hogdahl, A., Nilsson, L. & Rybo, G. (1966): Menstrual blood loss - a population study. *Acta Obstet. Gynaecol. Scand.* **45,** 320–351.
10. Hallberg, L., Hulten, L., Lindstedt, G., Lundberg, P., Mark, A., Purens, J., Svanberg, B. & Swolin, B. (1993): Prevalence of iron deficiency in Swedish adolescents. *Ped. Res.* **34,** 680–687.
11. National Research Council (1989): Recommended Dietary Allowances. 10th edn. Washington, DC: National Academy Press.
12. Fairweather-Tait, S.J. (1993): Iron. In Flair Concerted Action No 10 Status papers. *Int. J. Vit. Nutr. Res.* **63,** 296–301.
13. Kivivuori, S.M., Anttila, R., Viinikka, L., Pesonen, K. & Siimes, M.A. (1993): Serum transferrin receptor for assessment of iron status in healthy prepubertal and early pubertal boys. *Ped. Res.* **34,** 297–299.
14. Agha, F., Sadaruddin, A., Khan, R.A. & Ghafoor, A. (1992): Iron deficiency in adolescents. *J. Pak. Med. Assoc.* **42,** 3–5.
15. Bergstrom, E., Hernell, O., Lonnerdal, B. & Persson, L.A. (1995): Sex differences in iron stores of adolescents: what is normal? *J. Ped. Gastro. Nutr.* **20,** 215–224.
16. Olsson, K.S., Marsell, R., Ritter, B., Olander, B., Akerblom, A., Ostergard, H. & Larsson, O. (1995): Iron deficiency and iron overload in Swedish male adolescents. *J. Int. Med.* **237,** 187–194.
17. English, R.M. & Bennett, S.A. (1990): Iron status of Australian children. *Med. J. Aust.* **152,** 582–586.

18. Seoane, N.A., Roberge, A.G., Page, M., Allard, C. & Bouchard, C. (1985): Selected indices of iron status in adolescents. *J. Can. Diet. Assoc.* **46,** 293–303.

19. Health and Welfare Canada (1983): *Recommended nutrient intakes for Canadians.* Ottawa: Bureau of Nutritional Sciences.

20. Expert Scientific Working Group (1985): Summary of a report on assessment of the iron nutritional status of the United States population. *Am. J. Clin. Nutr.* **42,** 1318–1330.

21. Nelson, M., Bakaliou, F. & Trivedi, A. (1994): Iron-deficiency anaemia and physical performance in adolescent girls from different ethnic backgrounds. *Br. J. Nutr.* **72,** 427–433.

22. Nelson, M., White, J. & Rhodes, C. (1993): Haemoglobin, ferritin, and iron intakes in British children aged 12–14 years: a preliminary investigation. *Br. J. Nutr.* **70,** 147–155.

23. Southon, S., Wright, A.J.A., Finglas, P.M., Bailey, A.L. & Belsten, J.L. (1992): Micronutrient intake and psychological performance of schoolchildren: consideration of the value of calculated nutrient intakes for the assessment of micronutrient status in children. *Proc. Nutr. Soc.* **51,** 315–324.

24. Moynihan, P.J., Anderson, C., Adamson, A.J., Rugg-Gunn, A.J., Appleton, D.R. & Butler, T.J. (1994): Dietary sources of iron in English adolescents. *J. Hum. Nutr. Dietet.* **7,** 225–230.

25. Kerr, G.R., Lee, E.S., Lam, M.M., Lorimor, R.J., Randall, E., Forthofer, R.N., Davis, M.A. & Magnetti, S.M. (1982): Relationships between dietary and biochemical measures of nutritional status in HANES I data. *Am. J. Clin. Nutr.* **35,** 294–308.

26. Miles, C.W., Collins, J.S., Holbrook, J.T., Patterson, K.Y. & Bodwell, C.E. (1984): Iron intake and status of men and women consuming self-selected diets. *Am. J. Clin. Nutr.* **40,** 1393–1396.

27. British Nutrition Foundation. Report of the Task. (1995): Force. *Iron: Nutritional and Physiological Significance.* London: Chapman and Hall.

28. Soustre, Y., Dop, M.C., Galan, P. & Hercberg, S. (1986): Dietary determinants of the iron status in menstruating women. *Int. J. Vit. Nutr. Res.* **56,** 281–286.

29. Preziosi, P., Hercberg, S., Galan, P., Devanlay, M., Cherouvrier, F. & Dupin, H. (1994): Iron status of a healthy French population: factors determining biochemical markers. *Ann. Nutr. Metab.* **38,** 192–202.

30. Hallberg, L. & Rossander-Hulten, L. (1991): Iron requirements in menstruating women. *Am. J. Clin. Nutr.* **54,** 1047–1058.

31. Allen, L.H. (1993): Iron-deficiency anaemia increases risk of preterm delivery. *Nutr. Rev.* **51,** 49–52.

32. Beard, J.L. (1994): Iron deficiency: assessment during pregnancy and its importance in pregnant adolescents. *Am. J. Clin. Nutr.* **59,** (suppl) 502S–510S.

33. Gardner Merchant Educational Services (1994): *The Gardner Merchant School Meals Survey.* Kenley: Gardner Merchant.

34. Dwyer, J.T. (1991): Nutritional consequences of vegetarianism. *Ann. Rev. Nutr.* **11,** 61–91.

35. Bergan, J.G. & Brown, P.T. (1980): Nutritional status of 'new' vegetarians. *J. Am. Dietet. Assoc.* **76,** 151–155.

36. Nickerson, N.J., Stanitski, C.L., Dyment, P.G., Smith, R.E. & Strong, W.B. (1985): Decreased iron stores in high school female runners. *Am. J. Dis. Child* **139,** 1115–1119.

37. Cook, J.D. (1994): The effect of endurance training on iron metabolism. *Semin. Hematol.* **31,** 146–154.

38. Doyle, W., Jenkins, S., Crawford, M.A. & Puvandendran, K. (1994): Nutritional status of schoolchildren in an inner city area. *Arch. Dis. Child* **70,** 376–381.

39. Wright, A.J.A., Southon, S., Bailey, A.L. , Finglas, P.M., Maisey, S. & Fulch, R.A. (1995): Nutrient intake and biochemical status of non- institutionalized elderly subjects in Norwich: comparison with younger adults and adolescents from the same general community. *Br. J. Nutr.* (in press).

40. Armstrong, P.L. (1989): Iron deficiency in adolescents. *BMJ* **298,** 499.

41. Smith, N.J., Stanitski, C.L., Dyment, P.G., Smith, R.E. & Strong, W.B. (1985): Decreased iron stores in high school female runners. *Am. J. Dis. Child* **139,** 1115–1119.

42. Ballin, A., Berar, M., Rubinstein, U., Kleter, Y., Hershkovitz, A. & Meytes, D. (1992): Iron state in female adolescents. *Am. J. Dis. Child* **146,** 803–805.

Iron Nutrition in Health and Disease, edited by Leif Hallberg and Nils-Georg Asp
©1996 John Libbey & Company Ltd., pp. 149–156

Chapter 15

Prevalence of iron deficiency in adolescents

Lena Rossander-Hulthén and Leif Hallberg

Institute of Internal Medicine, Department of Clinical Nutrition, Göteborg University, Annedalsklinikerna, Sahlgrenska University Hospital, Göteborg, Sweden

Summary

Iron deficiency is defined as absence of iron stores, combined with signs of an iron deficient erythropoiesis. In an extensively studied random sample of women, all aged 38 years, a single criterion of serum ferritin (SF) ≤ 15 μg/l was found to discriminate best between iron deficient and iron replete women, based on absence/presence of stainable iron in bone marrow smears. The same criterion was used in the present studies in teenagers, since the relationship between SF and transferrin saturation (TS) was the same in the teenagers as in the adult women.

The prevalence of iron deficiency has been studied in two samples of teenagers.

In both studies low SF concentration was associated with significant decreases in haemoglobin concentration, MCH and MCV. The results showed that, with decreasing serum ferritin, the decrease of these measurements occurred already before SF had reached the level of 15 μg/l, suggesting that serum ferritin can be used as a single criterion of iron deficiency in teenagers, to indicate both empty iron stores and the presence of an iron deficient erythropoiesis.

In one study, comprising 220 girls and 207 boys, 15–16 years old, from four schools, the prevalence of iron deficiency was found to be 40 and 15 per cent, respectively.

A second more recent study was performed to obtain a more representative sample for the whole population. This study comprised 13 schools and included 620 boys and 624 girls, 15–16 years old. Design and size of this latter sample allowed more detailed analyses for factors associated with a low SF.

Infections are known to increase SF. In the second study, we examined the effect of occurrence of common cold during the preceeding month on SF. In boys with no history of infection ($N = 497$), 25.2 per cent had SF 15 μg/l, whereas those who had had common cold the previous month only 8.2 per cent had SF ≤ 15 μg/l. The corresponding figures for the girls were 39.6 per cent of those with no infection ($N = 502$) and 15.6 per cent among those with a common cold during the preceeding month ($N = 122$).

The prevalence of iron deficiency is in the process of being analysed in relation to factors that may influence iron balance such as growth rate, diet, physical activity and subjective assessment of menstruation. A reasonable explanation for the unexpectedly high prevalence of iron deficiency observed in the two samples may be high iron requirements combined with a low bioavailability of the dietary iron.

Introduction

Iron requirements are very high in adolescents of both sexes, especially during the growth spurt periods[1]. In girls, the menarche imposes further requirements to cover menstrual iron losses[2]. Girls have the main part of their growth spurt before menarche but growth usually continues up to the age of 16–17 years[3]. In boys, there are also additional needs relating to the increase in haemoglobin concentration at the time of puberty[4]. In boys, the high requirements persist for several years (Fig. 1). Thereafter there is a dramatic decrease at the age of 17–18. In analysing the prevalence of iron deficiency in teenagers, it is therefore important to consider these marked changes in requirements with age, especially in boys.

The first study was a pilot study mainly to estimate prevalence. The second study was made on a sample that was more representative of the whole population. This study was more comprehensive and included, besides measurements of iron status, bone density, physical endurance and peak performance, body composition, pubertal development and a series of biochemical measurements such as erythropoietin, sexual hormones, growth hormone indicators and biochemical bone markers. Studies on growth rate, assessments of diet, physical activity and other life-style factors were also included. Many of these measurements are not yet complete. The present paper is a preliminary report on factors related to iron status.

Methods and materials

The first study in teenagers was made in 1990, in a sample of 15–16-year-old boys and girls from four schools in Göteborg[5]. The study comprised 220 girls (86 per cent of those invited to the study) and 207 boys (80 per cent of those invited to the study) and whose parents had given permission for the drawing of blood samples. This sample represented one-tenth of all pupils in the 9th grade that year.

The second study was performed 1994/95, including both boys and girls, 15–16 years old, to obtain a more representative sample of the whole population. This study was carried out to get baseline knowledge about the iron situation in adolescents in Sweden before the general iron

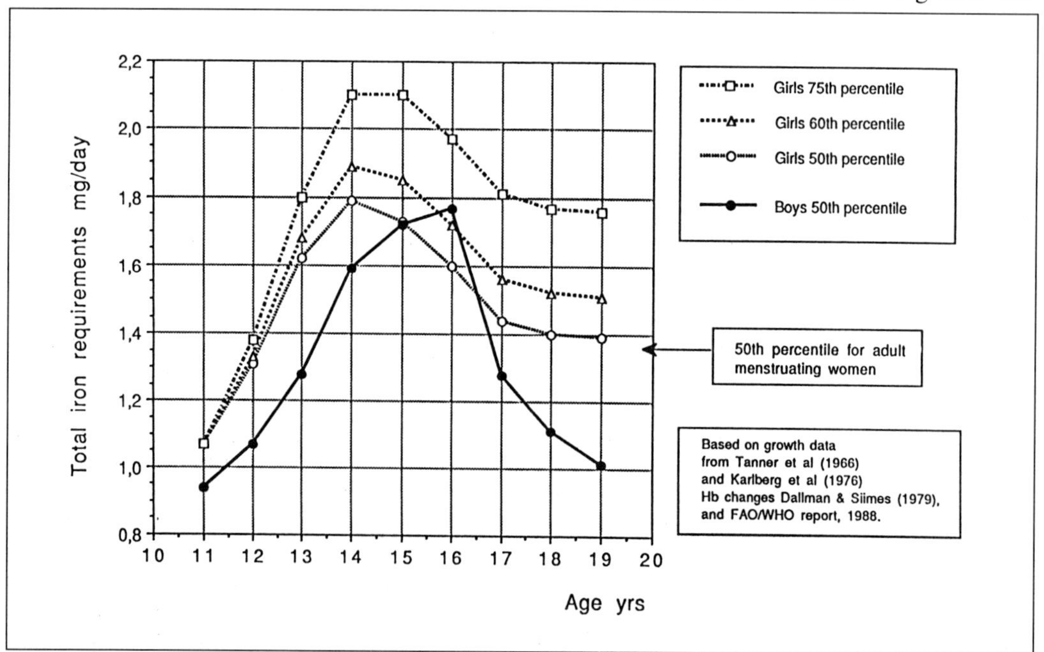

Fig. 1. Iron requirements in adolescents. Consideration is taken as to the fraction at different ages that had reached menarche.

fortification of white wheat flour was stopped (31 Dec. 1994). A new study is to be made in about 1999. This second study was more extensive and comprehensive, and comprised 13 schools chosen to represent areas with different socioeconomic and living conditions. All adolescents in grade nine at these schools were invited to participate. The study included 620 boys (87 per cent of those invited to the study) and 624 girls (89 per cent of those invited to the study), representing about 25 per cent of the total number of adolescent students in this age group in Göteborg.

The serum ferritin (SF) values, Hb concentration, MCV and MCH were analysed using the same methods as in the first study[5].

Results and discussion

The choice of diagnostic criteria for iron deficiency

Studies on the prevalence of iron deficiency were previously based mainly on haemoglobin determinations and focused on the prevalence of anaemia. The balance of evidence indicates that the main negative effects of iron deficiency are not related to a reduced supply of oxygen to tissues by a reduced concentration of haemoglobin in the blood, but rather to an insufficient content of iron in tissues, especially iron-containing or iron-dependent enzymes.

Iron is supplied to all tissues in the body bound to transferrin in plasma. The uptake of iron in different tissues is regulated by the number of transferrin receptors on the surface of the cells. The transferrin receptors on different cells are probably identical. Therefore, if the supply of iron to the erythron is compromised, then it can be predicted that the supply to other tissues that require iron is also compromised. The functional definition of iron deficiency would thus be a condition where no more iron can be mobilized from iron stores and where the first signs of a compromised supply of iron to the erythron appear. Different methods used alone or in different combinations have been used to try to establish suitable cut-off values for the diagnosis of iron deficiency[6–8]. Unfortunately, no independent methods such as absence/presence of stainable iron in bone-marrow smears or effects of iron and placebo supplementation have been used to establish the validity of the different criteria used.

In 203 adult menstruating women comprehensive studies on iron status were made in our laboratory including studies on stainable iron in bone marrow smears, measurements of iron absorption and menstrual blood losses, extensive haematological studies and also an iron/placebo supplementation trial. Thus, it was possible for the first time to evaluate the diagnostic efficiency of different methods used alone or in combinations to establish a diagnosis of iron deficiency[9,10]. Careful analyses showed that SF $\leq$ 15 μg/l used alone had the best predictive value to establish a diagnosis of iron deficiency with absent iron stores and signs of a compromised supply of iron to the erythron[9]. Further data from the same study population of adult women related various measurements to individual iron requirements. It was found that a SF $\leq$ 15 μg/l coincided with iron requirements of 1.7 mg/day and with a drastic increase in transferrin concentration (TIBC), a drastic decrease in haemoglobin concentration and disappearance of stainable iron in bone marrow smears[10]. In the therapeutic trial a significant increase in haemoglobin concentration was noted in 75 per cent of those women with no or trace amounts of stainable iron. No significant effect was seen in women having stainable iron. (It should be noted that those with trace amounts of iron were also included in the iron deficiency group). It can thus be concluded that the validity of the cut-off value for SF of $\leq$ 15 μg/l has been firmly established by several independent measurements. The main practical diagnostic problem using serum ferritin is to find suitable kits with sufficient accuracy and precision at low values and the use of the international standard for calibration.

In teenagers no such comprehensive study has been made as in adult women.

In studies on the adult woman we noted a close correlation between log SF and transferrin saturation. We found that the regression lines were the same for adult women and for teenage boys and girls. Moreover, signs of an iron deficient erythropoiesis appeared at the same SF level. These facts suggest that the same cut-off value for SF should be used in teenagers. The origin of serum ferritin is still unknown. The balance of evidence strongly suggests, however, that SF is related to the size of the main iron stores and to the state of the reticuloendothelial system influenced by, for example, infections and inflammations in the body. Transferrin saturation is related to plasma iron turnover and to the state of iron stores as reflected by the strong correlation to SF noted in the samples of both adults and teenagers. Present knowledge shows that there is a carefully controlled uptake of transferrin-bound iron in stores and tissues which strongly suggests that these fundamental mechanisms are the same at all ages. The fact that the relationship between SF and transferrin saturation was the same in adult women, girls and boys thus imply that the same cut-off values should be used in adults, teenagers and possibly also in younger children.

It is important to use independent criteria when searching for the distribution of normal values and to calculate the prevalence of disease. A normal distribution of laboratory values does not imply that the measurements included are normal. Also, pathological values may be normally distributed.

Haematological data

The distributions of log SF in boys and girls are shown in Figs 2–4.

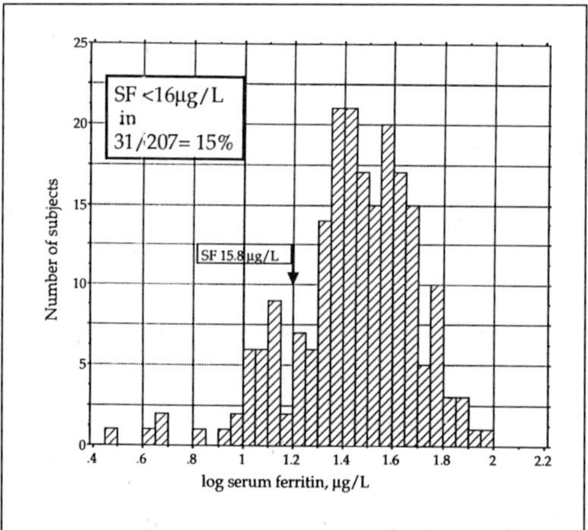

Fig. 2. Distribution of log serum ferritin concentration in 207 boys aged 15–16 years. Log serum ferritin; 15 = 1.2; 20 = 1.3; 30 = 1.48; 40 = 1.6.

Among the 207 boys in the first study, 31 (15 per cent) had SF ≤ 15 μg/l, and the corresponding values for the boys in the second study was 136 (21.9 per cent) out of 620. The prevalence of iron deficiency was higher in this second study ($P < 0.005$). It should be emphasized that the new sample was more representative for the general population of Göteborg.

Of the 220 girls in the first study, 88 (40 per cent) had SF ≤ 15 μg/l, and the corresponding values for the girls in the second study were 226 (36.2 per cent) out of 624. The prevalence of iron deficiency was not significantly lower in the second study.

For both boys and girls there was a high correlation between SF on the one hand, and Hb, MCV and MCH on the other ($P < 0.001$).

Serum ferritin (SF) and infection

An important factor to be considered in studies on prevalence of iron deficiency based on SF measurements is that SF values may be falsely too high due to recent infections, inflammatory diseases, liver diseases or starvation[11–13]. In our first study, made during March to April 1990, 25 per cent of both the boys and the girls had a history of upper respiratory infection during the preceeding month. The infection rate was significantly higher among those with higher SF, suggesting that a preceeding infection to some extent shifted SF toward higher values. In the

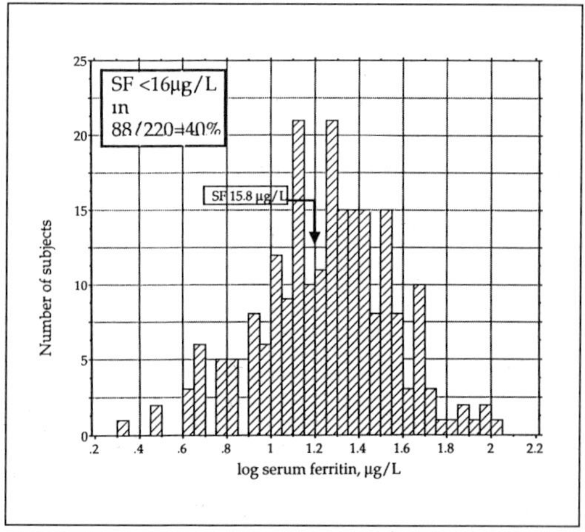

Fig. 3. Distribution of log serum ferritin concentration in 220 girls aged 15–16 years. Log serum ferritin: 15 = 1.2; 20 = 1.3; 30 = 1.48; 40 = 1.6.

second study, we also found a marked shift of SF towards higher values in those who reported an upper respiratory infection during the preceeding month ($P < 0.001$). Also in the second study made in October to December 1994 we found that 25 per cent had had a common cold the preceeding month. Among the girls with no history of infection ($N = 502$) we found 39.6 per cent with SF values ≤ 15 µg/l versus 15.6 per cent among those girls with a history of infection ($N = 122$)(Fig. 6). For the boys with no history of infection ($N = 497$) we found 25.2 per cent with SF values ≤15 µg/l versus 8.2 per cent among those boys with a history of infection (Fig. 6). Our findings imply that differences in prevalence of iron deficiency between different studies might actually be explained by differences in rate of simple respiratory infections such as a common cold for a couple of days. Our findings also imply that in studies on prevalence and causes of iron deficiency it is only meaningful to include subjects without known infections. Thus in analysing the present material we have limited our analyses to those subjects with no known infection. We have tested available acute phase reactants to identify those subjects who had increased SF due to common cold (e.g. haptoglobin, α-1-antitrypsin, α-1-antichymotrypsin, orosomucoid, ceruloplasmin, albumin, CRP [c-reactive protein]). None of available acute phase reactants could be used alone to identify those who had had an infection.

Growth

All the boys and girls were measured and weighed at the examination and their school health records were reviewed for height and weight during the whole school period to calculate the growth rate. For the boys, but not for the girls, we found a strong negative correlation between weight gain during the last year and serum ferritin but also between height gain the last year and serum ferritin ($P = 0.001$.)

Menstruation

Unfortunately it was not possible to measure menstrual iron losses for the girls in the two studies. The girls were asked about age for menarche, but also to estimate their menstrual losses (three alternatives for answers: heavy, small, not sure), number of days for menstruation and questions about bleeding through. Based on previous studies in our laboratory we know that it is very difficult for the individual woman to estimate her own menstrual losses. The main reason is the individual constancy of the menstrual blood losses. For the menstruating girls (98 per cent) we found a negative correlation between SF and estimated heavy losses and bleeding through ($p<0.01$). This was rather unexpected since it is difficult to estimate

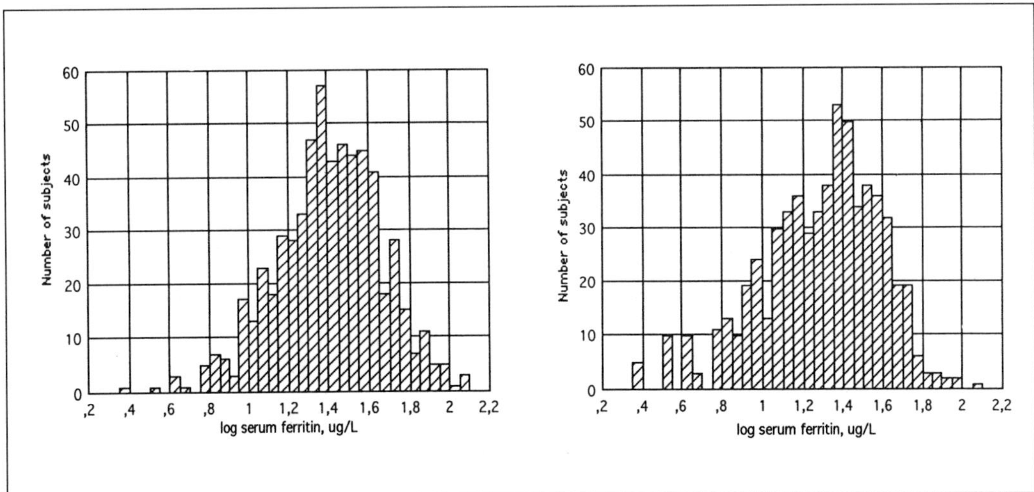

Fig. 4. Distribution of log serum ferritin concentration in 620 boys and 624 girls aged 15–16 years. Log serum ferritin: 15 = 1.2; 20 = 1.3; 30 = 1.48; 40 = 1.6.

menstrual losses by a history. Bleeding through is probably the most sensitive indicator of heavy menstruations.

Dietary intake

In the second study dietary information was collected on all individuals using a dietary history method. The questionnaire was filled out by the subjects and completed with an individual interview with a trained dietitian. In the dietary questionnaire special consideration was taken to the composition of the different meals. This design facilitated filling in the questionnaire. In this way meal composition could be considered in the analyses of individual dietary intake, not just the total intake of nutrients. The questionnaires about the diet are currently being analysed.

Statistical analyses of relationship between dietary factors and iron status

Statistical analyses of relationships between dietary factors and iron status are difficult to interprete. Iron status is determined by the balance between iron absorption and iron requirements.

The analysis thus far has shown no correlation between SF and the dietary factors analysed in the girls. For the boys, again with the dietary material only partly analysed, we have found a positive correlation between SF and the content of ascorbic acid in breakfast and dinner meals.

Furthermore, we have found a negative correlation between SF and intake of calcium at lunch and dinner meals.

Certain conditions are required to demonstrate a significant relationship between a dietary factor and iron status by statistical analyses. One obvious condition is that the factor is present in amounts expected to influence iron absorption. Another equally important condition is that the content of the factor in the main meals, containing most of the dietary iron, varies sufficiently to lead to detectable differences in iron absorption. For example, if most subjects have tea with

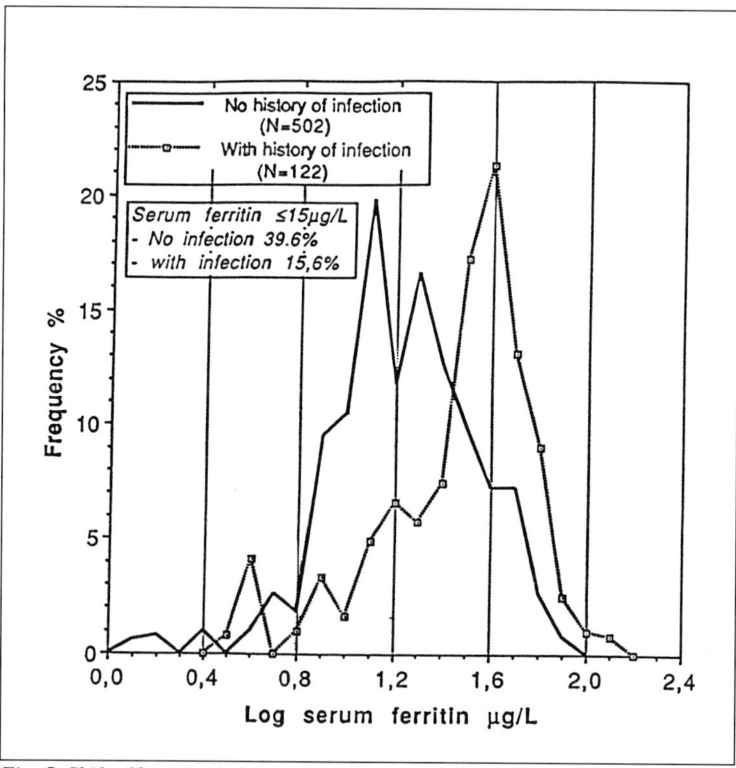

Fig. 5. Shift of log serum ferritin distribution by a mild respiratory infection in 15–16 year old girls.

their main meals, it would be difficult or even impossible to detect the marked effect of tea on iron absorption by this kind of analysis. Often the variation in iron requirements is much greater than the variation in dietary composition. Therefore, absence of a relationship between intake of certain dietary components and iron status should not, without further analysis, be used to suggest that the factor is without importance for iron status. A similar pitfall is the relationship between total iron intake and iron status. Differences in bioavailability of dietary iron may be more important than the absolute intake of iron.

Physical activity

The adolescents also answered a questionnaire about their habitual physical activity (physical training and exercise, transportation by foot or bicycle). A surprising fact was the observation from the first study that physical activity - with the exception of a small group with extremly high physical acyivity - was very low at this age both in boys and girls. Physical activity was higher for boys, 3.2 h per week, versus 2.2 h for the girls. There was no difference between those with low SF values and those with higher.

Comparing number of hours per week watching TV, a sedentary activity, we found that the boys watched TV more than girls (9.9 h per week versus 7.6 h; $t = 3.79$) and that girls with serum ferritin 15 ≤ µg/l watched more TV than girls with higher serum ferritin values (8.5 h versus 7.0 h; $t = 2.13$).

These observations do not imply that physical activity is without importance for iron nutrition. Our findings may simply be explained by the small variation in physical activity.

Conclusion

In two studies we have found a high prevalence of iron deficiency in teenage girls and boys. Iron deficiency was defined as absence of iron stores and signs of an iron deficient erythropoiesis. An explanation for the unexpectedly high prevalences observed may be a combination of high iron requirements and a low intake and/or low bioavailability of the dietary iron. To date, the consequences of iron deficiency in this

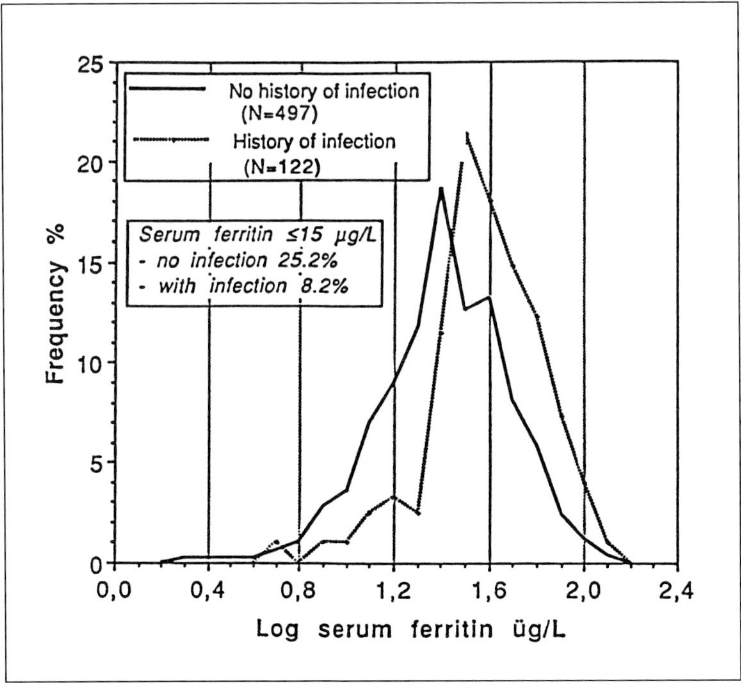

Fig. 6. Shift of log serum ferritin distribution by a mild respiratory infection preceeding month in a sample of 15–16 year old boys.

age group are not sufficiently well known. We know, however, that the observed insufficient supply of iron to the erythron leading, for example, to reductions in Hb, MCV and MCH, also implies that there is an insufficient supply of iron to all other tissues requiring iron for synthesis of various important compounds in the cells. This fact cannot be ignored by simply classifying different findings indicating the presence of iron deficiency as physiological effects of growth.

Acknowledgements

This work was supported by Swedish Medical Research Council Project B9519X–OH721–20B and Project B9619X0472121A.

References

1. FAO/WHO (1988): *Requirements of vitamin A, iron, folate and vitamin B_{12}*. Food and Nutrition series 23. Rome: FAO.
2. Hallberg, L. & Rossander-Hulthén, L. (1991): Iron requirements in menstruating women. *Am. J. Clin. Nutr.* **54,** 1047–1058.
3. Karlberg, P., Taranger, J., Engstrom, I., Lichtenstein, H. & Svennberg-Redegren, I. (1976): The somatic development of children in a Swedish urban community. A prospective longitudinal study. *Acta Paediat. Scand.* (Suppl. 258).
4. Dallman, P.R., Siimes, M.A. & Stekel, A. (1980): Iron deficiency in infancy and childhood. *Am. J. Clin. Nutr.* **33,** 86–118.
5. Hallberg, L., Hultén, L., Lindstedt, G., Lundberg, P.A., Mark, A, Purens, J., Svanberg, B. & Swolin, B. (1993): Prevalence of iron deficiency in Swedish adolescents. *Pediatr. Res.* **34,** 680–687.
6. Cook, J.D. & Finch, C.A. (1979): Assessing iron status of a population. *Am. J. Clin. Nutr.* **32,** 2115–2119.
7. Siimes, M.A., Addiego, J.E. & Dallman, P.R. (1974): Ferritin in serum: diagnosis of iron deficiency and iron overload in infants and children. *Blood* **43,** 581–590.
8. Lipschitz, D.A., Cook, J.D. & Finch, C.A. (1974): A clinical evaluation of serum ferritin as an index of iron stores. *N. Engl. J Med.* **290,** 1213–1216.
9. Hallberg, L., Bengtsson, C., Lapidus, L., Lundberg, P.-A. & Hulthén, L. (1993): Screening for iron deficiency: an analyses based on bonemarrow examinations and serum ferritin determinations in a population sample of women. *Brit. J. Haematol.* **85**, 787–98.
10. Hallberg, L., Hulthén, L., Bengtsson, C., Lapidus, L. & Lindstedt, G. (1995): Iron in menstruating women. *Eur. J. Clin. Nutr.* **49,** 200–207.
11. Birgegård, G., Hallgren, R., Killander, A., Stromberg, A., Venge, P. & Wide, L. (1978): Serum ferritin during infection. *Scand. J. Haematol.* **21,** 333–340.
12. Lundberg, P.-A., Lindstedt, G., Andersson, T., Branegard, B. & Lundquister, G. (1984): Increase in serum ferritin concentration induced by fasting. *Clin. Chem.* **30,** 161–163.
13. Worwood, H. Serum ferritin. CRC Critical Reviews in clinical Laboratory Sciences, **10**, 171–204, 1979

Iron Nutrition in Health and Disease, edited by Leif Hallberg and Nils-Georg Asp
©1996 John Libbey & Company Ltd., pp. 157–163

Chapter 16

Sex differences in iron stores of adolescents

Erik Bergström[1,2], Olle Hernell[1], Bo Lönnerdal[3] and Lars Åke Persson[2]

[1]*Department of Paediatrics, Umeå University, Sweden,* [2]*Department of Epidemiology and Public Health, Umeå University, Sweden* [3]*Department of Nutrition, University of California, Davis, CA, USA*

Summary

Iron deficiency anaemia is no longer a public health problem in most industrialized countries. There are, however, suggestions, supported by reported levels of serum ferritin, that there is a high prevalence of 'non-anaemic iron deficiency' in adolescents claimed to be caused by a too low iron intake. This chapter, based on data on iron status and dietary intake from 867 adolescents from northern Sweden, in the Umeå Youth Study, discusses the evidence in favour and against this suggestion. Our conclusion is that iron intakes in Swedish adolescents are adequate and that there is no convincing evidence, apart from the levels of serum ferritin, to support the suggestion that iron deficiency is prevalent among adolescents in industrialized countries. The suggested high prevalence of 'non-anaemic iron deficiency' is an effect of choosing too high a cut-off value for serum ferritin. We propose that there is a need to define separate reference values of serum ferritin for boys and girls at different ages. Furthermore, preliminary findings show that there seems to be an association between low physical fitness, high body mass index and high iron stores in adolescent boys. These findings may be important in view of the increasing concern regarding the reported associations between high iron stores and chronic diseases, such as cardiovascular disease and cancer.

Introduction

In adults, serum ferritin (SF) has been shown to be a reliable estimate of the amount of stored iron and is presently regarded as the best tool with which to evaluate iron status in individuals and the prevalence of iron deficiency in populations[1–3]. Iron stores, as measured by SF, are known to vary considerably with age and sex[4]. Recent epidemiological studies of SF values in adolescents in some industrialized countries have demonstrated quite similar SF distributions[5–9]. Figure 1 shows the distributions of SF values of 14- and 17-year-old boys and girls from the Umeå Youth Study[5], illustrating that the distribution of the 17-year-old boys differ strikingly from the other groups. We know that boys and girls before puberty have similar SF values and that the values increase during puberty in boys, but not in girls[5,6], but how these changes are regulated is not fully understood. It is clear, however, that sex hormones play a major role in the dramatic increase in SF in boys, and also in the absence of an increase in girls. The hormonal influence is also reflected in the variation of iron status during different menstrual phases[10,11], and by the increase in SF following menopause[4]. We do not know, however, what the 'normal' distribution of SF values of boys and girls at different ages in childhood and adolescence are.

Low iron stores

Non-anaemic iron deficiency

In Sweden, as in most industrialized countries, anaemia among children and adolescents due to iron deficiency is no longer a public health problem[12]. It has been suggested, however, that 'non-anaemic iron deficiency', i.e. the combination of low iron stores and normal haemoglobin concentration, is a prevalent problem among adolescents in industrialized countries, and that this justifies more emphasis on general prevention programmes, including iron fortification of food. Teenage girls are regarded to be at highest risk because of a combination of high iron requirements due to rapid growth during puberty, iron losses through menstruation, and a supposed insufficient iron intake[7]. This view, that iron deficiency is more prevalent in girls, has gained support from the fact that girls during puberty have lower iron stores than boys, as estimated by SF, and also that adult women have lower SF values than adult men[4]. When applying the generally accepted cut-off value of SF for low iron stores (12 µg/l)[13] to adolescent populations, this has resulted in a surprisingly high prevalence of 'iron deficiency', especially in girls. Even higher prevalence figures have been obtained by some investigators using higher cut-off limits (15 µg/l)[7]. These findings have, by some investigators, been interpreted as evidence for a high prevalence of iron deficiency in adolescents[7], although this interpretation has been questioned[5,14]. It should be noted that the potential long-term health hazard of non-anaemic iron deficiency remains to be verified[15–17]. It is important to mention that SF reflects only the amount of stored iron, i.e. excess iron, and not the iron necessary for normal cellular metabolism in different tissues. Assessment of circulating transferrin receptors may prove to be a more valid method to measure iron deficiency at the cellular level[18]. There is to date no conclusive evidence of any significant changes in other iron status parameters of adolescents, e.g. haemoglobin, transferrin saturation or transferrin receptors, at SF values above 10–12 µg/l[5,7,14].

Differences in haematological parameters between men and women

As SF reflects the total amount of storage iron in the body, it is reasonable to suggest that post-pubertal boys and adult men with their greater red cell and muscle mass are expected to have proportionally larger iron stores and, consequently, higher SF values than women. Different reference values for men and women are accepted and used for haemoglobin concentration. Another important difference between men

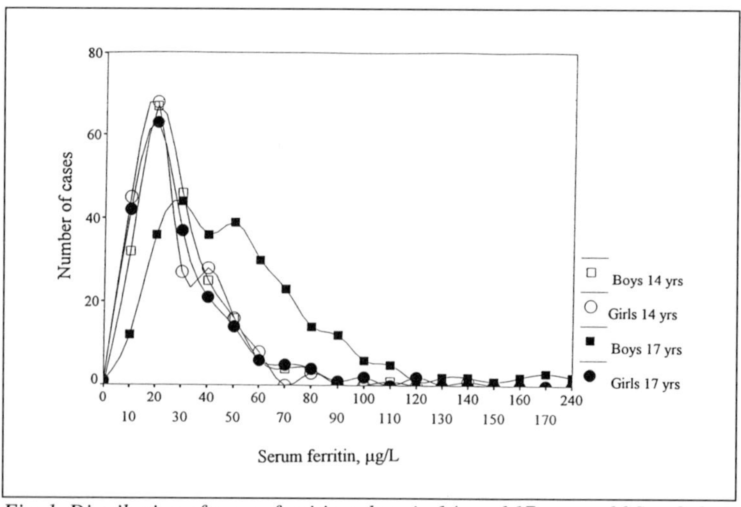

Fig. 1. Distribution of serum ferritin values in 14- and 17-year- old Swedish adolescents from the Umeå Youth Study .

and women is that women have been shown to have 2 to 2.5 times higher iron absorption than men[19].

Dietary iron intake

What would cause non-anaemic iron deficiency in adolescents? Are the dietary iron intakes inadequate and/or are there excess iron losses? There is no evidence to prove that either of these two possible causes of iron deficiency is prevalent in adolescents in industrialized countries today. It has been suggested that a sedentary lifestyle with low physical activity and subsequent low nutrient intake, including iron, causes iron deficiency in as much as 15 per cent of the boys and 40 per cent of the girls[7]. It is noteworthy that there are no suggestions of any other nutrient deficiencies in adolescents. In the Umeå Youth Study[5] we evaluated serum iron status of adolescents in relation to age, sex and dietary iron intake. We were able to demonstrate that the mean iron intake in Swedish adolescents is high in boys, 1.6 times recommended dietary allowances (RDA), and adequate in girls, 0.9 times RDA. No significant associations could be found between dietary iron intake and SF, except for an increased risk of low SF values in girls with low intake of haem iron. These iron intakes in adolescents have also been confirmed in two subsequent studies (Bergström, E. *et al.*, unpublished). It should be recognized, that the RDA is set at a high level (+2 SD of the mean intake of a normal population), thus covering the needs of 95 per cent in a population. It is also important to note that the absorbable iron, apart from amount and type of iron ingested, may also be regulated through variation in the absorption rate as iron absorption increases when iron stores are low[20]. Our conclusion is that Swedish adolescents have adequate iron intakes and that these results argue against a high prevalence of iron deficiency in adolescents.

Iron losses

Diseases, predominantly intestinal parasites and malaria with increased iron losses, being the major causes of iron deficiency in developing countries, are today very rare in adolescents in the industrialized world, implying that excessive iron losses should be equally rare. In individual cases with low SF values it is, however, appropriate to look for causes other than dietary iron deficiency, such as celiac disease and other malabsorption disorders[14]. In a follow-up of the adolescents from our survey in the Umeå Youth Study, the majority of the adolescents had normal SF values. Of those with persistently low SF values, one girl, on further examination, appeared to have a silent, previously unidentified, celiac disease. All the other adolescents with low SF values were clinically healthy and showed no signs of iron deficiency. They also appeared to be physically active above average (Bergström, E. *et al.*, unpublished).

Physical activity is known to reduce concentrations of haemoglobin and SF. This has been regarded mainly as consequence of increased iron losses leading to iron deficiency, the so-called sports anaemia, induced by the physical activity[21]. However, alternatively, the lower haemoglobin concentration and iron stores found in physically fit individuals could indicate a physiological adaptation, including a redistribution of body iron. That sports anaemia is not caused by iron deficiency, is suggested by the findings that iron supplements given to athletes with supposed iron deficiency have, in most studies, not been effective, unless the subjects were also anaemic[22].

It is difficult to accept that normal physical growth, or menstruation in girls, could cause significant iron deficiency in a large proportion of healthy adolescents with adequate, or even high, iron intakes and no other excess iron losses. An alternative explanation is that the criteria for iron deficiency is false, i.e. that SF, as a single criterion for iron deficiency, is not a proper measurement of iron deficiency in adolescents, at least not with adult cut-off values.

Reference values for serum ferritin in children and adolescents

Based on our studies we have suggested that, instead of using reference values for adult males, separate reference values of SF for boys and girls of different ages should be defined, also including cut-off values for low SF values[5]. An established way of setting reference values of different biochemical, physiological and anthropometric measurements in children and adolescents, is to use the distribution of a supposed normal population as a reference. The upper and lower normal cut-off limits are then usually set at ±2 SD of the mean, or the 2.5th and 97.5th percentile, thus covering 95 per cent of the population. If this method is employed on our relatively large sample (472 boys and 395 girls)[7], the lower cut-off values will be 8.0 and 6.1 µg/l for the 14-year-old boys and girls, respectively, and 11.1 and 5.5 µg/l for the 17-year-old boys and girls, respectively (Table 1). These cut-off limits would, of course, reduce the prevalence of 'low iron store' figures considerably for the 14-year- old boys and girls and the 17-year-old girls. For the 17-year-old boys, however, the new cut-off limit is close to the most commonly used cut-off limit for male adults (12 µg/l) and thus does not change the number of subjects that would be classified as having low iron stores. This group is, by definition, only 3 per cent (97th percentile). It is noteworthy that when multiple criteria for iron deficiency, i.e. both low SF (< 12 µg/l) and low transferrin saturation (< 16 per cent), were used in our study population (14- and 17-year-old boys and girls together), the prevalence of iron deficiency was 5 per cent.

Large iron stores

Risk of large iron stores

Although the risk for girls and women to be iron deficient is discussed, there is also an increasing concern that high levels of stored iron, especially in men, are potential health hazards. Large iron stores, estimated by SF, have been reported to be associated with an increased risk of myocardial infarction in men[23] and also cancer[24], although the evidence is still inconclusive[25,26]. There is, however, no evidence to support the notion that large iron stores are beneficial, unless a major blood loss is expected, and we do not know the safe upper limit. Free iron may induce oxidative processes, such as oxidation of LDL cholesterol in the arterial wall, thus contributing to the atherosclerotic process[27–29]. Sullivan claims that iron stores, in parallel to subcutaneous fat tissue, are signs of excess and he also claims that depletion of iron stores may have protective effect[30].

Interestingly, preliminary findings from the Umeå Youth Study suggest that high physical fitness, estimated with a running test, in boys, but not in girls, and a low body mass index (BMI) seem to be related to *small* iron stores in boys despite a higher dietary intake of iron (Bergström *et al.*, unpublished). This association may primarily be explained by differences in BMI. These findings are in accordance with a study of SF in adult men[31], where men with low levels of physical activity and high BMI showed higher SF values. An association between overweight and high SF values has also been noted in a recent study of adolescent boys[14].

It is tempting to speculate, that the lowering effect of physical activity and fitness on iron stores seen in boys and adult men may in fact be beneficial. If so, this further suggests that the higher ferritin levels found in adult men, compared to adult women, should not be regarded as 'normal', especially not for women. The larger iron stores in men may, apart from any biological sex difference, result at least partly from a sedentary life-style with low physical activity

Table 1. Mean and percentile values of serum ferritin (µg/l) in 14- and 17-year- old Swedish adolescents from the Umeå Youth Study

		Percentile						
Group	**Mean (SD)**	**3**	**5**	**10**	**50**	**90**	**95**	**97**
Boys 14 years (n = 201)	29.0 (16.4)	8.0	9.6	12.2	24.6	53.0	95.0	63.3
Girls 14 years (n = 197)	27.3 (17.6)	6.1	7.5	9.9	22.4	47.8	58.7	62.9
Boys 17 years (n = 271)	52.8 (34.8)	11.1	14.5	20.8	46.2	93.6	114.0	151.8
Girls 17 years (n = 198)	29.5 (20.9)	5.5	6.6	8.1	23.8	54.7	74.4	82.5

and high energy intakes, resulting in increased BMI, low physical fitness, and also large iron stores. This hypothesis is in accordance with the view that the health benefits of physical exercise could partly be a result of lower iron levels[32], but in contrast with the view that a sedentary life style is related to iron deficiency[7].

Conclusions

During sexual maturation the iron stores of boys increase, whereas the iron stores of girls remain unchanged as estimated by SF. There is no convincing evidence to say that these differences, among adolescents in industrialized countries such as Sweden, are explained by iron deficiency caused by insufficient dietary intake. This implies that the low SF values found in adolescents should be regarded as normal, in turn implying that adult reference values for SF can not be applied to children and adolescents. We propose that there is a need for separate reference values of SF for boys and girls at different ages; children are not small adults. Available data also indicate that the large iron stores of post-pubertal males, compared to post-pubertal females, reflect sex-related differences in iron status that are caused by normal hormonal differences between males and females. It is also important to further evaluate the associations between large iron stores in males and chronic diseases, such as cardiovascular diseases and cancer. The preliminary findings that physical inactivity and overweight seem to be related to large iron stores in boys, but not in girls, may also prove to be important. It is possible that the iron stores of girls and women in industrialized countries are not too small but, alternatively, that iron stores of adult males may be too large. The interpretation depends on who is regarded as the norm: males or females.

References

1. Jacobs, A. (1985): Ferritin: an interim review. *Current Topics in Hematol.* **5,** 25–62.
2. Worwood, M. (1990): Ferritin. *Blood Rev.* 259–269.
3. Cook, J.D., Baynes, R.D. & Skikne, B.S. (1992): Iron deficiency and the measurement of iron status. *Nutr. Res. Rev.* **5,** 189–202.
4. DeMaeyer, E.M., Dallman, P., Gurney, J.M., Hallberg, L., Sood, S.K. & Srikantia, S.G. (1989): *Preventing and controlling iron deficiency anemia through primary health care*, pp. 1–58. Geneva: WHO.
5. Bergström, E., Hernell, O., Lönnerdal, B. & Persson, L.Å. (1995): Sex differences in iron stores of adolescents: what is normal. *J. Pediatr. Gastroenterol. Nutr.* **20,** 215–224.
6. Milman, N., Backer, V., Mosfeldt-Laursen, E., Graudal, N., Ibsen, K.K. & Jordal, R. (1994): Serum Ferritin in children and adolescents. Results from population surveys in 1979 and 1986 comprising 1312 individuals. *Eur. J. Haematol.* **53,** 16–20.
7. Hallberg, L., Hultén, L., Lindstedt, G., Lundberg, P.A., Mark, A., Purens, J., Svanberg, B. & Swolin, B. (1993): Prevalence of iron deficiency in Swedish adolescents. *Pediatr. Res.* **34,** 680–687.
8. English, R.M. & Bennet, S.A. (1990): Iron status of Australian children. *Med. J. Aust.* **152,** 582–586.
9. Valberg, L.S., Sorbie, J., Ludwig, J. & Pelletier, O. (1976): SF and the Iron Status of Canadians. *Can. Med. Assoc. J.* **114,** 417–421.
10. Vellar, O.D. (1974): Changes in hemoglobin concentration and hematocrit during the menstrual cycle. I. A cross-sectional study. *Acta Obstet. Gynecol. Scand.* **53,** 243–246.
11. Kim, I., Yetley, E.A. & Calvo, M.S. (1993): Variations in iron-status measures during the menstrual cycle. *Am. J. Clin. Nutr.* **58,** 705–709.

12. Persson, L.Å., Samuelsson, G. & Sjölin, S. (1989): Nutrition and health in Sweden 1930–1980. *Acta Paediatr. Scand.* **78,** 865–872.

13. Finch, C.A., Bellotti, V., Stray, S., Lipschitz, D.A., Cook, J.D., Pippard, M.J. & Huebers, H.A. (1986): Plasma ferritin determination as a diagnostic tool. *West. J. Med.* **145,** 657–663.

14. Olsson, K.S., Marsell, R., Ritter, B., Olander, B., Åkerblom, Å., Östergård, H. & Larsson, O. (1995): Iron deficiency and iron overload in Swedsih male adolescents. *J. Intern. Med.* **237,** 187–194.

15. Beard, J.L., Connor, J.R. & Byron, C.J. (1993): Iron in the brain. *Nutr. Rev.* **51,** 157–170.

16. Idjradinata, P. & Pollitt, E. (1993): Reversal of developmental delays in iron-deficient anaemic infants treated with iron. *Lancet* **341,** 1–4.

17. Oski, F.A. (1993): Iron deficiency in infancy and childhood. *N. Engl. J. Med.* **329,** 190–193.

18. Cook, J.D., Baynes, R.D., Skikne, B.S. (1992): Iron deficiency and the measurement of iron status. *Nutr. Res. Rev.* **5,** 189–202.

19. Kuhn, I.N., Monsen, E.R., Cook, J.D. & Finch, C.A. (1968): Iron absorption in man. *J. Lab. Clin. Med.* **71,** 715–721.

20. Bezwoda, W.R., Bothwell, T.H., Torrance, J.D., Macphail, A.P., Charlton, R.W., Kay, G. & Levin, J. (1979): The relationship between marrow iron stores, plasma ferritin concentrations and iron absorption. *Scand. J. Haematol.* **22,** 113–120.

21. Newhouse, I.J. & Clement, D.B. (1988): Iron status in athletes - an update. *Sports Med.* **5,** 337–352.

22. Cook, J.D. (1994): The effect of endurance training on iron metabolism. *Semin. Hematol.* **31,** 146–154.

23. Salonen, J.T., Nyyssönen, K., Korpela, H., Tuomilehto. J., Seppänen, R. & Salonen, R. (1992): High stored iron levels are associated with excess risk of myocardial infarction in eastern Finnish men. *Circulation* **86,** 803–811.

24. Stevens, R.G., Jones, D.Y., Micozzi, M.S. & Taylor, P.R. (1988): Body iron stores and the risk of cancer. *N. Engl. J. Med.* **319,** 1047–1052.

25. Burt, M.J., Halliday, J.W. & Powell, L.W. (1993): Iron and coronary heart disease (editorial). *BMJ* **307,** 575–576.

26. Ascherio, A. & Willet, W.C. (1994): Are body iron related to the risk of coronary heart disease? *N. Engl. J. Med.* **330,** 1152–1153.

27. Cross, C.E., Halliwell, B., Borish, E.T., Pryor, W.A., Saul, R.L., McCord, J.M. & Harman, D. (1987): Oxygen radicals and human disease. *Ann. Intern. Med.* **107,** 526–545.

28. Salonen, J.T. (1993): The role of iron as a cardiovascular risk factor. *Current Opinion in Lipidology* **4,** 277–282.

29. Fuhrman, B., Oikne, J. & Aviram, M. (1994): Iron induces lipid peroxidation in cultured macrophages, increase their ability to oxidatively modify LDL, and affects their secretory properties. *Atherosclerosis* **111,** 65–78.

30. American Heart Association. Conference on cardiovascular disease epidermiology and prevention; Santa Fe (1993). *Food Chemical News* March **29**, 19.

31. Lakka, T.A., Nyyssönen, K. & Salonen, J.T. (1994): Higher levels of conditioning leisure time PA activity are associated with reduced levels of stored iron in Finnish men. *Am. J. Epidemiol.* **140,** 148–160.

32. Lauffer, R.B. (1991): Exercise as prevention: Do the health benefits derive in part from lower iron levels? *Medical Hypothesis* **35,** 103–107.

Iron Nutrition in Health and Disease, edited by Leif Hallberg and Nils-Georg Asp
©1996 John Libbey & Company Ltd., pp. 165–182

Chapter 17

Iron requirements, iron balance and iron deficiency in menstruating and pregnant women

Leif Hallberg and Lena Hultén

Department of Internal Medicine, Section of Clinical Nutrition, University of Göteborg, Annedalsklinikerna, Sahlgrens Hospital, S-413 45 Göteborg, Sweden

Summary

Menstrual iron losses are the main souce of variation in iron requirements in adult menstruating women. The distribution of their iron requirements is well-known based on a study in 476 randomly selected women. Different contraceptive methods may greatly influence iron requirements. The effect of the variation in iron requirements in menstruating women on iron balance and iron status depends on the properties of the diet and the efficacy of the regulatory systems controlling iron absorption. The interrelationship between different factors influencing iron balance has been examined in a few recent studies. In a sample of 203 menstruating women, all aged 38 years, it was found that with increasing iron requirements, due to increasing menstrual losses, serum ferritin was gradually decreasing suggesting decreasing amounts of stored iron. At the same time iron absorption was increasing. Above a certain level of iron losses, in the range of 1.6–1.8 mg/day, iron balance could no longer be maintained in an iron replete state. Haemoglobin concentration and the content of stainable iron in bone-marrow smears then started to decrease. About 30 per cent of the women were below this critical balance level as judged from the distribution of iron requirements in the earlier sample of 476 menstruating women. The critical level observed is only valid for the average diet consumed by these women. The prevalence of iron deficiency based on absence of stainable iron in bone-marrow smears or a serum ferritin ≤ 15 µg/l in the sample of 203 women was 34 and 33 per cent, respectively.

Studies on iron absorption from the whole diet in two other samples of women showed that a diet with a higher iron content or a higher bioavailability of its iron would balance the physiological iron requirements in a considerably greater fraction of women. Women with lower iron requirements would then get more iron in their stores, in turn leading to a reduction in the absorption of iron. In normal subjects the down-regulation of the absorption with increasing iron stores seems to be very efficient, thus setting an upper limit for the amount of stored iron. This down-regulation has been noted in previous studies by several investigators.

Iron requirements and their unequal distribution in pregnancy are well known. The dietary iron absorption increases markedly in the second half of pregnancy and roughly parallel to the increasing iron requirements. Even if the diet had the most optimal properties for iron absorption there will still be a considerable deficit (about 500 mg), however, between requirements and absorption of iron.This deficit would physiologically be covered from iron stores. Few women today, with present low energy expenditure and present diet, have iron stores of this magnitude and most women therefore need iron supplementation.

Pregnancy is a non-steady state which influences the validity of most laboratory measurements of iron status. Moreover, there are systematic changes in Hb, transferrin, red cell indices and serum ferritin at different stages of pregnancy. All these facts make it difficult to diagnose the individual woman in need of iron and to determine the true prevalence of especially mild iron deficiency. Several well-controlled studies show that iron supplementation is required in most women and even in those who are iron replete in early pregnancy.

Introduction

The iron situation is critical in many women in the fertile age period. This is assignable to both the high menstrual iron losses in many women and the very high iron requirements in pregnancy. The body tries to balance high iron requirements by adjusting the absorption of iron from the diet and by utilizing iron stores if present, for example, in pregnancy.

Iron balance means that absorption equals requirements. Thus, in a state of iron deficiency a balance can be achieved by increasing the absorption and by a reduction of menstrual iron losses due to a lowering of the haemoglobin concentration. In an iron replete state, iron stores can be formed leading to a reduction of the absorption down to a point when no more iron is absorbed than needed to cover basal losses. There are thus an infinite number of iron balance states from severe iron deficiency to a state of iron repletion.

The relationships between iron requirements, iron balance, iron absorption and iron status are outlined in Fig. 1. These relationships have been studied in detail by many investigators. What is less well established is the sequence of these events and at what critical point iron deficiency can be considered to be present.

The purpose of this paper is to examine the distribution of the iron requirements in women, the physiological adaptations in the body that take place to meet the requirements and the probability for iron deficiency to develop.

Iron requirements in menstruating women

In healthy, adult menstruating women iron is required to cover basal iron losses, mainly derived from losses of cells from the body surfaces and menstrual iron losses. The average basal iron losses have been estimated from body weight (14 µg iron per kilogram body weight per day) by following the decrease in specific activity of radioactive iron in red cells for a long time in adult men after administration of ^{55}Fe[1]. The true interindividual variation in basal iron losses including experimental errors is not known but has been estimated at ± 15 per cent (coefficient of variation)[2]. It is well established that there is a marked variation in menstrual blood losses between different women[3–6]. Menstrual losses of iron are thus the main source of variation in the iron requirements in non-pregnant, menstruating women. Menstrual losses in individual women are very constant from menarche and throughout fertile life[7]. It is therefore possible to calculate the distribution of the menstrual blood losses and the total iron requirements in random samples of women. The methods used for conversion of menstrual blood losses into iron losses in iron replete women and for the addition of the distribution of basal iron

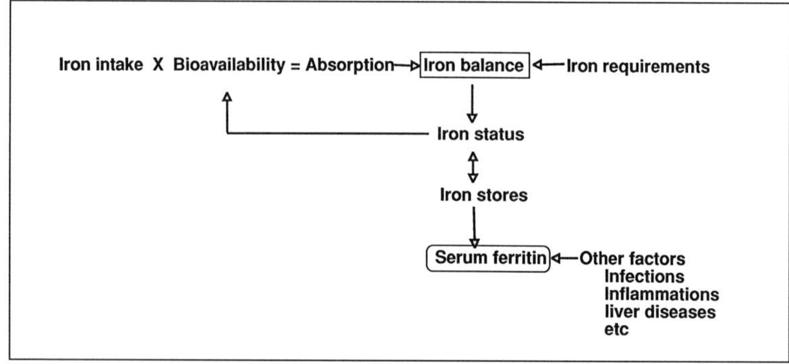

Fig. 1. Interrelationships between factors influencing iron balance.

losses to obtain the distribution of total iron losses have been described previously[8].

In 1963 the menstrual blood losses were measured in a sample of 476 women randomly selected from the population in Göteborg, Sweden[3]. In this sample there was no-one using contraceptive pills, which are known to reduce menstrual losses by about half[9]. The distribution of iron requirements are graphed in Fig. 2. This graph is an inverse cumulative distribution curve describing the probability of inadequacy at different amounts of iron absorbed.

In 1968–69 a new sample of 203 women was examined[10,11]. These women were all aged 38 years and were also randomly selected from the census register in Göteborg. Menstrual blood losses were measured and the distribution of iron requirements was calculated as in the 1963 sample. This distribution is also graphed in Fig. 2. In this sample drawn 5–6 years later, contraceptive pills were now used by 56 of the 203 women (28 per cent). It was evident that there was a small shift of the distribution curve towards lower values and a less pronounced tail to the right. Such a change in the distribution curve was anticipated in a previous paper[8].

Studies on menstrual blood losses were made in several populations in different parts of the world. All studies showed the same skewed distribution. Considering the differences in body size, mean values and median values are very similar. Differences between studies are mainly related to the tail. A smaller tail may be due to an incomplete sampling of menstrual blood, for example, by not using tampons and towels simultaneously. Calculation of iron losses without considering the often lowered haemoglobin concentration in those with heavy losses will also reduce the tail.

It is important to emphasize that the choice of anticonceptional method used has a marked effect on iron requirements. The most used intrauterine devices (IUD), such as cupper-7, doubles menstrual iron losses[12]. The most recently approved IUD releasing laevo-norgestrel, however, reduces menstrual losses after one year by 97 per cent (!) both in those with small and those with heavy menstrual losses[13]. In a study on 17 women with menorrhagia, followed for 12 months after inserting this new IUD, the concentration of SF was doubled. Differences in the use of contraceptive methods must thus be considered when evaluating iron requirements in different populations.

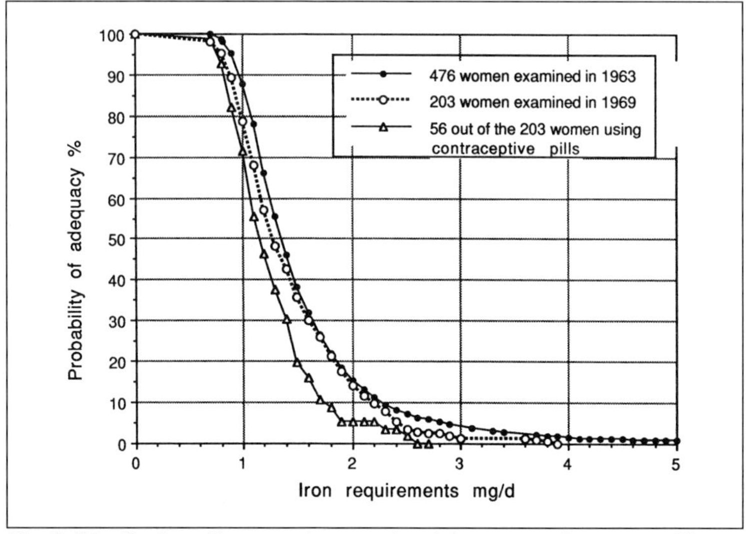

Fig. 2. Distribution of iron requirements in adult menstruating women. The graphs are inverse cumulative distribution curves giving the probability for iron deficiency to occur at different amounts of iron absorbed (for further explanations see text).

Relationship between iron requirements, iron absorption and iron status

Several investigators have clearly shown that there is a strong relationship between iron status and iron absorption[14–21]. The nature of this regulator is not known. In our sample of 203 menstruating women, several independent measurements were made which allowed further analyses of these relationships. Iron absorption from a small dose of an inorganic iron salt (0.56 mg Fe^{2+}) was used as a measure of the 'setting' of the mucosal cells to absorb iron. Previous studies have shown that there is a close correlation between the absorption from this dose and the absorption from the frequently used so-called reference dose which contains 3 mg Fe^{2+}, and which in turn is closely related to food iron absorption[21,22]. The absorption of iron from this dose was also related to the iron requirements in these women determined from measurements of menstrual iron losses, individual haemoglobin concentrations and estimated basal iron losses (Fig. 3).

It was evident that with increasing iron requirements there is a decreasing concentration of serum ferritin (SF) and an increasing absorption from the small iron dose The flattening of the absorption curve in Fig. 4 at higher iron requirements suggests that the absorption from this dose might have reached a ceiling at about 80 per cent. In spite of the increased absorption of iron at increasing iron requirements this increase did not compensate the increasing requirements. Before this maximal absorption had been reached there were clear signs of depleted iron stores and signs of an iron deficient erythropoiesis.

Transferrin (TIBC) and transferrin saturation (TS) in relation to iron requirements and serum ferritin (SF)

As shown in Fig. 4 there is a continuous and parallell decrease in TS with decreasing SF suggesting a close relationship between iron stores and transferrin saturation. A similar close relationships between TS and SF was also seen in other studies[21,23]. TIBC, however, stays constant at lower iron requirements but suddenly increases when iron requirements have reached a point almost coinciding with the decrease in Hb and the decrease in stainable marrow iron (Fig. 5). These findings imply that the rate of release of iron to transferrin becomes successively slower with decreasing iron stores and increas-

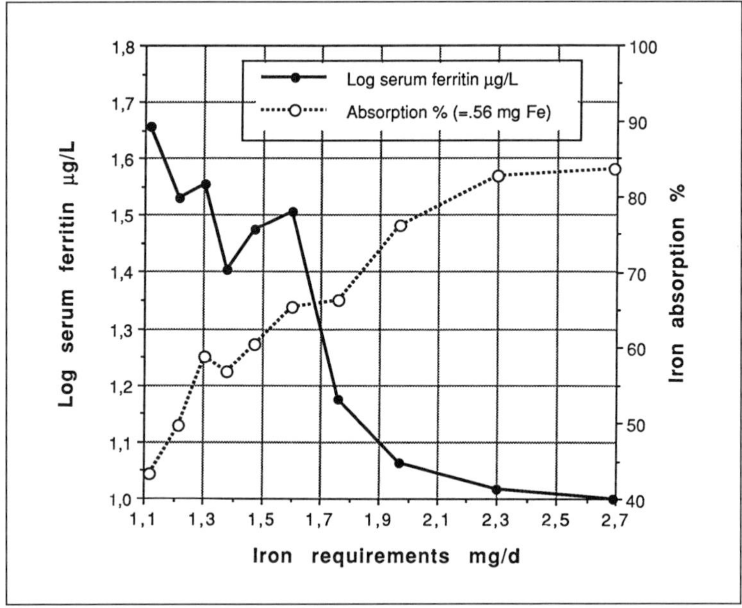

Fig. 3. Mean values of iron absorption from ferrous sulphate (0.56 mg Fe) and log serum ferritin at different decil values of iron requirements.

ing iron requirements. At a certain point in this development, possibly when iron stores are depleted, some signal initiates the increase in TIBC which counteracts the rate of decrease in TS. It is well known that the concentration of transferrin in plasma (TIBC) is mainly determined by the production and release of transferrin from liver cells which are transcriptionally regulated and responsive to iron status. For a review see Ref. 24. It is tempting to see these changes as rational mechanisms to facilitate the delivery of iron to tissues.

At this critical point the average transferrin saturation was about 25 per cent. (Figs. 5 & 6). This finding may seem to be incompatible with the often quoted cut-off value of 16 per cent for TS[25]. It should be remembered, however, that the figure 16 per cent was obtained in a carefully studied clinical group of patients with an established iron deficiency anaemia, with a median TS value of 7 per cent, and who responded to iron therapy with a haemoglobin increase of at least 20 g/l. In two random samples of women in whom the presence/absence of iron deficiency was based on presence/absence of stainable iron in bone marrow smears the mean value of TS in the iron deficient groups were also about 25 per cent and the overlap of the distributions was very marked[10,26]. A TS below 60 per cent, as a criterion for iron deficiency, may be useful in clinical diagnosis in patients with anaemia. The validity of using this low cut-off value in epidemiological studies on ID can thus be seriously questioned.

At what point during a negative iron balance does iron deficiency develop?

Iron status can be considered as a continuous variable from a severe iron deficiency anaemia over the normal iron status with varying amounts of stored iron, to iron overload. During a hypothetical slow development of a negative iron balance in a normal subject, iron stores are first successively diminished. At the point when

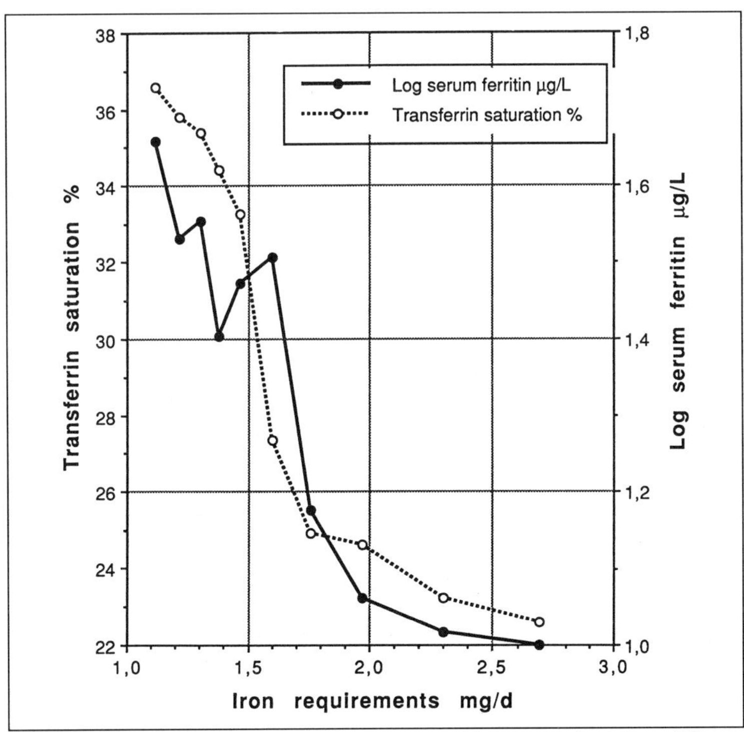

Fig. 4. Mean values of transferrin saturation and log serum ferritin at different decile values of iron requirements.

no more iron can be mobilized and the negative iron balance remains, the state of iron deficiency has been reached. From this critical point onwards the supply of iron is compromised to transferrin and further on to transferrin receptors on different tissues, including the erythron, leading to a decreased formation of haemoglobin. Sooner or later this will result in detectable changes in the simple, classical laboratory tests (Hb, MCH, MCV, TIBC or transferrin saturation). Functionally, therefore, the stage of iron deficient erythropoiesis starts as soon as no more iron can be mobilized from the iron stores. When Hb has been lowered to a point below minus 2 standard deviations of the distribution of Hb in otherwise normal subjects of the same sex and age and living at the same altitude the stage of iron deficiency anaemia (IDA) has been reached. IDA is thus a statistical definition and not a stage that is functionally different from iron deficiency or iron deficient erythropoiesis. In more severe IDA oxygen transport is compromised. In otherwise healthy subjects with normal cerebral and myocardial circulation, symptoms related to a slowly developing anaemia do appear late.

In this sample of women it is thus of great interest to observe when signs of an impaired supply of iron to tissues can be noted. As seen in Fig. 5 there is a rather sudden decrease both in Hb and in the fraction of subjects lacking stainable iron in their bone-marrow smears. As mentioned above, this point coincides with the increase in TIBC. There are thus three independent measurements showing that these changes occurred at about the same time and at iron requirements of about 1.6–1.8 mg iron/day. It is also worth noting that in this range serum ferritin drops to about 15 µg/l. The critical absorption where iron needs cannot be covered by absorption from the diet was about 1.7 mg/day in the present study. A diet with a higher bioavailability or containing more iron would accordingly cover higher iron requirements and balance iron requirements in a greater proportion of women. Similarly, a diet with lower iron content or a lower bioavailability can be expected to increase the prevalence of iron deficiency. It is a matter of fact that this reasoning is valid for the average women. The individual variation between women in dietary bioavailability and iron intake is disregarded. The present findings clearly show that there is no obvious intermediate stage between depletion of the iron stores and appearence of signs of an iron deficient erythropoiesis.

Iron balance in relation to iron stores and bioavailability

As mentioned above the relationship between iron absorption and iron status is well established. The efficacy of this regulator to balance increasing iron requirements by increasing the dietary iron absorption depends on (1) the content of dietary haem and non-haem iron and (2) the bioavailability of iron, which in turn is determined by the composition of the meals.

It has been suggested that the size of iron stores rather than the bioavailability of the dietary iron is the main determinant of iron absorption at least from Western-type diets[27]. Since both factors influence the amount of iron absorbed, however, it may be hard to compare their relative importance. In two recent studies the total amounts of iron absorbed over periods of 5–10 days were measured from four diets with different bioavailability in two groups of subjects[28,29]. Non-haem iron absorption from all meals was measured by homogenously labelling all meals with an extrinsic radioiron tracer to the same specific activity. Haem iron absorption from the meals was calculated from their haem iron content and the known relationship between haem iron absorption and iron absorption from reference iron doses. By relating iron absorption to serum ferritin it was thus possible to examine both the effect of differences in bioavailability of the four diets and differences in iron status expressed as serum ferritin. The slopes of the four regression lines in Fig. 7 show the marked effect of iron status on iron absorption and the differences in the slopes for the four diets show that differences in bioavailability also markedly influence the amount of iron absorbed. The conclusion is thus that both iron status and bioavailability are strong determinants of iron absorption, but that there is an upper level of iron status where there is no further effect neither of iron status nor of bioavailability.

Down-regulation of iron absorption at increasing iron stores

The fact that the regression lines converge and intersect with the horizontal line representing basal iron losses at points corresponding to serum ferritin values of about 40–60 μg/l (95 per cent confidence limits) implies that the down-regulation of iron absorption is very effective. Based on studies on the relationship between iron stores and SF these findings would suggest that iron stores in women would not amount to more than about 500 mg. This is consistent with the highest figures for iron stores estimated in women in phlebotomy studies. The obvious objection will be that this interpretaion cannot be true since many women in the general population actually have higher SF levels. The distribution of serum ferritin in women in the general population shows that even higher figures than 60 μg/l are seen in a considerable fraction. In our sample of 203 women, 15.6 per cent had SF values above 60 μg/l and, in the NHANES II study, 19 per cent of white women 20–44 years of age exceeded 60 μg/l. In the 45–64 year group of women 50 per cent exceeded 60 μg/l and even more in those between 65–74 years.

If we disregard the few who are homozygotes for hereditary haemochromatosis, how can the observed, very powerful control of iron absorption be compatible with the observed high prevalence of considerably higher serum ferritin values with increasing age? This is seen both in men and women but especially in women.

One traditional obvious explanation, besides an effect of a reduction in iron requirements with age in women, would be that inflammatory processes and even simple infections, which markedly influence the concentration of SF, might increase with age. Causes for the high SF other than high iron stores should always be looked for but it is hard to believe that inflammatory

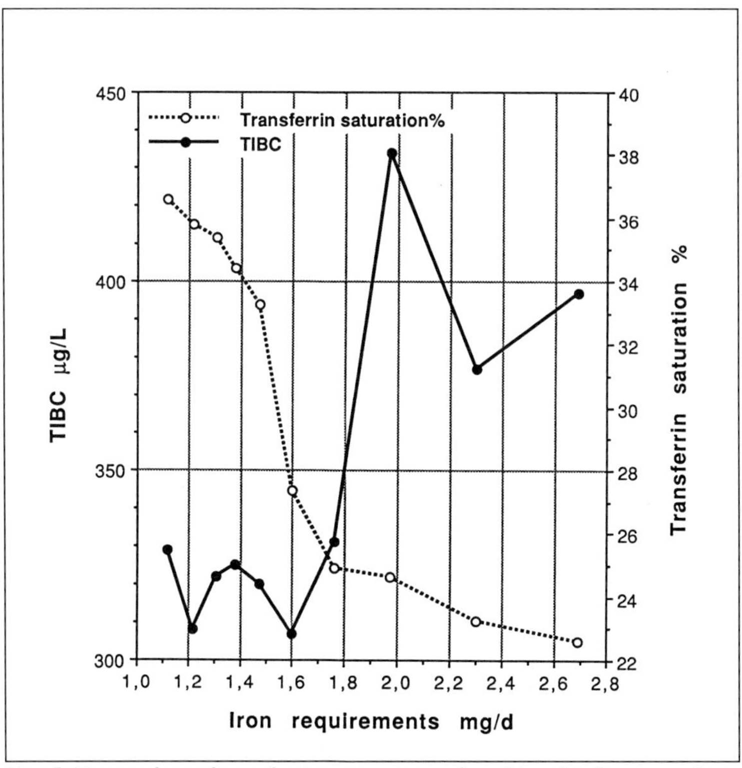

Fig. 5. Mean values of transferrin saturation and total iron binding capacity (TIBC) at different decile values of iron requirement.

disorders could be a main explanation for the observed rather large proportions of middle-aged and elderly women in the population having SF above 60. A similar reasoning is valid for men. Other explanations should be looked for. One factor seems not to have been considered. With increasing age, and starting already at the age of 20, there is a continous reduction in red cell mass, so-called metabolic active mass and total content of ^{40}K in the body which parallels the decrease in physical activity. There is also reduction in oxygen consumption, both overall consumption at rest. In a review by Munro[30] it was pointed out that there is a 40 per cent reduction in muscle mass in a 70 year subject in relation to those around 20 years of age. Much data are available about these continuous changes with age from 20 years and upwards. The present changes in life-style would rather exaggerate these physiological age changes.

If we assume that iron stores have reached such a level at a certain time and that no more iron will accumulate by absorption from the diet, due to this effective regulator in the intestines, it would still be possible for iron stores to increase by being provided with iron 'from behind'; that is, from catabolized red cells, effected by a shift of iron from circulating red cell mass to iron stores.

For example, a 25 per cent reduction of the red cell mass in a 65 kg woman, having originally about 1600 mg of circulating red cell iron, would imply a 400 mg increase in stored iron. A similar change in a 75 kg man would have an even greater effect since both blood volume and Hb concentration decrease with age – a reduction of the red cell mass corresponding to a shift of 500–600 mg iron may be expected. There may, of course, be marked individual dif-

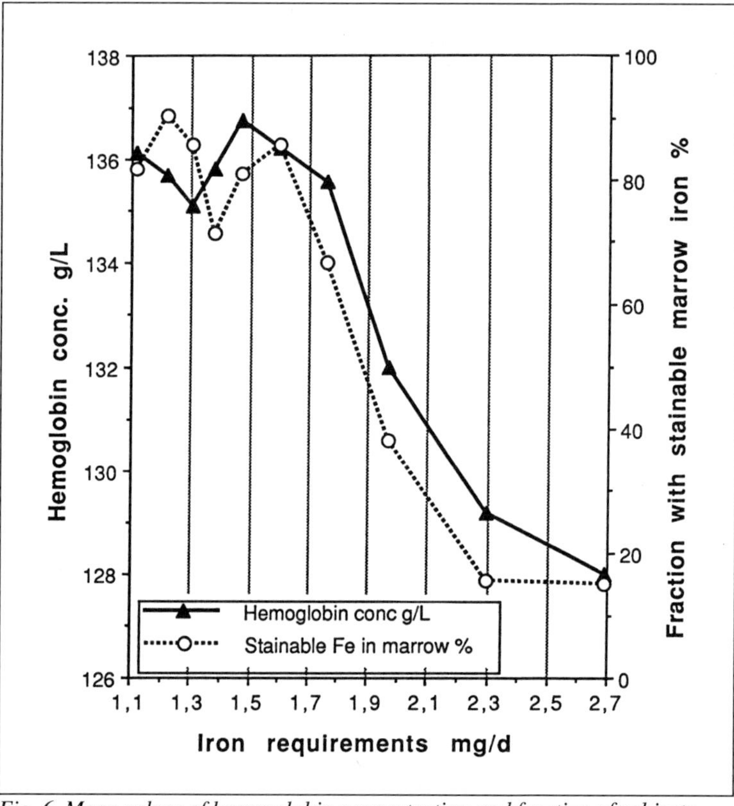

Fig. 6. Mean values of haemoglobin concentration and fraction of subjects with stainable iron in bone marrow smears at different decil values of iron requirements.

ferences. A general rule would be that the more sedentary the life-style the greater would be the expected change in iron stores and SF. This should also be considered as a confounding factors in the discussion on a relationship between SF and coronary heart disease.

These considerations are based on the two facts that the body cannot excrete iron, and that absorption is never zero, which means that being middle aged and older will lead to a redistribution of iron from circulation to stores. The rate of redistribution would then depend on rate of change in life-style. It might be worthwhile to examine this hypothesis.

Meal composition and bioavailability of iron

In the studies on the total amounts of iron absorbed from the whole diet, calculations were also made of the total amounts of iron absorbed in borderline iron deficient/iron replete subjects[29]. Non-haem iron absorption was adjusted to a serum ferritin of 15 μg/l and haem iron to a reference dose absorption of 40 per cent. Figure 8 shows the total amounts of iron absorbed from the four diets studied. These amounts are the maximal amounts estimated to be absorbed by a subject still being iron replete. The horizontal lines show the iron requirements in different proportions of women based on our previous studies on the distribution of iron requirements in women[8]. It is quite evident that the composition of the meals has a marked effect on the probability for iron deficiency to develop.

The diet showing the highest absorption contained about three times more haem iron (1.6 mg/day) than the diet with medium bioavailability (0.5 mg haem iron). Out of the 10 main meals served in the high bioavailability diet eight contained meat and two meals fish. The meat meals contained red meat in 7 and chicken in one meal. In the medium bioavailability diet four meals out of the 10 main meals were vegetarian (two of these were based on youghurt and muesli, one cottage cheese and one just vegetables). The diet contained one fish meal, one chicken meal, two meals with ham and two meals with small amounts of mixed ham and red meat. The phytate content was considerably higher in the medium bioavailability diet (185 versus 73 mg phytate-P per meal). The total

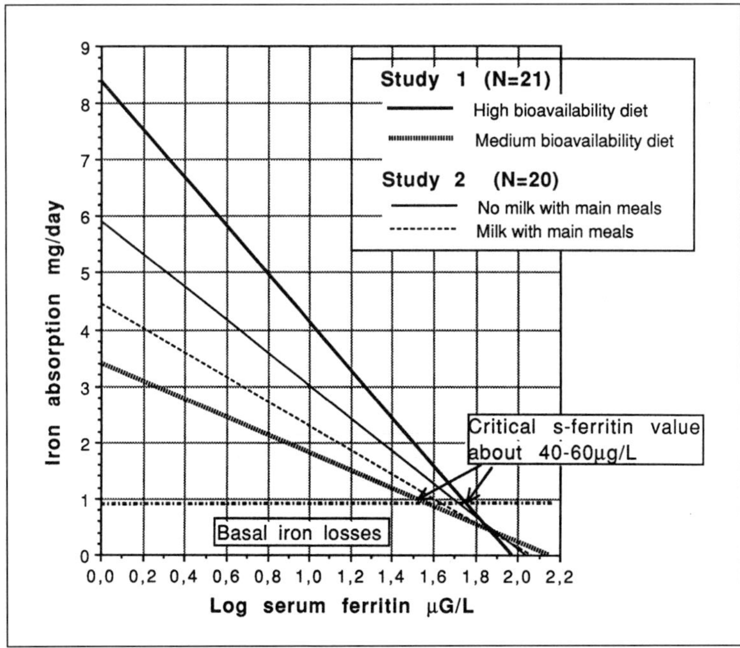

Fig. 7. Regression lines for the relationship between total amounts of iron absorbed and log serum ferritin in two studies.

amount of calcium was about the same but the diet of medium bioavailability had more main meals with a high calcium content. The average bioavailability in borderline iron replete/iron deficient subjects were 19.3 and 11.8 per cent for the two diets. The corresponding figure in an average Swedish diet has been calculated to be about 14 per cent and the figures for the other two diets in Fig. 9 were 17.6 per cent and 13.4 per cent, respectively. These two diets were identical except that calcium was distributed in two ways, with more calcium in main meals showing the lowest bioavailability.

The medium bioavailability diet was designed to reflect a common dict in young women in Sweden. Actually, several of the volunteers in the two studies, who were dieticians, had diets similar to this one. The factor explaining most of the difference between the high and medium bioavailability diets was the content of meat. Another main conclusion of the present studies is that diets can be designed that cover 90–95 per cent of physiological iron requirements in adult menstruating women in spite of present low energy and iron intakes. In practice that would, for example, mean a considerably higher meat intake.

Prevalence of iron deficiency

There is no doubt that the prevalence figures obtained in studies on iron deficiency very much depend on the criteria used. Therefore, in our group of 203 women who were all examined using a great number of independent measurements, we calculated the prevalence of iron deficiency in different ways and using different crteria. This is illustrated in Table 1.

The prevalence based on the absence of stainable iron in bone smears was 34 per cent. If SF $\leq$ 15 μg/l was used the prevalence was 34 per cent. If this criterion was combined with the criterion TS $<$ 16 per cent only one third of those classified as iron deficient would be included. This was discussed in a previous paper[10]. If we used both conditions, absence of stainable iron together with SF $\leq$ 15 μg/l, the

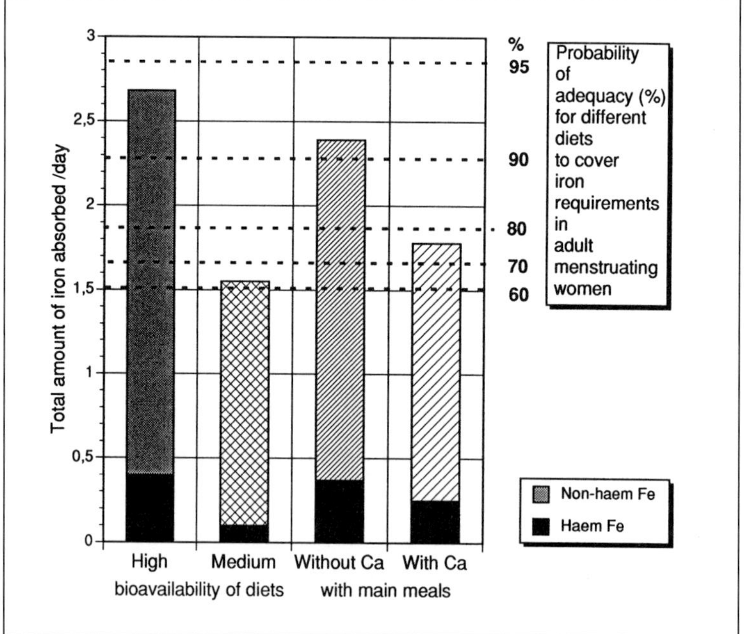

Fig. 8. Total amounts of iron absorbed in two studies (four diets). Absorption of haem and nonhaem iron is adjusted to a borderline iron replete/iron deficient state. Horizontal lines show iron requirements in different proportions of menstruating women, so as to be able to relate iron absorption from different diets to iron requirements.

prevalence dropped to 25.6 per cent, because some of those lacking iron in their smears had somewhat higher SF than 15. If we were to use a cut-off value of ≤ 12 µg/l for SF in stead of ≤ 15 µg/l, the prevalence would be 20.7 per cent. In the latter estimation, however, only 61 per cent of those lacking stainable bone marrow iron would be included among those classified as iron deficient. The prevalence would be the same, 20.7 per cent, if two conditions were used, namely absence of stainable iron together with SF ≤ 12 µg/l. It should be noted that the similar prevalence of 34 per cent above did not include exactly the same individuals, due to existing overlaps in distributions.

If we estimate the prevalence of iron deficiency from the studies already presented on the 203 women, and basing the estimations on changes in different parameters (Hb, TIBC and stainable iron in bone- marrow smears) at different deciles of the distribution of iron requirements, we observed a significant decrease in Hb and stainable iron in bone-marrow smears and a significant increase in TIBC in the range between the 6th and 7th decile values. All data thus suggested that the true prevalence of iron deficiency in this group would be in the range between 30 and 40 per cent.

In our studies on the 38-year-old women we also made a double blind supplementation study, measuring changes in Hb when giving placebo and iron tablets (37 mg t.i.d.) to two groups of women (*N* = 44 and 45, respectively). The 203 women analysed in the present paper were selected from an original sample comprising 372 women. In the 203 were only included those where all kinds of measurements were available[10]. In 286 women a bone marrow examination was made and from this sample 99 women were selected with no or only trace amounts of iron in their bone marrow smears. There was a significant haemoglobin response in 75 per cent of those given iron in spite of the fact that only 20 per cent had Hb < 120 g/l. There was no significant response in the placebo group. The methodology and interpretaion of results have been discussed in a previous paper[31].

Table 1. Prevelance of iron deficiency in menstruating women in Sweden

Diagnostic criteria	Prevalence (%)
Serum ferritin (SF) ≤ 15 ±/l	34
SF ≤ 15 µg/l + TS <16%	7.9
SF≤12 µg/l	20.7
Absence of stainable bone-marrow[a]	34
Absence + SF ≤ 15 µg/L	25.6
Absence + SF ≤ 12 µg/L	20.7
Prevalence percentage based on sudden change in parameter in relation to the distribution of iron requirments.	
• TIBC increase	6–7th decile=30–40%
• Hb decrease	6–7th decile=30–40%
• Stainable iron decrease	6–7th decile=30–40%

[a] Significant Hb response in 75 per cent of those with absence or trace amounts of stainable iron in bone marrow smears (Fe/placebo).

Conclusions

The prevalence of iron deficiency in women in the fertile age period in Sweden is about 30 per cent. There are reasons to believe that the prevalence is significantly lower in countries such as France where among other things the dietary composition is more favourable for iron nutrition. A prevalence figure of 16 per cent was reported by Hercberg *et al.* and his group for 476 native mainly nulliparous French women aged 17–42 years[32]. The diagnostic criterion used was SF <12 µg/l.

Iron requirements in pregnancy

The iron requirements in pregnancy are well known and are estimated by adding up iron requirements for the fetus, the placenta, the increase of the maternal red cell mass and basal iron losses by the mother. For reviews see Refs 33 and 34. The total amounts vary with the body size of the mother but can be estimated at about 1000 mg. It is also well known that the requirements are not evenly distributed in time. In the first trimester iron requirements are actually lower than in the nonpregnant state, due to the cessation of menstrual iron losses. The requirements increase almost continuously during the latter half of pregnancy due to the linear growth of the red cell mass and the exponential growth of placenta and fetus.

A series of physiological adaptations take place already early in pregnancy. There is a marked vasodilatation and a reduction of the total peripheral resistance in the vascular bed. Blood volume increases, mainly by an increase in plasma volume. The red cell mass increases in proportion to the need for total oxygen transport to mother and fetus. Early in pregnancy there is an increase in the content of 2,3-DPG in the red cells of the mother which later on will facilitate the oxygen delivery to the fetus. It has the immediate effect that the red cell mass does not increase in proportion to the need for oxygen transport[35]. In fact, the blood volume can be kept about 500 ml lower than would have been required otherwise. An obvious and well known effect of these changes is the physiological anaemia of pregnancy. The new setting of the Hb concentration in early pregnancy is thus not primarily an effect of a plasma volume increase but an effect of 2,3-DPG.

During pregnancy significant changes takes place in most haematological measurements. Some of these changes are related to the marked negative iron balance and the utilization of iron stores if present. Marked changes are also observed in women who are iron supplemented. There is thus a decrease in Hb, packed cell volume, plasma iron and transferrin saturation and an increase in total iron- binding capacity (TIBC) in both iron replete and iron deficient women. In studies comparing supplemented and unsupplemented women the increase in TIBC was higher in unsupplemented women already from the 16 week. From about the 24th week higher values were seen in the supplemented women in Hb, Hct, MCV, plasma iron and TS. A significant decrease in SF in both supplemented and unsupplemented pregnant women is seen from about the 20th week. A selection of the numerous studies on this topic are Refs 36–43.

Iron balance in pregnancy is determined on one side by the unevenly distributed and marked iron requirements and on the other by the amounts of available iron stores at the start of pregnancy and the amounts of iron absorbed from the diet. The amounts absorbed are determined by the intakes of haem and non-haem iron, the meal composition and by the changes in the iron absorption induced by the pregnancy.

In the first trimester we found that iron absorption from a test meal was significantly reduced compared with non-pregnant women. Mean absorption was only 0.7 per cent. A probable explanation is the lowered iron requirements[44]. A 100 ml reduction of the red cell mass has been observed at 12 weeks of gestation[37]. A reduction in the number of reticulocytes has also been noted. These changes are compatible with the seemingly paradoxical observation of an increase in serum ferritin in early pregnancy noted in a study in 30 women where Hb and SF were carefully followed from early pregnancy onwards[45]. In a study of 114 women we also found a marked shift of SF towards higher values at about the 10th week of gestation compared to non-pregnant women in the same population and age group (Fig. 9). All these findings suggest that erythropoiesis is reduced in the first trimester.

In the second and third trimester we found an increase in the iron absorption from the same test meal in unsupplemented women. Iron absorption increased to 4.5 per cent at 24th week and to 13.5 per cent at 36th week. The absorption from this test meal show the *relative* changes in absorption that occur during pregnancy. The absorption figures are thus not representative for the true absorption of iron from the whole diet[44]. Based on studies of iron absorption from a hamburger meal in another group of pregnant women[46] who had been granted legal abortion and who also were examined at the same time in the first trimester, it can be calculated that the absorption from a hamburger meal was 3.1 times higher than from the test meal used in our first study at 12, 24, and 36 weeks of gestation. In our recent studies on iron absorption from the whole diet[29], serving a diet which had a very high bioavailability we found that the highest fractional non-haem iron absorption observed in a woman with iron deficiency anaemia due to heavy menstrual blood losses was 42 per cent. The maximum haem iron absorption was 32 per cent. Applying these figures to the iron absorption in the last trimester, assuming an intake of 12 mg non-haem iron (no fortification iron) and 1 mg haem iron, the total daily amounts of iron that might be absorbed in the three trimesters from a diet with a very high bioavailability would be 0.4, 1.9 and 5 mg. The amounts of haem iron absorbed during pregnancy included in these three figures was obtained using the formula given in our recent paper on iron absorption from the whole diet and was based on the known relationship between haem iron absorption and absorption from a small dose of inorganic iron[29]. The iron absorption frominorganic iron during pregnancy was recently reported[47]. Using stable isotopes, 7.2, 21.1, 36.3 and 26.3 per cent of iron was absorbed from a 5 mg iron dose of ferrous sulfate given at weeks 12, 24 and 36 of gestation and at 12 weeks post partum, respectively.

In a recent study, non-haem iron absorption from a test meal was measured at the 12th, 24th and 36th week of gestation and at 16–24 weeks after delivery[48]. The test meal contained 3.2 mg native iron and 2.83 mg iron added as stable isotopes to label the food. The geometric mean absorption figures were 7.2, 36.3, 66.1 and 11.3 per cent for the four occasions. The test meal was considered to have medium bioavailability. In spite of that, the absorption figures reported were thus much higher than would be expected from different absorption studies made in our laboratory, for both pregnant women and non-pregnant women with iron deficiency anaemia mentioned above. The fractional absorption figures were also considerably higher than from 5 mg ferrous iron at different stages of pregnancy reported by the same authors[47]. These considerations thus suggest that for some reason these figures based on absorption measurements using stable isotopes might be systematically much too high.

The increase in iron absorption during pregnancy roughly parallels the change in iron requirements. The increased amounts of iron absorbed, however, do not always cover the increase in iron requirements. This would be true for even the most optimal diet. Table 2 shows calculations of daily iron requirements during pregnancy and daily amounts of iron that may be absorbed from a diet with good bioavailability. Our original absorption data in pregnancy were used to estimate the *relative* changes in iron absorption during pregnancy. The *absolute* total absorption figures (haem and non-haem) shown in the graph were calculated from our absorption studies on different meals and were

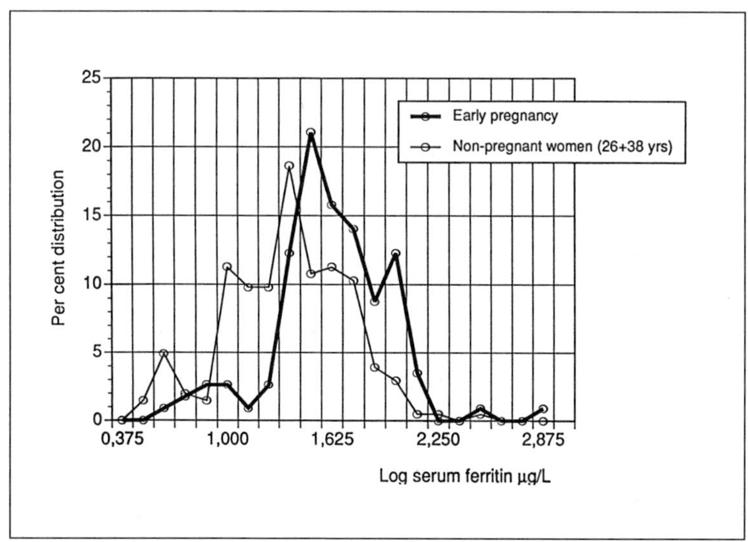

Fig. 9. Distribution of serum ferritin in 114 pregnant women at the 11th week of pregnancy (range 8–13 weeks) compared with 122 non-pregnant controls of about same age range, 26–38 years.

now checked with our most recent studies on total iron absorption from the whole diet as mentioned above.

It is evident from Table 2 that there will be a deficit between requirements and absorption of iron that has to be covered either from iron stores, if present, or from supplementation with iron. The existence of such a deficit is also evident from the numerous studies showing lower Hb in the last trimester in unsupplemented versus supplemented women. It has been postulated that the fetus will always gets the iron it needs. In a well controlled Finnish study of new-born babies and of infants at 6 months of age, SF was significantly lower if the mothers had a low serum ferritin concentration at term than for those born to mothers with a normal ferritin concentration and having been given iron supplements[41]. Recently, determinations of transferrin receptor were made in the third trimester in a sample of 176 pregnant women where a majority were taking iron supplements regularly. Results suggested that such measurements might be useful to detect those few who are iron deficent in spite of iron supplementation[49].

In our early ancestors the diet was probably better, with respect to iron with high amounts of animal protein and ascorbic acid[50]. Considering these facts it is probable that early woman had sufficient amounts of iron in their stores and sufficient high bioavailability of their dietary iron to balance the high iron requirements in pregnancy. Their main problem would have been to restitute their iron stores between pregnancies. It is of interest, however, that in lactating women at 8–10 weeks post partum we found that iron absorption from our test meal was twice that in the control group of nonpregnant women. To make valid comparisons, absortion in the two groups were related to iron stores expressed as the degree of stainable bone-marrow iron. The increased absorption during the lactation period is thus well adapted to the purpose of restituting iron stores in preparation for the next pregnancy. So far no explanations for the increased absorption during lactation can be offered. It would be reasonable to assume that some hormonal factor might be responsible for a different 'setting' of the mechanisms responsible for control of iron absorption[34]. The restitution ability of iron stores depends on dietary iron intake and its bioavailability. Present low energy life style in young women and their often low meat intake makes it difficult to achive sufficient iron stores between pregnancies.

Studies on iron balance in pregnancy and a great number of well controlled studies comparing the effects of giving iron supplementation and placebo certainly indicate that iron supplementation is required in most women. It should also be emphasized that it is hard to identify those few *not* requiring iron supplementation.

It may seem hard to accept teleologically that there is an obvious need to give extra iron to most women in a physiological, natural state such as pregnancy. The present low energy life style and present traditional composition of the diet may, however, also be considered as unphysiological looking at the development of man and his diet in a longer time perspective.

Table 2. Iron requirements and iron absorption in different trimesters in pregnancy and post partum. Iron requirements and caclulated iron absorption were reported previously[33,34]

	1st trimester	2nd trimester	3rd trimester	Post partum	Reference
Fe requirements	0.8 mg	5.8 mg	9.8 mg	1.1 mg	
Calculated total dietary absorption	0.4 mg 6.3%	2.0 mg 12%	5.0 mg 30%	3.5 mg 24%	
Absorption from:					
Test meal	0.7%	4.5%	13.5%	7.2%	Svanberg *et al*[43]
5 mg Fe^{2+}	7.2%	21.1%	36.3%	26.3%	Wittaker & Lind[47]
Test meal	7.2%	36.3%	66.1%	11.3%	Barrett *et al*[48]

Concluding remarks

It is obvious that the body possesses ingenious mechanisms aimed at the maintainance of iron balance in an iron replete state both in menstruating women and in pregnancy. In spite of these biological features, however, iron deficiency remains the most common deficiency disorder in the world and is the main deficiency disorder in developed countries especially in teenagers and women in the fertile age period. The principal general explanation for this paradoxical situation - of a nutritional deficiency in populations where almost no-one is starving and where everyone gets sufficient food to cover their energy requirements - is the dramatic, continuous reduction in energy expenditure and energy intake over time, and especially in the last few generations.

Acknowledgement

This work is supported by Swedish Medical Research Council Project B95-19X-04721-20B, and by Swedish Council for Forestry and Agriculture Research Project 50.0267-93.

References

1. Green, R., Charlton, R.W., Seftel, H. *et al.* (1968): Body iron excretion in man. A colloborative study. *Amer. J. Med.* 336–353.
2. FAO/WHO (1988): *Requirements of vitamin A, iron, folate and vitamin B12.* Food and Nutrition Series 23. Rome: FAO.
3. Hallberg, L., Högdahl, A.-M., Nilson, L. & Rybo, G. (1966): Menstrual blood loss a population study. Variation at different ages and attempts to define normality. *Acta Obstet. Gynaecol. Scand.* **45,** 320–351.
4. Cole, S.K., Billewica, W.Z. & Thomson, A.M. (1971): Sources of variation in menstrual blood loss. *J. Obstet. Gynaecol. Br. Comm.* **78,** 933–939.
5. Hefnawi, F., El-Zayat, A.F. & Yacout, M.M. (1980): Physiological studies of menstrual blood loss. *Int. J. Gynaecol. Obstet.* **17,** 343–352.
6. Beaton, G.H., Myo Thein, Milne, H. & Veen, M.J. (1970): Iron requirements of menstruating women. *Am. J. Clin. Nutr.* **23,** 275–283.
7. Hallberg, L. & Nilsson, L. (1964): Constancy of individual menstrual blood loss. *Acta Obstet. Gynaecol. Scand.* **43,** 352–359.
8. Hallberg, L. & Rossander-Hultén, L. (1991): Iron requirements in menstruating women. *Am. J. Clin. Nutr.* **54,** 1047–1058.
9. Nilsson, L. & Sölvell, L. (1967): Clinical studies on oral contraceptives - a randomized, double blind, crossover study of 4 different preparations. *Acta Obstet. Gynaec. Scand.* **46,** Suppl 8, 1–31.
10. Hallberg, L., Bengtsson, C., Lapidus, L., Lundberg, P.-A. & Hultén, L. (1993): Screening for iron deficiency: an analysis based on bone-marrow examinations and serum ferritin determinations in a population sample of women. *Brit. J. Haematol.* **85,** 787–798.
11. Hallberg, L., Hultén, L., Bengtsson, C., Lapidus, L. & Lindstedt, G. (1995): Iron balance in menstruating women. *Europ. J. Clin. Nutr.* **49,** 200–207.
12. Guillebaud, J., Bonnar, J., Morehead, J. & Matthews, A. (1976): Menstrual blood-loss with intrauterine devices. *Lancet* **1,** 387–390.
13. Andersson, J.K. & Rybo, G. (1990): Levonorgestrel- releasing intrauterine device in the treatment of menorrhagia. *Br. J. Obstet. Gynecol.* **97,** 690–694.
14. Cook, J.D., Lipschitz, D.A., Miles, L.E.M. & Finch, C.A. (1974): Serum ferritin as a measure of iron stores in normal subjects. *Am. J. Clin. Nutr.* **27,** 681–687.

15. Heinrich, H.C., Brüggemann, J., Gabbe, E.E. & Gläser, M. (1977): Correlation between diagnostic $^{59}Fe^{2+}$-absorption and serum ferritin concentration in man. *Z. Naturforsch.* **32,** 1023.

16. Walters, G.O., Jacobs, A., Worwood, M., Trevett, D. & Thomson, W. (1975): Iron absorption in normal subjects and patients with idiopathic haemachromatosis: relationship with serum ferritin concentration. *Gut* **16,** 188–192

17. Bezwoda, W., Bothwell, T.H., Torrance, J.D. *et al.* (1979): The relationship between marrow iron stores, plasma ferritin concentrations and iron absorption. *Scand. J. Haematol.* **22,** 113–120.

18. Baynes, R.D., Bothwell, T.H., Bezwoda, W.R., MacPhail, A.P. & Derman, D.P. (1987): Relationship between absorption of inorganic and food iron in field studies. *Ann. Nutr. Metab.* **31,** 109–116.

19. Lynch, S.R., Skikne, B.S. & Cook, J.D. (1989): Food iron absorption in idiopathic hemochromatosis. *Blood* **74,** 2187–2193.

20. Cook, J.D., Dassenko, S. & Skikne, B.S. (1990): Serum transferrin receptor as an index of iron absorption. *Brit. J. Haematol.* **75,** 603–609.

21. Taylor, P., Martinez-Torres, C., Leets, I., Ramirez, J., Garcia-Casal, M.N. & Layrisse, M. (1988): Relationships among iron absorption, percent saturation of plasma transferrin and serum ferritin concentration in humans. *J. Nutr.* **118,** 1110–1115.

22. Magnusson, B., Björn-Rasmussen, E., Hallberg, L. & Rossander, L. (1981): Iron absorption in relation to iron status. Model proposed to express results of food iron absorption measurements. *Scand. J. Haematol.* **27,** 201–208.

23. Hallberg, L., Hultén, L., Lindstedt, G. *et al.* (1993): Prevalence of iron deficiency in Swedish adolescents. *Pediatric Research* **34,** 680–687.

24. Aisen, P. (1994): Iron metabolism: An evolutionary perspective. In: *Iron metabolism in health and disease*, eds. J.H. Brock, J.W. Halliday, M.J. Pippard & L.W. Powell, pp. 1–30. London: W.B. Saunders.

25. Bainton, D.F. & Finch, C.A. (1964): The diagnosis of iron deficiency anemia. *Am. J. Med.* **37,** 62–70.

26. Hallberg, L., Hallgren, J., Hollender, A., Högdal, A.-M. & Tibblin, G. (1968): Occurrence of iron deficiency anemia in Sweden. In: *Occurrence, causes and prevention of nutritional anaemias*, ed, Blix, G., pp. 19–25. Uppsala: Almqvist & Wiksell,

27. Cook, J.D., Dassenko, S.A. & Lynch, S.R. (1991): Assessment of the role of non heme-iron availability in iron balance. *Am. J. Clin. Nutr.* **54,** 717–722.

28. Gleerup, A., Rossander-Hultén, L., Gramatkowski, E. & Hallberg, L. (1995): Iron absorption from the whole diet: Comparison of the effect of two different distributions of daily calcium intake. *Am. J. Clin. Nutr.* **61,** 97–104.

29. Hultén, L., Gramatkovski, E., Gleerup, A. & Hallberg, L. (1995): Iron absorption from whole diet. Relation to meal composition, iron requirements and iron status. *Europ. J. Clin. Nutr.* **49,**. 794–808.

30. Munro, H.N. (1981): Nutrition and ageing. *Br. Med. Bull.* **37,** 83–88.

31. Rybo, E., Bengtsson, C., Hallberg, L. & Odén, A. (1985): Effect of iron supplementation to women with iron deficiency. *Scand. J. Haematol.* **34,** Suppl. 43, 103–114.

32. Galan, P., Hercberg, S., Soustre, Y., Dop, M.C. & Dupin, H. (1985): Factors affecting iron stores in French female students. *Human Nutr. Clin. Nutr.* **39C,** 279–287.

33. Hallberg, L. (1988): Iron balance in pregnancy. In: *Vitamins and minerals in pregnancy and lactation*, ed., Berger, H. New York: Raven Press.

34. Hallberg, L. (1992): Iron balance in pregnancy and lactation. In: *Nutritional anemias*, pp. 13–25. (Nestlé Nutrition Workshop Series; vol 30). New York: Raven Press.

35. Flanagan, B., Muddowney, F.P. & Cannon, P.J. (1966): The relationship of circulating red cell mass, basal oxygen consuption and lean body mass during normal human pregnancy. *Clin. Sci.* **30,** 439–451.

36. deLeeuw, N.K.M., Lowenstein, L. & Hsieh, Y.-S. (1966): Iron deficiency and hydremia in normal pregnancy. *Medicine* **45,** 291–315.

37. Taylor, D.J. & Lind, T. (1979): Red cell mass during and after normal pregnancy. *Br. J. Obstet. Gynecol.* **86,** 364–370.

38. Dawson, E.B. & McGanity, W.J. (1987): Protection of maternal iron stores in pregnancy. *J. Reprod. Med.* **32,** 478–487.

39. Romslo, I., Haram, K., Sagen, N. & Augensen, K. (1983): Iron requirements in normal pregnancy as assessed by serum ferritin, serum transferrin saturation and erythrocyte protoporphyrin determinations. *Brit. J. Obstet. Gynecol.* **90,** 101–107.

40. Buytaert, G., Wallenburg, H.C.S., van Eijck, H.G. & Buytaert, P. (1983): Iron supplementation during pregnancy. *Europ. J. Obstet. Gynec. Reprod. Biol.* **15,** 11–16.

41. Puolakka, J., Jänne, O. & Vihko, R. (1980): Evaluation by serum ferritin assay of the influence of maternal iron stores on the iron status of newborns and infants. *Acta Obstet. Gynecol. Scand.* **Suppl. 95,** 53–56.

42. Taylor, D.J., Mallen, C. & Lind, T. (1982): Effect of iron supplementation on serum ferritin levels during and after pregnancy. *Brit. J. Obstet. Gynecol.* **89,** 1011–1017.

43. Svanberg, B. (1975): Absorption of iron in pregnancy. *Acta Obstet. Gynecol. Scand.* **Suppl. 48,** 7–27.

44. Svanberg, B., Arvidsson, B., Björn-Rasmussen, E., Hallberg, L., Rossander, L. & Swolin, B. (1975): Dietary iron absorption in pregnancy. A longitudinal study with repeated measurements of non-haeme iron absorption from whole diet. *Acta Obstet. Gynecol. Scand.* **Suppl. 48,** 43–68.

45. Kaufer, M. & Casanueva, E. (1990): Relation of prepregnancy serum ferritin levels to hemoglobin levels throughout pregnancy. *Europ. J. Clin. Nutr.* **44,** 709–715.

46. Svanberg, B. (1975): Iron absorption in early pregnancy. A study of the absorption of non-haem iron and ferroud iron in early pregnancy. *Acta Obstet. Gynecol. Scand.* **Suppl. 48,** 69–85.

47. Whittaker, P.G. & Lind, T. (1991): Iron absorption during normal human pregnancy: a study using stable isotopes. *Br. J. Nutr.* **65,** 457–463.

48. Barrett, J.F.R., Whittaker, P.G., Williams, J.G. & Lind, T. (1994): Absorption of non-haem iron from food during normal pregnancy. *BMJ* **309,** 79–82.

49. Carriaga, M.T., Skikne, B.S., Finley, B., Cutler, B. & Cook, J.D. (1991): Serum transferrin receptor for the detection of iron deficiency in pregnancy. *Am. J. Clin. Nutr.* **54,** 1077–1081.

50. Eaton, S.B. & Konner, M. (1985): Paleolithic nutrition: A consideration of its nature and current implications. *New Engl. J. Med.* **312,** 283–289.

Iron Nutrition in Health and Disease, edited by Leif Hallberg and Nils-Georg Asp
©1996 John Libbey & Company Ltd., pp. 183–194

Chapter 18

Iron deficiency and physical performance: Experimental studies

George A. Brooks

Exercise Physiology Laboratory, Department of Human Biodynamics, 103 Harmon, University of California, Berkeley, CA 94720- 4480, USA

Summary

With laboratory rats we have manipulated components of oxygen transport and utilization, using dietary manipulation, exchange transfusion of plasma or packed erythrocytes, pharmacological blockade, and endurance as well as sprint exercise training. Results lead us to conclude that although dietary iron deficiency leads to both central (i.e. O_2 transport) and peripheral (e.g. metabolic) deficits, in terms of the ability to sustain submaximal effort, the peripheral consequences of dietary iron deficiency are likely more severe. We further conclude that in terms of sustained effort, alterations in energy substrate utilization are equally or more detrimental to endurance than are the consequences of iron deficiency on the apparent V_{max} of muscle mitochondrial for O_2 consumption.

We find that in the face of limitations in oxygen transport and utilization, the body possesses remarkable plasticity in terms of adaptation so that reasonable levels of physical exertion can be maintained. A major adaptation appears to be an enhanced dependence on glucose as a fuel. This adaptation is understandable because in contrast to lipid, carbohydrate is a more oxygen-efficient fuel. Further, the adaptive response appears to be mediated by catecholamines, which on one hand (by epinephrine) stimulate peripheral glycogenolyis and lactate production, while on the other hand (by norepinephrine) stimulate hepatic glucose production. Thus, the consequences of iron deficiency are shifted from the more impacted periphery, to the lesser effected central gluconeogenic organs. Moreover, at the peripheral muscle cell level, subtle compensatory adaptations occur which include elevated GLUT 4 levels as well as in ratios of mitochondrial TCA cycle constituents.

Finally, although unproven, there occur similar metabolic compensations to a variety of situations in which the ability to consume and utilize oxygen is affected. The commonalty of these adaptations suggests presence of general cross-adaptive responses.

Introduction

The capacities for sustained high power output during exercise and recovery from exercise are dependent upon the consumption, transport, and use of oxygen[1]. Concomitantly, the demands for high rates of cell respiration associated with sustained exertions require elevations in the supply of oxidizable substrates, particularly endogenous carbohydrate sources (i.e. glucose, glycogen and lactate). During exercise, there must be a high degree of coordination among neuromuscular, cardiovascular, endocrine and cell metabolic systems. Further, the fluxes of oxygen and energy substrates must be graded precisely to the exercise load. These requirements of controlling high flux rates make physical exercise and exercise training powerful tools in studying metabolism in normal and pathophysiology.

In an effort to determine the interrelationships among the maximal capacities to transport and use oxygen and exercise endurance, as well as to determine the limitations and compensations associated variations in the resistances to oxygen transport and use, we have employed the following manipulations with laboratory rats: dietary iron deficiency, dietary iron deficiency followed by refeeding or exchange-transfusion of plasma or packed erythrocytes for whole blood, pharmacological blockade, and sprint as well as endurance exercise training. A coordinated series of hormonal, morphological, and enzymatic adaptations to iron insufficiency have been observed. Moreover, the results obtained on laboratory animals have provided a basis to approach understanding and resolution of a number of chronic conditions which affect functional capacities and metabolic responses in humans. Thus, the work on animals has led to identification of a set of general adaptive responses to conditions associated with limitations in the capacity to transport and utilize oxygen.

An example of the ability to manipulate, by means of diet, body iron stores is found in the work of Perkkio *et al.*[2]. Figure 1 illustrates the ability to titrate levels of haemoglobin and skeletal muscle mitochondrial cytochrome c by dietary manipulation. Figure 2 from the same study shows how variations in arterial oxygen transport (i.e. haemoglobin) and muscle mitochondrial respiratory capacity (i.e. cytochrome c) affect maximal oxygen consumption (V_{O_2max}) and exercise endurance. Note in particular, the decline in exercise endurance when haemoglobin falls below 10 g/dl.

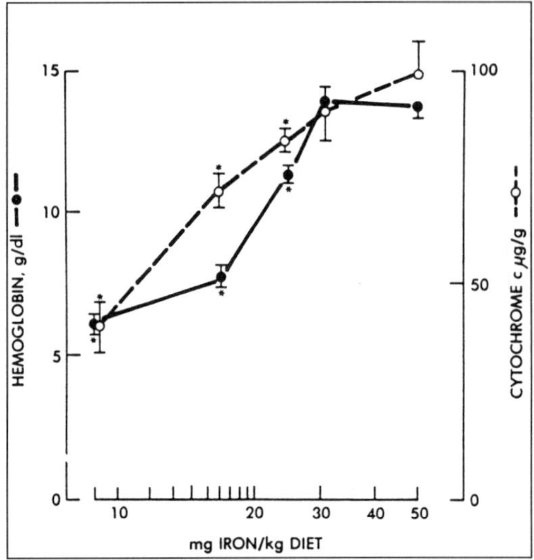

*Fig. 1. Blood haemoglobin and gastrocnemius cytochrome c contents in adult rats can be manipulated by varying the dietary iron content provided to weanling fats. The * symbol indicates where values differ from control rats fed a normal (50 mg iron/kg food) diet. Data from Perkkio et al.*[2].

Mitochondrial adaptations to endurance training

With iron-sufficient and otherwise well-nourished female rats, we determined the relationships among exercise endurance and the capacity to consume and utilize oxygen. Ten weeks of endurance training improved both V_{O_2max} (+15 per cent) and muscle mitochondrial content (+100 per cent) in laboratory rats[3] (Table 1). Endurance to a standard exercise challenge (i.e. time to fatigue at constant running speed) improved 300 per cent, and endurance correlated significantly better with muscle respiratory capacity ($r = 0.92$) than with V_{O_2max} ($r = 0.74$) (Table 2). In contrast to the effects of

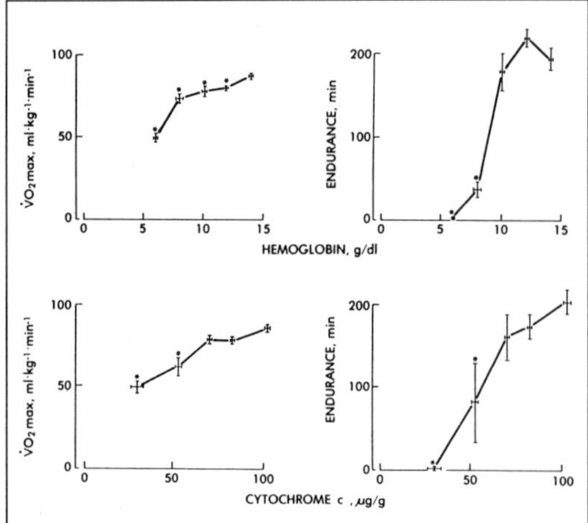

*Fig. 2. Maximal oxygen consumption (V_{O_2max}) and treadmill endurance capacity of rats plotted as functions of blood haemoglobin and gastrocnemius cytochrome c contents. The * symbol indicates where values differ from control rats fed a normal (50 mg iron per kg food) diet. Data from Perkkio et al.*[2].

endurance training, sprint training of laboratory rats improves V_{O_2max} similarly (≈ 15 per cent), but muscle mitochondrial respiratory capacity is little affected. Consequently, endurance capacity of sprint trained rats is little improved in comparison to untrained controls[4] (Table 3). From these experiments on the effects of different types of training on muscle mitochondrial content, V_{O_2max}, and running endurance, we concluded that both the capacity to transport and use oxygen are important determinants of exercise endurance. However, we demonstrated the relative importance of peripheral adaptations on capacity to sustain high rates of muscle cell respiration.

Work performance impairment and the extent of anaemia and tissue iron deficiency

According to Dallman[1], in sedentary individuals the manifestations of iron deficiency are subtle, whereas in the physically active iron deficiency results in impaired performance. As already noted, adult rats raised from weaning on an iron deficient diet are both anemic and have peripheral (e.g. mitochondrial) deficits (Fig. 1)[2,5]. Consequently, iron deficient rats display both low capacities to transport and use oxygen as well as depressed exercise endurance with the handicap for activity related to the severity of the deficiency (Fig. 2)[2,5–7]. In response to iron deficiency, there occur adaptations in levels of both iron-containing and other enzymes in liver and muscle mitochondria[7–9], and correction of anaemia by exchange transfusion of packed erythrocytes or short-term iron refeeding improves V_{O_2max}. However, even after correction of anaemia by refeeding (Fig. 3) or transfusion of packed erythrocytes (Fig. 4), mitochondrial deficits persist and endurance capacity is little improved until peripheral deficits are repaired (Fig. 2). These results again show the importance of iron adequacy for peripheral (mitochondria) adaptations in supporting sustained, submaximal exercise.

Table 1. Mitochondrial content of muscle, maximal oxygen consumption (vo_2max), and running endurance of endurance trained rats

		Endurance	
Paremeter	**Control group (n = 9)**	**Group (n = 9)[a]**	**Percentage difference**
Pyruvate-malate oxidase	15.5 ± 0.7	25.1 ± 1.2	+62
Succinate oxidase	20.1 ± 1.0	43.6 ± 1.2	+117
Palmitol carnitine oxidase	21.1 ± 2.6	50.4 ± 4.7	+138
Cytochrome oxidase	19.2 ± 0.8	38.3 ± 1.8	+99
Succinate dehydrogenase	14.9 ± 0.8	30.9 ± 1.8	+108
NADH dehydrogenase	17.5 ± 0.8	27.9 ± 1.7	+59
Choline dehydrogenase	25.9 ± 1.7	55.7 ± 3.8	+115
Cytochrome c (and C_1)	16.2 ± 0.6	31.6 ± 1.2	+95
Cytochrome a	18.2 ± 0.7	36.5 ± 1.6	+101
Average mitochondrial parameters			+99
V_{O_2max} (ml/kg/min)	76.6 ± 1.2	87.7 ± 2.0	+14.5
Maximal endurance (max)	36.3 ± 2.2	182.6 ± 10.4	+408

[a]All endurance-trained values higher than controls,($P < 0.01$)
*$P < 0.01$ control *vs* endurance trained .
Data from Davies *et al.*[2]

Table 2. Correlation matrix for muscle oxidases V_{O_2max}, and maximal endurance[a]

Paremeter	Pyruvate-malate oxidase	Palmitol carnitine oxidase	$V_{O_2}max$ (weight normalized)	Maximal endurance
Cytochrome oxidase	0.95	0.93	0.74	0.92
Pyruvate-malate oxidase	–	0.89	0.68	0.89
Palmitol carnitine oxidase	–	–	0.71	0.91
V_{O_2max} (weight normalized)	–	–	–	0.70

[a]All correlations reported were statistically significant (P <0.01).
Data from Davies *et al.*[3].

Table 3. Muscle cytochrome content

Parameter	Control	Sprint trained	Percent change
Cytochrome c+c_1	13.6 ± 0.6	14.4 ± 0.5	0
Cytochrome a	6.5 ± 0.4	7.1 ± 0.6	0
Cytochrome	2.1 ± 0.09	2.0 ± 0.10	0
V_{O_2max} (ml/kg/min)	61.1 ± 0.4	70.5 ± 1.7	15.4[a]
Endurance	32.9 ± 1.8	35.9 ± 1.5	0

[a]P < 0.01 controls *versus.* endurance trained.
Data from Davies *et al*[3].

To further explore relationships between anaemia and tissue iron deficiency on exercise endurance, we made endurance-trained rats acutely anaemic. Exchange transfusion of plasma for whole-blood in previously endurance trained rats significantly decreased V_{O_2max}, but these acutely anaemic, but previously endurance-trained rats with elevated mitochondrial and tissue iron contents displayed far superior endurance than did iron-sufficient, but untrained rats[6]. Again, the importance of tissue iron adequacy for exercise endurance was indicated.

Increased glucose dependency and gluconeogenesis

It has long been known that, during exercise, anaemic individuals display elevated circulating glucose and lactate levels, and so there was suspicion that iron deficiency increased glycolytic metabolism. Further, in recognition that lactacidemia in iron deficient individuals during exertion could have been due to decreased clearance as well as increased production, we conducted studies utilizing primed-continuous infusion of [^{3}H]- and [^{14}C]-glucose in rats during rest and exercise. Isotope infusion was accomplished through previously implanted jugular catheters, and arterial blood was sampled from a left carotid artery catheter. Rates of oxygen consumption, carbon dioxide production, and glucose oxidation were determined by means of a computerized, rapid flow open-circuit calorimetry system. Our results indicate that even at rest iron deficient rats with anaemia and mitochondrial lesions display increased blood glucose flux (Fig. 5) and oxidation as well as increased glucose recycling, a measure of gluconeogenesis (Fig. 6)[11]. Additionally, using [^{14}C]-lactate we observed that rats made

Fig. 3. Parameters of arterial oxygen transport (haematocrit), muscle respiratory capacity (pyruvate oxidase), and physical performance during treadmill running ($\dot{V}O_{2max}$, and endurance) following dietary iron repletion in deficient rats. Note that $\dot{V}O_{2max}$ tracks the marker for arterial O_2 transport, whereas endurance tracks the mitochondrial marker. Data from Davies et al.[5].

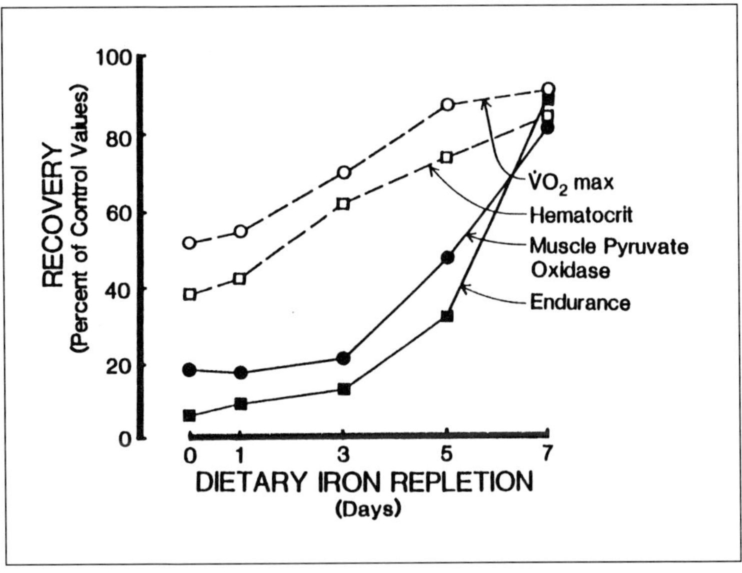

Fig. 4. $\dot{V}O_{2max}$, maximal treadmill running speed achieved during assessment of $\dot{V}O_{2max}$, and endurance during a standardized, continuous treadmill running test in control and iron deficient rats. Half the deficient rats had anaemia repaired by exchange transfusion of packed donor erythrocytes for whole (anaemic) blood. Sham animals had blood withdrawn and immediately replaced. Note the improvement in $\dot{V}O_{2max}$, but not running endurance in transfused iron deficient rats which retain mitochondrial and other peripheral iron deficits. From Davies et al.[6].

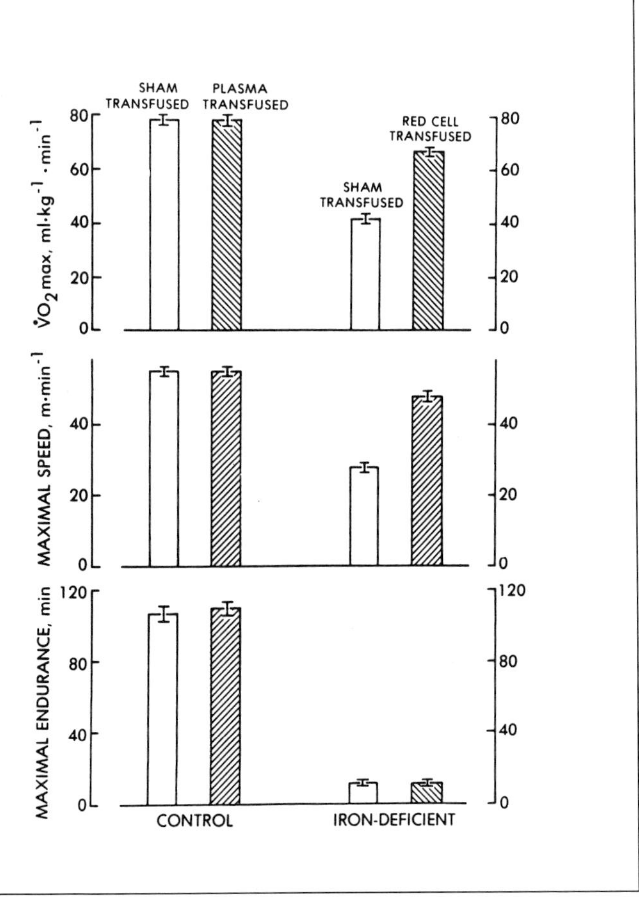

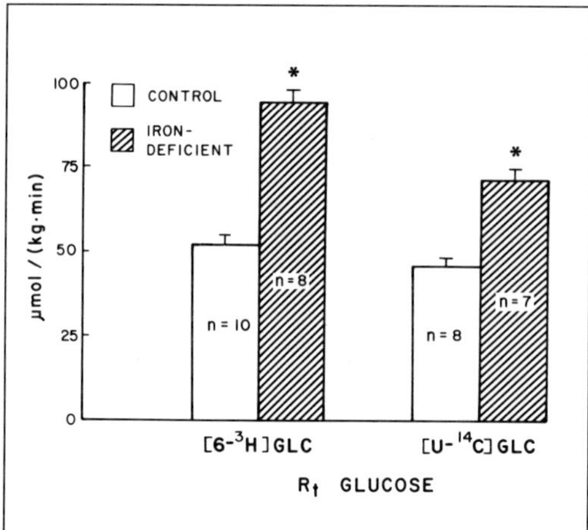

*Fig. 5. Glucose turnover (R_t) determined on resting control and iron deficient rats studied by primed continuous infusion of irreversible [6-^{3}H]- and reversible [U-^{14}C]glucose tracers. * Indicates significant differences between iron deficient and sufficient rats. Note significant increases determined by both tracers ($p<0.05$). From Henderson et al.[11].*

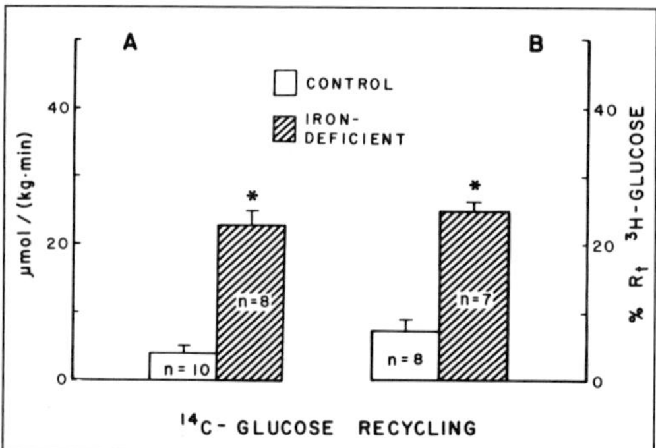

*Fig. 6. Glucose recycling rates determined on resting control and iron deficient rats determined from differences in the fluxes of [6-^{3}H]- and [U-^{14}C]glucose. Data given in absolute terms (A, left) and as per cent of the irreversible (^{3}H) glucose flux * Indicates significant differences between iron deficient and sufficient rats.(B, right). From Henderson et al.[11].*

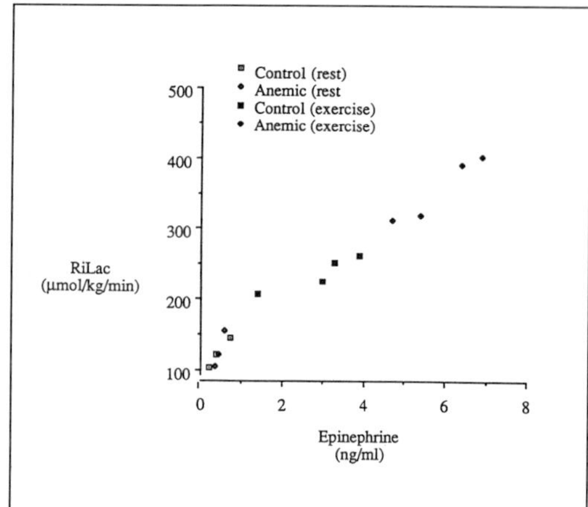

Fig. 7. Blood lactate flux (RiLac), determined from primed-continuous infusion of [U-^{14}C]lactate, as a function of arterial (epinephrine) in adult rats studied at rest and during exercise. Some rats were made acutely anaemic by exchange transfusion of plasma for whole blood, r = 0.99. From Gregg et al.[14].

acutely anaemic by exchange-transfusion of plasma for whole blood displayed increased lactate flux, even at rest[12].

In terms of endocrine signaling, the shifts in patterns of substrate utilization involving increased glucose disposal and lactate production associated with anaemia and iron deficiency appear to be associated with sympathoadrenal responses and elevated levels of circulating catecholamines. In contrast, insulin and glucagon levels are little affected[13]. Because increasing the precursor (lactate) supply for gluconeogenesis could be considered a partial compensation to metabolic consequences of iron deficiency, we explored aspects of lactic acidosis on glucose homeostasis in iron deficient and anaemic rats using a variety of techniques[14–18]. These technical approaches involved studies on intact exercising anaemic and iron sufficient rats using isotopic tracers, studies on hepatocytes isolated from iron sufficient and iron deficient rats, and studies on intact exercising iron deficient rats using pharmacological blocking agents.

With [^{3}H]- and [^{14}C]-glucose tracers we confirmed that gluconeogenesis is increased in acutely anaemic rats during treadmill running[14]. Also, we showed using primed continuous infusions of [^{14}C]-lactate and [^{3}H]-glucose in acutely anaemic rats that while glucose disposal (R_d) is increased, lactate production (R_a) is elevated and lactate clearance is decreased during exercise[15]. Thus, lactic acidosis in exercising anaemic rats is due to both increased lactate production and decreased clearance. We further showed that the rate of lactate production was highly correlated with the circulating epinephrine level (Fig. 7). An association between lactate and catecholamines in anaemic individuals has been a frequent observation. Further, it is an observation in well-nourished humans exercising at sea level and high altitude (*vide infra*).

To determine if iron deficiency affected the intrinsic capacity for gluconeogenesis, we compared the abilities of hepatocytes isolated from iron sufficient and iron deficient rats for gluconeogenesis from lactate plus pyruvate. We focused on lactate as it is acknowledged to be the most important gluconeogenic precursor, and because elevated circulating lactate is commonly observed in exercising iron deficient and anaemic individuals[1]. However, we also studied the effects of iron deficiency on gluconeogenesis from alanine and glycerol. We found that whereas all hepatocytes responded in a dose-response manner to the three carbon precursors (Fig. 8) as well as norepinephrine, iron deficiency *decreased* the intrinsic capacity of hepatocytes for gluconeogenesis. Thus, we concluded that the elevated rates of gluconeogenesis observed in iron deficient[11,12] and anaemic[14,15] rats during exercise must be attributable to changed hormonal signaling or precursor supply.

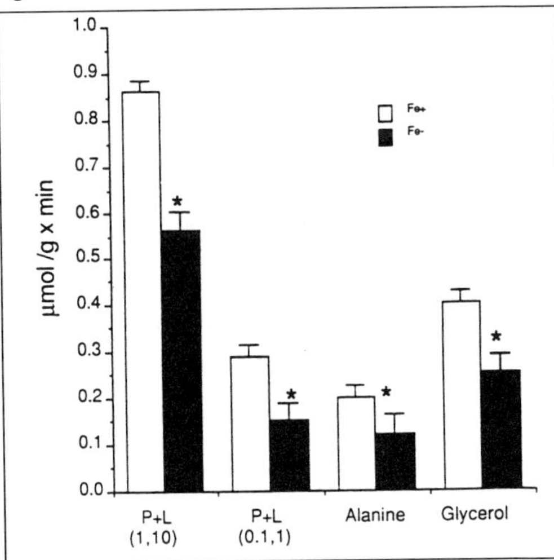

*Fig. 8. Capacities for gluconeogenesis from 3-carbon precursors (lactate (L), pyruvate (P), alanine and glycerol) in hepatocytes isolated from iron sufficient (Fe+) and -deficient (Fe–) rats. * Indicates significant differences between iron deficient and sufficient rats.Depressed capacities for gluconeogenesis were observed in hepatocytes from deficient rats studied with all precursors and precursor concentrations. Data from Klempa et al.*[16].

To further explore the mechanism of increased gluconeogenesis in iron deficiency, we used the selective β_2-adrenergic blockade on lactate production and gluconeogenesis from lactate; in exercising iron deficient rats we utilized the selective blocker ICI 118,551[17]. In both iron sufficient and iron deficient rats, β_2 blockade resulted in decreased circulating lactate levels during rest and treadmill running. However, the effects were most pronounced in iron deficient animals, who suffered decreased blood glucose levels as a result of decreased lactate precursor supply for gluconeogenesis during exercise (Fig. 9)[17]. We interpreted the results to indicate that iron-deficient rats are dependent on gluconeogenesis to maintain blood glucose homeostasis.

To verify the importance of gluconeogenesis as compensation for iron deficiency, in another series of experiments we utilized mercaptopicolinic acid (MPA) to inhibit phosphoenolpyruvate carboxykinase (PEPCK) and block gluconeogenesis. We observed that gluconeogenic blockade with MPA resulted in elevated lactate, but low blood glucose in exercising iron deficient rats (Fig. 10)[18]. Thus, it is revealed from the results of studies using β_2 and gluconeogenic blockade that sympathetic responses can be extremely important in minimizing the effects of effects of iron deficiency on glucose homeostasis. Again, as pointed out by Dallman[1], dietary iron deficiency has greater effects on peripheral (e.g. muscle), than central (e.g. hepatic) iron stores. Thus, the coordinated effects of catecholamines, with epinephrine stimulating muscle glycogenolysis and glycolysis with concomitant lactate production, can be mitigated by the liver in which the capacity for glyconeogenesis can be maintained because of increased precursor supply and norepinephrine stimulation.

These adaptations in glucose flux and oxidation, and lactate production and gluconeogenesis are interpreted to represent *a shift towards use of more oxygen-efficient pathways* as more energy is available for a given oxygen flux is carbohydrate, rather than lipid is oxidized.

Tissue adaptations to iron deficiency

Because exercise training can improve muscle mitochondrial content (Table 1), we hypothesized that training may enable rats to partially compensate for the effects of dietary iron deficiency. Our initial attempts (Fig. 11), were at least partially successful and indicated that regular exercise could improve muscle mito-

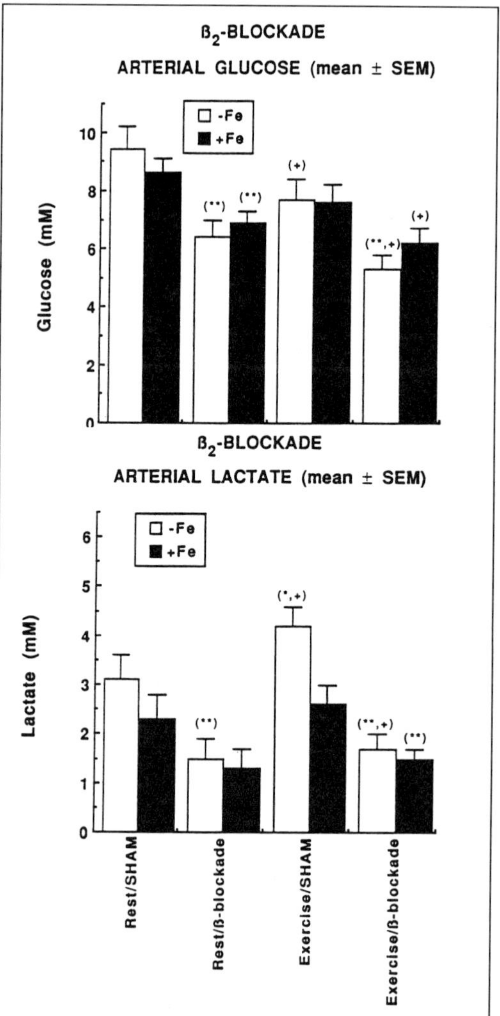

*Fig. 9. Arterial glucose (top) and lactate concentrations (bottom) in resting and exercising control (solid histogram bars) and iron deficient rats (open bars) with β_2-adrenergic blockade using ICI 118,551. Reducing muscle glycogenolysis by β_2 blockade causes a decline in gluconeogenic precursor (lactate) supply, and a concomitant fall in blood glucose, particularly in iron deficient rats. Data from Linderman et al.[17]. * Indicates significant differences between iron deficient and sufficient rats.. Sham animals injected with the same vehicle, but without drug.*

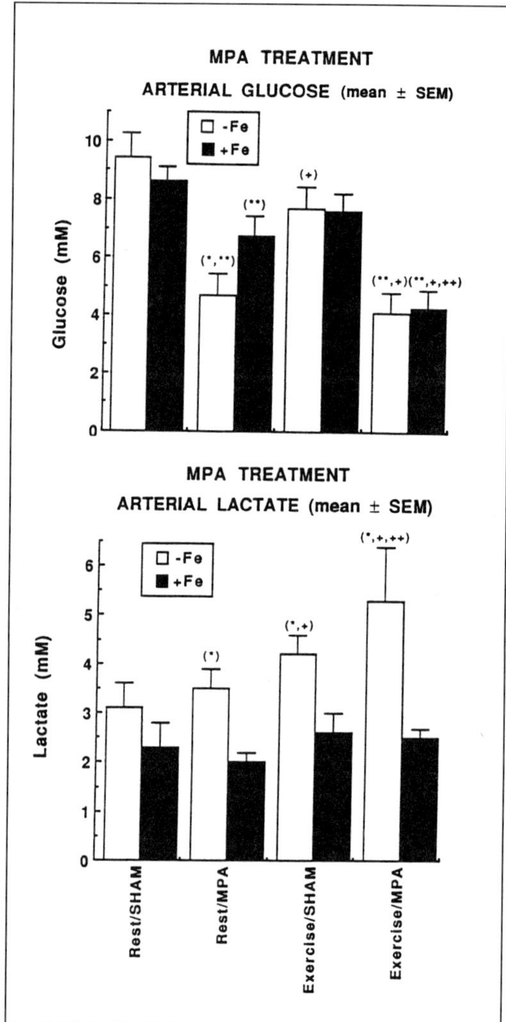

*Fig. 10. Arterial glucose (top) and lactate concentrations (bottom) in resting and exercising control (solid histogram bars) and iron deficient rats (open bars) injected with the blocker of gluconeogenesis, mercaptopicolinic acid (MPA). Blocking lactate removal by gluconeogenic blockade results in blood lactate accumulation, and a concomitant fall in blood glucose, particularly in iron deficient rats. Data from Linderman et al.[18]. * Indicates significant differences between iron deficient and sufficient rats.. Sham animals injected with the same vehicle, but without drug.*

chondrial content and, with it, exercise endurance[7]. Subsequently, we demonstrated that, whereas the proportionality among mitochondrial components is maintained in many circumstances (e.g. endurance training, Table 1), in iron deficiency, the proportionality is not maintained. For instance, we found that, whereas iron containing cytochrome c of the electron transport chain (ETC) is depressed, the iron-containing TCA cycle enzymes citrate synthase and isocitrate dehydrogenase were maintained[9]. Further, we found that endurance training exaggerated the disproportionality between ETC and TCA cycle components of skeletal muscle mitochondria[10]. The relative increase in TCA cycle enzymes probably serves to compensate for the handicap in ETC components by correcting the mitochondrial redox potential towards normal.

Already, we have noted a shift towards glucose as a fuel accompanied iron deficiency. Whereas catecholamine stimulation signals peripheral glycogenolysis and hepatic gluconeogenesis, relative levels of insulin and glucagon are unaffected and apparent insulin action is increased. Because this latter effect could be associated with increased muscle levels of the insulin (and contraction) regulatable cell membrane glucose transport protein GLUT-4, we determined the

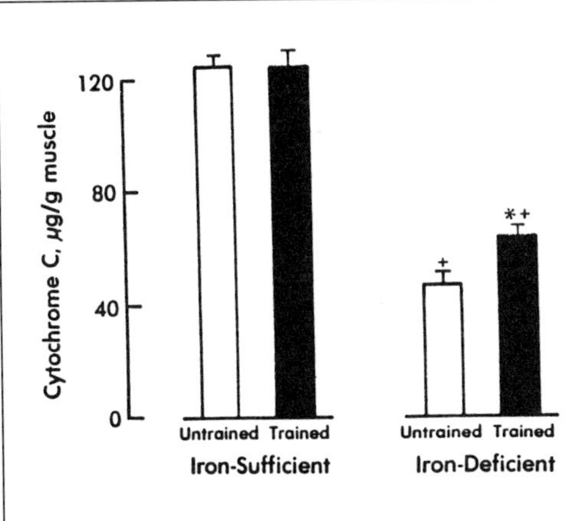

*Fig. 11. Dietary iron deficiency reduces gastrocnemius cytochrome c content, but mild endurance training allows for compensations in cytochrome c, and several other mitochondrial constituents. Data from Perkkio, et al.[7]. *Significantly different from iron-sufficient groups, + significantly different from untrained iron-deficient group, P<0.05.*

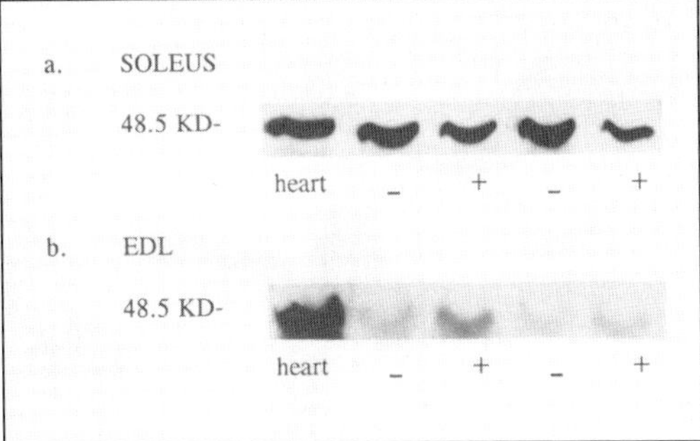

Fig. 12. Western blot analysis of GLUT 4 protein content using the polyclonal antibody ECU4 in soleus (a) and extensor digitorum longus (b) muscles form iron-deficient (–) and -sufficient (+) control rats. The insulin (and contraction) regulatable muscle cell glucose transport protein (GLUT 4) appears to increase in response to dietary iron deficiency, particularly in soleus (slow-oxidative) skeletal muscle. From Kern et al (unpublished).

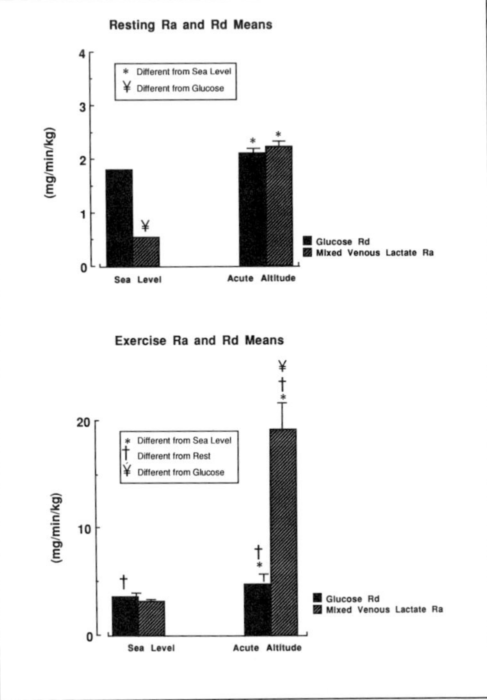

Fig. 13. Blood glucose and lactate kinetics at sea level (SL) and 4,300 m altitude in 6 men measured by primed-continuous infusion of [6,6-^{2}H]glucose and [3–^{13}C]lactate during rest and exercise at the same power output which elicited 50 per cent of the sea level VO_{2max}. Exercise and altitude exposure cause significant increases in blood glucose (R_a) and lactate (R_d) fluxes. Data from Brooks et al.[19].

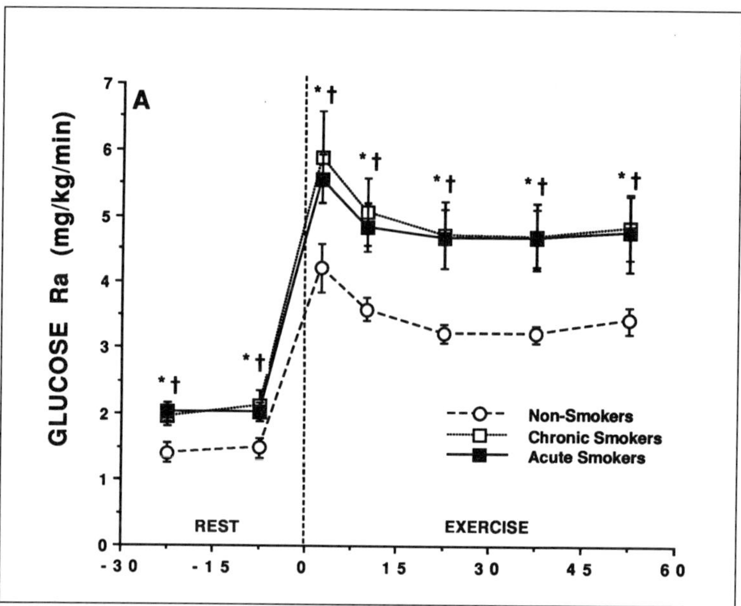

*Fig. 14. Glucose rate of appearance (R_a) determined by primed-continuous infusion of [6,6-^{2}H]glucose rest and exercise at 50 per cent of $Vo_{2max.}$ in non smokers (open circles) and in chronic smokers who had abstained for 12 h (open squares) or just smoked two cigarettes (closed squares). Smoking increases the blood glucose flux. * Significant difference between non-smokers and acute smokers; † significant difference between non-smokers and chronic smokers, $P<0.05$. Data from Colberg et al.*[20]

effect of dietary iron deficiency on muscle GLUT-4 content (Fig. 12). This result of increased soleus (predominantly slow-oxidative fibre type) GLUT-4 is one possible explanation of how in iron deficiency unchanged levels of insulin could be accompanied by increased glucose disposal rates.

Cross-adaptive responses

We conclude by reiterating that these studies using laboratory rats as models of dietary iron deficiency and anaemia are of interest because they provide means to probe and understand the consequences of developmental and chronic iron deficiency in humans. Further, the results also are relevant to human adaptations to other conditions that stress oxygen transport and utilization, such as intense physical exercise, altitude exposure and cigarette smoking. For instance, we have observed that altitude results in hypoxia, catecholamine signalling, lactacidaemia, increased glucose dependence, elevated circulating lactate, increased gluconeogenesis from lactate, and increased apparent insulin action (Fig. 13)[19]. In fact, our previous experiments using the iron deficient rat model provided good insight into the design and conduct of studies on men exposed to 4300 m altitude on Pikes Peak. Similarly, by stimulating catecholamine secretion and biasing metabolism towards increased glucose dependence, cigarette smoking has some effects similar to iron deficiency (Fig. 14)[21]. Again, use of the iron deficient and anaemic rat model offers the means to manipulate and understand many of these cross-adaptive responses common to conditions in which capacities of oxygen transport and utilization are stressed.

References

1. Dallman, P.R. (1982): Manifestations of iron deficiency. *Serum Hematol.* **19,** 19–30.
2. Perkkio, M.V., Jansson, L.T., Brooks, G.A., Refino, C.J. & Dallman, P.R. (1985): Work performance in iron deficiency or increasing severity. *J. Appl. Physiol.* **58,** 1477–1480.
3. Davies, K.J.A., Packer, L. & Brooks, G.A. (1981): Biochemical adaptation of mitochondria, muscle, and whole animal respiration to endurance training. *Arch. Biochem. Biophys.* **209,** 539–559.
4. Davies, K.J.A., Packer, L. & Brooks, G.A. (1982): Exercise bioenergetics following sprint training. *Arch. Biochem. Biophys.* **215,** 260–265.
5. Davies, K.J.A., Maguire, J.J., Brooks, G.A., Dallman, P.R. & Packer, L. (1982): Muscle mitochondrial bioenergetics, oxygen supply and work capacity during iron deficiency and repletion. *Am. J. Physiol.* (Endocrinol. Metab. 5) **242,** E418–E427.
6. Davies, K.J.A., Donovan, C.M., Refino, C.J., Brooks, G.A., Packer, L. & Dallman, P.R. (1984): Distinguishing effects of anemia and muscle iron deficiency on exercise bioenergetics in the rat. *Am. J. Physiol.* (Endocrinol. Metab. 9) **246,** E535–E543.
7. Perkkio, M.V., Jansson, L.T., Henderson, S.A., Refino, C.J., Brooks, G.A. & Dallman, P.R. (1985): Work performance in the iron deficient rat: Improved endurance with exercise training. *Am. J. Physiol.* (Endocrinol. Metab. 12) **249,** E306–E311.
8. Azevedo, J.L., Willis, W.T., Brooks, G.A., Turcotte, L.P., Rovner, A.S. & Dallman, P.R. (1989): Reciprocal changes of muscle oxidases and liver enzymes to iron repletion. *Am. J. Physiol.* (Endocrinol. Metab. 19) **256,** E401–E405.
9. Willis, W.T., Henderson, S.A., Brooks, G.A. & Dallman, P.R. (1987): Effects of iron deficiency and training on mitochondrial enzymes in skeletal muscle. *J. Appl. Physiol.* **62,** 2442–2446.
10. Willis, W.T., Dallman, P.R. & Brooks, G.A. (1988): Physiological and biochemical correlates of increased work performance in trained iron-deficient rats. *J. Appl. Physiol.* **65,** 256–263.
11. Henderson, S.A., Dallman, P.R. & Brooks, G.A. (1986): Glucose turnover and oxidation are increased in the iron deficient rat. *Am. J. Physiol.* (Endocrinol. Metab. 13) **250,** E414–E421.
12. Brooks, G.A., Henderson, S.A. & Dallman, P.R. (1987): Increased glucose dependence in resting, iron-deficient rats. *Am. J. Physiol.* **253,** (Endocrinol. Metab. 16) E461–E466.
13. Zinker, B.A., Dallman, P.R. & Brooks, G.A. (1993): Augmented glucoregulatory hormone concentrations during exhausting exercise in mildly iron-deficient rats. *Am. J. Physiol.* (Regulatory Integrative Comp Physiol 34) **265,** R863–R871.
14. Gregg, S.G., Kern, M. & Brooks, G.A. (1989): Acute anemic increases glucose dependence during endurance exercise. *J. Appl. Physiol.* **66,** 1874–1880.
15. Gregg, S.G., Mazzeo, R.S., Budinger. T.F. & Brooks, G.A. (1989): Acute anemia increases lactate production and decreases clearance during exercise. *J. Appl. Physiol.* **67,** 756–764.
16. Klempa, K.L., Willis, W.T., Chengson, R., Dallman, P.R. & Brooks, G.A. (1989): Iron deficiency decreases gluconeogenesis in isolated rat hepatocytes. *J. Appl. Physiol.* **67,** 1868–1872.
17. Linderman, J.K., Dallman, P.R., Rodriguez, R.E. & Brooks, G.A. (1993): Lactate is essential for the maintenance of euglycemia in iron deficient rats at rest and during exercise. *Am. J. Physiol.* (Endocrinol. Metab. 27) E662–E667.

18. Linderman, J.K., Brooks, G.A., Rodriguez, R.E. & Dallman, P.R. (1994): Glucoregulation in gluconeogenesis-inhibited iron deficient rats. *J. Nutr.* **124,** 2131–2138.

19. Brooks, G., Wolfel, E.E., Groves, B.M., Bender, P.R., Butterfield, G.E., Cymerman, A., Mazzeo, R.S., Sutton, J.R., Wolfe, R.R. & Reeves, J.T. (1992): Muscle accounts for glucose disposal but not lactate release during exercise after acclimatization to 4,300 m. *J. Appl. Physiol.* **72,** 2435–2445.

20. Colberg, S.R., Casazza, G.A., Horning, M.A. & Brooks, G.A. (1994): Increased dependence on blood glucose in smokers during rest and exercise. *J. Appl. Physiol.* **76,** 26–32.

Iron Nutrition in Health and Disease, edited by Leif Hallberg and Nils-Georg Asp
 pp. 195–203

Chapter 19

Iron deficiency, anaemia and physical performance

Björn Ekblom

Department of Physiology and Pharmacology, Karolinska Institute, P.O. Box 5626 S-11486, Stockholm, Sweden

Summary

Endurance physical exercise increases the losses of iron through sweat, urine and gastrointestinal bleedings. This will increase the iron metabolism. Added to the basal iron requirement it might increase the risk of obtaining iron deficiency and even anaemia in endurance athletes, specifically women athletes. However, the frequency of iron deficiency and anaemia in endurance athletes is no greater than in the general Western population.

There seems to be no major negative effect on physical performance and related physiological factors in athletes with non-anaemic iron deficiency. This does not, however, exclude possible negative effects on mental performance[54] and other functions.

Iron supplementation to non-anaemic iron deficient althletes is without major effect, which is in disagreement with corresponding studies in animals[75]. However, it must be emphasized that a status of non-anaemic iron deficiency may easily lead to a relative anaemia, which has a negative influence on performance.

Introduction

Iron and iron metabolism during exercise have been areas of interest for many years and excellent reviews have been published[16,27,30,47].

This chapter focuses on the effects of supplementation of iron and variation of iron stores on physical performance and the physiological adaptation to exercise in man. However, one important point in this discussion is the role of the haemoglobin concentration ([Hb]).

Previous studies have shown that even a small increase or decrease in [Hb] - either acutely[13,24–26,32,33] or over several weeks[3,23] - can influence maximal aerobic power (V_{O_2max}), physical performance and the physiological adaptation to exercise.

The results from these studies show that there is no compensation for a decreased oxygen carrying capacity within the oxygen transport system chain to keep V_{O_2max} unchanged. Physical performance, evaluated i.e. as time to exhaustion in a standardized heavy rate of work, changes in a corresponding way.

Even a small change in [Hb] within 'normal'ranges will have an effect on physical performance and V_{O_2max}. This is especially important to keep in mind when discussing the effect of iron supplementation in iron deficient subjects. Subjects in some studies[37,39] were iron deficient but, more importantly, relatively anaemic. That is, their [Hb] was lowered but remained above the lower limit of the normal distribution for respective genders. In this situation iron supplementation increases [Hb] and, as expected, the V_{O_2max} and physical performance.

Exercise and iron balance

Over 100 years ago, and as confirmed in many later studies[17,19,45,55], Kast[34] showed that there is a traumatic intravascular haemolysis during running and walking. However, the amount of haemolysis is fairly small compared to the daily normal turnover of RBC, so this factor cannot acount for any larger loss of iron, especially since most of this iron is taken care of[22].

Studies[8,36] have shown that the amount of iron lost in cell free sweat during exercise is in the range of 0.1–0.2 mg/l. Although athletes may sweat a lot this factor alone cannot cause a condition of iron deficiency in athletes.

However, a relatively more severe problem might be the loss of iron from bleeding in the gastrointestinal tract and the bladder. This is not an uncommon condition in endurance training athletes, especially if they are on some kind of medication, such as aspirin[58]. It has been estimated that in some athletes up to 0.7–1.0 mg of iron per day can be lost due to gastrointestinal bleeding[30,44,63] and from the bladder[4]. This must be of importance for the iron balance in those athletes, who experience such problems.

Thus, Haymes and Lamanca have estimated that the iron loss in endurance training athletes is on average 1.5–1.7 mg/day for men and 2.2–2.3 for women[30], the latter subjected to some variations due to amount of blood lost in menses[29]. During extreme situations, such as long-distance competitions, greater losses can occur[62].

Apart from the above-mentioned losses of iron another need of iron in athletes is the increased total Hb and myoglobin mass, induced by physical training. However, this increase per day is very small and can easily be accounted for by the normal diet.

Although intensive training has been reported to cause a reduction in haematological parameters[40,41], other studies have not found this[6,38,46,56]. There are several possible explanations for these differences, such as different type of athletes, different amounts and types of training, and differences in diets. It seem to be a common view, however, that the reduction in [Hb], Hct and RBC during a racing season in most athletes is not a consequence of a reduction of iron stores[18,28].

Iron status in athletes

It is obvious that iron metabolism is enhanced with intense physical training. However, will intense training increase the need for iron above the content provided by a well balanced diet and, thus, contribute to iron deficiency in athletes?

Iron deficiency (i.e. serum ferritin < 12 g/l, transferrin saturation < 18 per cent) and anaemia are frequently reported to occur in athletes at a frequency of a few per cent and higher[9,14,30,21,38,42,49,52,53,59,68,71]. Although there are some inconsistent data, a large majority of well designed studies have also shown that the prevalence of iron depletion and anaemia in athletes is no higher than in the general population[1,7,15,18,20,31,52,53,55,57,64,70,71,74]. Thus, even if some athletes do experience iron deficiency with or without anaemia, this condition does not occur more frequently than in the general population and probably occurs for the same reasons as in the general population.

One of the most important reasons for iron deficiency is a low intake of diatary iron. In athletes with a large energy intake this factor should not be a problem, since the intake of essential nutrients follows the total energy intake, at least in the Scandinavian diet, and thus is a guarantee for high a intake of iron in the athlete[5].

However, recent studies have shown an inverse relationship between iron indices and the amount of carbohydrate in the diet of athletes[67]. A carbohydrate-rich diet is important for restoring muscle and liver glycogen stores after training and competitions. Even if it can be compensated for by a higher intake of protein (mainly meat) it is possible that a high carbohydrate diet may cause a subnormal uptake of iron in some athletes. Despite this, it must be concluded that most athletes can keep a positive iron balance through a well-balanced diet[65,66,68].

Effects of iron supplementation

The problem here is in determining whether or not iron supplementation will increase physical performance and/or affect key physiological functions and parameters. Here there are some inconsistent data.

As expected, iron supplementation can increase maximal aerobic power and physical performance in anaemic subjects[37,39,51,61]. Magazanik *et al.*[41] studied the effect of iron supplementation and placebo in 28 latent iron deficient/mild anaemic young women during training. The increase in maximal aerobic power over a 7 week training programme was the same in the iron and placebo groups, despite the fact that [Hb] increased more in the treatment group.

Physical performance and related physiological factors in non-anaemic, non-iron deficient athletes are not affected by iron supplementation[65,72,73]. The interesting question relates to the effect of iron supplementation in non-anaemic but iron deficient athletes. Below, a brief summary is given of studies in which iron supplementation has been given to latent iron deficient but non-anaemic athletes, often in training. The important result is that [Hb] was more or less unchanged, whereas serum ferritin and other indices of iron status improved in comparison to levels before the supplementation period.

Ballin *et al.*[2] found some positive effects on lassitude, mood and concentration after iron supplementation in 29 female adolescents with initially low iron stores, but there were no effects on physical performance. Risser *et al.*[57] did not find any positive effects of iron supplementation on subjective ratings of physical performance or mood in a total of 100 female athletes from different sports.

Klingshirn *et al.*[35] studied non-anaemic iron deficient female runners in a double blind, 8 week, iron supplementation and training study. There were minor increases in V_{O_2max} and [Hb], and a substantial increase in treadmil endurance time, but with no difference between groups.

Matter *et al.*[43] studied 27 female runners in a double blind, supplementation-placebo fashion. No effect of iron supplementation on performance or V_{O_2max} was noted.

Newhouse *et al.*[48] studied 40 prelatent iron deficient female runners. After 8 weeks of supplementation there were no effects on anaerobic and aerobic performance tests, V_{O_2max}, ventilatory threshold or muscle enzyme data.

Nilsson *et al.*[50] studied 7 non-anaemic iron deficient athletes. After the supplementation period endurance time and V_{O_2max} were unchanged, while peak blood lactate concentration after maximal exercise decreased.

Rowland *et al.*[60] conducted a double blind, cross-over study for 4 weeks of iron supplementation in 14 initially iron deficient female runners (serum ferritin <20 g/l) but [Hb] values remained above lower normal limits (120 g/l). There was an increase in treadmill endurance time in the treatment compared to the placebo group, while V_{O_2max} was unchanged in treatment but increased in the placebo group. However, some minor changes in [Hb] occurred in the treatment but not the placebo group, which could explain part of the different results in the two groups. Schoene *et al.*[61] could not find any difference in maximal aerobic power or time to exhaustion after 2 weeks of iron supplementation in nine latent anaemic female athletes despite a marginal increase in [Hb] in both the treatment and the placebo groups.

The conclusion is that there seems to be no study showing any clear positive effects on performance or different physiological parameters after iron supplementation in iron deficient, non-anaemic subjects.

Experimental evidences of the role of iron in humans

Celsing and co-workers[11,12] studied nine young healthy, physically active males (mean age 28 years, height 183 cm and weight 77 kg), who were made anaemic by serial blood venesection for during 6–8 weeks. [Hb] decreased from on average from 146 to 106 g/l. The subjects were given a diet low in iron. After the anaemic period blood retransfusions of red blood cells restored the Hb concentration to pre-experimental level. Conventional laboratory parameters, such as serum ferritin and iron-binding capacity, showed that the subjects were iron deficient both before and after the reinfusion (Table 1). V_{O_2} and other physiological data were measured with conventional methods. Endurance was evaluated using a running test on the treadmill

Table 1. Laboratory values (mean ± SD) for three conditions.

Condition	Serum Iron (μmol/l)	Serum ferretin (μg/l)	Iron sat (%)	Hb (gl)
Control	18.4 ± 5.1	59.8 ± 41.7	40.1 ± 15.3	146 ± 9.6
Anaemic	4.3 ± 1.4	7.3 ± 1.7	7.1 ± 4.7	110 ± 7.1
Reinfusion	6.8 ± 3.8	9.1 ± 6.5	11.0 ± 6.0	145 ± 8.7
(Normal range)	(11-32)	(30-200)	(10-60)	(130-170)

Table 2. Values (mean ± SD) during the endurance test in control (C) and after reinfusion (R)

Parameter		At 25 min	At 35 min	At exhaustion
Respiratory Quote	C	0.99 ± 0.02	0.99 ± 0.02	0.99 ± 0.03
	R	0.98 ± 0.03	0.99 ± 0.03	0.99 ± 0.02
Blood lactate concentration (mM)	C	4.0 ± 1.0	6.7 ± 1.4	7.3 ± 1.6
	R	4.6 ± 1.2	7.5 ± 1.7	7.7 ± 1.9
Heart Rate (b min)	C	161 ± 8	176 ± 10	178 ± 7
	R	161 ± 10	176 ± 14	177 ± 14
RPE[a] (points)	C	14.4 ± 0.7	17.5 ± 1.6	18.7 ± 0.8
	R	14.8 ± 0.6	16.6 ± 1.0	18.6 ± 1.2

[a] RPE = rate or perceived exertion[3].

(work time about 45 min in the control test) at a speed corresponding to and above the anaerobic threshold[11,12].

After the transfusion of the red blood cells maximal aerobic power and physical performance were not different from pre-experimental levels. Blood lactate concentration during the submaximal endurance test were not different after the reinfusion (the non-anaemic, iron deficient test) compared to the control test before the start of the venesections (Table 2).

Muscle biopsies revealed that there was no difference between pre- and post-experimental values on either iron dependent and non-dependent glycolytic and oxidative muscle enzymes or on myoglobin concentration (Table 3).

Thus, 6–8 weeks of severe anaemia and some weeks of iron deficiency did not impair the physical performance as long as the Hb concentration was kept normal.

In order to study the effect of a longer period of iron deficiency on the peripheral factors mentioned above, Celsing *et al.*[10] took muscle biopsies from eight anaemic and iron deficient and nine haematological normal Indonesian subjects. It was concluded that chronic iron deficient anaemia with Hb concentration of 80–100 g/l or less did not impair the biological function of the skeletal muscle, since there was no relationship between the different enzymes or myoglobin and the Hb concentration, ferritin or other markers of the iron content of the body.

The conclusion from these experiments is that the peripheral metabolism system is not affected by iron deficiency without anaemia and is in agreement with the data of Thompson *et al.*[69] and Newhouse *et al.*[48].

Table 3. Data on enzyme activities (mean ± SD) in m. vastus lateralis and m. delteoideus for three conditions: C = control, A = anaemia, R = reinfusion

Muscle	Condition	6-Phosphate fructokinase	Hexokinase	Oxoglutarate dehydrogenase	Citrate synthase	Cytochrome c oxidase 30°C (μmol O_2/min/g wet wt)
Vastus lateralis	C	35 ± 12	1.6 ± 0.6	1.0 ± 0.2[b]	14 ± 4.7[c]	4.4 ± 1.8
(N=9)[a]	A	35 ± 5.9	1.4 ± 0.2	1.1 ± 0.3[b]	13 ± 2.2[c]	4.4 ± 1.1
	R	31 ± 5.8	1.6 ± 0.4	1.0 ± 3.6[b]	13 ± 3.6[c]	3.6 ± 1.7
Deltoidues	C	35 ± 4.9	1.5 ± 0.2	1.1 ± 0.3	11 ± 2.9	3.3 ± 1.0
(*n*=6)	A	34 ± 9.4	1.6 ± 0.4	1.1 ± 0.3	12 ± 4.9	3.7 ± 1.6
	R	25 ± 4.0	1.3 ± 0.3	0.8 ± 0.3	8.9 ± 3.3	2.7 ± 1.0

[a]N, number of subjects
[b]N=7
[c]N=8

References

1. Balaban, E.P., Cox, J.V., Snell, P., Vaughan, R.H. & Frenkel, E.P. (1989): The frequency of anemia and iron deficiency in the runner. *Med. Sci. Sports Exerc.* **21,** 643–648.
2. Ballin, A., Berar, M., Rubinstein, U., Kleter, Y., Hershkovitz, A. & Meyters, D. (1992): Iron state in female athletes. *Am. J. Dis. Child* **146,** 803–805.
3. Berglund, B. & Ekblom, B. (1991): Effect of recombinant human erythropoietin treatment on blood pressue and some hematological parameters in healthy males. *J. Int. Med.* **229,** 125–130.
4. Blacklock, N.J. (1977): Bladder trauma in the long distance runner - 10 000 metre haematouria. *Br. J. Chol.* **49,** 129–32.
5. Blixt, G. (1965): A study on the relation between total calories and single nutrients in Swedish food. *Acta Soc. Med. Upsala* **70,** 117.
6. Blum, S.M., Sherman, A.R. & Boileau, R.A. (1986): The effects of fitness-type exercise on iron status in adult woman. *Am. J. Clin. Nutr.* **43,** 456–63.
7. Brotherhood, J., Brozovic, B. & Pugh, L.G.C. (1975): Haematological status of middle- and longdistance runners. *Clin. Sci. Molecul. Med. **48,** 139–145.*
8. Brune, M., Magnusson, B., Persson, H. & Hallberg, L. (1986): Iron losses in sweat. *Am. J. Clin. Nutr.* **43,** 438–443.
9. Casoni, I., Borsetto, Cavicchi, A., Marnitelli, S. & Conconi, F. (1985): Reduced haemoglobin concentration and red cell haemoglobinization in Italian marathon and ultramarathon runners. *Int. J. Sports Med.* **6,** 176–179.
10. Celsing, F., Ekblom, B., Sylvén, C., Everett, J. & Åstrand, P.O. (1988): Effect of chronic iron deficiency anaemia on myoglobin content, enzyme activity and capillary density in human skeletal muscle. *Acta Med. Scand.* **223,** 451–457.
11. Celsing, F., Blomstrand, E., Werner, B., Pihlstedt, P. & Ekblom, B. (1986): Effects of iron deficiency on endurance and muscle enzyme activity in man. *Med. Sci. Sports Exerc.* **18,** 156–161.
12. Celsing, F., Nyström, J., Pihlstedt, P., Werner, B. & Ekblom, B. (1986): Effect of long-term anaemia and retransfusion on central circulation during exercise. *J. Appl. Physiol.* **61,** 1358–1362.

13. Celsing, F., Svedenhag, J., Pihlstedt, P. & Ekblom, B. (1987): Effect of anaemia and stepwise-induced polycythemia on maximal aerobic power in individuals with high and low haemoglobin concentration. *Acta Physiol. Scand.* **29,** 47–54.

14. Clement, D.B. & Asmundson, R.C. (1982): Nutritional intake and hematologiscal parameters in endurance runners. *Phys. Sportsmed.* **10,** 37–43.

15. Clement, D., Asmundson, B. & Medhurst, C. (1977): Hemoglobin values: comparative study of the 1976 Canadian Olympic team. *Can. Med. As. J.* **117,** 614–616.

16. Cook, J.D. (1994): The effect of endurance training on iron metabolism. *Semin. Hematol.* **31,** 146–154.

17. Davidsson, R.L.J. (1964): Exertional heamoglobinuria. *J. Clin. Path.* **17,** 536–540.

18. Douglas, P.D. (1989): Effect of a season of competition and training on hematological status of women field hockey and soccer players. *J. Sports Med. Phys. Fitness* **29,** 179–183.

19. Dressendorfer, R.H., Wade, C.E., Keen, C.L. & Scaff, J.H. (1982): Plasma mineral levels in marathon runners during a 20-day road race. *Phys. Sportsmed.* **10,** 113–118.

20. Dufaux, B., Hoederath, A., Streitberger, A., Hollman, W. & Assmann, G. (1981): Serum ferritin, trasferrin, haptoglobin and iron in middle-and longdistance runners. *Int. J. Sports Med.* **2,** 43–46.

21. Ehn, L., Carlmark, B. & Höglund, S. (1980): Iron status of athletes involved in intense physical activity. *Med. Sci. Sports Exerc.* **12,** 61–64.

22. Eichner, E.R. (1992): Sports anaemia, iron supplements and blood doping. *Med. Sci. Sports Exerc.* **24,** 315–318.

23. Ekblom, B. & Berglund, B. (1991): Effect of erythropoietin administration on maximal aerobic power in man. *Scand. J. Med. Sci. Sports* **1,** 125–30.

24. Ekblom, B., Huot, R., Stein, E.M. & Thorstensson, A. (1975): Effect of changes in arterial oxygen content on circulation and physical performance. *J. Appl. Physiol.* **39,** 71–75.

25. Ekblom, B., Goldbarg, A.N., Gullbring, B. (1972): Response to exercise after blood loss and reinfusion. *J. Appl. Physiol.* **33,** 175–180.

26. Ekblom, B., Wilson, G. & Åstrand, P.-O. (1976): Central circulation during exercise after venesection and reinfusion of red blood cells. *J. Appl. Physiol.* **40,** 379–383.

27. Fogelholm, M. (1992): *Vitamin and mineral status of physically active people. Dietary intake and blood chemistry in athletes and young people*. p. 227. Finland, ML: Turku, Publications of the Social Insurance Institution.

28. Gugleilmini, C., Casoni, I., Patracchini, M., Manfredini, F., Grazzi, G., Ferrari, M. & Conconi, F. (1989): Reduction of Hb levels during the racing season in nonsideropenic professional cyclists. *Int. J. Sports Med.* **10,** 352–356.

29. Hallberg, L., Hogdahl, A.M., Nilsson, L., Rybo, G. (1966): Menstrual blood loss – a population study. *Acta Obst. Gyn. Scand.* **45,** 320–351.

30. Haymes, E.M. & Lamanca, J.J. (1989): Iron loss in runners during exercise. Implications and recommendations. *Sports Med.* **7,** 277–285.

31. Haymes, E.M. & Spillman, D.M. (Iron status of women distance runners, sprinters and control women. *Int. J. Sports Med.* **9,** 430–33.

32. Kanstrup, I.-L. & Ekblom, B. (1982): Acute hypervolemia, cardiac performance and aerobic power during exercise. *J. Appl. Physiol.* **52,** 1186–1191.

33. Kanstrup, I.-L. & Ekblom, B. (1984): Blood volume and hemoglobin concentration as determinants of maximal aerobic power. *Med. Sci. Sports Exerc.* **16,** 256–262.

34. Kast, A. (1966): (Title unknown). *Dtsch. Med. Wschr.* 1884; 10: 840. as referenced by Payne BB. Low plasma haptoglobin in march haemoglobinuria. *J. Clin. Path.* **19,** 170–72.

35. Klingshirn, L.A., Pate, R.R., Bourque, S.P., Davis, J.M. & Sargent, R.G. (1992): Effect of iron supplementation on endurance capacity in iron-depleted female runners. *Med. Sci. Sports Exerc.* **24,** 819–824.

36. Lamanca, J.J., Haymes, E.M., Daly, J.A., Mofatt, R.J. & Waller, M.F. (1984): Sweat iron loss of male and female runners during exercise. *Acta Med. Scand.* **216,** 149–155.

37. LaManca, J.J. & Haymes, E.M. (1993): Effects of iron repletion on V_{O_2max}, endurance and blood lactate in women. *Med. Sci. Sports Exerc.* **25,** 1386–1392.

38. Lampe, J.W., Slavin, J.L. & Apple, F.S. (1986): Poor iron status of women runners training for a marathon. *Int. J. Sports Nutr.* **7,** 111–117.

39. Lukaski, H.C., Hall, C.B. & Siders, W.A. (1991): Altered metabolic response of iron-deficient women during graded, maximal exercise. *Eur. J. Appl. Physiol.* **63,** 140–145.

40. Magazanik, A., Weinstein, Y., Dlin, R.A., Derin, M., Schwartzman, S. & Allalouf, D. (1988): Iron deficiency caused by 7 weeks of intensive physical exercise. *Eur. J. Appl. Physiol.* **57,** 198–202.

41. Magazanik, A., Weinstein, Y., Abarbanel, J., Lewinski, U., Shapiro, Y., Inbar, O. & Epstein, S. (1991): Effect of an iron supplement on body iron status and aerobic capacity of young training women. *Eur. J. Appl. Physiol.* **62,** 317–323.

42. Magnussion, B., Hallberg, L., Rossander, L. & Swolin, B. (1984): Iron metabolism and 'sports anaemia' – a hematological comparison elite humans and control subjects. *Acta Med. Scand.* **216,** 157–164.

43. Matter, M., Stittfall, T., Graves, J., Myburgh, K., Adams, B., Jacobs, P. & Noakes, T.D. (1987): The effect of iron and folate therapy on maximal exercise performance in female marathon runners with iron and folate deficiency. *Clin. Sci.* **72,** 415–422.

44. McMahan, F.L., Ryan, M.J., Larson, D. & Fisher, R.L. (1984): Occult gastrointestinal blood loss in marathon runners. *Ann. Intern. Med.* **100,** 846–847.

45. Miller, B.J., Pate, R.R. & Burgess, W. (1988): Foot impact force and intravascular hemolysis during distance running. *Int. J. Sports Med.* **9,** 56–60.

46. Moore, R.J., Friedl, K.E., Tulley, R.T. & Askew, E.W. (1993): Maintenance of iron status in healthy men during an extended period of stress and physical activity. *Am. J. Clin. Nutr.* **58,** 923–927.

47. Newhouse, I.J. & Clement, D.B. (1988): Iron status in athletes. An update. *Sports Med.* **5,** 337–352.

48. Newhouse, J.J., Clement, D.B., Taunton, J.E. & McKenzie, D.C. (1989): The effects of prelatent/latent iron deficiency on physical work capacity. *Med. Sci. Sports Exerc.* **21,** 263–268.

49. Nickerson, H.J., Holuberts, M., Tripp, A.D. *et al.* (1985): Decreased iron stores in high school female runners. *Am. J. Dis. Child* **139,** 1115–1119.

50. Nilson, K., Schoene, R.B., Robertsson, H.T., Escourrou, P. & Smith, N.J. (1981): The effect of iron repletion on exercise-induced lactate production in minimally iron-deficient subjects. *Med. Sci. Sports Exerc.* **13,** 92.

51. Ohira, Y., Edgerton, V.R., Gardner, G.W., Senewiratne, B., Barnard, R.J. & Simpson, D.R. (1979): Work capacity, heart rate and blood lactate responses to iron treatment. *Br. J. Haematol.* **41,** 365–372.

52. O'Toole, M.L., Iwane, H., Douglas, P.S., Applegate, E.A. & Hiller, W.D.B. (1989): Iron status in ultraendurance triathletes. *Phys. Sportsmed.* **17,** 90–102.

53. Plowman, S.A. & McSwegin, P.C. (1981): The effect of iron supplementation on female cross country runners. *J. Sports Med.* **21,** 407–416.

54. Pollitt, E., Hathirat, P., Kotchabhkdi, N.J., Missell, L. & Valyasevi, A. (1989): Iron defieciency and educational achievement in Thailand. *Am. J. Clin. Nutr.* **50,** 687–697.

55. Resina, A., Gatteschi, L., Giamberardino, M.A., Rubenni, M.G., Trabassi, E. & Troni, M.G. (1988): Comparison of RBC indices and serum iron parameters in trained runners and control subjects. *Hematologia* **73,** 449–454.

56. Ricci, G., Masotti, M., Depaoli Vitali, E., Vedovato, M. & Zanotti, G. (1988): Effects of exercise on hematological parameters, serum iron, serum ferritin, red cell 2,3-diphosphoglycerate and creatin content and serum erythropoietin in long-distance runners during basal training. *Acta Haematol.* **80,** 95–98.

57. Risser, W.L., Lee, E.J., Poindexter, H.B.W., West, M.S., Pivarnik, J.M., Rissner, J.M.H. & Hickson, J.F. (1988): Iron deficiency in female athletes: its prevalence and impact on performance. *Med. Sci. Sports Exerc.* **20,** 116–121.

58. Robertsson, J.D., Maughan, R.J. & Davidsson, R.L.J. (1987): Faecal blood loss in response to exercise. *Br. Med. J.* **295,** 303–305.

59. Rowland, T.W., Black, S.A. & Kelleher, J.K. (1987): Iron deficiency in adolescent endurance athletes. *J. Adol. Health Care* **8,** 322–326.

60. Rowland, T.W., Molly, B.D., Green, G.M. & Kelleher, J.F. (1988): The effect of iron therapy on the exercise capacity of nonanemic iron-deficient adolescent runners. *Am. J. Dis. Child* **142,** 165–169.

61. Schoene, R.B., Escourrou, P., Robertsson, H.T., Nilson, K.L., Parsons, J.R. & Smith, N.J. (1983): Iron repletion decreases maximal exercise lactate concentrations in female athletes with minimal iron-deficient anemia. *J. Lab. Clin. Med.* **102,** 306–312.

62. Seiler, D., Nagel, D., Franz, H., Hellstern, P., Leitzmann, C. & Jung, K. (1989): Effects of long-distance running on iron metabolism and hematological parameters. *Int. J. Sports Med.* **10,** 357–362.

63. Stewart, J.G., Ahlquist, D.A., McGill, D.B., Ilstrup, Swartz, S. & Owen, R.A. (1984): Gastrointestinal blood loss and anemia in runners. *Ann. Intern. Med.* **100,** 843–845.

64. Stewart, G.A., Steel, J.E., Toyne, A.H. & Stewart, M.J. (1972): Observations on the hematology and the iron and protein intake of Australian Olympic athletes. *Med. J. Austral.* **2,** 1339–1343.

65. Telford, R.D., Catchpole, E.A., Deakin, V., Hahn, A.G. & Plank, A.W. (1992): The effect of 7 to 8 months of vitamin/mineral supplementation on athletic performance. *Int. J. Sports Nutr.* **2,** 135–153.

66. Telford, R.D., Catchpole, E.A., Deakin, V., McLeay, A.C. & Plank, A.W. (1992): The effect of 7 to 8 months of vitamin/mineral supplementation on the vitamin and mineral status of athletes. *Int. J. Sports Nutr.* **2,** 123–134.

67. Telford, R.D., Cunningham, R.B., Deakin, V. & Kerr, D.A. (1993): Iron status and diet in athletes. *Med. Sci. Sports Exerc.* **25,** 796–800.

68. Telford, R.D., Bunney, C.J., Catchpole, E.A., Catchpole, W.R., Deakin, V., Gray, B., Hahn, A.G. & Kerr, D.A. (1992): Plasma ferritin concentration and physical work capacity in athletes. *Int. J. Sports Nutr.* **2,** 335–342.

69. Thompson, C.H., Kemp, G.J., Taylor, D.J., Radda, G.K. & Rajagopalan, B. (1993): No evidence of mitochondrial abnormality in skeletal muscle of patients with iron-deficient anaemia. *A. Int. Med.* **234,** 149–154.

70. Watts, E. (1989): Athletes anaemia. *Br. J. Sp. Med.* **23,** 81–83.

71. Weight, L.M., Klein, M., Noakes, T.D. & Jacobs, P. (1992): 'Sports anemia' – A real or apparent phenomenon in endurance- trained athletes. *Int. J. Sports Med.* **13,** 344–347.

72. Weight, L.M., Myburgh, K.H. & Nakes, T.D. (1988): Vitamin and mineral supplementation. Effect on running performance in trained athletes. *Am. J. Clin. Nutr.* **47,** 192–195.

73. Weight, L.M., Noakes, T.D., Labadaros, D., Graves, J., Jacobs, P. & Berman, P.A. (1988): Vitamin and mineral status of trained athletes including the effects of supplementation. *Am. J. Clin. Nutr.* **47,** 186–191.

74. de Wijn, J.F., de Jongste, J.L., Mosterd, W. & Willebrand, D. (1971): Hemoglobin, paced cell volume, serum iron and iron binding capacity of selected athletes during training. *J. Sports Med. Phys. Fitn.* **11,** 42–51.

75. Willis, W.W., Gohil, K., Brooks, G.A. & Dallman, P.R. (1990): Iron deficiency: Improved exercise performance within 15 hours of iron treatment in rats. *J. Nutr.* **120,** 909–916.

Iron Nutrition in Health and Disease, edited by Leif Hallberg and Nils-Georg Asp
©1996 John Libbey & Company Ltd., pp. 205–217

Chapter 20

Brain iron: Function and dysfunction in relation to cognitive processes

S. Shoham[1], Y. Glinka[2], Z. Tanne[2] and M.B.H. Youdim[2]

[1]*Department of Research, Herzog Hospital, Jerusalem, Israel 91351;* [2]*Department of Pharmacology, Technion-Israel Institute of Technology, Israel 31096*

Summary

The histochemical distribution of iron (Perl's) and immunohistochemical distribution of ferritin (Fer), transferrin (Tf) and transferrin-receptor (TfR) in the hippocampus in iron deficiency have been documented for rats. In adults (over 6 months old), intense histochemical staining of iron was observed in the CA3 region. In young iron-supplemented rats (8 weeks old) this region did not stain for iron. In adults, ferritin-immunoreactive (Fer-ir) microglia formed a pattern overlapping the CA3–4 region and dentate gyrus. In young rats, Fer-ir microglia were observed in CA3 but their density was lower in CA4 compared to adult rats and there were no Fer-ir microglia in their dentate gyrus. In iron deficient rats, Fer-ir microglia appeared at CA3 but were not present at all in CA4 or dentate gyrus. To the best of our knowledge this is the first description of such an anatomical spread of ferritin-expression in hippocampal microglia in early development in rats and of retardation of this process in iron deficiency.

In both adults and young, Tf-ir oligodendrocytes were distributed throughout the hippocampus. Their lower numbers in iron deficiency may reflect poor myelination. However, TfR immunoreactivity changed from staining of both nerve cells and blood vessels in CA1–3 in early development to exclusive staining of blood vessels in adults.

In iron deficient rats neurons were TfR-ir but blood-vessels were generally not stained. These distribution patterns converge to produce a picture of retardation in hippocampal development in iron deficiency and thus a site of possible mechanisms of cognitive deficits.

Since the blood-brain barrier (BBB) is disrupted in iron deficient rats, the danger of dietary EAAs in iron deficiency should be considered. The present study explores hippocampal neurotoxicity after systemic injection of kainate, an agonist at glutamate receptors.

Six hours after administration of kainic acid, morphologic damage to nerve cells was observed in the hippocampal CA3 field of iron deficient rats, whereas in iron-supplemented rats, this region remained intact. Damage to the CA3 field after such a short time interval parallels the effect of kainate administration into the lateral cerebral ventricle. Thus, the vulnerability of the CA3 region of iron deficient rats may reflect disruption of the BBB to kainate. This possibility is currently being investigated and may lead to insights for prevention of dietary induced neurotoxicity in human iron deficiency. At 6 days after systemic kainate injection, damage to CA1–2 was observed in iron-supplemented rats, whereas in iron deficient rats this region was protected. This result may reflect the hazardous effects of iron in oxidative stress which has been shown to be one of the mechanisms of glutamate neurotoxicity.

Introduction

Iron is essential for several biochemical reactions in normal cell function[93]. The importance of iron at higher levels of function, such as learning and memory, has been suggested by the consequences of iron deficiency in humans. Children with iron deficiency suffer from apathy, short attention span, inability to concentrate, and they generally achieve low scores on intelligence tests[22,23,36]. This suggests that adequate supply of iron may place some constraints on cognitive function through the contribution of iron to normal development. To explore this question, animal models of nutritional iron deficiency have been developed and cognitive deficits have been demonstrated[38]. This chapter focuses first on studies which explored involvement of neurotransmitter systems in cognitive dysfunction in iron deficiency and then reviews work on proteins for iron regulation in the hippocampus of iron deficient rats.

Effects of iron deficiency on neurotransmitter systems

For a short time (1–15 min) after storage of new information in memory the ability to remember this information can be enhanced or diminished by a variety of treatments[18]. Several neurotransmitters or their agonists, including norepinephrine, dopamine, acetylcholine and several neuropeptides have been administered to rats after learning a new task and 24 h later rats that received the treatment have displayed better performance than controls who received a vehicle. The amygdala, septum, and hippocampus have been shown to be most important in mediation of these modulatory mechanisms[18]. Evidence was presented that in many cases of post-training neurotransmitter modulation of learning and memory is associated with modulation of emotional processes[20].

Since iron is essential for biosynthesis and metabolism of several neurotransmitters including peptides[2], and since emotional changes have been proposed as contributing factors in cognitive dysfunction in human iron deficiency in early childhood[22], there is reason to consider reports on alterations to neurotransmitter systems in iron deficiency as possible causal factors in cognitive dysfunction and indeed several studies have been conducted on this subject[2].

We have reported on the impairment of dopaminergic neurotransmission due to subsensitivity of the D2 receptor[6]. Several other lines of evidence support a relationship between iron metabolism and the D2 receptor and dopamine D2 receptor functions and behavior[38]. Although dopamine receptors are mostly associated with motor function, there is evidence that the D2 receptor has a role in consolidation of memory. After training in a new learning task (conditioned emotional response), microinjection of amphetamine or of a specific D2 receptor agonist (quinpirole) but not of a D1 agonist (SK&F38393) into the ventral striatum enhances performance 24 h after training[19].

There is evidence that several peptide neurotransmitters modulate learning and memory in a similar fashion[18]. Since there is elevation of some opio-peptide neurotransmitter levels in iron deficiency[38] this may also contribute to modulation of learning and memory in iron deficiency syndrome.

However, in iron deficiency, reduction in D2 receptors or any other neurotransmitter system is not likely to account for all aspects of cognitive dysfunction. If deprivation of iron is initiated post-weaning, then nutritional iron replacement normalizes the quantity of D2 receptors[6] and all other reported alterations in neurotransmitter systems[2]. Under the same conditions, it has been found that cognitive dysfunction persists, despite iron replacement[37]. Furthermore, in several cases of human iron deficiency in early childhood, cognitive function was not completely restored after iron replacement therapy[23]. Therefore, mechanisms aditional to changes in modulatory neurotransmitter systems must be involved. Since iron is essential for DNA and protein synthesis[2], its deprivation may disrupt normal development of anatomical systems in brain which are essential for learning.

Effects of iron deficiency on hippocampal development

Several anatomical systems are probably involved in cognition. However, the hippocampus, has been of particular interest because of its specialization in learning associations between stimuli. The ability of the hippocampal circuitry to learn associations has been demonstrated in the paradigm of long term potentiation (LTP) using slices of a hippocampus *in vitro*[16]. Stimuli in the form of electrical potentials are administered to specific subregions of the hippocampal slice. Subsequently, electrophysiological recordings demonstrate that the hippocampal neuronal circuitry has learned the association between the stimuli. There is evidence that these hippocampal processes are essential for normal learning and memory of the whole organism[1]. In addition, hippocampal circuitry is involved in modulation of affective responses which contribute to performance in various learning and memory tasks[20].

In early development, hippocampal neuronal circuitry is susceptible to interference. Thus, at the age of weaning, exposure of rats to impoverished or enriched environments can modulate hippocampal learning as demonstrated by the LTP paradigm[14]. It is conceivable that deprivation of iron at post-weaning age, may also interfere with normal hippocampal development, which might then contribute to the cognitive dysfunction associated with iron deficiency.

As a first step, we asked whether deprivation of iron alters the anatomical distribution of proteins of iron regulation in the hippocampus. Such alterations, if discovered, may point to sites where further investigation may reveal interference with the development of synaptic mechanisms essential for learning.

To explore this question systematically it is necessary to briefly review the flow of information in the hippocampus. The hippocampus is conventionally divided into zones labelled CA1, CA2, CA3, CA4 and the dentate gyrus. The flow of information from the entorhinal cortex passes first through the dentate gyrus and then to the CA3–4 region. Then information flows out from the hippocampus through the fornix but some information continues to flow within the hippocampus from CA3 to CA1–2.

In both adult rats and humans, iron accumulates in the dentate gyrus and CA3–4[4,17]. The anatomical distribution of proteins regulating iron has been explored in the hippocampus of developing[12,32], adult and ageing[4] rats. These proteins include transferrin, transferrin receptor, and ferritin. Transferrin is the mobilization protein for iron and is expressed mainly in oligodendrocytes[2,10]. Transferrin- receptor is the protein which enables the transport of the transferrin-iron complex from the extracellular environment into a cell and is located on neurons, glia and on blood vessels[2] where it controls transport of iron from blood. Ferritin is considered as the storage protein of iron and is expressed mainly in oligodendrocytes but also in microglia and under some conditions in astrocytes[2].

The present study compares the anatomical distribution of cells in the hippocampus, expressing the above proteins in three groups of rats: adult (over 6 months old), young on iron-supplemented diet and young on iron deficient diet.

Experiment 1

Effects of nutritional iron deficiency on the anatomical distribution of iron and of proteins of iron regulation in the hippocampus were studied.

Methods

Sprague-Dawley rats (21 days old) had access to food and distilled water *ad libitum*. The iron deficient group received a diet low in iron (5 ppm) for 5 weeks, whereas control rats were given the same diet with added ferrous sulfate. The experimental diet was as described by Tanne *et al.*[33]. The extent of iron deficiency was established by measuring the haemoglobin level which was in the iron deficient group and in the iron-supplemented group.

After 5 weeks rats were anaesthetized with pentobarbital sodium. The brain was fixed by transcardial perfusion of 4 per cent paraformaldehyde then by further immersion fixation for 1 h at 4 °C. After immersion in 10 per cent sucrose PBS brains were cut on a cryostat. Thaw-mounted sections (15 µm thick) were used for histochemical staining of iron and floating sections (30 µm thick) were used for immunohistochemistry.

The histochemical staining for iron was a modification of that used by Hill and Switzer[17]. The modification was the addition of 0.1 per cent sodium dodecyl sulfate to the reaction medium to enhance penetration[21].

Polyclonal antibodies to human ferritin and transferrin were provided by Sigma (Rehovot, Israel). A monoclonal antibody to transferrin receptor (clone OX26) was purchased from Chemicon, USA. Dilution of all antibodies was 1:500. Standard biotin-avidin-peroxidase staining was performed.

Results and discussion

Perl's histochemical stain

In adult rats, intense staining was obtained in the inner layer of the far lateral CA3 region (Fig. 1b). Staining of neuropil was observed along with staining of oligodendrocytes. This pattern replicates earlier observations by others[17,32]. In young rats, iron-supplemented or iron deficient, no histochemical staining of iron was obtained in the hippocampus (Fig. 1d). However, in the globus pallidus, in iron-supplemented rats, clusters of oligodendrocytes and the perimeter of some blood vessels in the globus pallidus were stained (Figs 2b and 2c) thus showing that at some regions iron accumulation was already present but not in the hippocampus.

Ferritin

In adult rats, ferritin-immunoreactive (Fer-ir) oligodendrocytes and microglia were scattered

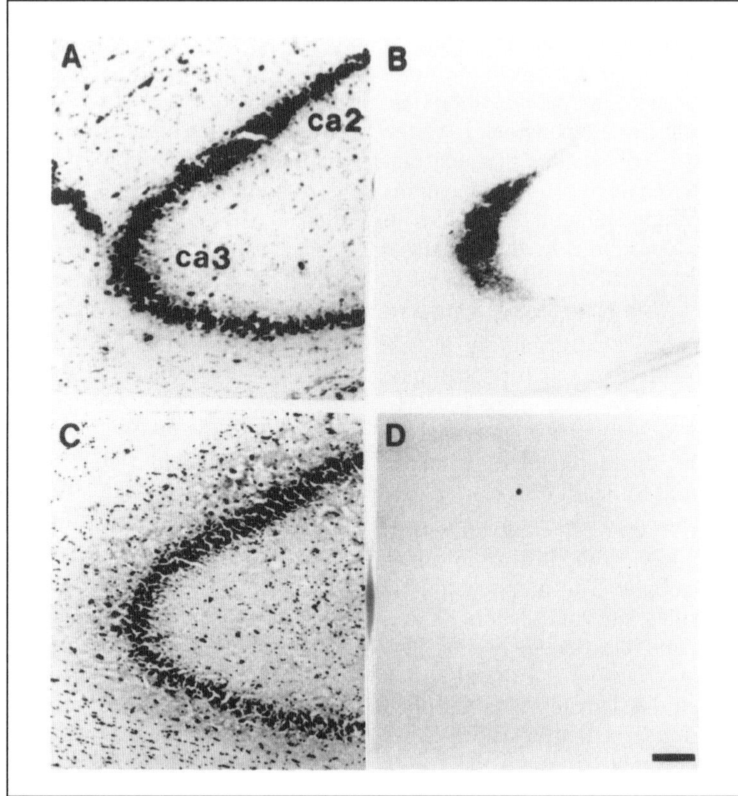

Fig. 1. Perl's iron histochemistry, comparing the CA3 region in adult and young rats. (a) Adult rat, cresyl violet staining demonstrates the organization of the CA3 region. (b) In an adjacent section from the same rat, Perl's iron histochemistry demonstrates accumulation of iron in CA3. (c) Young rat; cresyl violet staining demonstrates the CA3 region. (d), In an adjacent section from the same rat, no iron accumulation is detected. Calibration bar is 100 μm.

along the extent of CA3, CA4, and dentate gyrus (Fig. 2f and Fig. 4). Ferritin-ir microglia were more numerous and were dispersed with more or less fixed intervals. In young iron-supplemented rats, ferritin-ir microglia were arranged similar to the adult pattern from the CA3 region up to a distance towards CA4 (Fig. 4). This suggests that the organization of ferritin-ir microglia parallels development in the rat hippocampus. As the rat matures, the field of dispersion of Fer-ir microglia advancess from CA3 toward the dentate gyrus. In a study comparing adult and aged rats, a general increase in the number of Fer-ir microglia was described[4]. To our knowledge, the present report is first to describe a developmental trend in the anatomical organization of Fer-ir microglia. However, the functional significance of this pattern remains unknown.

Normally, oligodendrocytes and not microglia are thought to be mainly responsible for iron-storage[2], although under some conditions, such as in myelin-deficient mice, microglia appear to be recruited for iron storage[8]. In the present study, hippocampal microglia were not stained by Perl's iron histochemistry (Fig. 1d). Thus, the functional significance of the developmental spread of ferritin expression in hippocampal microglia (Fig. 4) does not seem related to iron storage.

Another functional interpretation may be based on the fact that microglia respond to changes in the status of synaptic innervation. In the hippocampus, microglia become active in response to denervation of the entorhinal input[13]. Perhaps the spread of ferritin expression in hippocampal microglia along the course of normal develop-

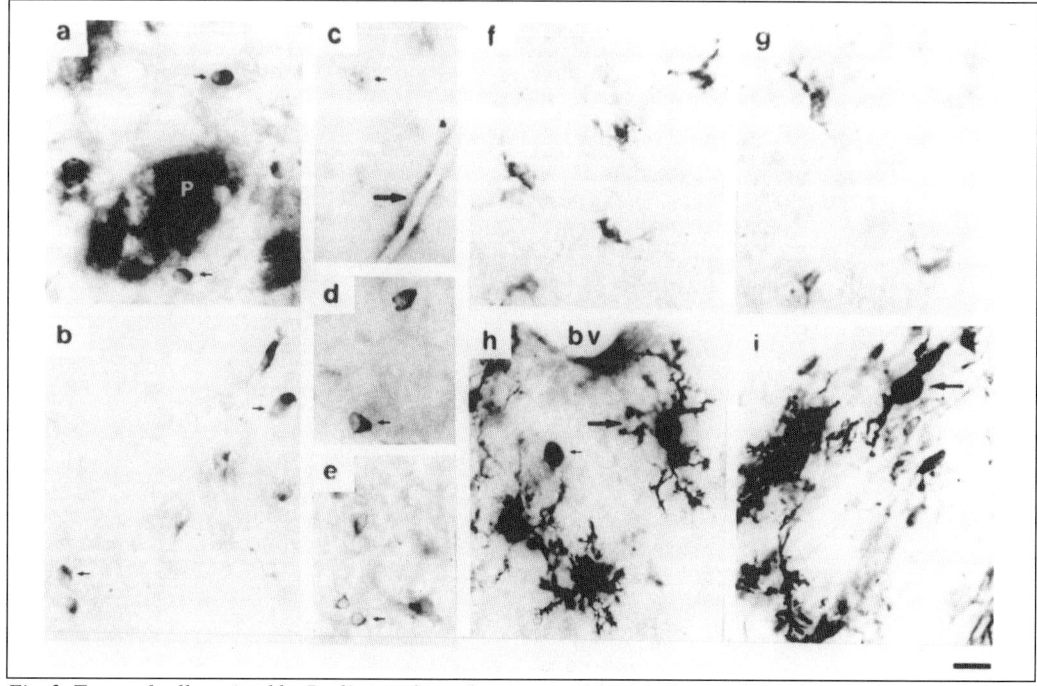

Fig. 2. Types of cells stained by Perl's iron histochemistry and ferritin immunohistochemistry. (a) In adults, Perl's stain demonstrates both oligodendrocytes and myelin patches (P). (b) In young rats, only oligodendrocytes are stained. (c) In young rats, on iron-supplemented diet, Perl's stain demonstrated iron along the wall of blood vessels in the globus pallidus. (d) and (e) display ferritin immunoreactive oligodendrocytes in iron-supplemented and iron-deficient rats, respectively. (f), and (g) demonstrate hippocampal ferritin-ir microglia in both iron-supplemented and iron-deficient rats respectively. (h) In young animals, some ferritin-ir oligodendrocytes near blood vessels (bv) displayed a full dendritic tree (arrow). This was not seen in adult rats except at the site of excitatory amino acid injection (i). Calibration bar is 10 μm in all frames except for (c), in which it is 100 μm.

ment parallels the normal development of synaptic innervation patterns in the hippocampus, which are necessary for the normal imprinting of experience, i.e. learning and memory. The functional state of microglia in the course of development may be neurotrophic[28]. Direct evidence for activation of microglia in relation to 'synaptic stripping' has been demonstrated in a paradigm employing transient trauma to the facial nerve[28]. As in several other cells, expression of ferritin may reflect a functional state in which iron is required[35]. As hippocampal synaptic organization matures, microglia may be gradually recruited in a progression from CA3 towards CA4 and dentate gyrus. The recruited microglia may express ferritin since they require iron to mobilize some neurotrophic actions on synapses.

In iron deficient rats Fer-ir microglia were present in the far lateral CA3 region but their dispersion did not extend into CA4 or dentate gyrus (Fig. 4). If the spread of the field of Fer-ir microglia parallels development of synaptic innervation of the hippocampus, then there may be retardation in the normal development of synaptic innervation of the hippocampus in iron deficient animals. Currently we are exploring this question using various markers of synaptic innervation.

Transferrin

In adult rats, transferrin immunoreactive (Tf) oligodendrocytes were scattered throughout the hippocampus with no apparent overlap with a specific hippocampal subregion. In young iron-supplemented rats, the density of Tf. oligodendrocytes was lower than in the adults (Fig. 5). It has been suggested that the emergence of Tf-ir oligodendrocytes in development parallels the development of myelination[10]. Thus, it is

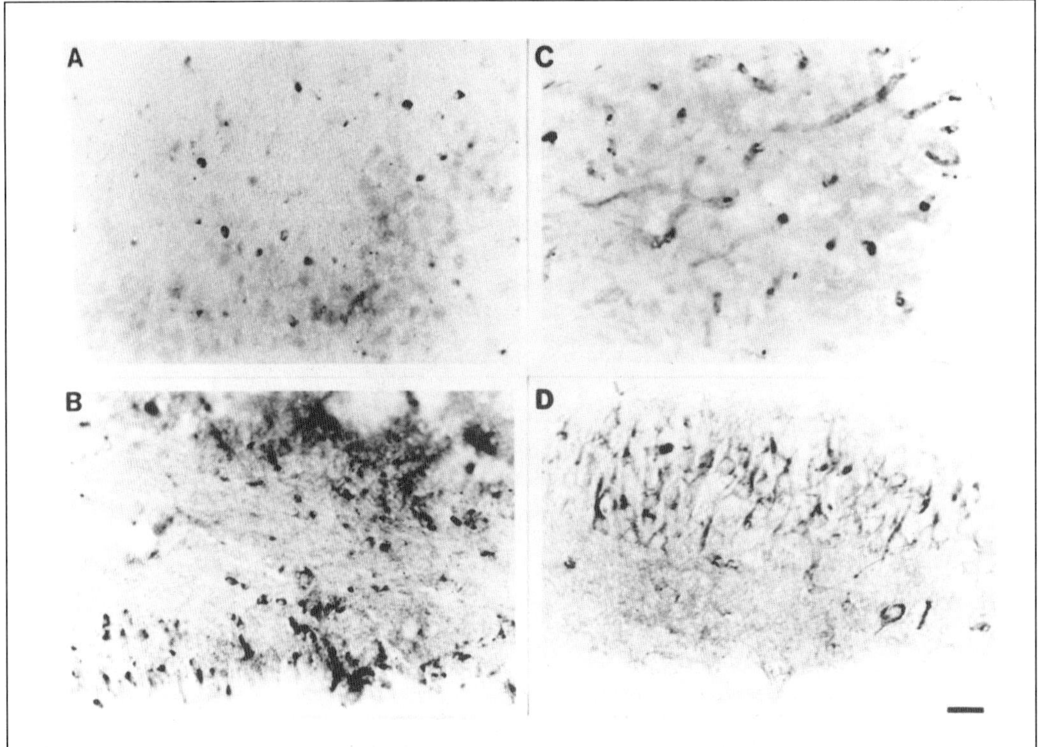

Fig. 3. (a) Transferrin-immunoreactive oligodendrocytes in the hippocamapl grey matter and (b) in white matter. (c) Transferrin receptor immunoreactive cells appeared in the hippocampus of iron-deficient animals, (b) but in iron-supplemented and adult animals blood vessels were stained and not cells. Calibration mark is 25 μm.

possible that the difference in density of Tf-ir oligodendrocytes reflects, in part, differences in the extent of myelination.

In iron deficient rats, very few Tf-ir oligodendrocytes were observed. Thus, it appears that in iron deficient rats the process of myelination was retarded. This observation is in agreement with the hypothesis of Connor and Fine[10], suggesting that the development of myelination requires mobilization of iron. It is however surprising that Tf-ir was lower in iron deficient rats in light of earlier reports on elevation of transferrin expression in iron deficiency[34]. Since Tf-ir oligodendrocytes were abundant in the striatum of our iron deficient animals, it is possible that the lowered number of Tf-ir oligodendrocytes in the hippocampus is a feature specific to this region at this developmental stage. Earlier developmental studies did not focus on transferrin in the hippocampus[10,32] but provided general quantitative trends of transferrin in development. Our immunohistochemical technique is qualitative and does not allow quantitative assessment of transferrin expression per cell. It is also conceivable that in order to compensate for the lack of iron, the fewer Tf-ir oligodendrocytes in iron deficient rats make more transferrin per cell than Tf-ir oligodendrocytes in iron-supplemented rats.

Transferrin receptor

In adult rats, transferrin receptor (TfR) immunoreactivity was observed in blood vessels, mostly in CA3–4 and in the dentate gyrus (Fig. 3c, Fig. 6). In young iron-supplemented rats, TfR-ir blood vessels were visualized in CA3 (Fig. 6). In iron deficient rats, very little TfR-ir was observed in blood vessels in the vicinity of the CA3 region (Fig. 6) but staining of nerve cells was prominent (Fig. 3d). Typically, the immunoreactivity was restricted to the outline of the cell body leaving the nucleus unstained.

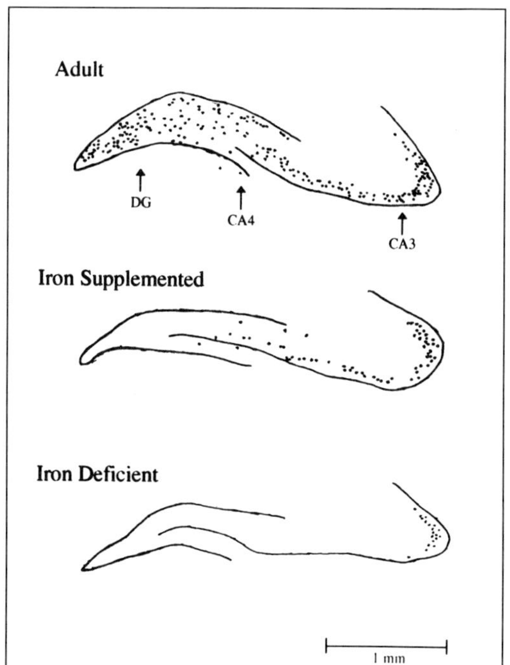

Fig. 4. Spread of ferritin-immunoreactive microglia in the hippocampus. In iron-supplemented young rats, microglia spread from CA3 into CA4, whereas in adults the whole region including CA3, CA4 and dentate gyrus contains Ferritin-ir microglia. In iron deficient rats, this spread is retarded.

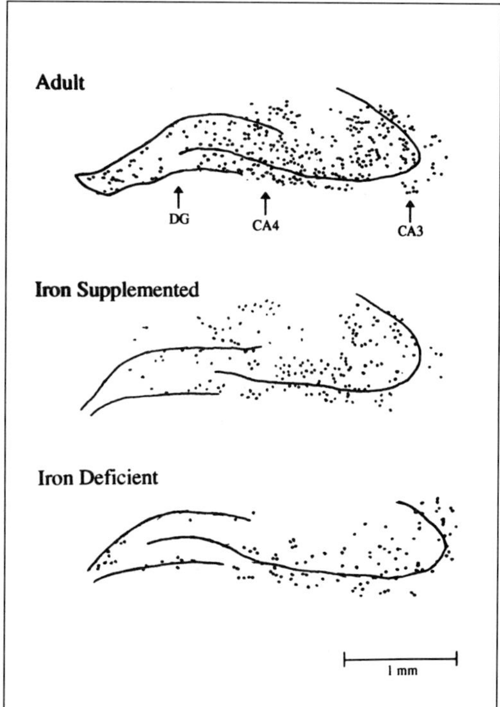

Fig. 5. Distribution of transferrin-immunoreactive oligodendrocytes. Tf-ir oligodendrocytes were more numberous in the adult compared to the young iron-supplemented rats. In iron deficiency there was less Tf-ir oligodendrocytes than in controls.

This pattern is also typical of pyramidal neurons in the motor cortex of the rat. Since expression of TfR on the pyramidal neurons of motor cortex is associated with their metabolic demands, it may be speculated that in iron deficient rats, the increased expression of TfR on hippocampal nerve cells reflects an attempt to maximize utilization of the little iron which is available in these animals.

Other investigators have reported increased overall expression of TfR in iron deficiency[24]. We find that the increase in hippocampus is selective to nerve cells in CA1–4. This is puzzling since it makes sense that in iron deficiency TfR expression should be increased in blood vessels to maximize transport of iron into brain. Perhaps the fact that the blood-brain barrier to iron remains open in iron deficiency[7] leaves the only site for additional increase in efficiency of iron mobilization at the neuronal expression of transferrin receptor.

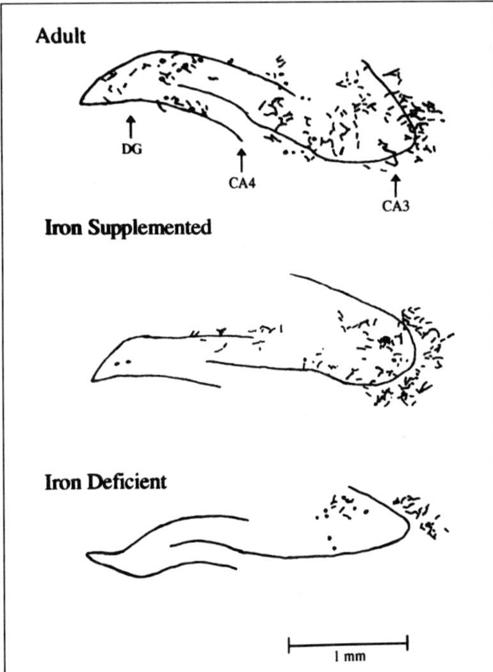

Fig. 6. Transferrin receptor immunoreactivity on blood vessels. In adults, blood vessels were stained throughout the extent of CA3 to the dentate gyrus. In young, iron-supplemented rats, blood vessels were stained in CA3 but their density decreased towards CA4. In iron deficiency the density of TfR-ir blood vessels in CA3 was less than in controls.

In summary, deprivation of iron in young rats retards development of the histochemical distribution of proteins for iron regulation in the hippocampus. This may reflect a general retardation of hippocampal development. Retardation in hippocampal development should be manifested in learning tasks which tap spatial orientation ability[1]. Indeed, in a study which employed a water maze in which rats had to employ spatial discrimination, iron deficient rats displayed more errors than controls[37]. Furthermore, dietary iron replacement failed to bring the level of performance to that of normal controls. Thus, the possible retardation in hippocampal maturation in iron deficiency is an imporant question which is currently being investigated in our laboratories.

Experiment 2

Vulnerability of hippocampal neurons to excitotoxic neurodegeneration in iron deficiency was investigated.

Introduction

One of the mechanisms which are known to cause neurodegeneration in a wide spectrum of human conditions involves excessive activation of excitatory amino acid receptors[11,26]. Such activation leads to various biochemical processes which damage cells, for example the opening of sodium channels which is followed by excessive water inflow and cell swelling, and the opening of calcium channels which disrupts calcium homeostasis, leading to impairment of many vital elements of cell function including increased oxidative stress[11].

The brain is protected from excitatory amino acids which may be found in foods by the blood-brain barrier (BBB), but early in development glutamate and other EAAs obtained from foods cross the BBB and, if they are administered at sufficiently high doses, they cause damage to central nervous system cells[29,30].

Iron deficiency retards maturation of the BBB to iron and alters the BBB to insulin[6]. Perhaps in iron deficiency there is also alteration in the BBB to EAAs which may enhance vulnerability to EAAs obtained with food. In the present study we explore toxicity of kainic acid in iron deficiency. This EAA activates a subset of glutamate receptors and its toxicity to the hippocampus in the rat has been amply documented[25–27]. It is of particular relevance here, that the distribution of kainate-induced damage to the hippocampus depends on the route of administration: systemic injection leads to damage of the CA1–2 fields[26], whereas intracerebro-ventricular (ICV) injection[27], a treatment which bypasses the BBB to kainate[3], leads to damage of the CA3 region. In the present study we examined the distribution of damage in the hippocampus after systemic administration of kainate.

Methods

Two groups of rats ($N = 8$ each) were prepared as described above, one iron deficient and one iron-supplemented. After the 4 weeks of dietary treatment, rats were injected subcutaneously with kainate dissolved in 0.1M phosphate buffered saline, pH 7.4. Two survival intervals were set. For the short survival interval (6 h), the dose of kainate was 15 mg/kg ($N = 6$ in each group) and for the long survival interval (5 days) the dose was 10 mg/kg ($N = 2$ in each group). Rats were sacrificed and brains processed as described above.

Results and discussion

Behavioural seizures

Similar to previous studies in which kainate was injected systemically[3,26], seizures developed within 2 h after injection and subsided around 6 h post-injection. Iron-supplemented and iron deficient rats displayed seizures of similar form and intensity. Apparently, the deprivation of iron has not affected the maturation of kainate-induced seizures since this maturation takes place before the 21st day of life in the rat[26].

Distribution of damage

At 6 h after kainate injection, the CA3 region in iron deficient animals was clearly damaged (Fig. 7b). In contrast, in the iron-supplemented group, the CA3 region remained intact (Fig. 7a). This finding suggests that in iron deficiency, systemically injected kainate has direct access to kainate receptors in the CA3 region, similar to studies in which kainate is injected into the

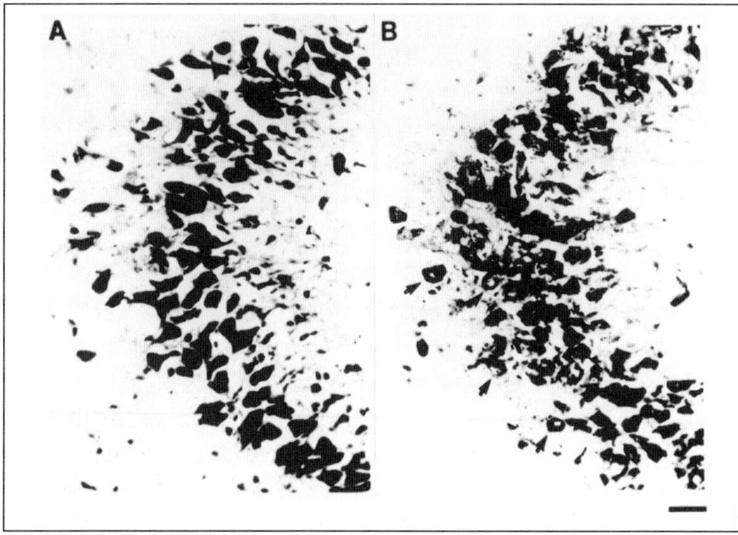

Fig. 7. Cresyl violet staining of the CA3 region at 6 h after systemic kainate injection. (a) iron-supplemented, (b) iron deficient. In iron-supplemented rats, the CA3 region remained largely intact, whereas in iron deficient rats there were nerve cells with vacuolation (arrows in B), and shrinkage of neurons and of the spaces between neurons. In addition, there was some loss of glial cells (small round cells in a) in iron deficient rats. Calibration bar is 25 µm.

cerebral ventricles thus bypassing the BBB to kainate[27]. Currently we are investigating the effects of iron deficiency on the BBB to kainate. If indeed iron deficiency alters the BBB to systemically circulating EAAs, then some of the severe irreversible cognitive impairments in nutritional iron deficiency may be related to EAA neurotoxicity.

At 5 days after systemic injection of kainate, the hippocampus of iron deficient rats was not further injured beyond some shrinkage of neurons in CA3 (Figs. 8a and 8b). However, in the iron-supplemented group the CA1–2 region was damaged while the CA3 region was still intact (Figs 8c and 8d). This pattern of damage in the iron- supplemented group suggests involvement of slow, calcium-mediated processes[26]. The fact that iron deficient rats were relatively protected from this type of damage is in agreement with the hypothesis of the contribution of iron to calcium-mediated neurodegeneration[39].

There are additional mechanisms by which the CA1–2 region in iron deficiency may be protected. One possibility is that damage to CA3, which occurs early in the iron deficient group, protects the CA1–2 region from further excitatory stimulation. Another possibility is that the lower levels of available iron diminish the risks of oxidative stress. Oxidative stress has been suggested to participate in EAA neurotoxicity[11] and iron has been suggested to contribute to the oxidative stress in several conditions[5,39]. In stroke, for example, in which EAAs are known to contribute to ischaemia- reperfusion damage, deprivation of iron protects from damage[31]. Thus, under some conditions, lack of iron may have some beneficial effects through protection against oxidative stress.

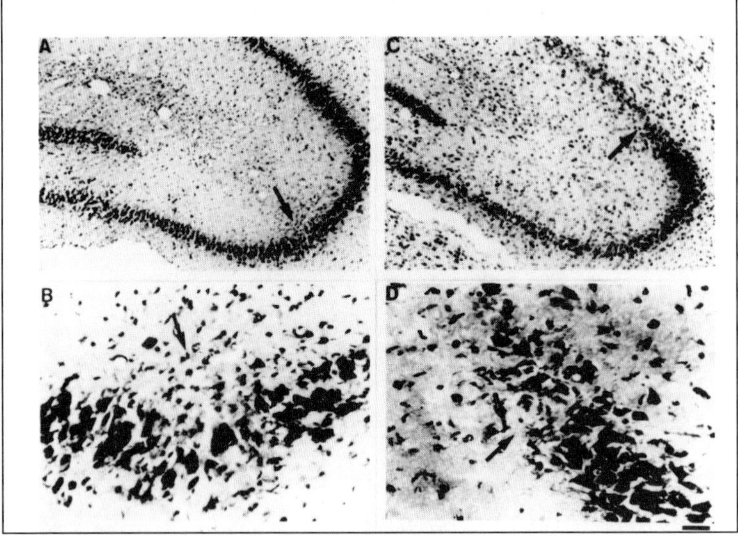

Fig. 8. Cresyl violet staining of the CA2 and CA3 regions at 5 days after systemic kainate injection. A, In an iron deficient rat, the CA2 region is largely intact but there is some damage to CA3 (arrow) and magnification in B. C, In an iron-supplemented rat, the CA2 region was severely damaged (arrow pointing at the border between CA2 and CA3) and magnification in D. Note in D, the sharp border between CA3 which is preserved in iron-supplemented rats and the loss of nerve cells in CA2. Calibration bar is 100 μm in A and C, and 25 μm in B and D.

References

1. Barnes, C.A. (1988): Spatial learning and memory processes: the search for their neurobiological mechanisms in the rat. *Trends Neurosci.* **11,** 163–169.

2. Beard, J.L., Connor, J.D. & Jones, B.C. (1993): Brain iron: location and function. *Prog. Food Nutr. Science* **17,** 183–221.

3. Ben-Ari, Y. (1985): Limbic seizure and brain damage produced by kainic acid: Mechanisms and relevance to human temporal lobe epilepsy. *Neuroscience* **14,** 375–403.

4. Benkovic, S.A. & Connor, J.R. (1993): Ferritin, transferrin and iron in selected regions of the adult and aged rat brain. *J. Comp. Neurol.* **338,** 97–113.

5. Ben-Shachar, D., Eshel, G., Finberg, J.P.M. & Youdim, M.B.H. (1991): The iron chelator desferrioxamine (Desferal) retards 6-hydroxydopamine-induced degeneration of nigrostriatal dopamine neurons. *J. Neurochem.* **56,** 1441–1444.

6. Ben-Shachar, D., Ashkenazi, R. & Youdim, M.B.H. (1986): Long-term consequence of early iron-deficiency on dopaminergic neurotransmission in rats. *Int. J. Dev. Neurosci.* **4,** 81–88.

7. Ben-Shachar D., Yehuda S., Finberg J.P.M., Spanier, I. & Youdim, M.B.H. (1988): Selective alteration in blood-brain barrier and insulin transport in iron-deficient rats. *J. Neurochem.* **50,** 1434–1437.

8. Connor, J.R. & Menzies, S.L. (1990): Altered cellular distribution of iron in the CNS of myelin deficient rats. *Neuroscience* **34,** 265–271.

9. Connor, J.R., Boeshore, K.L., Benkovic, S.A. & Menzies, S.L. (1994): Isoforms of ferritin have a specific cellular distribution in the brain. *J. Neurosci. Res.* **37,** 461–465.

10. Connor, J.R. & Fine, R.E. (1987): Development of transferrin-positive oligodendrocytes in the rat central nervous system. *J. Neurosci. Res.* **17,** 51–59.

11. Coyle, J.T. & Puttfarcken, P. (1993): Oxidative stress, glutamate, and neurodegenerative disorders. *Science* **262,** 689–695.

12. Dwork, A.J., Lawler, G., Zybert, P.A., Durkin, M., Osman, M., Willson, N. & Barkai, A.I. (1990): An autoradiographic study of the uptake and distribution of iron by the brain of the young rat. *Brain Res.* **518,** 31–39.

13. Fagan, A.M. & Gage, F.H. (1990): Cholinergic sprouting in the hippocampus: A proposed role for IL-1. *Exp. Neurol.* **110,** 105–120.

14. Green, E.J. & Greenough, W.T. (1986): Altered synaptic transmission in dentate gyrus of rats reared in complex environments: Evidence from hippocampal slices maintained *in vitro*. *J. Neurophysiol.* **55,** 739–750.

15. Greenough, W.T. & Bailey, C.H. (1988): The anatomy of memory: convergence of results across a diversity of tests. *Trends Neurosci.* **11,** 142–147.

16. Gustafsson, B. & Wigstrom, H. (1988): Physiological mechanisms underlying long-term potentiation. *Trends Neurosci.* **11,** 156–162.

17. Hill, J.M. & Switzer, R.R. III (1984): The regional distribution and cellular localization of iron in the rat brain. *Neuroscience* **11,** 595–603.

18. Izquierdo I. (1989): Different forms of post-training memory processing. *Behav. Neur. Biol.* **51,** 171–202.

19. Izquierdo I. (1992): Dopamine receptors in the caudate nucleus and memory processes. *Trends Neuroscience.* **13,** 7–8.

20. Izquierdo, I. & Medina, J.H. (1991): $GABA_A$ receptor modulation of memory: the role of endogenous benzodiazepines. *Trends Pharmacol. Sci.* **12,** 260–265.

21. LeVine, S.M. & Macklin, W.B. (1990): Iron-enriched oligodendrocytes: A reexamination of their spatial distribution. *J. Neurosci. Res.* **26,** 508–512.

22. Lozoff, B., Brittenham, G.M., Viteri, F.E., Wolf, A.W. & Urrutia JJ. (1982): Developmental deficits in iron deficient infants: Effects of age and severity of iron lack. *J. Pediatr.* **100,** 35–17.

23. Lozoff, B. (1989): Behavioural aspects of iron deficiency in infancy. *Am. J. Clin. Nutr.* **50,** (Suppl), 641–55.

24. Lu, J.P., Hayashi, K. & Awai, M. (1989): Transferrin receptor expression in normal, iron-deficient and iron-overloaded rats. *Acta Pathol. Jpn.* **39,** 759–764.

25. Lothman, E.W. & Collins, R.C. (1981): Kainic acid induced limbic seizures: metabolic, behavioral, electroencephalographic and neuropathological correlates. *Brain Res.* **218,** 299–318.

26. McDonald, J.W. & Johnston, M.V. (1990): Physiological and pathophysiological roles of excitatory amino acids during central nervous system development. *Brain Res. Rev.* **15,** 41–70.

27. Nadler, J.V., Perry, B.W., Gentry, C. & Cotman, C.W. (1980): Degeneration of hippocampal CA3 pyramidal cells induced by intraventricular kainic acid. *J. Comp. Neurol.* **192,** 333–359.

28. Nadajima, K. & Kohsaka, S. (1993): Functional roles of microglia in the brain. *Neurosci. Res.* **17,** 187–203.

29. Olney, J.W. & Ho, O.L. (1970): Brain damage in infant mice following oral intake of glutamate, aspartate or cysteine. *Nature* **227,** 609–610.

30. Olney, J.W. & Sharpe, I.G. (1969): Brain lesions in an infant rhesus monkey treated with monosodium glutamate. *Science* **166,** 386–388.

31. Patt, A., Horesh, I.R., Berger, E.M., Harken, A.H. & Repine, J.E. (1990): Iron depletion or chelation reduces ischemia/reperfusion-induced edema in gerbil brain. *J. Pediatr. Surg.* **25,** 224–227.

32. Roskams, A.J.I. & Connor, J.R. (1994): Iron, transferrin, and ferritin in the rat brain during development and aging. *J. Neurochem.* **63,** 709–716.

33. Tanne, Z., Coleman, R., Nahir, M., Shomrat, D., Finberg, J.P.M. & Youdim, M.B.H. (1994): Ultrastructural and cytochemical changes in the heart of iron-deficient rats. *Bioch. Pharmac.* **47,** 1759–1766.

34. Taylor, E.M., Crowe, A. & Morgan, E.H. (1991): Transferrin and iron uptake by the brain: effects of altered iron status. *J. Neurochem.* **57,** 1584–1592.

35. Theil, E.C. (1987): Ferritin, structure, gene regulation, and cellular function in animals, plants, and microorganisms. *Ann. Rev. Biochem.* **56,** 289–315.

36. Walter, T., Kowalskys, J. & Stekel, A. (1983): Effect of mild iron deficiency on infant mental development scores. *J. Pediatr.* **102,** 519–522.

37. Yehuda, S., Youdim, M.B.H. & Mostofsky, D.I. (1986): Brain iron-deficiency causes reduced learning capacity in rats. *Pharmacol. Biochem. & Behav.* **25,** 141–144.

38. Youdim, M.B.H., Ben-Shachar, D. & Yehuda, S. (1989): Putative biological mechanisms of the effect of iron deficiency on brain biochemistry and behavior. *Am. J. Clin. Nutr.* **50,** 607–617.

39. Youdim, M.B.H., Ben-Shachar, D. & Riederer, P. (1990): The role of monoamine oxidase, ironmelanin interaction, and intracellular calcium in Parkinson's disease. *J. Neural Transm.* **32,** (Suppl.), 239–248.

Iron Nutrition in Health and Disease, edited by Leif Hallberg and Nils-Georg Asp

Chapter 21

Effect of iron deficiency anaemia on cognitive skills in infancy and childhood

Tomas Walter

Hemotology Unit, Institute of Nutrition and Food Technology, University of Chile, Santiago 138-11, Chile

Summary

Animal experimentation has shown that early iron deficiency irreversibly affects brain iron content and distribution, which results in neurotransmitter and behavioural alterations. Even though extrapolation of animal data is often misleading, iron deficiency anaemia has been consistently shown to be associated with psychomotor delays in infancy. The areas most involved are language and body balance. In these infants iron therapy, in most cases, was not sufficient to reverse psychological effects even after complete correction of haematological measures.

These findings may imply that the impact of iron deficiency anaemia during infancy may be associated with irreversible adverse effects on cognitive performance. Careful follow-up studies of these infants at 5–6 years of age and preliminary data at ten years, has shown that cognitive disadvantages persist, now assessed with a comprehensive set of psychological tests that reliably predict future competence.

Thus, if once anaemia ensues, even timely and adequate iron therapy seems to be ineffective in reversing these behavioural and cognitive disadvantages; the only feasible way to approach this problem is by prevention of iron deficiency in infancy. Health authorities, having shown that treatment of iron deficiency anaemia is already too late to revert potential deficits, should strive to prevent iron deficiency with adequate fortification food strategies or supplementing targeted population groups.

Introduction

Iron has played an important and fascinating role in the history of mankind. Apart from the effect of anaemia severe enough to compromise cardiovascular function, the consequences of iron lack have been usually ignored. In spite of the long history of study and well understood treatment, iron deficiency remains the most common nutritional deficiency worldwide[1,2].

Animal studies have made an important contribution to understanding how the brain and iron interact. In animal studies it is possible to make certain that iron deficient animals differ from controls only in their dietary iron intake; adequate intake of other nutrients can be controlled, and genetic endowment and rearing conditions can be made the same.

Non-haem iron is unevenly distributed in the mammalian brain, with very high levels in some areas, such as the extrapyramidal basal ganglia.

Biochemical work has been conducted mostly with rats, because it is remarkable that the distribution of brain iron is similar in rats and humans. Brain iron accumulates from gestation to early adulthood, and brain iron levels are more sensitive to iron deficiency in very young animals than in adults. For example, rats made iron deficient between gestation and 21 days of age do not normalize their brain iron content even after long term iron therapy, whereas rats made iron deficient approaching adulthood do so after only 1–3 weeks[3,4]: rats with iron deficiency also have persistent behavioural and learning deficits[5]. Although these lasting changes have yet to be explained, it is possible that they relate to altered central nervous system neurotransmission, as has been demonstrated in altered cortical nerve conduction[6]. Thus far, alterations in iron deficient animals have been identified in the dopamine, serotonin and γ- aminobutyric acid (GABA) systems. Details of these biochemical neurotransmitter changes induced by iron deficiency in experimental animals are given elsewhere in this publication.

Research on neurotransmitters is fruitful ground, where findings in the next few years may assist in the orientation towards the mechanisms whereby the changes observed in human studies may be explained, leading to further clarification of iron's role in the CNS[7,8]. Bearing this model in mind, experimental animals have been shown to have behavioural[9], electroneurophysiologic[6] and neurotransmitter alterations[10].

Although the behavioural changes in iron deficient humans may be compatible with alterations in neurotransmitters, linking specific biochemical changes in iron deficient animals to specific behavioural alterations in iron deficient humans must be made with caution. Furthermore, altered behaviour in iron deficiency may be due to changes in the peripheral as well as in the central nervous system. Although extrapolating animal studies to man is often misleading, studies in infancy and childhood have supported the association of iron deficiency anaemia with behavioural and cognitive impairments conceptually recognizing a 'window of vulnerability'. This window in the infant should be placed between 6 months and 23 months, precisely when iron deficiency anaemia is more prevalent and during which the latter part of the brain growth spurt and the unfolding of fundamental mental and motor processes occur[11].

When iron deficiency anaemia develops during the first 2 years of life it has been shown to be associated with detained psychomotor development and changes in behaviour. These effects have been shown to endure after several months of iron therapy, despite complete correction of iron nutritional measures. Moreover, it is still unsettled as to whether or to what extent they are reversible after a longer period of observation, since the long term prospective follow-up studies reported to date, to be discussed, show the persistence of cognitive deficits at 5–6 and even as far as 10 years of age in those who during infancy had anaemia and were adequately treated.

Iron deficiency in infancy

In human populations, nutritional deficits are not uniformly distributed. They are more likely to occur in the context of poverty, environmental deprivation, and handicapped social conditions, all of which can adversely influence behaviour and development. Recent studies of the behavioural outcome of iron deficiency have addressed these methodological challenges by broadening attention to the social, environmental, and other factors associated with iron deficiency.

During the past decade, heralded by the inceptive work of Oski and Honig[12], several studies have addressed the cognitive effects of iron deficiency in infants[13–16]. The inherent difficulties of identifying intervening variables in the complex field of mental development, coupled in some cases with suboptimum design, have prevented significant progress in the investigation of iron deficiency. However, three more recent studies, one conducted in Costa Rica[17], the other in Santiago, Chile[18], and the last in Indonesia[19] are perhaps the least contaminated with the uncertainties that precluded firm conclusions arising from previous work.

The Santiago study was performed in association with a field trial of fortified infant foods. One hundred ninety-six healthy, full-term infants from a community clinic in the city of

Santiago were included in a food fortification study at 3 months of age and followed up to age 12 months with monthly clinic well-child visits and weekly house calls by a nurse. Because the assignment to the fortified foods was random, and fortification turned out to be the strongest determinant of the infants' iron status, all other intervening factors were essentially offset with this study design.

At age 12, 121/2 and 15 months, the infants' behavioural and cognitive development were assessed with the Bayley scales of infant development[20]. This well-known and accepted tool is used to determine psychomotor development from ages 3 to 30 months. It consists of a mental scale to evaluate cognitive skills, such as language acquisition and abstract thinking, and a motor or psychomotor scale to evaluate gross motor abilities, such as coordination, body balance and walking. Most studies use the Bayley scales of infant development even though this tool is not ideal because it is non-specific and it poorly predicts future IQ[21]. However, it is a reproducible and reliable measure of behaviour in infancy. Additionally, the almost universal use of this test allows for useful comparisons.

The Costa Rica study enrolled 191 12–23-month-old otherwise healthy infants with heterogeneous iron status. These children were recruited in a cross-sectional survey, as opposed to the longitudinal follow-up of the infants in the Santiago study. The infants were divided into groups ranging from most to least iron deficient. The Bayley scales of infant development were administered before, and after one week and after three months of intramuscular or oral iron treatment with appropriate placebo controls.

The study from Indonesia enrolled 141 infants 12–18 months of age and separated iron status classes as anaemic, non-anaemic iron deficient and iron sufficient. Each of these groups was randomized to receive iron or placebo during 4 months. Bayley scales were administered before and after. The remarkable aspect of this design is the presence of an anaemic placebo group. Aukett also conformed an anaemic placebo group but the Bayley scales were not used, thus no comparisons are possible.

At what stage of iron deficiency is infant behaviour adversely affected?

It was clear in the Santiago, Costa Rica and the Indonesian study that a decrease in haemoglobin leading to overt anaemia was necessary to significantly affect mental and psychomotor development scores. The performance of the non-anaemic iron deficient infants as a whole was indistinguishable from that of the controls. Even non-anaemic infants who responded to a therapeutic trial of iron with a significant elevation of haemoglobin (> 10 g/l) who had a decrease in haemoglobin below their own normal level (but had not yet reached the lower limit for the population) and could be thus technically defined as 'anaemic' showed no tendency toward lower scores.

In the Chilean study, when the mental and psychomotor development indices were based only on haemoglobin (the most common indicator of iron status) three groups could be identified: those with haemoglobin levels < 105 g/l., those with haemoglobin levels of 110 g/l and an intermediate group with haemoglobin levels of 105–109 g/l. Each group was statistically distinct from each other. Among anaemic infants, haemoglobin concentration was correlated with performance: infants with moderate anaemia (haemoglobin 84–104 g/l) had significantly lower scores than those with mild degrees of anaemia (Hb 105–109 g/l). These infants, in turn, had poorer development indices than those with haemoglobin levels > 110 g/l with no graded improvement seen at higher haemoglobin levels (Fig. 1).

Similarly, in the Costa Rica study infants with moderate iron deficiency anaemia (Hb < 110 g/l) had lower mental and motor test scores than appropriate controls and infants with mild anaemia (Hb 101–105 g/l) received lower motor but not mental scores.

In the Indonesian study there were also statistically significant lower scores in the anaemic group compared with the iron sufficient thus the non-anaemic iron deficient group, confirming that anaemia is necessary to elicit lower developmental scores.

The Chilean study also evaluated the *effect of chronic anaemia* on infant development. Infants who were anaemic at both 9 and 12 months of

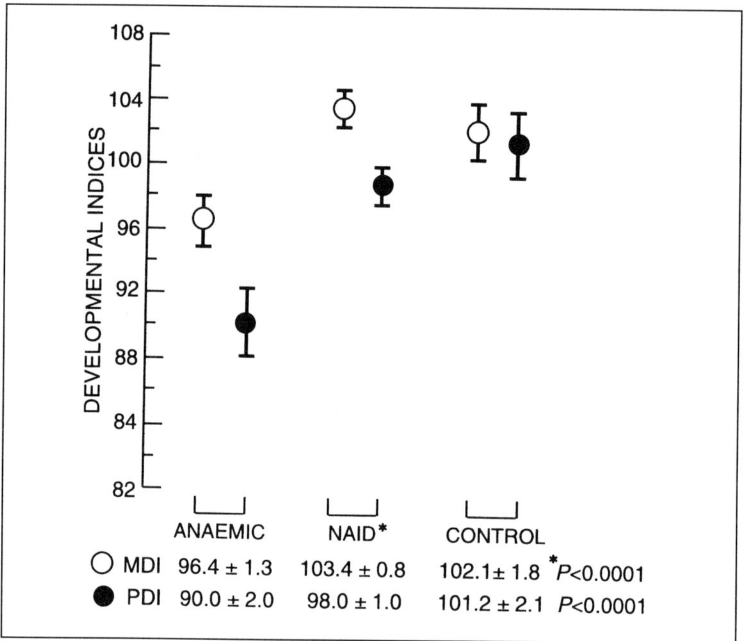

*Fig. 1. Effect of anaemia age 12 months on development indices. Anaemics show a significant fall in PDI and MDE, whereas non-anaemic iron-deficient subjects (NAID) and controls are not significantly different. *, one-way analysis of variance.*

age and whose anaemia had a duration of 3 or more months were compared with those who were anaemic at 12 but not at 9 months of age (i.e. those whose anaemia was presumed to be present for less than 3 months). Infants who were anaemic for more than 3 months had significantly lower mental and motor development indices than those anaemic for less than 3 months.

In a recent study by Walter *et al.* (unpublished) we made an attempt to determine whether the appearance of anaemia lowered the Bayley scores of infants. Rather than looking at infants already anaemic, we performed Bayley tests at 6 months of age in infants enrolled in a trial of fortified infant cereals. These infants had a haematologic assessment at 4 months, assuring their normality. It is unlikely that full term infants who are normal at 4 months of age would become anaemic at 6 months. We presumed this to be the case, so we did not perform iron status measurements at 6 months, only the Bayley test. Two months later, at 8 months of age, an iron status evaluation was performed. Infants with a haemoglobin under 105 g/l were removed from the study and treated. Before iron treatment the anaemic and an equal number of iron sufficient controls from the same cohort were tested with the Bayley scales. Those who had become anaemic from 6 to 8 months were compared to those who remained iron sufficient. In the iron sufficient the Mental Development Index (MDI) did not change from 6 to 8 months, however the Psychomotor Development Index (PDI) decreased significantly. In the anaemic group, both indices fell significantly. It is still uncertain what these preliminary results mean, but continued trials of this sort may eventually clarify the real role of iron in development.

Why is anaemia necessary for an effect to be detected?

If the effect of iron deficiency on behaviour were mediated by metabolic processes that depend on the presence of iron, then overt anaemia may be necessary to disclose these effects. Siimes *et al.*[22] demonstrated in animals fed graded amounts of iron that tissue haem proteins were not affected until saturation of transferrin fell significantly. Haemoglobin, as well as tissue cytochrome C and myoglobin decreased steadily thereafter, demonstrating that the availability of iron to the erythroid marrow is limited concomitantly to other tissues.

In humans, iron-restricted erythropoiesis (when iron availability becomes a limiting factor for haemoglobin synthesis) corresponds to the moment when haemoglobin concentration begins to decrease, presumably along with other tissue iron proteins. However, manifest anaemia supervenes weeks or months later when haemoglobin values fall below 110 g/l. Anaemia becomes evident, therefore, after considerable decrease of tissue iron proteins. A milder iron deficit may not generate sufficient tissue depletion to be reflected in behaviour, although the psychological tests available for infants may be too crude to identify subtle deficits.

The results of other research published to date support the conclusion of the Santiago, Costa Rica and Indonesian studies - iron deficiency severe enough to produce anaemia is associated with deteriorated achievement in developmental tests in infancy and as anaemia progresses in severity and duration, deficits become more intense.

Effect of iron treatment

Until recentlty most studies examining the behavioural effects of iron deficiency were designed to detect changes in developmental test performance within 5–11 days of starting iron therapy. This emphasis on short-term treatment effects was guided by two considerations. Clinicians describing iron deficient anaemic infants as irritable, apathetic and distractible have commented that these characteristics seem to disappear within a few days of iron treatment, and early retesting might allow any behavioural changes to be attributed to altered central nervous system function rather than to correction of anaemia.

Consistent results have been obtained in studies that included a placebo treatment, indicating that short-term increases in test scores observed among iron-treated anaemic infants are not significantly greater than those among placebo-treated anaemic infants, and thus probably related to a practice effect.

Although separating the effects of iron deficiency from those of anaemia is important, a more pertinent question from a clinical perspective is whether iron therapy completely corrects behavioural abnormalities regardless of how soon the changes are detectable.

Studies in Costa Rica[13], Chile[18] and the UK[23] included an iron treatment period of three months after which psychomotor development tests were repeated. The long-term iron therapy was planned to provide complete or near complete correction of iron status, thus permitting the correction of anaemia and other tissue-iron-dependent functional components. Despite the improved iron status most of the formerly anaemic infants were unable to improve their psychomotor performance. Only a small group of Costa Rican infants who achieved total correction of iron measures showed improvement of the motor development index, a finding that was not reproduced in the Santiago study.

The UK study, using a different test of psychomotor development showed that a greater proportion of infants with marked haematological responses to iron therapy had an improvement in their psychomotor achievements (passing 50 per cent of expected marks for age). However, this study is difficult to compare with other results because the developmental tool used was unlike that used in other studies. The analyses of mean developmental scores revealed no significant effects of treatment and the decision to consider an increase in haemoglobin of > 20 mg/l is an arbitrary cut-off point that has no counterpart in other studies.

Only the well designed protocol in Indonesia[19] shows an unequivocal recovery in psychomotor scores after therapy in anaemics given iron compared to anaemics receiving 4 months of placebo. The improvements in the anaemics given iron were remarkable, with rises of 19 to 24 points in the Bayley scales, bringing their levels to those of the non-anaemic infants for both MDI and PDI. This goes to prove that studies in this field may give conflicting results and that newer and more imaginative techniques must be used to interpret current controversies.

Specific patterns of failure

The Chilean study found that when examining the mental scale, items that required comprehension of language but did not involve a visual demonstration were passed by fewer anaemic infants than controls. Language development in this age group was best marked by vocalization of disyllabic words imitation of words (mama, dada), saying two words with meaning and pointing to own clothing or toys. In the psychomotor scale balance in the standing position and walking (sits from standing stands alone and stands up) were accomplished by significantly fewer anaemic infants than controls. Similar findings were reported in the Costa Rica study.

Because the follow-up period in the Costa Rican, Chilean, Indonesian and UK studies was only 2–4 months, these studies could not resolve whether the adverse effects of iron deficiency anaemia on behaviour continued beyond infancy. The lower mental and motor test scores among many of the iron deficient anaemic infants might have responded to a more extended course of iron therapy. A study of such a treatment course was completed in Costa Rica; however, the 6 months of therapy in pursuit of full correction of iron nutrition measures have proven to be of no avail in the search for improvement of developmental scores (B. Lozoff, personal communication, 1990). It is also possible that the deficit might persist even if there is no laboratory evidence of iron deficiency. This outcome would indicate that iron deficiency anaemia in infants of a certain age, perhaps of a particular severity or chronicity, has irreversible effects. The age of 12 months was the lower limit in the study from Indonesia, but younger infants affected with anaemia may not show such unprecedented recovery.

Long term effects of iron deficiency anaemia

Effect at 5 years

Cognitive performance of children who were anaemic during infancy

The long term persistence issue has been addressed by two follow-up studies recently described in 5-year-old Costa Rican[17] and Chilean children[24] who had been well characterized as infants in iron status environmental variables and their psychomotor development. These children were the subjects of respective reports during their infancy as described above. At 5 years of age an evaluation with a comprehensive set of psychometric tests showed that those who as infants had presented with iron deficiency anaemia had lower scores on many of these tests compared to children with higher haemoglobins in infancy. These disadvantages persisted after statistical control of many potentially confounding variables.

The Chilean children studied were part of a cohort followed longitudinally from birth to 12 months of age in a field trial of iron fortified food as previously described. This study[24] included only the formerly anaemic infants and the iron sufficient controls, thus excluding all effects of intermediate stages of iron deficit. The study by Lozoff *et al.*[17] in Costa Rica included most of the infants seen at an earlier age with various grades of iron nutrition. The children were separated into formerly anaemics and non-anaemics for all comparisons.

The battery of psychological tests available for this age group is more comprehensive and better predictive of future cognitive performance, unlike the well recognized poor predictability of measures of psychomotor tests.

Stanford-Binet intelligence test. This test was selected by Walter's group. It provides an index of general intelligence (IQ) with an average of 100 ± 16[25].

Illinois psycholinguistic abilities test. This test evaluates cognitive functions that play a role in the communication process. It is composed of 10 subtests assessing mainly receptive and expressive processes. Each subtest provides an equivalent age and standard score and subtest scores together provide a language measure that can be expressed as psycholinguistic quotient and/or standard score average[26].

Woodcock-Johnson psychoeducational abilities test. Short pre-school cluster. This pre-school scale provides an age score of broad cognitive ability. It also allows the estimation of percentile ranks, standard scores and relative performance indices[27].

Bruininks-Oseretsky test of motor proficiency. This provides a comprehensive index of general motor proficiency as well as separate measures of gross and fine motor skills. Normative data include standard scores for age groups percentiles ranks and age equivalent scores are also provided[28].

Developmental test of visual motor integration (VMI). Raw scores obtained after copying 24 geometrical forms are compared with normative data allowing estimation of age equivalence and standard scores[29].

Lozoff performed the same tests but used the Wechsler intelligence scale[30] and the Goodenough draw-a-man test[31] and did not perform the Illinois psycholinguistic test.

The haematological status of these children was very adequate, confirming the fact that after therapy is given to achieve full correction of iron deficit during infancy the introduction of table foods in addition to the decreased demands for growth pose preschool children at low risk of iron deficiency.

In both long term studies the children who as infants had iron deficiency anaemia scored lower than the formerly non-anaemic control children in tests of mental and motor functioning at 5 years of age. Statistically significant differences in scores were found for all tests, the only exceptions being the Goodenough test in the Costa Rican children and, in the Chilean study, the gross motor aspect of the Bruininks-Oseretsky test of motor proficiency where differences were borderline.

Lozoff *et al*[17]. used linear regression and covariate analysis models to adjust for confounders. After these procedures they were able to show significant differences in the adjusted means for several subtests of the Woodcock-Johnson psychoeducational battery, the Beery visual motor integration, all parts of the Bruininks-Oseretsky motor proficiency and the performance IQ of the Wechsler intelligence scale.

Walter *et al*[16]., in an effort to give an appreciation of relative risk of poorer performance when the infant had been exposed to anaemia, used a logistic regression approach. The confounders included in the regression model were those identified as being associated statistically both with the exposure variable and the outcome, such as neurologic maturity[32], maternal education, a modified Home inventory for Measurement of the Environment (HOME) inventory[33] height:age ratio, attendance at nursery school, and duration of breast feeding.

Initially the unadjusted logistic regression showed a higher risk of lower performances in the event of iron deficiency anaemia during infancy for virtually all the outcome tests. After adjusting for this comprehensive and reliable set of potential confounders the very high odds ratio persisted for the fine motor section of the Bruininks- Oseretsky test of motor proficiency, the Woodcock-Johnson pre-school cluster score, and the Illinois test of psycholinguistic abilities. However, neuroimmaturity became a significant predictor of risk for the Standford-Binet IQ scale and the Bruininks-Oseretsky test of motor proficiency at odd ratios even stronger than for anaemia. For the visual motor integration the mother's education was the only significant risk predictor, and for the Woodcock-Johnson and Illinois, apart from the potent effect of anaemia, the modified Home inventory was a weaker, albeit significant, predictor of poorer performances.

The striking prevalence of neurologic immaturity or 'soft signs' in the formerly anaemic children in the Chilean population is suggestive of an additional factor which poses these children at high risk of lower cognitive achievement. This finding was not reported for the Costa Rican children. The association between soft neurologic signs and cognitive risk is well documented, mostly linked to adverse neonatal events or prematurity[34]. A study by Cantwell[35] reports on 61 full-term infants followed developmentally from birth to 7 years of age. Of these, 32 developed anaemia and 9 who were given iron dextran injections as neonates served as non-anaemic controls. A blinded neurological evaluation was done at 6–7 years. The group of former anaemics had a higher incidence of soft signs and Binet IQ scores were 6 points lower on average. Unfortunately, this communication in abstract form was not followed by a full report. However, it is surprisingly similar to our findings and is the only previous information linking neuroimmaturity as a long term effect of anaemia. Nevertheless, in our study the fact that these infants were seen from birth and followed thereafter, quite clearly puts to rest other plausible causes to explain neurologic immaturity based on adverse medical events other that anaemia during infancy. It is not known, however, how a poor home environment may affect neurologic maturation but there do not seem to exist reports of an association of this nature. A tempting hypothesis is that this neurologic syndrome may be the mediator between anaemia and poor cognitive performance.

Since iron deficiency anaemia is most prevalent in disadvantaged populations, usually associated with poverty, it is very difficult to separate the effect of the environment from the nutritional deficiency. Nonetheless, some of the results of this study are similar to those of two other follow-up studies of children who had anaemia as infants. Studies by Palti[36,37] based on data from a comprehensive health programme in Israel found that lower haemoglobin levels at 9 months of age were associated with lower developmental IQ scores and less desirable behaviour in the preschool years and at school age, even alter other important factors such as maternal education, socioeconomic status and birth weight were considered. The second study by Dommergues *et al.*[38] in France found that children who had anaemia at 2 years of age continued to have lower test scores at 4 years of age. Although these results are congruent with ours, these studies were retrospective, used more limited measures of iron status and/or development and lacked data on response to iron therapy.

Despite the consistency in the findings, the biggest challenge continues to be to demonstrate that the alleged decreased cognitive abilities are in fact caused by the early exposure to iron deficiency anaemia[39]. The well demonstrated plasticity of the neural system in the face of gross insults occurring during early life is not congruent with the apparent inability to compensate for the comparatively much milder impact of the low tissue availability of iron during the first few months of age. It is also worth noting that the differences shown here are quite subtle. They are impossible to demonstrate without the presence of carefully selected control subjects because the scores of the formerly anaemic children fall well within the normal range.

The follow-up of these children into the school period is of paramount importance, as well as other intervention field studies to link IDA causally to psychomotor delay

Effect at 10 years

The cohort of 196 infants studied in 1985 was reduced to 74 seen at 5 years, because only the anaemic and the iron sufficient controls were recalled. Currently, these children are 10 years of age and have been recalled for further study (Walter *et al.*, unpublished). Besides a haematological control and a general physical exam, they underwent a battery of psychometric tests and their school marks were reviewed. These studies are at a preliminary stage of analysis; however, we can mention several facts. The Stanford-Binet IQ scale shows no statistical differences between groups, as does the visual motor integration test. The Woodcock-Johnson test subscales of oral language and general abilities show significantly lower performances in the formerly anaemic. The Bruininks motor abilities test scales show no differences except for the subtest of the 'ruler catch' time response velocity. Neurologic immaturity continued to affect over one-third of the children but the difference between the groups disappeared.

School grades in language, mathematics, physical education and general grade averages were examined. To avoid common differences between schools, teachers and other confounders and recognizing the problems affecting school achievements measured in grades, we compared the marks with the average of the class in the way growth is measured, i.e. *Z* scores. Thus a *Z* of 0 is equal to the average of the class. There

*Table 1. School grades compared to the average of the class (*P < 0.05) at 10 years*

	Former Iron status	
	non anaemic	**Anaemic**
Language	no difference	
Math	no difference	
Physical Ed	+ 0.22 ± 0.6	− 0.03 ± 0.5*
All subjects	+ 0.29 ± 0.6	− 0.1 ± 0.4*

were significant differences between the groups in physical education and the general grade average score (Table 1). This preliminary analysis shows that, though differences are attenuated by time, they may still present a handicap to cognitive achievement in basic education. Again, we cannot confirm these effects are due causally to iron deficiency; however, they do serve as a marker of higher risk.

References

1. DeMaeyer, E. & Adlels-Tegman, M. (1985): The prevalence of anaemia in the world. *World Health Stat. Q.* **38,** 302–316.

2. Florentino, R.F. & Guirries, R.M. (1984): Prevalence of nutritional anemia in infancy and childhood with emphasis on developing countries. In: *Iron nutrition in infancy and childhood,* ed. A. Stekel, pp. 61–74. New York: Raven Press.

3. Dallman, P.R., Siimes, M.A., Manies, E.C. (1975): Brain iron: Persistent deficiency following short-term iron deprivation in the young rat. *Br. J. Haematol.* **31,** 209–215.

4. Dallman, P.R. & Spirito, R.A. (1977): Brain iron in the rat: Extremely slow turnover in normal rats may explain long-lasting effects of early iron deficiency. *J. Nutr.* **107,** 1075–1981.

5. Weinberg, J., Brett, L.P., Levine, S. & Dallman, P.R. (1981): Long-term effects of early iron deficiency on consummatory behavior in the rat. *Pharmacol. Biochem. Behav.* **4,** 447–453.

6. Ruiz, S., Walter, T., Pérez, H., Stekel, A., Hernández, A. & Soto-Moyano, R. (1984): Effect of early iron deficiency on the rat parietal associate cortex. *Intern. J. Neurosci.* **23,** 161–168.

7. Leibel, R.I., Greenfield, D.B. & Pollit, E. (1979): Iron deficiency: behavior and brain biochemistry. In: *Nutrition: Pre and post natal development,* pp. 383–439. New York: Plenum Press.

8. Dallman, P.R. (1986): Biochemical basis for the manifestations of iron deficiency. *Ann. Rev. Nutr.* **6,** 13–40.

9. Yehuda, S. (1990): Neuro-chemical basis of behavioural effects of brain iron deficiency. In: *Brain behavior and iron in the infant diet,* ed. J. Dobbing, pp. 63–81. London: Springer Verlag.

10. Youdim, M.B.H. (1990): Neuro-pharmachological and Neuro-biochemical Aspects of Iron Deficiency. In: *Brain behavior and iron in the infant diet,* ed. J. Dobbing, pp. 83–105. London: Springer Verlag.

11. Dobbing, J. (1990): Vulnerable periods in the developing brain. In: *Brain, behavior, and iron in the infant diet,* ed. J. Dobbing, pp. 1–7. London: Springer Verlag.

12. Oski, F.A. & Honig, A.S. (1978): The effects of therapy on the developmental scores of iron-deficient infants. *J. Pediatr.* **92,** 21–25.

13. Lozoff, B., Brittenham, G.M. & Wolf, A.W. (1987): Iron deficiency anemia and iron therapy: Effect on infant developmental test performance. *Pediatrics* **79,** 981–995.

14. Lozoff, B., Brittenham, G.M., Viteri, F.E., Wolf, A.W. & Urrutia, J.J. (1982): The effects of short-term oral iron therapy on developmental deficits in iron-deficient anemia infants. *J. Pediatr.* **100,** 351–357.

15. Oski, F.A., Honig, A.S., Helu, B. & Howanitz, P. (1983): Effect of iron therapy on behavior performance in non anemic, iron-deficient infants. *Pediatrics* **71,** 877–880.

16. Walter, T., Kovalsky, J. & Stekel, A. (1983): Effect of mild iron deficiency on infant mental development scores. *J. Pediatr.* **102,** 519–527.

17. Lozoff, B., Jimenez, E. & Wolf, A. (1991): Long-term developmental outcome of infants with iron deficiency. *N. Engl. J. Med.* **325,** 687–694.

18. Walter, T., De Andraca, I., Chadud, P. & Perales, C.G. (1989): Iron deficiency anemia: Adverse effects on infant psychomotor development. *Pediatrics* **84,** 7–17.

19. Idjradinata, P. & Pollitt, E. (1993): Reversal of developmental delays in iron-deficient anemic infants treated with iron. *Lancet* **341,** 1–4.

20. Bayley, N. (1969): Bayley scales of infant development. New York: Psychological Corporation.

21. McCall, R.B. (1979): The development of intellectual functioning in infancy and the prediction of later IQ. In: *Handbook of infant development,* pp. 707–741. New York: John Wiley.

22. Siimes, M.A., Refino, C. & Dallman, P.R. (1980): Manifestations of iron deficiency at various levels of dietary iron intake. *Am. J. Clin. Nutr.* **33,** 570–574.

23. Aukett, M.A., Parks, Y.A., Scott, P.H. & Wharton, B.A. (1986): Treatment with iron increases weight gain and psychomotor development. *Arch. Dis. Child.* **61,** 849–857.

24. De Andraca, I., Walter, T., Castillo, M., Pino, P., Rivera, P. & Cobo, C. (1991): Iron deficiency anemia and its effects upon psychological development at preschool age: a longitudinal study. *Nestle Nutrition Annals* 53–62.

25. Terman, C. & Merril, M. (1975): Medida de la Intelligencia Método para el empleo de las pruebas del Stanford Binet. Tercera Revision (1975), Formas L-M 1972. Madrid: Espasa Calpe.

26. Kirk, S.A., MacCarthy, Y.Y. & Kork, W.D. (1978): *Illinois Test of Psycholinguistic Abilities,* revised edn. Los Angeles, CA: Western Psychological Services.

27. Woodcock, R.W. (1982): *Bateria Woodcock Psicoeducativa en Español.* Teaching Resources Corporation.

28. Bruininks, R. (1978): *Bruininks–Oseretsky Test of Motor Proficiency.* Minesota, MN: American Guidance Service.

29. Beery, K.E. (1982): *Administration, scoring and teaching manual for the developmental test of visual integration.* Cleveland: Modern Curriculum Press.

30. Wechsler, D. (1967): *Manual for the Wechsler preschool and primary scale of intelligence.* New York: Psychological Corporation.

31. Harris, D.B. (1963): Childrens drawings as measures of intellectual maturity: a revision and extension of the Goodenough draw-a-man test. New York: Harcout Brace and Worlds.

32. Scheinberg, L.C., Taylor, J.M. & Schaumberg, H.H. (1977): Examen neurologico. In *Manual practico de diagnostico neurológico,* pp. 8–65. Fondo Educativo Interamericano SA.

33. Caldwell, B.M. (1975): *Instruction Manual. Home inventory for infants.* Little Rock: University of Arkansas.

34. Huttenlocher, P.R., Levine, S.C., Huttenlocher, J. & Gates, J. (1990): Discrimination of Normal and at Risk Preschool Children on the Basis of Neurolofical Tests. *Develop. Med. and Child Neurol.* **32,** 394–402.

35. Cantwell, R.J. (1974): The long term neurological sequelae of anemia in infancy. *Ped. Res.* **8,** 342(A).

36. Palti, H., Meijer, A. & Adler, B. (1985): Learning achievement and behavior at school of anemic and iron-anemic infants. *Early Hum. Dev.* **10,** 217–223.

37. Palti, H., Pevsner, B. & Adler, B. (1983): Does anemia in infancy affect achievement on developmental and intelligence tests? *Hum. Biol.* **55,** 183–194.

38. Dommergues, J.P., Archambeaud, M.P., Ducot, B., Gerval, C., Hiard, C., Rossignol, C. & Tchernia, G. (1989): Carence en fer et tests de developpment psychomoteur etude longitudinale entre lage de 10 mois et l'age de 4 ans. *Arch. Fr. Pediatr.* **46,** 487–490.

39. Lozoff, B. (1990): Has iron deficiency been shown to cause altered behavior in infants? In: *Brain behavior and iron in the infant diet*, ed. J. Dobbing. pp. 107–131. London: Springer Verlag.

Iron Nutrition in Health and Disease, edited by Leif Hallberg and Nils-Georg Asp
©1996 John Libbey & Company Ltd., pp. 231–238

Chapter 22

Iron and infection

Chaim Hershko

Department of Medicine, Shaare Zedek Medical Center, Department of Human Nutrition and Metabolism, Hebrew University Hadassah Medical School, Jerusalem, Israel

Summary

Since iron deprevation in bacterial cultures is regularly associated with inhibition of growth, it has been suggested that iron deficiency may represent an important defense mechanism. Because of the paucity of clinical data supporting the significance of iron deficiency or overload in determining the severity of infectious disease in man, the nutritional immunity hypothesis has remained a topic of continued controversy. This controversy is of more than academic interest, since both iron deficiency and infectious diseases are common conditions, and iron supplementation in some populations may resolve one problem while aggravating the other. Clinical studies, in which the incidence and severity of infectious diseases are correlated with iron status, are of great value in assessing the validity of the nutritional immunity hypothesis. Because of the inherent limitations of studying the infectious complications of pre-existent iron deficiency, it is preferable to study the effect of iron administration on the incidence and severity of infection, comparing the results with untreated controls with an identical background. Most of the carefully designed prospective randomized trials show no conclusive evidence of an increased risk of infection following oral iron treatment. In view of the possible beneficial effects of selective iron depletion, the iron chelating drug deferoxamine (DF) has been evaluated as a potential antimalarial agent. DF inhibits the growth of *P. falciparum* cultures, rats infected with *P. berghei*, mice with *P. vinckei* and Aotus monkeys with P. *falciparum*. Clinical studies in tropical countries leave no doubt as to the ability of DF to hasten recovery from malaria, presumably by inhibiting parasite growth in a similar fashion to its effect in experimental *in vitro* and *in vivo* systems. However, additional large-scale carefully controlled studies are needed, with particular emphasis on mortality and neurological sequelae, before DF could be recommended for the treatment of cerebral malaria. These intriguing observations on the antimicrobial effects of DF and other iron chelators lend new meaning to the term 'nutritional immunity' and open new channels for exploring the possibility of controlling infection by means of selective intracellular iron deprivation.

Introduction

Iron is a trace metal essential for life, and plays a key role in oxygen transport, deoxyribonucleotide synthesis and redox reactions. Consequently, living organisms from bacteria to man have developed elaborate mechanisms for its acquisition, transport and storage. Most microorganisms obtain iron by producing their own iron-binding compounds, siderophores, classified chemically as either phenolates or hydroxamates[1]. These siderophores are able to compete successfully with the iron-binding proteins of the host. Since iron deprivation in bacterial cultures is regularly associated with inhibition of growth, it has been suggested that iron deficiency may represent an important defense mechanism[2]. The term nutritional immunity was introduced by Kochan in 1973 to emphasize the importance of iron deprivation as a key mechanism limiting the growth of invading organisms[3].

If iron deprivation inhibits bacterial growth, it may be assumed that clinical conditions associated with iron excess in the host may increase the risk of infection and, conversely, that iron deficiency may have a protective effect. This issue has important practical implications since iron deficiency is a very common condition in underprivileged populations with a high incidence of infectious disease, and measures taken to prevent iron deficiency may aggravate the risk of infection. However, at present there is a shortage of well-controlled studies addressing this issue, and the nutritional immunity hypothesis remains a topic of continued controversy[4,5]. This chapter addresses some of the key questions related to iron and infection: the importance of iron for the ability of microorganisms to induce clinical disease; the clinical evidence supporting the role of iron status in determining the severity of infection in the host; the effect of iron status on mechanisms of host resistance; the possibility that selective iron depletion in relevant compartments may be an effective mechanism for the control of infection.

Iron and bacterial virulence

The acquisition of sufficient iron is an essential requirement of bacteria for their continued multiplication in the host. This is illustrated by the close correlation between the availability of iron and bacterial virulence[6]. For example in both *E. coli* and *Vibrio*, plasmids encoding for iron-sequestration systems are also determinants of virulence[7,8]. Virulent isolates of *Vibrio vulnificus* differ from non-virulent ones by their ability to produce phenolate siderophores and to utilize transferrin iron[9]. The presence of a siderophore binding protein on the cell surface of *Pseudomonas aeruginosa* is essential for its virulence[10]. *Neisseriae* are able to develop surface receptors specific for human transferrin and lactoferrin in response to iron starvation, and only *Neisseriae* utilizing transferrin iron are pathogenic[11]. Finally, injection of inorganic iron to rodent models of bacterial infection enhances the *in vivo* virulence of *Klebsiella, Pseudomonas, E. coli* and a large number of other bacteria[12].

Collectively, these studies demonstrate the correlation between bacterial virulence and their ability to acquire iron through endogenous iron-acquisition system or by the existance of easily available iron compartments in the host.

Infection and the iron-overloaded host

A number of clinical observations indicate that under conditions of extreme iron overload microorganisms of limited pathogenicity may produce severe infection. For example, *Yersinia enterocolitica*, an organism usually causing mild enteric infections, may be associated with severe sepsis, intestinal perforation or multiple liver abscesses in patients with transfusional iron overload or hereditary haemochromatosis[13–15]. This may be further aggravated by deferoxamine therapy, because *Yersinia* is unable to produce its own siderophore but is able to utilize iron bound to desferrioxamine. Another microorganism whose pathogenicity is greatly increased by iron overload is *Vibrio vulnificus* which is completely inhibited by normal human serum, but grows readily in serum from haemochromatotic patients or in normal blood with saturated transferrin[16].

Other clinical observations imply that even moderate iron excess may lead to aggravation of infection. In patients with pneumococcal pneumonia, mortality was higher in subjects with low unsaturated iron-binding capacity implying that insufficient unsaturated transferrin may facilitate bacteremia[17]. In patients with *Shigella septicaemia*, the ability of serum to inhibit bacterial growth was lower in subjects with higher trasnferrin saturation[18]. Likewise, in haemodialysis patients, increased serum ferritin was associated with increased susceptibility to bacterial infection[19]. All of these correlations are indirect and could be a reflection of other compounding factors such as combined nutritional deficiencies. They also may have represented the effects of overwhelming infection rather than its cause.

However, experimental animal models clearly indicate that iron loading aggravates the severity of infection. In *Staphylococcus aureus*-induced experimental pyelonephritis in mice, parenteral iron administration resulted in increased severity of disease, as documented by bacterial growth and severity of pathological lesions in the kidneys[20]. Likewise, in thalassemic iron-loaded mice, resistance to infection with *Listeria monocytogenes* was greatly impaired by the combination of iron overload and deferoxamine treatment, but not by deferoxamine without iron overload[21].

All of these observations indicate that severe iron overload or parenteral iron therapy, in particular with coexistent deferoxamine administration, may increase the severity of infection with some microorganisms, in particular in those with an inadequate mechanism of iron acquisition. However, the importance of moderate or mild iron excess in determining the severity of infection remains at present controversial.

Infection and the iron deficient host

In order to assess the impact of iron deficiency on infection it must be isolated from other variables that may be coexistent with, but independent of iron deficiency. For instance, poverty is closely correlated with iron deficiency because haem iron, the most readily absorbable food iron, is also the most expensive dietary item. Poverty, in turn, is also associated with poor housing conditions, unavailability of refrigerators and other necessary sanitary conditions which may have a profound effect on the risk of infectious disease. Hence, documentation of a simple correlation between iron deficiency and infection may be misleading[22]. A much more useful approach is studying the impact of iron administration on infection, since in this manner the only variable affected by the therapeutic intervention is the iron status of the host. Care should be exercised to restrict studies to those employing oral iron, since parenteral iron is unphysiological and has already been shown in animal studies to be harmful when administered during infection.

Some of the earlier studies of this category have been reviewed in our previous publication on iron and infection[5]. In the present discussion we shall focus on prospective controlled studies in tropical and third-world countries, as they represent a special category wherein the incidence and severity of infectious diseases may be much greater than in Western countries, and since most of the preliminary uncontrolled reports of parenteral iron treatment aggravating infection originated from the tropics. One of the first, and most often quoted studies was conducted by Murray *et al.*[23]. In this prospective randomized study of adult Somali nomads with iron deficiency anaemia, oral iron therapy resulted in a 12-fold increase in infectious episodes compared to untreated controls. The most striking differences were in malaria, brucellosis and tuberculosis. Unfortunately, none of the subsequent studies has been able to confirm such a dramatic effect of oral iron treatment on infectious disease. Thus, in a study conducted among preschool village children in India, no significant increase in the frequency or duration of respiratory and enteric infections has been found after 12 months of iron supplementation despite careful follow-up by weekly home visits[24]. Likewise, in a prospective randomized study of prepubescent schoolchildren in Papua New Guinea treated by oral iron, there was no difference in malarial parasite rate, parasite density, or levels of antimalarial IgG between children receiving oral iron and the control group[25]. Similarly in a study of Pakistani infants randomized to receive a milk cereal diet with or without iron fortification, there was no effect of iron on the incidence of infections[26]. In another study among Guam infants with salmonellosis, infants on a high-iron formula were more likely to develop salmonellosis than breast-fed controls, but the design of the study made it impossible to distinguish the protective effect of breast feeding from the possible deleterious effect of iron[27]. In contrast, in patients with recurrent *Staphylococcal furunculosis* and laboratory evidence of iron deficiency, oral iron therapy resulted in a striking clinical improvement[28].

Thus, the simplistic view that iron deficiency may be beneficial and that its correction may involve an increased risk of infection cannot be supported by clinical evidence. In order to understand this seemingly contradictory situation, one must bear in mind that iron deficiency may not only interfere with bacterial growth but, at the same time interfere with host resistance. Iron deficiency results is a wide range of abnormalities in host resistance[29] including impaired lymphocyte mitogenic response, abnormal delayed hypersensitivity and impaired development of germinal centres[30,31]. In addition, a wide range of abnormalities in granulocyte function have also been demonstrated in iron deficiency such as impaired phagocytic function, abnormal bactericidal activity, respiratory burst, and myeloperoxidase acivity[31–33]. Hence, any possible beneficial effect that iron deficiency may have in limiting the proliferation of infective agents may be counterbalanced by impaired host resistance caused by iron deficiency.

In summary, available data do not support the notion that oral iron is harmful, and at present there is no justification for witholding oral iron treatment intended for the correction of iron deficiency anaemia.

Control of infection by selective iron depletion

If the unavailability of iron limits microbial growth but at the same time impairs host resistance, an optimal way of infection control would be the selective depletion of iron in compartments relevant to microbial growth. Surprisingly, this is exactly what one may observe in studying the anomalous distribution of iron in the host elicited by the inflammatory response.

The chain of events occurring during the inflammatory response is described in Fig. 1. This process is mediated by a number of important cytokines including IFN-gamma, IL–1 and TNF. In response to these cytokines, the cell depletes its intracellular labile, metabolically active iron pool by three parallel mechanisms: (a) enhancement of ferritin synthesis by a non-iron-mediated mechanism, resulting in a shift of cellular iron into the relatively inert ferritin storage compartment[34,35]; (b) down-regulation of transferrin receptor production resulting in a decrease in cellular iron uptake and limiting iron availability for the intracellular pathogen[36,37]; and (c) activation of the synthesis of nitric oxide from L-arginine and the formation of reactive nitrogen intermediates which inactivate the iron-sulfur centres of vital cellular enzymes by the formation of iron-sulfur-nitric oxide complexes[38]. That the antibacterial effect of cytokines is mediated by iron depletion is elegantly demonstrated by the reversal of this effect by iron treatment and its potentiation by deferoxamine[39].

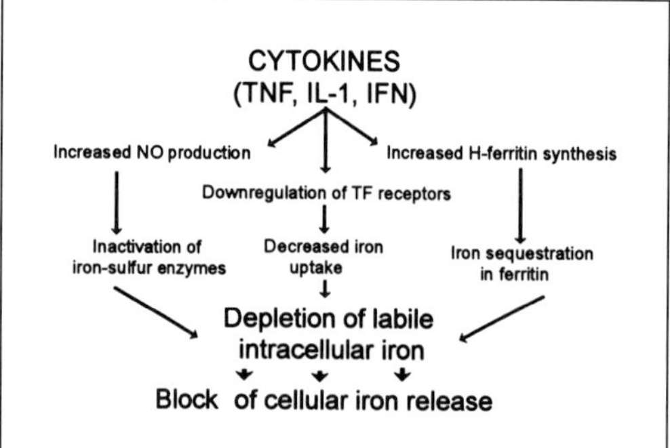

Fig. 1. Depletion of the labile intracellular iron pool results in a block of iron release from the cell.

If deferoxamine (DF) simulates the antimicrobial effect of cytokines on intracellular pathogens, it would be worthwhile to exploit this action for antimicrobial therapy. Malaria has been the first model to test the antimicrobial potential of DF. DF inhibits the growth of *P. falciparum* cultures at concentrations above 20 μM[40]. *In vivo* studies in rats infected with *P. berghei*, mice with *P. vinckei* and monkeys with *P. falciparum* have shown that DF is able to suppress malaria if a continuous supply of the chelator is assured by frequent (8 hourly) subcutaneous injections[41,42], or by osmotic pumps.

Encouraged by these studies in experimental animals, several investigators have tested the antimalarial effect of DF in humans. Traore *et al.*[43] have studied the effect of DF 0.5 g i.m. given twice daily for 3 days on the rate of clearance of parasitaemia in patients with *P. falciparum* malaria who were also receiving chloroquine. In another clinical study by Bunnag *et al.*[44] 14 patients with symptomatic *P. vivax* and 14 with uncomplicated *P. falciparum* malaria received continuous i.v. DF 100 mg/kg for 72 h. In addition, two controlled studies of DF in human malaria have been conducted by Gordeuk *et al.* In the first of these, the effect of DF therapy in partially immune adults with asymptomatic *P. falciparum* parasitaemia has been tested[45]. In the second randomized, double-blind, placebo-controlled trial by Gordeuk *et al.*[46] the effect of DF 100 mg/kg/day given by intravenous infusion for 72 h was studied in 83 children with cerebral (*P. falciparum*) malaria. All patients were receiving, in addition, standard therapy consisting of quinine and sulfadoxine pyrimethamine. Among 50 patients with deep coma, median recovery time was decreased by DF from 68 to 24 h. The rate of parasite clearance was 2 times faster in the DF-treated group. However, there was no significant difference in rates of mortality.

Collectively, these studies leave no doubt as to the ability of DF to hasten recovery from malaria, presumably by inhibiting parasite growth in a similar fashion to its effect in experimental *in vitro* and *in vivo* systems. In cerebral malaria, an additional beneficial effect could be inhibition of oxidative brain damage by preventing the formation of toxic free radicals through the iron-driven Fenton reaction. However, as emphasized in a recent editorial[47], additional large-scale carefully controlled studies are needed, with particular emphasis on mortality and neurological sequelae, before DF could be recommended for the treatment of cerebral malaria.

We and others[48,49] have studied other, orally effective iron chelating compounds, some of which have already been shown to be more effective iron chelators than DF. In a study of a group of phenolic iron chelators, we have found that the most powerful iron chelator in this group, with an increased affinity to iron and increased lipid solubility, was also the most effective antimalarial agent[50]. Consequently, we postulated that both affinity to iron and increased lipophilicity may contribute to the antimalarial activity of an iron chelator. Recent studies by Shanzer *et al.*[51] employing a series of synthetic iron chelators have confirmed our conclusions that the antimalarial effect of iron chelators is determined by their lipophilicity as well as their affinity to iron.

In addition to malaria, DF was also shown to inhibit the proliferation *in vitro* and *in vivo* of *Leishmania donovani*[52], *Trypanosoma cruzi*[53], *Pneumocystis carinii*[54], and *Leqionella pneumophila*[36]. These intriguing observations on the antimicrobial effects of DF and other iron chelators lend new meaning to the term 'nutritional immunity'[3] and open new channels for exploring the possibility of controlling infection by means of selective intracellular iron deprivation. Packaging the chelator in liposomes or red cell ghosts, or manipulating their lipid solubility to improve their delivery to appropriate target organs, such as the macrophage system, may greatly improve their efficiency. In view of the short half-life and poor oral effectiveness of DF, it is unlikely that this drug will be suitable for clinical use as a practical antimicrobial agent. However, with the introduction of simple, orally effective new chelators, it is reasonable to expect that future research may lead to the identification of iron chelators with considerable usefulness in the control of infectious disease.

References

1. Neilands, J.B. (1981): Microbial iron compounds. *Ann. Rev. Biochem.* **50,** 715–731.
2. Weinberg, E.D. (1992): Iron depletion: a defense against intracellular infection and neoplasia. *Life Sci.* **50,** 1289– 1297.
3. Kochan, I. (1973): The role of iron in bacterial infections with special considerations of host-tubercle bacillus interaction. *Curr. Top. Microbiol. Immunol.* **60,** 1–30.
4. Keusch, G.T. (1990): Micronutrients and susceptibility to infection. *Ann. NY Acad. Sci.* **587,** 181–188.
5. Hershko, C. (1993): Iron, infection and immune function. *Proc. Nutr. Soc.* **52,** 165–174.
6. Payne, S.M. (1988): Iron and virulence in the family of Enterobacteriaceae. *Crit. Rev. Microbiol.* **16,** 81–111.
7. Crosa, J.H. (1984): The relationship of plasmid mediated iron transport and bacterial virulence. *Ann. Rev. Microbiol.* **38,** 69–89.
8. Ike, K., Kawahara, K., Danbara, H. & Kume, K. (1992): Serum resistance and aerobactin iron uptake in avian Escherichia coli mediated by conjugative 100-megadalton plasmid. *J. Vet. Med. Sci.* **54,** 1091–1098.

9. Stelma, G.N., Reyes, A.L., Peeler, J.T., Johnson, C.H. & Spaulding, P.L. (1992): Virulence characteristics of clinical and environmental isolates of Vibrio vulnificus. *Appl. Environ. Microbiol.* **58,** 2776–2782.

10. Sokol, P.A. (1987): Surface expression of ferripyochelin-binding protein is required for virulence of Pseudomonas aeruginosa. *Infect. Immun.* **55,** 2021–2025.

11. Schryvers, A.B. & Gonzalez, G.C. (1989): Comparison of the abilities of different protein sources of iron to enhance Neisseria meningitidis infection in mice. *Infect. Immun.* **57,** 2425–2429.

12. Sussman, M. (1974): Iron and infection. In: *Iron in Biochemistry and Medicine*, eds. A. Jacobs & M. Worwood, pp. 649–679. New York: Academic Press.

13. Vadillo, M., Corbella, X., Pac, V., Fernandez-Viladrich, P. & Pujol, R. (1994): Multiple liver abscesses due to Yersinia enterocolitica discloses primary hemochromatosis. *Clin. Infect. Dis.* **18,** 938–941.

14. Green, N.S. (1992): Yersinia infections in patients with homozygous beta-thalassemia associated with iron overload and its treatment. *Pediatr. Hematol. Oncol.* **9,** 247–254.

15. Mazzoleni, G., deSa, D., Gately, J. & Riddell, R.H. (1991): Yersinia enterocolitica infection with ileal perforation associated with iron overload and deferoxamine therapy. *Dig. Dis. Sci.* **36,** 1154–1160.

16. Bullen, J.J., Spalding, P.B., Ward, C.G. & Gutteridge, G.M. (1991): Hemochromatosis, iron and septicemia caused by Vibrio vulnificus. *Arch. Intern. Med.* **151,** 1606–1609.

17. Lambert, C.C. & Hunter, R.L. (1990): Low levels of unsaturated transferrin as a predictor of survival in pneumococcal pneumonia. *Ann. Clin. Lab. Sci.* **20,** 140–146.

18. Struelens, M.J., Mondal, G., Roberts, M. & Williams, P.H. (1990): Role of bacterial and host factors in the pathogenesis of Shigella septicemia. *Eur. J. Clin. Microbiol. Infect. Dis.* **9,** 337–344.

19. Seifert, A., von Herrath, D. & Schaefer, K. (1987): Iron overload, but not treatment with desferrioxamine favours the development of septicemia in patients on maintenance hemodialysis. *Quart. J. Med.* **65,** 1015–1024.

20. Ang, O., Gungor, M., Aricioglu, F., Inanc, D. *et al.* (1990): The effect of parenteral iron administration on the development of staphylococcus aureus-induced experimental pyelonephritis in rats. *Int. J. Exp. Pathol.* **71,** 507–511.

21. Ampel, N.M., Bejarano, G.C. & Saavedra, M. (1992): Deferoxamine increases the susceptibility of beta-thalassemic, iron-overloaded mice to infection with Listeria monocytogenes. *Life Sci.* **50,** 1327–1332.

22. Dallman, P.R. (1987): Iron deficiency and the immune response. *Amer. J. Clin. Nutr.* **46,** 329–334.

23. Murray, M.J., Murray, A.B., Murray, M.B. & Murray, C.J. (1978): The adverse effect of iron repletion on the course of certain infections. *Brit. Med. J.* **2,** 1113–1115.

24. Damsdaran, M., Naidu, A.N. & Sarma, K.V.R. (1979): Anemia and morbidity in rural preschool children. *Ind. J. Med. Res.* **69,** 448–456.

25. Harvey, P.W., Heywood, P.F., Nesheim, M.C. *et al.* (1989): The effect of iron therapy on malarial infection in Papua New Guinean schoolchildren. *Amer. J. Trop. Med. Hyg.* **40,** 12–18.

26. Javaid, N., Haschke, F., Pietschnig, B., Schuster, E. *et al.* Interaction between infections, malnutrition and iron nutritional status in Pakistani infants. A longitudinal study. *Acta Paediat. Scand. Suppl.* **374,** 141–150.

27. Haddock, R.L., Cousens, S.N. & Guzman, C.C. (1991): Infant diet and salmonellosis. *Amer. J. Publ. Health* **81,** 997–1000.

28. Weijmer, M.C., Neering, H. & Welten, C. (1990): Preliminary report: furunculosis and hypoferremia. *Lancet* **336,** 464–466.

29. Prasad, A.N. & Prasad, C. (1991): Iron deficiency: non-hematological manifestations. *Prog. Food. Nutr. Sci.* **15,** 255–283.

30. Brock, J.H. & Mainou-Fowler, T. (1983): The role of iron and transferrin in lymphocyte transformation. *Immunol. Today* **4,** 347–351.

31. Gygax, M., Hirni, H., Zwahken, R., Lazary, S. & Blum, J.W. (1993): Immune functions of weal calves fed low amounts of iron. *Zentralbl. Veterinarmed. A.* **40,** 345–358.

32. Walter, T., Arredondo, S., Arevalo, M. & Stekel, A. (1986): Effect of iron therapy on phagocytosis and bactericidal activity in neutrophils of iron-deficient infants. *Amer. J. Clin. Nutr.* **44,** 877–882.

33. Murakawa, H., Bland, C.E., Willis, W.T. & Dallman, P.R. (1987): Iron deficiency and neutrophil function: different rates of correction of the depressions in oxidative burst and myeloperoxidase activity after iron treatment. *Blood* **69,** 1464–1468.

34. Konijn A.M. & Hershko C. (1977): Ferritin synthesis in inflammation: I. Pathogenesis of impaired iron release. *Brit. J. Haemat.* **37,** 7–16.

35. Fahmy, M. & Young, S.P. (1993): Modulation of iron metabolism in monocyte cell line U937 by inflammatory cytokines: changes in transferin uptake, iron handling and ferritin mRNA. *Biochem. J.* **296,** 175–181.

36. Byrd, T.F. & Horwitz, M.A. (1989): Interferon gamma-activated human monocytes downregulate transferrin receptors and inhibit the intracellular multiplication of Legionella pneumophila by limiting the availability of iron. *J. Clin. Invest.* **83,** 1457–1465.

37. Lane, T.E., Wu-Hsieh, B.A. & Howard, D.H. (1991): Iron limitation and the gamma interferon-mediated antihistoplasma state of murine macrophages. *Infect. Immun.* **59,** 2274–2278.

38. Lancaster, J.R. & Hibbs, J.B. (1990): EPR demonstration of iron-nitrosyl complex formation by cytotoxic activated macrophages. *Proc. Natl. Acad. Sci. USA* **87,** 1223–1227.

39. Barnewall, R.E. & Rikihisa, Y. (1994): Abrogation of gamma iterferon-induced inhibition of Ehrlichia chaffeensis infection in human monocytes with iron transferrin. *Infect. Immun.* **62,** 4804–4810.

40. Raventos-Suarez, C., Pollack, S. & Nagel, R.L. (1982): Plasmodium falciparum: inhibition of *in vitro* growth by desferrioxamine. *Amer. J. Trop. Med. Hyg.* **31,** 919–922.

41. Hershko, C. & Peto, T.E.A. (1988): Deferoxamine inhibition of malaria is independent of host iron status. *J. Exper. Med.* **168,** 375–387.

42. Fritch, G., Treumer, J., Spira, D.T. & Jung, A. (1985): Plasmodium vinckei: Suppression of mouse infections with desferrioxamine B. *Exper. Path* **60,** 171–174.

43. Traore, O., Carnevale, P., Kaptue-Noche, L. *et al.* (1991): Preliminary report on the use of desferrioxamine in the treatment of Plasmodium falciparum malaria. *Amer. J. Hem.* **37,** 206–208.

44. Bunnag, D., Poltera, A.A., Viravan, C. *et al.* (1992): Plasmodicidal effect of desferrioxamine B in human vivax and falciparum malaria from Thailand. *Acta Trop. Basel.* **52,** 59–67.

45. Gordeuk, V.R., Thuma, P.E., Brittenham, G.M. *et al.* (1992): Iron chelation with desferrioxamine B in adults with asymptomatic Plasmodium falciparum parasitemia. *Blood* **79,** 308–312.

46. Gordeuk, V.R., Thuma, P., Brittenham, G.M. *et al.* (1992): Effect of iron chelation therapy on recovery from deep coma in children with cerebral malaria. *New Engl. J. Med.* **327,** 1473–1477.

47. Wyler, D.J. (1992): Bark, weeds, and iron chelators - Drugs for malaria. *New Engl. J. Med.* **327,** 1519–1521.

48. Hershko, C., Theanacho, E.N., Spira, D.T. *et al.* (1991): The effect of N-alkyl modification on the antimalarial activity of 3-hydroxypyrid-4-one oral iron chelators. *Blood* **77,** 637–643.

49. Heppner, D.G., Hallaway, P.E., Kontoghiorghes, G.J. & Eaton, J.W. (1988): Antimalarial properties of orally active iron chelators. *Blood* **72,** 358–363.

50. Yinnon, A.M., Theanacho, E.N., Grady, R.W. *et al.* (1989): Antimalarial effect of HBED and other phenolic and catecholic iron chelators. *Blood* **74,** 2166–2171.

51. Shanzer, A., Libman, J., Lytton, S., Glickstein, H. & Cabantchik, Z.I. (1991): Reversed siderophores act as antimalarial agents. *Proc. Nat. Acad. Sci. USA* **88,** 6585–6589.

52. Segovia, M., Navarro, A. & Artero, J.M. (1989): The effect of liposome-entrapped desferrioxamine on Leishmania donovani *in vitro. Ann. Trop. Med. Parasitol.* **83,** 357–360.

53. Lalonde, R.G. & Holbein, B.E. (1984): Role of iron in Trypanosoma cruzi infection in mice. *J. Clin. Invest.* **73,** 470–476.

54. Clarkson, A.B., Saric, S. & Grady, R.W. (1990): Deferoxamine and eflornitine (DL-α-difluoromethylornithine) in a rat model of Pneumocystis carinii pneumonia. *Antimic. Ag. Chemoth.* **34,** 1833–1835.

Iron Nutrition in Health and Disease, edited by Leif Hallberg and Nils-Georg Asp

Chapter 23

Iron and free radicals

John M.C. Gutteridge

Oxygen Chemistry Laboratory, Unit of Critical Care, Department of Anaesthesia and Intensive Care, Royal Brompton Hospital NHS Trust and National Heart & Lung Institute, Sydney Street, London, SW3 6NP, UK

The highly reactive and damaging hydroxyl radical (•OH) can be formed in biological systems by the radiolysis of water, by transition metal-dependent Fenton-type reactions, by the interaction of two endogenous free radical gases, namely superoxide (O_2^-) and by nitric oxide ($NO^•$), and by the reaction of superoxide with hypochlorous acid (HOCl). The high, almost diffusion controlled, reactivity of the hydroxyl radical means that damage by •OH generated in free solution by radiolysis is random and non-specific. When •OH is generated by Fenton chemistry, however, the site of iron complexation largely determines the site of •OH damage. Thus, although the chemical reactivity of •OH remains unchanged, the target for biological damage can be greatly influenced by Fenton chemistry.

To limit the participation of iron in reactions leading to aggressive oxidant formation, the body takes great care to sequester iron, in poorly or non-reactive storage and transport forms such as ferritin, haemosiderin transferrin and lactoferrin. Further protection is provided by structural compartmentalization of iron complexes. Tissue injury, by whatever mechanism, has the potential to stimulate free radical reactions by releasing intracellular iron and stimulating neutrophil activation.

Many metalloproteins can become damaged during severe oxidative stress and release their metal ions into solution. Thus, hydrogen peroxide can release cheletable iron from haem proteins, superoxide can release a small amount of iron from ferritin (non-core iron), and peroxynitrite ($ONOO^-$) formed by the reactive of O_2^- with $NO^•$ can release copper from caeruloplasmin. Released reactive metal ions act as triggers for further oxidative damage, and in the case of copper damage to low density lipoproteins can signal non-regulated lipid uptake by the macrophage scavenger receptor, which may ultimately lead to the development of atherosclerosis.

Life in an oxygen-rich atmosphere has necessitated an absolute requirement for antioxidant protection against reactive forms of oxygen. The intracellular reduction of oxygen to water involves the addition of four electrons, and when these are added one at a time three reactive forms of oxygen are made, two of which are free radicals. Addition of the first electron makes the superoxide (O_2^-) radical, and almost every normal aerobic cell contains superoxide dismutase enzymes to destroy it. These enzymes are either copper-zinc or manganese containing proteins. The product of the dismutation reaction is hydrogen peroxide (H_2O_2), and two enzymes exist to destroy it, namely catalase and the glutathione peroxidases (GSHPx). These proteins are predominantly intracellular, and by removing oxygen intermediates allow a small pool of low molecular mass iron to exist with cells for DNA and protein synthesis, and for signalling.

Extracellular fluids do not handle oxygen in the same way and require entirely different antioxidant defences to those found intracellularly. Here, we find proteins that efficiently bind or inactivate transition metal ions or their complexes. Thus, transferrin and lactoferrin bind, and transport iron, ferritin and haemosiderin store iron, and haemopexin and the haptoglobins bind haem and haemoglobin, respectively, decreasing their ability to stimulate peroxide decompositions. If reactive iron and copper are removed from extracellular fluids, oxygen intermediates such as O_2^-, H_2O_2, lipid peroxides (LOOH) and nitric oxide ($NO^\bullet$) can survive, and act as important signal, messenger and trigger molecules.

Oxygen radicals

The most reactive and damaging oxidant formed in biological systems is the hydroxyl radical •OH. Almost all of our knowledge concerning the chemistry of •OH comes from radiation studies, since it is a major product of the radiolysis (homolysis) of water. By the early 1970s it was clear that •OH radicals were formed in biological systems during normal aerobic metabolism[1]. The unusual chemistry of the oxygen molecule (it has two unpaired electrons) make it prefer accepting electrons (reduction) one at a time. When molecular oxygen (dioxygen) is completely reduced to water four electrons (e) are added, and when these are added singly two free radical intermediates are formed:

[1] $O_2 + e + H^+ \rightarrow HO_2^\bullet \xrightarrow{pH\ 7.4} H^+ + O_2^-$

[2] $O_2^- + e + 2H^+ \rightarrow H_2O_2$

[3] $H_2O_2 + e \rightarrow OH^- + {}^\bullet OH$

[4] ${}^\bullet OH + e + H^+ \rightarrow H_2O$

A free radical has an unpaired electron which is shown as a bold dot.

The importance of reactive iron species (RIS) in free radical reactions.

Until recently, the biological reactions that led to •OH formation were considered to be almost entirely dependent on the presence of trace amounts of transition metal ions, particularly iron[2]. Thus, a reaction between superoxide (O_2^-) and hydrogen peroxide (H_2O_2) requires an iron catalyst as first proposed by Haber and Weiss in 1934[3]. Equations 5–7 summarize how •OH radicals can be formed by iron catalysis:

[5] $O_2^- + Fe^{3+} \leftrightarrow O_2 + Fe^{2+}$

[6] $2O_2^- + 2H^+ \rightarrow H_2O_2 + O_2$

[7] $H_2O_2 + Fe^{2+} \rightarrow OH^- + {}^\bullet OH\ Fe^{3+}$

Equation 7 is known as the Fenton reaction[4], and a combination of equations 5–7 as 'superoxide-driven' Fenton chemistry. The possibility that RIS can also react with hypochlorous acid (HOCl) to generate •OH has recently been proposed[6]:

[8] $HOCl + Fe^{2+} \rightarrow {}^\bullet OH + Cl^- + Fe^{3+}$

Superoxide may also react with HOCl, and with nitric oxide ($NO^\bullet$) to form hydroxyl radicals in reactions that are iron-independent:[7,8]

[9] $O_2^- + HOCl \rightarrow {}^\bullet OH + O_2 + Cl^-$

[10] $O_2^- + NO^\bullet \rightarrow ONOO^- \rightarrow {}^\bullet OH + NO_2^\bullet$

The intermediate in equation 10 is peroxynitrite ($ONOO^-$) which is itself a powerful oxidant. There is still considerable ongoing debate concerning the reaction intermediates involved in equations 7–10.

The acceptance that redox-active forms of iron were required in biological systems to make hydroxyl radicals from hydrogen peroxide prompted a search among many groups, including our own, to develop methods to detect and measure biological iron that could participate *in vivo* in superoxide-driven Fenton chemistry[5].

Free radicals beget radicals, and so when •OH attacks another biological molecule to abstract a hydrogen atom it leaves behind an unpaired electron. Equations 11–13 show what happens when an •OH radical attacks an unsaturated lipid molecule (LH). Hydrogen abstraction leaves behind a carbon-centred lipid molecule ($L^\bullet$) which reacts rapidly with dioxygen to form a peroxyl radical ($LO_2^\bullet$). The peroxyl radical attacks another unsaturated lipid forming a lipid hydroperoxide (LOOH) and a lipid radical ($L^\bullet$) to propagate the chain reaction.

[11] $LH + {}^\bullet OH \rightarrow LO_2^\bullet$

[12] $L^\bullet + O_2 \rightarrow LO_2^\bullet$

[13] $LO^{\bullet}_2 + LH \rightarrow LOOH + L^{\bullet}$

A complex mixture of lipid peroxides are formed by free radicals in this way. However, it should also be appreciated that stereospecific lipid peroxides are constantly formed by purposeful biochemistry in the body using enzymes such as cyclooxygenase and lipoxygenases. In the presence of reactive iron complexes, lipid peroxides will decompose to form alkoxyl ($LO^{\bullet}$) and peroxyl radicals

[14] $2LOOH \rightarrow LO^{\bullet} + LO^{\bullet}_2 + H_2O$

and eventually yield a complex mixture of cytotoxic aldehydic molecules. Such a sequence of chemistry involving the peroxidation of low density lipoproteins[9] is at present thought to play a major role in the development of atherosclerosis.

What are the potential sources of reactive low molecular mass iron?

Cells contain a small pool of low molecular mass (low Mr) iron essential for the synthesis of DNA and iron-containing proteins. The exact size and nature of this iron pool remains an enigma, however. Any form of tissue injury can cause release of low Mr iron and one major cause is microbleeding whereby iron is released in the form of haemoglobin. Organic peroxides and hydrogen peroxide are able to release low Mr iron from the haemoglobin molecule[10] that can be chelated by bleomycin. The chelation of iron by bleomycin and its ability to undergo redox cycling to damage DNA forms the basis of an assay to detect and measure low Mr iron in biological materials[5]. In Table 1 are listed some of the clinical conditions in which bleomycin-chelatable iron has been detected in biological fluids and cell extracts.

In normal human plasma, mononuclear iron is firmly bound to transferrin which retains a considerable iron-binding potential. This available iron-binding capacity (about 75 per cent of the total) provides an important antioxidant defense against iron-driven free radical reactions[11]. In combination with the iron-oxidizing (ferroxidase) protein caeruloplasmin, transferrin provides an essential primary antioxidant defence against iron-driven radical chemistry[12]. As implied above, iron correctly loaded onto transferrin, or lactoferrin, does not stimulate free radical reactions, unless of course iron is first released at low pH, or by the presence of iron reductants and iron chelators. Similar considerations also apply to the iron storage protein ferritin with the following qualifications: iron replete ferritin does appear to stimulate lipid peroxide decompositions, and around 10 per cent of ferritin iron appears to be able to stimulate superoxide-driven Fenton chemistry. It has been suggested that this is due to a fraction of iron not loaded into the central core of the protein[13].

Of the body's total iron (approximately 4.5 g), two thirds is present as haemoglobin and myoglobin, and so haem iron is a major potential source of reactive iron. Native haemoglobin is not a Fenton catalyst, although it does stimulate lipid peroxidation possibly through reaction with lipid hydroperoxides to generate ferryl haemoglobin (iron(IV)), or as mentioned above through release of low Mr iron.

In spite of the body's tight control over iron homeostasis, reactive forms of iron do become available during iron overload, and as a result of tissue injury. Such forms of iron are able to stimulate free radical reactions and convert poorly reactive oxygen species into highly reactive and damaging molecules. Iron chelation strategies are likely to be more succesful than non-specific radical scavenging in preventing site-specific radical damage during tissue injury.

Acknowledgements

The British Lung Foundation and the British Oxygen Group are thanked for their for their generous support.

Table 1. Bleomycin-detectable iron in biological samples

Fluid	Bleomycin chelatable iron µmol/l (unless otherwise stated)	Comments	Refs
Blood Serum/Plasma			
Normal healthy controls[25]	0		14
Arthritis (osteo, rheumatoid)[31]	0		14,15
Haemochromatosis[7]	4.3 ± 6.7		16,17
Fulminant hepatic failure[20]	2.2 ± 2.2	only 2 patients did not show BLM iron	18
Myeloid leukaemia			
before chemotherapy[6]	1.0 ± 1.8	only 2 patients showed BLM iron	19
after chemotherapy[4]	9.5 ± 8.5	all showed BLM iron	
Non-lymphocytic leukaemia			
before chemotherapy[9]	0.4 ± 1.0	only 2 patients showed BLM-iron	20
1–6 days after chemotherapy[9]	2.6 ± 2.6	3 patients did not show BLM iron	
Adult respiratory distress syndrome (ARDS) patients with multi-organ failure[5]	0.46 ± 0.22	represents 33% of ARDS patients managed during the period of study	21
Cardiopulmonary bypass			
extracorporeal blood circulation[4]	0.27 ± 0.9	mock bypass; BLM iron present in 2 samples	22
blood cardioplegia	0.24 ± 0.26	BLM iron present in 27% of patients receiving warm blood cardioplegia	23
Hypotransferrinaemic mice[8]	16.0 ± 5.0	both the control and hpx/hpx mice had NTA-detectable iron (1.5 and 1.3 µM) present	24
control mice[5]	0		
Newborn infants (cord)[25]	0.27 ± 0.56	only 6 samples showed BLM iron	25,26
Newborn infants 1–5 days[13]	0.33 ± 0.72	only 3 samples showed BLM iron	25
Kwashiorkor patients[50]	up to 19.5	58% of patients with kwashiorkor had BLM iron in their plasma	27
Marasmus patients[6]	0		
Sweat fluids			
Arm fluid[12]	0.72 ± 2.5	BLM-iron present in only 1 sample	28
Trunk fluid[10]	4.62 ± 2.9	BLM-iron present in all samples	
Synovial Fluids			
Rheumatoid arthritis[21]	3.1 ± 1.9	approximately 40% of synovial fluids from patients show BLM iron	
Osteoarthritis[22]	0.37 ± 1.1	when stressed at a pH value of 5.3	15,29
Pleural exudate			
Rat (inflammatory)[2]	0.85*	collection conditions unknown	
Colostrum			
Bovine[4]	4.1 ± 8.2*	BLM iron present in only one sample; collection condition unknown	
Eye vitreous humor			
Rabbit (3 pooled samples)	4.80*	collection conditions unknown	

Cont...

Table 1. Bleomycin-detectable iron in biological samples (cont.)

Fluid	Bleomycin Chelatable iron **μmol/l (unless otherwise stated)**	**Comments**	**Refs**
Cerebrospinal fluids cont.			
Normal human[12]	1.8 ± 1.3	unbuffered assay reagents	30
Normal human[15]	0.55 ± 0.27	pH 7.0	31
Neuronal ceriod lipofucinoses[15]	5.37 ± 2.0	unbuffered assay reagents	30
Neuronal ceriod lipofuciness[7]	1.6 ± 0.8	pH 5.3	32
Encephalopathy[9]	1.0 ± 0.4	pH 5.3	32
Multiple sclerosis[6]	1.75 ± 0.8	unbuffered assay reagents	30
Epilepsy[5]	2.48 ± 0.8	unbuffered assay reagents	30
Meningism due to treatment with iron-dextran[1]	36.0		33
Cerebral and ocular toxicity due to treatment with desferrioxamine and prochloperazine[1]	0	sample showed an iron-binding capacity	34
Urine			
Renal reperfusion injury			
control[8]	138 ± 54 pmol/30 min		35
15–45 min reperfusion[8]	1590 ± 776 pmol/30 min		
45–75 min reperfusion[6]	1249 ± 506 pmol/30 min		
Cellular ultrafiltrates			
10,000 Da exclusion			
Brain tissue, gerbil[8]	20.5 ± 3.5 nmol/wet wt		36
Red blood cells human[1]	0.65 nmol/l		
Red blood cells human + malarial parasites (falciparium)[1]	129 nmol/l		
Red blood cells, rat[10]	0		
Red blood cells, rat + *P. bergheii*[8]	0.91 ± 0.39 nmol/l		
30, 000 Da exclusion			
Kidney tissue control[15]	18 nmol/g/wet wt		37
Kidney tissue after ischaemia reperfusion[15]	57 nmol/g/wet wt		
Cellular homogenates			
Bacteria (5 different strains)	0.003-1.046 μmol/mg protein		38
Liver tissue (C3H/Hej, fatty streak resistant mice)			39
- normal diet	120–149 nmol/mg		
- atherogenic diet	57–78 nmoles/mg		

*Unpublished data samples provided by Drs Armstrong, Griffiths and Peto. Mean values are shown (± SEM or SD as derived in appropriate references)
BLM = bleomycin, NTA = nitrilotriacetate. Number of samples studied shown in superscript.

References

1. Halliwell, B. & Gutteridge, J.M.C. (1989): *Free Radicals in Biology and Medicine*, pp. 22–85. Oxford: Oxford University Press.
2. Gutteridge, J.M.C. & Halliwell, B. (1989): Iron toxicity and oxygen radicals. In: *Clinical haematology, international practice and research. Iron chelating therapy*, ed. C. Hershko, pp. 195–256. London: Baillière Tindall.
3. Haber, F. & Weiss, J. (1934): The catalytic decomposition of hydrogen peroxide by iron salts. *Proc. R. Soc. London* **147,** 332–351.
4. Fenton, H.J.H. (1894): Oxidation of tartaric acid in presence of iron. *J. Chem. Soc.* **64,** 899–909.
5. Gutteridge, J.M.C., Rowley, D.A. & Halliwell, B. (1981): Superoxide-dependent formation of hydroxyl radicals in the presence of iron salts. Detection of 'free' iron in biological systems by using bleomycin-dependent degradation of DNA. *Biochem. J.* **199,** 263–265.
6. Candeias, L.P., Stratford, M.R.L. & Wardman, P. (1994): Formation of hydroxyl radicals on reaction of hypochlorous acid with ferrocyanide, a model iron (II) complex. *Free Rad. Res.* **20,** 241–249.
7. Candeias, L.P., Patel, K.B., Stratford, M.R.L. & Wardman, P. (1989): Free hydroxyl radicals are formed on reaction between the neutrophil-derived species superoxide anion and hypochlorous acid. *FEBS Lett.* **333,** 151–153.
8. Beckman, J.S., Beckman, T.W., Chen, J., Marshall, P.A. & Freeman, B.A. (1990): Apparent hydroxyl radical production by peroxynitrite: Implications for endothelial injury from nitric oxide and superoxide. *Proc. Natl. Acad. Sci. USA* **87,** 1620–1624.
9. Steinberg, D., Pathasarathy, S., Carew, T.E. *et al.* (1989): Beyond cholesterol. Modifications of low-density lipoprotein that increases its atherogenicity. *N. Engl. J. Med.* **320,** 915–24.
10. Gutteridge, J.M.C. (1986): Iron promoters of the Fenton reaction and lipid peroxidation can be released from haemoglobin by peroxides. *FEBS Lett.* **201,** 291–295.
11. Gutteridge, J.M.C., Paterson, S.K., Segal, A.W. & Halliwell, B. (1981): Inhibition of lipid peroxidation by the iron-binding protein lactoferrin. *Biochem. J.* **199,** 259–261.
12. Gutteridge, J.M.C. & Quinlan, G.J. (1993): Antioxidant protection against organic and inorganic oxygen radicals by normal human plasma: the primary role for iron-binding and iron-oxidizing proteins. *Biochim. Biophys. Acta* **1156,** 144–150.
13. Bolann, B.J. & Ulvik, R.J. (1990): On the limited ability of superoxide to release iron from ferritin. *Eur. J. Biochem.* **193,** 899–904.
14. Gutteridge, J.M.C. (1986): Antioxidant properties of the proteins caeruloplasmin, albumin and transferrin. A study of their activity in serum and synovial fluid from patients with rheumatoid arthritis. *Biochim. Biophys. Acta.* **869,** 119–127.
15. Gutteridge, J.M.C. (1987): Bleomycin-detectable iron in knee-joint synovial fluid from arthritic patients and its relationship to the extracellular antioxidant activities of caeruloplasmin, transferrin and lactoferrin. *Biochem. J.* **245,** 415–421.
16. Gutteridge, J.M.C., Rowley. D.A., Griffiths. E. & Halliwell, B. (1985): Low molecular weight iron complexes and oxygen radical reactions in idiopathic haemochromatisis. *Clin. Sci.* **68,** 463–467.
17. Bullen, J.J., Spalding, P.B., Ward, C.G. & Gutteridge, J.M.C. (1991): Hemochromatosis, iron, and septicemia caused by Vibrio vulnificus. *Arch. Int. Med.* **1511,** 1606–1609.

18. Evans, P.J., Evans, R.W., Bomford, A., Williams, R. & Halliwell, B. (1994): Metal ions catalytic for free radical reactions in the plasma of patients wilth fulminant hepatic failure. *Free Rad. Res.* **20,** 139–144.

19. Halliwell, B., Aruoma, O.I., Mufti, G. & Bomford, A. (1988): Bleomycin-detectable iron in serum from leukaemic patients before and after chemotherapy. *FEBS Lett.* **241,** 202–204.

20. Gordeuk, V.R. & Brittenham, G.M. (1992): Bleomycin-reactive iron in patients with acute non-lymphocytic leukaemia. *FEBS Lett.* **308,** 4–6.

21. Gutteridge, J.M.C., Quinlan, G.J. & Evans, T.W. (1994): Transient iron overload with bleomycin-detectable iron in the plasma of patients with adult respiratory distress syndrome. *Thorax.* **49,** 707–710.

22. Moat, N.E., Evans, T.W., Quinlan, G.J. & Gutteridge, J.M.C. (1993): Chelatable iron and copper can be released from extracorporeally circulated blood during cardiopulmonary bypass. *FEBS Lett.* **328,** 103–106.

23. Pepper, J.R., Mumby, S. & Gutteridge, J.M.C. (1994): Transient iron-overload with bleomycin-detectable iron present during cardiopulmonary bypass surgery. *Free Rad. Res.* **21,** 53–58.

24. Simpson, R.J., Cooper, C.E., Raja, K.B., Halliwell, B. *et al.* (1992): Non-transferrin-bound iron species in the serum of hypotransferrinaemic mice. *Biochim. Biophys. Acta* **1156,** 19–26.

25. Evans, P.J., Evans, R., Kovar, I.Z., Holton, A.F. *et al.* (1992): Bleomycin-detectable iron in the plasma of premature and full term neonates. *FEBS Lett.* **303,** 210–212.

26. Lindeman, J.H.N., Houdkamp, E., Lentjev, E.G.W., Poorthuis, B.J.H. *et al.* (1992): Limited protection against iron induced lipid peroxidation by cord blood plasma. *Free Rad. Res. Commun.* **16,** 285–294.

27. Dempster, W.S., Sive, A.A., Rosseau, S., Malan, H. *et al.* (1995): Misplaced iron in Kwashiokor. *Eur. Clin. Nutr.* **49,** 208–210.

28. Gutteridge, J.M.C., Rowley, D.A., Halliwell, B., Cooper, D.F. *et al.* (1985): Copper and iron complexes catalytic for oxygen radical reactions in sweat from human athletes. *Clin. Chim. Acta* **145,** 267–273.

29. Rowley, D.A., Gutteridge, J.M.C., Blake, D.R., Farr, M. *et al.* (1985): Lipid peroxidation in rheumatoid arthritis. thiobarbituric acid-reactive material and catalytic iron salts in synovial fluid from rheumatoid patients. *Clin. Sci.* **66,** 691–695.

30. Gutteridge, J.M.C., Rowley, D.A., Halliwell, B. & Westermarck, T. (1988): Increased non-protein-bound iron and decreased protection against superoxide radical damage in cerebrospinal fluids from patients with neuronal ceroid lipofuscinosis. *Lancet* **5,** 459–460.

31. Gutteridge, J.M.C. (1992): Ferrous ions detected in cerebrospinal fluid by using bleomycin and DNA damage. *Clin. Sci.* **82,** 315–320.

32. Heiskala, H., Gutteridge, J.M.C., Westermarck, T., Alanen, J. *et al.* (1988): Bleomycin-detectable iron and phenanthroline-detectable copper in the cerebrospinal fluid of patients with neuonal ceroid-lipofuscinoses. *Am. J. Med. Genetics (Suppl).* **2,** 459–460.

33. Shuttleworth, D., Spence, C. & Slade, R. (1983): Meningism due to intravenous iron dextran. *Lancet* **2,** 435.

34. Blake, D.R., Winyard, P., Lunec, J., Williams, A. *et al.* (1985): Cerebral and ocular toxicity induced by desferrioxamine. *Quart. J. Med.* **219,** 345–355.

35. Paller, M.S. & Hedlund, B.E. (1988): Role of iron in post-ischaemic renal injury in the rat. *Kidney Internat.* **34,** 474–480.

36. Gutteridge, J.M.C., Cao, W. & Chevion, M. (1991): Bleomycin-detectable iron in brain tissue. *Free Rad. Res. Commun.* **11,** 317–320.

37. Baliga, R., Veda, N. & Shah, S.V. (1993): Increase in bleomycin-detectable iron in ischaemia/reperfusion to rat kidneys. *Biochem, J.* **391,** 901–905.

38. Gutteridge, J.M.C. & Wilkins, S. (1984): Non-protein bound iron within bacterial cells and the action of bleomycin. *Biochem. Internat.* **8,** 89–94.

39. Van Lenten, B.J., Prieve, J., Navab, M., Hama, S. *et al.* (1995): Lipid-induced changes in intracellular iron homeostasis *in vitro* and *in vivo. J. Clin. Invest.* **95,** 2104–2110.

Iron Nutrition in Health and Disease, edited by Leif Hallberg and Nils-Georg Asp

Chapter 24

Hereditary haemochromatosis - an overview

June W. Halliday

Liver Unit, Queensland Institute of Medical Research, The Bancroft Centre, P.O. Royal Brisbane Hospital, Brisbane, Queensland 4029, Australia

Summary

The term haemochromatosis (hereditary or genetic haemochromatosis) is now used to describe a genetic disorder in which a progressive increase in body iron stores results in the deposition of excessive amounts of iron in the parenchymal cells of the liver, pancreas, heart and other organs. The increase in iron stores results from an inappropriate increase in intestinal iron absorption. The excess iron deposition eventually results in cellular damage and functional insufficiency of the involved organs. A similar degree of iron overload may be associated with ineffective erythropoiesis (as in thalassaemia).

Genetic haemochromatosis is inherited as an autosomal recessive trait and the susceptibility locus is lightly linked to the HLA locus on chromosome 6. The gene frequency is appropriately 1 in 10 to 1 in 20 with a homozygote frequency in Caucasian populations (particularly of Celtic ancestry) of 1 in 300. In Australia the great majority of relatives predicted by HLA typing to be homozygous for the disease will exhibit full biochemical and clinical expression of the disease. Heterozygotes do not develop a progressive increase in iron stores to the extent seen in homozygotes but 25 per cent of these show some biochemical abnormality, such as an increase in transferrin saturation.

The diagnosis is now frequently made in asymptomatic subjects in whom an elevated serum iron, serum transferrin saturation and serum ferritin concentration have been detected. A liver biopsy with chemical determination of the hepatic iron concentration permits the hepatic iron index to be calculated (hepatic iron concentration in μmol/g dry wt ÷ age in years). An index greater than 1.9 is usually present in homozygous subjects. The relative risk of hepatocellular carcinoma in patients with iron overload who are already cirrhotic is 200-fold but phlebotomy therapy in pre-cirrhotic patients to remove the excess iron prevents the subsequent development of cirrhosis and of hepatocellular carcinoma. Early detection is thus very important and all first-degree relatives should be offered screening by transferrin saturation and serum ferritin. HLA typing of the family can often detect those at risk of developing iron overload.

The underlying biochemical defect leading to the high iron absorption in haemochromatosis is unknown. Theoretically the defect could lie in the intestinal mucosal cells of the upper small intestine, in the liver, the RE system or a more generalized defect. It could be a defective iron-binding protein, a transport protein or a receptor or it could be a defect in the regulation of an iron transport protein, a transport 'channel' or a receptor.

There is increasing evidence that haemochromatosis results from a generalized membrane transport or other defect in multiple organs. The inappropriately high iron absorption from the gut could result from an increased rate of uptake from the mucosal cell or an inappropriate compartmentalization or oxidation state of the intracellular iron pool leading to inappropriate binding of an iron regulatory protein (IRP) to RNA, resulting in a decreased ferritin and increased transferrin receptor levels. The elucidation of the basic defect still awaits the cloning and sequencing of the HLA-A linked gene on the short arm of chromosome 6.

The use of microsatellites (CA repeats) to determine the precise location of the haemochromatosis gene has revealed that the microsatellite D6S105 is the closest marker so far reported. A specific combination of alleles of HLA-A, D6S105, HLA-F, D6S248 and D6S265 forms the predominant ancestral haplotype in the Australian haemochromatosis population and may be associated with a single mutation of the haemochromatosis gene. Recent studies have shown that homozygosity for this ancestral haplotype is associated with an increased rate of iron accumulation. The high prevalence of the haemochromatosis gene may result from a selective advantage conferred against iron deficiency, especially in females.

Introduction

The body of a healthy adult male normally contains approximately 90 mmol (5 g) of iron and a female somewhat less. Of this iron, some 80 per cent is present in compounds such as haemoglobin, myoglobin and tissue enzymes, while the remainder represents storage iron. Approximately one third of these iron stores are in the liver and the remainder largely in the reticuloendothelial system. Storage iron exists in two forms: in the large iron-storage protein, ferritin, and as haemosiderin, a poorly defined molecule which consists of iron aggregates and protein derived from ferritin. As the iron concentration in the tissue rises the concentration of haemosiderin relative to that of ferritin also increases[1].

The amount of iron in the body is controlled largely at the point of entry, i.e. the intestinal mucosa. The lack of a major excretory pathway for iron in man means than any increase in iron intake, either by a prolonged increase in iron absorption or as a consequence of the administration of parenteral iron will produce an increase in iron stores in the body unless there is a concomitant pathological increase in iron losses, such as by blood loss.

The term haemochromatosis (HC), sometimes called hereditary or genetic haemochromatosis, is now used to describe a genetic disorder in which a progressive increase in body iron stores results in the deposition of excessive amounts of iron in the parenchymal cells of the liver, pancreas, heart and other organs. The increase in iron stores results from an inappropriate increase in intestinal iron absorption. The excess iron deposition eventually results in cellular damage and functional insufficiency of the involved organs. A similar degree of iron overload may arise as a consequence of ineffective erythropoiesis (as in thalassaemia).

Genetic or hereditary HC is inherited as an autosomal recessive trait and the susceptibility locus is tightly linked to the HLA locus on chromosome 6[2,3]. The gene frequency is approximately 1 in 10 to 1 in 20 with a homozygote frequency in Caucasian populations (particularly of Celtic ancestry) of 1 in 300[4]. In Australia the great majority of relatives predicted by HLA typing to be homozygous for the gene will exhibit full biochemical and clinical expression of the disease[5]. Heterozygotes do not develop a progressive increase in iron stores to the extent seen in homozygotes, but 25 per cent of these show some biochemical abnormality, such as an increase in transferrin saturation.

Until recent times a diagnosis of HC was made only in patients who presented with clinical signs and symptoms of the disease. These included the classic triad of skin pigmentation, hepatomegaly and diabetes as described by Sheldon in 1935[6]. Loss of libido and testicular atrophy were common and cardiac manifestations occurred in 5–15 per cent of symptomatic patients[7]. The diagnosis is now frequently made in asymptomatic subjects in whom an elevated serum iron, serum transferrin saturation and serum ferritin concentration have been detected[8,9]. A liver biopsy with chemical determination of the hepatic iron concentration permits the hepatic iron index to be calculated (hepatic iron concentration in μmol/g dry wt ÷ age in years; Figs 1a and 1b). An index greater than 1.9 is usually present in homozygous subjects and should read dry weight ÷ age and less than 1.5 in heterozygotes[10,11]. The relative risk of hepatocellular cancer in patients nearwith iron overload who are already cirrhotic is 200-fold[12], but phlebotomy therapy in pre-herecirrhotic patients to remove the excess iron prevents the

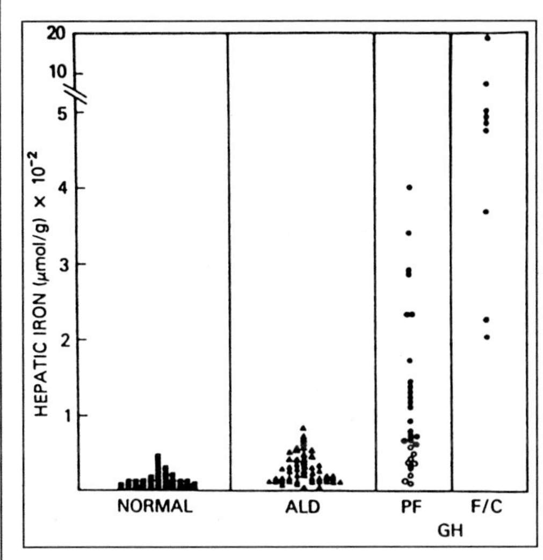

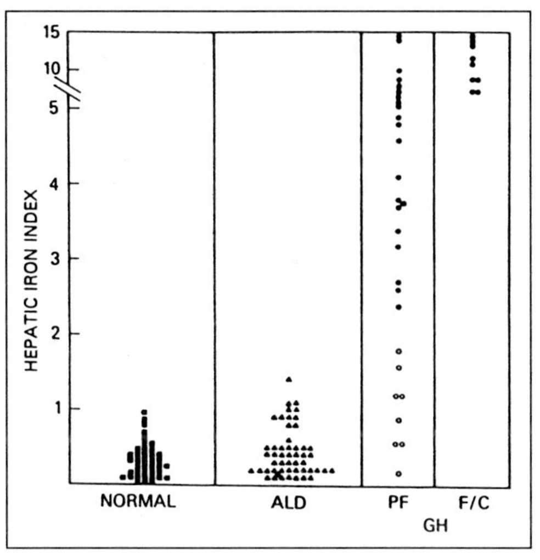

Fig. 1 (a). Hepatic iron concentrations and (b) hepatic iron index (ratio of iron concentration to age) in normal subjects, patients with alcoholic liver disease (ALD) and HC subjects: PF = prefibrotic; F/C = fibrotic or cirrhotic; HC heterozygotes are shown by open circles; homozygotes are shown by closed circles. (From Ref. 10 with permission)

subsequent development of cirrhosis and of hepatocellular carcinoma. Early detection is thus very important and all first-degree relatives should be offered screening by transferrin saturation and serum ferritin. HLA typing of the family can often detect those relatives of a proband who are at risk of developing iron overload.

Diagnosis

Although the classical clinical features of the disease are diagnostic in advanced iron overload, in the early stages laboratory investigations are often the first indicators of excess iron stores. These include an elevated serum iron level >30 μmol/l (>170 μg/100 ml) associated with an elevated transferrin saturation (50 per cent) and an elevated serum ferritin concentration[9,13,14]. Transferrin saturation and serum ferritin concentration are the best screening tests for asymptomatic, precirrhotic HC. When hepatic iron stores are more than twice the normal level, the serum ferritin rises above the normal range and transferrin saturation is usually greater than 50 per cent[8]. The serum ferritin usually rises in proportion to total body iron stores until it reaches levels of 1000 ng/ml or more[15]. The serum ferritin may be elevated out of proportion to body iron stores by hepatocellular necrosis, especially in alcoholic liver disease, or by other inflammatory processes, and several families in which the serum ferritin concentration has been normal despite unequivocal increases in body iron stores have been reported[16–18]. Despite these exceptional situations serum ferritin remains a useful screening test in family studies and transferrin saturation in population studies.

Liver biopsy allows definition of the extent of tissue damage and both histochemical and biochemical assessments of tissue iron. An attempt should be made to quantify the degree of iron excess as demonstration of increased body iron stores is essential for the diagnosis and also gives a guide to duration of venesection. Serum ferritin concentration, hepatic iron concentration and retrospective calculation of iron removed are all useful in calculating the degree of excess iron stores[19,20]. Hepatic iron concentrations in excess of 40 μmol/g dry weight are seen in early untreated HC and values may exceed 400 μmol/g in advanced symptomatic disease. Measurement of urinary iron excretion after administration of chelating agents is cumbersome and has largely been replaced by these other methods. Promising attempts have been made to measure hepatic density in iron overload indirectly by computed tomography[21–23] and magnetic resonance imaging[24]. These may become useful non-invasive screening tests, but liver biopsy will remain the definitive test for assessing the histological pattern and the degree of tissue damage, especially in early disease.

Screening of families

HLA typing is of no use as a screening test in the general population. It is extremely useful, however, in families and particularly in siblings of a proband to predict the risk of developing iron overload[25]. Physical examination and measurement of transferrin saturation and serum ferritin should be used to screen first-degree relatives of patients with HC. If both these indices are normal, the subject has a low probability of having increased iron stores[26]. If either test is abnormal, liver biopsy should be performed to quantify the tissue iron concentration and the degree, if any, of liver damage.

Pathology

The major pathological findings in *advanced* HC relate to the massive amounts of iron found in the parenchymal cells of most organs, particularly liver, pancreas, heart and endocrine glands. The liver is enlarged and nodular and, along with the pancreas, presents a striking reddish-brown colour. On histological examination, iron is found in large amounts in the parenchymal cells. Only in the late stages of the disease is iron also seen in Kupffer cells, macrophages and biliary epithelial cells - a useful factor in the differential diagnosis. This extensive iron deposition is associated with dense fibrosis in the liver and pancreas; in the liver the fibrosis leads eventually to a mixed macro-micronodular cirrhosis. Cell necrosis and inflammation are usually absent and the parenchymal cells otherwise usually appear normal. Iron appears first within the periportal hepatocytes and in a pericanalicular distribution within lysosomes. With increasing iron loading, hepatocytes in zones 2 and 3 (moving towards the central vein) become iron-loaded until the whole liver appears blue on a Perl's stain. This is followed by fibrosis in the portal areas eventually linking up to form a 'holly-leaf' pattern but with large areas of preserved parenchyma[27]. The mechanism of fibrosis in iron overload, in the apparent absence of inflammation remains controversial.

Histological examination of the pancreas usually shows heavy deposits of haemosiderin in the acinar cells. Haemosiderin is also found in the heart muscle fibres in advanced HC but fibrosis is rare. It is also deposited in the conducting fibres of the atrioventricular node which probably accounts for the cardiac arhythmias which may occur in this disease. The pituitary, adrenal, thyroid and parathyroid glands may also contain extensive iron as haemosiderin deposits, although evidence of functional impairment is usually confined to the pituitary. The characteristic metallic grey hue of the skin results from increased melanin (with or without iron) in the dermis in association with an atrophic epidermis. Increased iron deposition in the skin is very variable and tends to occur around the sweat glands[27].

The biochemical defect

The underlying biochemical defect in HC is unknown. One incontrovertible fact is that in HC, iron absorption is inappropriately high in relation to the body iron stores. Various hypotheses have been advanced to account for this. Theoretically, it could be a defect in the intestinal mucosal cells of the upper small intestine, a defect in the known iron-proteins transferrin or ferritin, or their receptors, or in a hitherto unknown transport protein. It could also be an abnormality in the regulation of a transport protein. The defect could be present in the liver, the reticuloendothelial system or as a more generalized defect.

The intestinal mucosal cell

It is a well-known fact that iron absorption is increased soon after stimulation of the bone marrow to increase erythropoiesis, as occurs after haemorrhage and hypoxia and also in iron deficiency; however, in each situation, the mechanism remains unclear. Several observations have suggested that the intestinal mucosal cell itself functions abnormally in HC and that the cell is behaving as if the body is iron deficient[28,29].

Two new membrane iron-binding proteins have been recently described, one by Teichmann and Stremmel[30] and one by Conrad and colleagues[31]. The former is a 160 kDa iron-binding protein (a trimer of 54 kDa monomers) prepared from solubilized human microvillous membrane proteins. It was localized to brushborder plasma membranes and was present in human intestinal mucosa, liver and heart but not in the oesophagus. An antibody against this protein inhibited Fe^{3+} uptake by more than 50 per cent. These data suggested that the transport of Fe^{3+} across human microvillous membranes represents a facilitated transport mechanism which may be mediated, at least in part, by this membrane iron-binding protein. Studies from this group also indicated that the protein was upregulated in HC and remained so after phlebotomy therapy[32]. The iron-binding protein described by Conrad *et al.*[31] is a 56 kDa molecule seen in the apical cytoplasm of rat duodenal mucosa. These two iron-binding proteins remain as potentially important sources of the defect but their biological significance remains to be confirmed.

Because of the technical difficulties in studying low-molecular weight iron-carriers there are few data available and the results to date have been inconclusive. It has been suggested that, whereas in normal subjects, iron chelators such as citrate and ascorbate may act on iron-regulatory element binding proteins (IRP) in the intestinal mucosa, resulting in upregulation of intracellular ferritin synthesis in response to increased cellular iron content, in HC the iron content of these cells is inappropriately low which is reflected in a low ferritin content.

At least two *in vivo* studies have provided data which indicate that the defective control of iron absorption in this disease is mediated at the level of intestinal cell transfer to the plasma (i.e. serosal transfer as opposed to mucosal uptake). In a recent study by McLaren *et al.*[33] mucosal iron kinetics were analysed using a compartmental model of intestinal iron absorption and systemic ferrokinetics. In subjects with HC, the transfer of mucosal iron to the plasma was inappropriately high, although still inversely related to body iron stores as in normal subjects. This increase in mucosal iron transfer rate appeared to be the major determinant of increased iron absorption.

There have been major recent advances in the elucidation of the coordinate regulation by iron of both ferritin synthesis and transferrin receptor (TfR) expression[34–37]. These proteins have now been shown to be regulated by means of binding proteins (the IRP) which bind to the iron regulatory elements in the mRNA of both TfR and ferritin. This coordinate regulation appears to be intact in HC and the gene for the protein lies on chromosome 9, not 6 as for the HC gene. However, in subjects with HC, intestinal mucosal H and L ferritin as well as immunohistochemically detectable ferritin fail to rise in parallel with the serum ferritin levels[38,39]. It has also been shown that the steady-state mRNA for both H and L ferritin is inappropriately low, whereas the mRNA for TfR is inappropriately increased[40] and there is sustained activity of an iron-regulatory factor[41]. These results could be interpreted as indicating a primary defect in ferritin transcription in the intestinal mucosal cells. However, it is more reasonable to suppose that these observations merely indicator: (1) that the coordinate regulation of the genes for TfR and for ferritin in the gut is still intact; (2) that the levels of iron in the gut cells are inappropriately low for reasons not clear; and (3) that the demonstrated abnormality in intestinal ferritin in HC is secondary to a primary abnormality elsewhere in the mucosal cell, to a more remote defect (for example in the liver or the monocyte-macrophage system), or to a more generalized cellular or membrane defect.

Numerous studies have concluded that both transferrin and its receptor function normally in HC[40,42]. Recent work supports the hypothesis that the TfR on the gut cells is concerned more with the transport of iron *from* the plasma to the mucosal cell, presumably for use within the cell especially during cell growth[43,44]. Moreover, the genes for each of these proteins are on chromosome 3.

It has been suggested that HC relates to a failure to 'switch' from neonatal to adult control of iron absorption[45,46]. The hypothesis is attractive but so far unsubstantiated. Anderson *et al.*[44]. showed that the intestine of the pre-term rat demonstrated a high level of duodenal TfR along the full length of the crypt-villus axis but soon after birth it was reduced in the area towards the villus tip. There was no correlation between iron absorption and TfR expression in either neonates or adult animals and the crypt receptor density remained high at all ages.

Recent mapping and linkage studies[47] place at least one of the H ferritin pseudogenes on chromosome 6, centromeric to the HC locus which makes this unlikely to be a candidate gene for the disease, as had been suggested.

Thus, the available evidence suggests that ferritin synthesis and function in the gut and liver are normal in HC. It is possible that the ferritin receptor is involved in the pathobiology of HC but evidence for this must await elucidation of its structure and physiological role.

The liver

In HC, in contrast to secondary iron overload, the abnormal iron accumulation occurs in the hepatocytes and it is only late in the disease that Kupffer cells, macrophages and biliary epithelial cells of the liver contain stainable iron. In addition, the high percentage saturation of circulating transferrin with iron is observed long before the accumulation of large amounts of iron in the liver. The deposition of iron in hepatocytes and parenchymal cells of other organs could occur by other means. There are at least three mechanisms of iron delivery to hepatocytes in normal animals[48]. In conditions of iron overload, iron is also delivered to hepatocyctes by non-transferrin-bound iron. The nature of this iron is ill defined but it probably includes a low-molecular-weight form and it could also include ferritin iron[49]. Thus, a primary role for hepatocytes in the control of iron accumulation seems unlikely. However, the production of a circulating regulator of iron absorption has never been excluded. Rat transplantation experiments have been used in attempts to provide some answers[50,51]. The available results would be consistent with a role for the intestinal mucosal cell in regulating iron uptake and body absorption according to its iron content. However, a further role for a humoral factor in regulating iron transfer across the intestinal cell remains a possibility.

Human liver transplantation has also provided some insight into this problem. The available data, which include some 22 subjects with HC successfully transplanted for end-stage liver disease, and a further four instances where a liver from an HC subject was inadvertently transplanted into a non-HC recipient, have recently been reviewed[52]. It was concluded that the combined data could best be explained by a combination of an hepatic and an extrahepatic defect before the disease is fully expressed.

Non-transferrin-bound iron and hepatocyte membrane transport

Hepatic transferrin receptors are reportedly reduced in HC[53] suggesting that hepatic iron overload is not due to increased clearance of transferrin-bound iron from the plasma. In contrast, recent attention has focussed on the low-molecular-weight iron complexes referred to collectively as 'non-transferrin-bound' iron (NTBI). Although the NTBI accounts normally for less than 1 per cent of the total serum iron, it may account for up to 35 per cent of serum iron in subjects with HC[49]. Hepatic clearance of this form of iron is remarkably efficient[54] and is not reduced by hepatic iron loading[55]. Thus, NTBI may be quantitatively much more important than transferrin-bound iron in hepatic iron accumulation in HC. Using the isolated perfused liver model, Wright and colleagues[56] provided evidence that the hepatic uptake of NTBI is mediated by a membrane carrier and occurs by an electron transfer mechanism in which there is a net movement of positive charge into the cell. These authors concluded that, since there is evidence that copper, zinc and manganese share a common carrier with iron, hepatic uptake and accumulation of these metal ions may be driven by similar transmembrane gradients[54,55]. However, uptake of NTBI did not appear to depend on the presence of transmembrane gradients for sodium, chloride or bicarbonate.

The early investigators Sheldon[6] and MacDonald[57] reported that the concentrations of other elements, specifically calcium, copper, lead and sulfur (but not zinc or manganese), were also increased in the liver and other organs affected in HC. If this is so, then other transition metal ions might compete with NTBI for incorporation into a cytosolic binding site[55,58].

Against this background, the recent demonstration of a membrane transport protein for copper that is defective in a disorder resulting from copper deficiency, Menke's disease, is of particular interest[59].

The reticuloendothelial system

The observation that Kupffer cells and intestinal macrophages contain little iron in subjects with HC has led to the suggestion that reticuloendothelial cells have a primary defect in iron metabolism, leading to reduced iron storage and the delivery of increased amounts of iron via the plasma to hepatocytes and other parenchymal cells. Kinetic studies involving reticuloendothelial function in HC lend support to this concept. A defect in storing iron, which is common to the two cell types, is certainly compatible with a number of observations in HC including the paucity of iron present in these cells, the increased iron absorption, and the early rise in transferrin saturation.

To date studies have failed to reveal any defect in the ferritin synthetic capabilities of these cells nor in their ability to take up iron. However, increased release of iron from these cells in the form of ferritin has been observed in mononuclear cells of both treated and untreated patients with HC. Fillet *et al.*[60] showed that the early release phase of iron from reticuloendothelial cells was considerably enhanced in patients with HC. The mechanism by which this enhanced release occurs has not been elucidated but may be related to the basic defect in HC.

A widespread parenchymal cell defect?

As discussed above, there is increasing evidence that HC results from a generalized membrane transport or other defect in multiple organs as occurs in cystic fibrosis and other disorders. It is possible that a membrane iron-transport protein or proteins could reside on parenchymal cells of a number of organs and, if defective, lead to iron accumulation in those tissues. Alternatively, if confined to the intestine and monocyte-macrophage system (e.g.

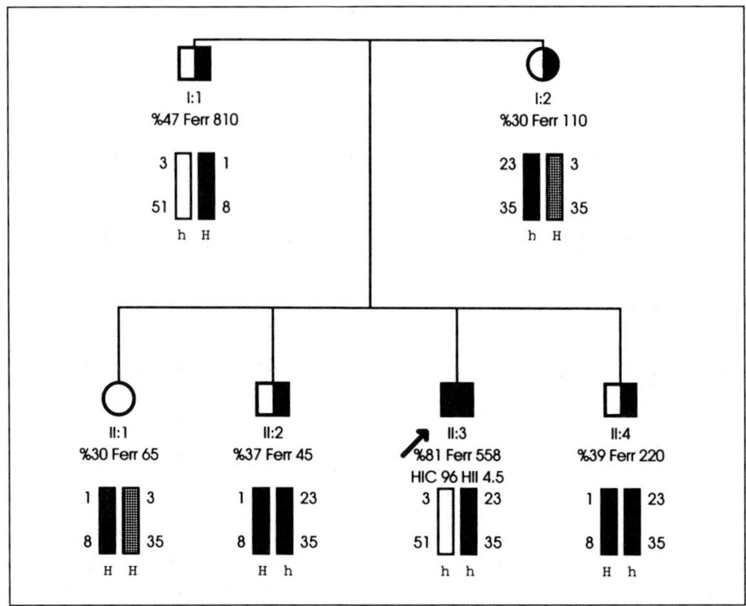

Fig. 2. HLA typing in a family illustrating a heterozygous mating resulting in iron overload in generation II. H = normal allele, h = HC allele, %= transferrin saturation, Ferr = ferritin (μg/l), HIC = hepatic iron concentration (μmol/g dry wt), HII = hepatic iron index, arrow = proband.

Kupffer cells of the liver), such a protein could be responsible for the rapid removal of iron from these cells so that the cells respond to an apparent iron deficient state, leading to a relative deficiency in ferritin and the concomitant increase in TfR concentration and sustained, inappropriately increased iron absorption.

Genetics of haemochromatosis

The gene responsible for HC has not yet been identified but it is known to be located on the short arm of chromosome 6 (6p) in close proximity to HLA-A. The linkage to HLA was first reported by Simon *et al.*[61]. HLA linkage has been used successfully to track the gene in affected pedigrees.

The pattern of inheritance of HC within a particular family can be traced by HLA typing of first-degree relatives of the proband (Fig. 2). Affected siblings of the proband usually have two HLA haplotypes identical to those of the proband, whereas unaffected siblings have one or neither haplotype identical to the proband[1,2,3,5,25]. In siblings resulting from a homozygous-heterozygous mating, affected individuals share the HLA haplotype from the unaffected (heterozygous) parent but may inherit either haplotype from the affected (homozygous) parent[62,63] (Fig 3).

The majority of homozygous relatives will eventually exhibit full clinical and biochemical expression of the disease although this depends on oral iron intake and physiological (and pathological) blood loss. In a recent study[5] 47 of 50 homozygous relatives (as determined by HLA studies) expressed the disease, either at first assessment or during a follow-up period of up to 8 years. In contrast, heterozygotes may demonstrate minor biochemical abnormalities of iron status, but do not develop a progressive increase in body iron stores of the order seen in homozygotes. In rare putative heterozygotes who appear to develop progressive iron overload, the possibility of either a chromosomal recombination, or a homozygous-heterozygous mating resulting in misclassification of ho-

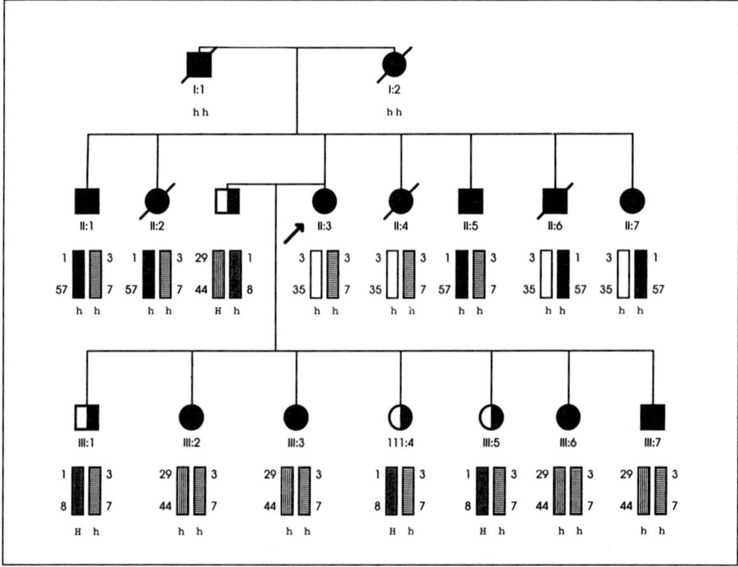

Fig. 3. A complex family tree illustrating the inheritance of HC in three generations (I,II,III) in which all offspring in generation II appear to have inherited an HC allele from each parent and all developed iron overload. Subject II:3 appeared to marry a heterozygote so that siblings III:2, III:3, III:6 and III:7 also developed iron overload. Black symbols = homozygotes, half colour = heterozygotes (male and female) HLA markers shown. Numbers refer to alleles. PD = presumed disease, h= HC allele, H = normal allele.

mozygotes as heterozygotes, must be considered[1–3,5,61].

Several theories have been proposed to account for the origin of the susceptibility gene for HC. One interesting hypothesis, proposed by Simon *et al.*[64], is that HC is basically a disease of Celtic peoples because a review of the relevant literature has revealed a similarity in geographic distribution of case reports and the current settlements of Celtic peoples. It has been suggested that the HC mutation arose on a chromosome carrying HLA-A3 and B7, and spread among European populations by migration[64]. A strong selection pressure during the evolution of the founder and/or derived populations must be invoked to account for the high frequency of the HC gene.

The precise location of the HC gene on chromosome 6 has been difficult to ascertain but the identification of short tandem repeat sequences (microsatellites) has now furnished a number of highly polymorphic markers (Fig. 4). In 13 large pedigrees studied in an Australian population, there was a clear association between HC and specific alleles at HLA-A and D6S105, i.e. HLA-A3 and D6S105 allele 8. In an analysis of 82 unrelated HC patients and 82 unrelated healthy controls D6S105–8 was present in 93 per cent of patients and 21 per cent of controls ($\chi^2 = 86.46$; $P < 0.0001$). The approximate relative risk for this allele was 48.4. HLA–A3 was present in 62 per cent of patients and 26 per cent of controls ($\chi^2 = 22.8, P < 0.001$). Approximate relative risk for A3 was 4.8. These results indicate that D6S105 is the closest marker to the HC gene so far reported[65]. A more recent haplotype analysis of chromosomes from 26 HC pedigrees containing multiply affected subjects was carried out in Australia[66]. HC status was assigned to 109 chromosomes of which 64 were affected and 43 were unaffected. The polymorphic markers HLA-A (serological) and microsatellites D6S248, D6S265, HLA-F and D6S105 were examined. All of these showed a highly significant allelic association with HC and no evidence of recombinations between the disease locus and the marker. A predominant ancestral haplotype allele 5–1–3–2–8 (marker order D6S248–D6S265-HLA-A-HLA-F-D6S105) was exclusively associated with HC (relative risk 903 for this haplotype) and was present in 33 per cent of the 64 affected chromosomes. This provides strong evidence for a common mutation associated with HC in Australian patients and the probable introduction of HC into the population on an ancestral haplotype. An analysis of hepatic iron stores as assessed by chemical determination of the liver iron concentration and determination of the hepatic iron index between siblings was carried out in 22 sibling pairs with HC[67]. A wide range of hepatic iron concentration (32–833 μmol/g dry wt) was found and the hepatic iron index ranged from 1.65 to 14.4. These differences could not be accounted for by differing expo-

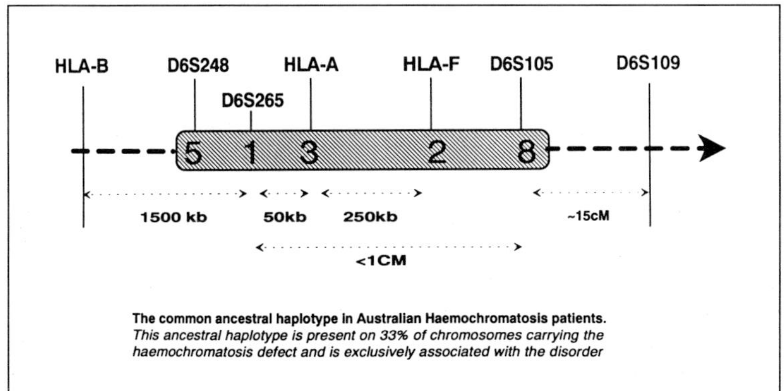

Fig. 4. Part of chromosome 6 showing the common ancestral haplotype in Australian HC patients. This ancestral haplotype is present on 33 per cent of chromosomes carrying the HC defect and is exclusively associated with the disorder. Numbers represent alleles of markers shown.

sure to the environmental factors that influence iron stores. However, a highly significant correlation for hepatic iron concentration ($r = 0.81$) and also for hepatic iron index ($r = 0.7$) was found between siblings of the same sex. These data provide strong evidence that genetic factors are the principal determinants of the amount of iron that accumulates in genetic HC. Recent evidence also suggests that HC patients with two copies of the ancestral haplotype show significantly more severe expression of the disorder[68].

The fact that the iron-loading gene in HC is tightly linked to the HLA loci and displays linkage disequilibrium with HLA-A suggests that abnormalities of a key protein coded at a single locus results in overt disease. A number of genes have been considered potential candidates for the HC gene on the basis of the function of their gene product. However, modern genetic techniques such as genetic linkage analysis, *in situ* hybridization, and somatic cell hybrid deletion mapping panel analysis have demonstrated that most of these can be excluded on the basis of incorrect chromosomal location. Despite all the evidence cited above, the elucidation of the basic metabolic defect still awaits the cloning and sequencing of the HLA-A linked gene on the short arm of chromosome 6, and then the identification and characterization of the gene product.

Treatment and prognosis

There is now strong circumstantial evidence that venesection therapy prolongs life and at least partly reverses established tissue damage[68]. This treatment should be undertaken as rapidly as possible to minimize the risk of complications. Up to 1000 ml per week (in two sessions) may be removed without significant problems occurring. Since 360–720 mmol (20–40 g) of stored iron may be present in the average patient, this schedule often has to be continued for 2–3 years. Plasma iron levels fall only when iron stores are depleted. After iron has been successfully removed, bleeding should be continued as required to keep the serum iron level below 27 μmol/l (150 μg/100 ml) and ferritin in the low normal range. Usually four 500 ml collections are required yearly. Therapy with desferrioxamine is not usually practical because the amount of iron excreted, 270–360 μmol/day (15–20 mg/day) does not compare with that removed by phlebotomy. However, in HC secondary to chronic anaemia, or in patients with severe heart failure who do not tolerate repeated venesection, iron-chelating agents should be used. In the follow-up of patients during phlebotomy the best guide to iron stores is the serum ferritin, provided there are no other concomitant disorders that elevate serum ferritin, such as active arthritis. The transferrin saturation remains elevated until iron stores fall, and finally the haemoglobin falls when iron stores are insufficient to allow for haemoglobin synthesis. Therefore the most cost-effective method of follow-up during therapy is to determine haemoglobin frequently with intermittent ferritin and transferrin saturation determinations.

Except for diabetes, testicular atrophy and chondrocalcinosis, manifestations of the disease improve or disappear as excess iron is progressively removed. Insulin requirements in diabetic patients usually decrease following depletion of iron stores. Replacement therapy with testosterone may also be useful but oral methyl testosterone should be avoided because of its possible relation to the development of hepatocellular carcinoma.

In 1935, when treatment was limited to supportive measures for diabetes, liver disease and heart failure, the mean survival after diagnosis was 4.4 years[7]. Primary liver cell cancer developed in 14 per cent of patients at that time. By 1969, phlebotomy had improved the 5 year survival rate to 89 per cent[69]. Although there is no absolute proof, strong evidence exists that the disease may be prevented by removal of excessive iron before tissue damage has occurred, provided that reaccumulation of iron is prevented[1,70]. Hepatocellular cancer does not appear to develop if the disease is treated before cirrhosis is present. The complications and natural course of the disease should thus be entirely preventable in patients and relatives with early overload (Figs 5 and 6)[71].

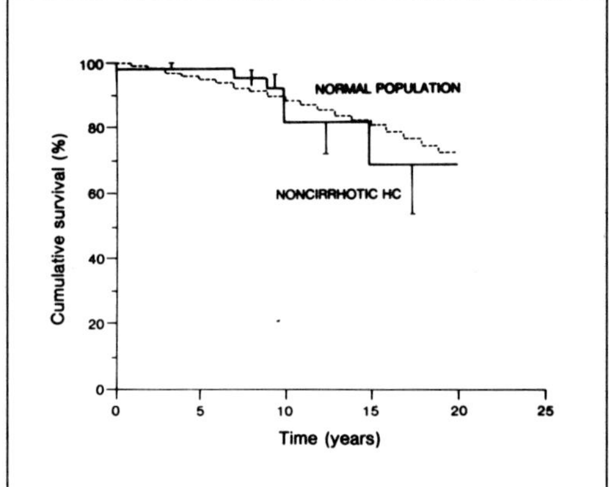

Fig. 5. Cumulative survival in 51 non-cirrhotic patients with HC. The survival rate in the non-cirrhotic patients was not significantly different from the rate expected; the confidence interval calculated for their survival always overlapped the rates expected in the normal population. (From Ref. 71 with permission)

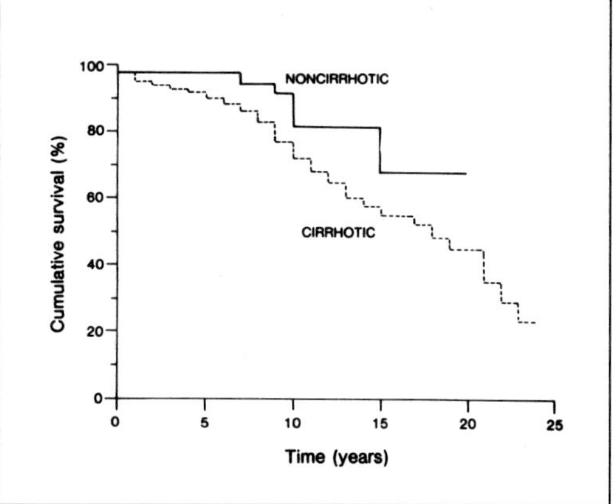

Fig. 6. Cumulative survival in 112 cirrhotic patients and 51 non-cirrhotic patients. Survival was significantly reduced in the cirrhotic patients as compared with the non-cirrhotic patients ($P < 0.05$, log rank test). The mean age and distribution of age were similar in both groups (46.7 ± 9.7 years ($\pm$S.D.) (range 24 to 77) in cirrhotic patients versus 45.4 ± 12.0 (18 to 75) in non-cirrhotic patients). (From Ref. 71 with permission)

References

1. Bassett, M.L., Halliday, J.W. & Powell, L.W. (1981): HLA typing in idiopathic haemochromatosis: distinction between homozygotes and heterozygotes with biochemical expression. *Hepatology* **1,** 120–126.
2. Simon, M., Alexandre, J.L., Bourel, M., Le Marec, B. & Scordia, C. (1977): Heredity of idiopathic hemochromatosis: a study of 106 families. *Clin. Genet.* **11,** 327–341.
3. Simon, M., Bourel, M., Genetet, B. & Fauchet, R. (1977): Idiopathic hemochromatosis: demonstration of recessive transmission and early detection by family HLA typing. *N. Engl. J. Med.* **297,** 1017–1021.
4. Leggett, B.A., Halliday, J.W., Brown, N.N., Bryant, S. & Powell, L.W. (1990): Prevalence of haemochromatosis amongst asymptomatic Australians. *Br. J. Haematol.* **74,** 525–530.
5. Powell, L.W., Summers, K.M., Board, P.G., Axelsen, E., Webb, S. & Halliday, J.W. (1990): Expression of hemochromatosis in homozygous subjects - Implication for early diagnosis and prevention. *Gastroenterology* **98,** 1625–1632.
6. Sheldon, J.H. (1935): *Haemochromatosis.* London: Oxford University Press.
7. Finch, S.C. & Finch, C.A. (1955): Idiopathic hemochromatosis, an iron storage disease. A. Iron metabolism in hemochromatosis. *Medicine* **34,** 381.
8. Halliday, J.W., Russo, A., Cowlishaw, J. & Powell, L.W. (1977): Serum ferritin in the diagnosis of early haemochromatosis: a study of 43 families. *Lancet* **ii,** 621–623.
9. Bassett, M.L., Halliday, J.W., Bryan, S., Dent, O. & Powell, L.W. (1988): Screening for hemochromatosis. *Ann. NY Acad. Sci.* **526,** 274–289.

10. Bassett, M.L., Halliday, J.W. & Powell, L.W. (1986): Value of hepatic iron measurement in early hemochromatosis and determination of the critical iron level associated with fibrosis. *Hepatology* **6,** 24–29.

11. Summers, K.M., Halliday, J.W. & Powell, L.W. (1990): Identification of homozygous hemochromatosis subjects by measurement of hepatic iron index. *Hepatology* **12,** 20–25.

12. Bradbear, R.A., Bain, C., Siskind, V., Schofield, F.D., Webb, S., Axelsen, E.M., Halliday, J.W., Bassett, M.L. & Powell, L.W. (1985): Cohort study of internal malignancy in genetic hemochromatosis and other chronic nonalcoholic liver diseases. *J. Natl. Cancer Inst.* **75,** 81–84.

13. Halliday, J.W. & Powell, L.W. (1988): Ferritin and cellular iron metabolism. *Ann. NY Acad. Sci.* **526,** 101–112.

14. Powell, L.W., Bassett, M.L., Axelsen, E., Ferluga, J. & Halliday, J.W. (1988): Is all genetic (hereditary) haemochromatosis HLA-related? *Ann. NY Acad. Sci.* **526,** 23–33.

15. Edwards, C.Q., Carroll, M., Bray, P. & Cartwright, G.E. (1977): Hereditary hemochromatosis. *N. Engl. J. Med.* **297,** 7–13.

16. Powell, L.W. & Halliday, J.W. (1976): Serum ferritin in haemochromatosis. *N. Engl. J. Med.* **294,** 1185.

17. Wands, J.R., Rowe, J.A., Mezey, S.E., Waterbury, L.A., Wright, J.R., Halliday, J.W., Isselbacher, K.J. & Powell, L.W. (1976): Normal serum ferritin concentrations in pre-cirrhotic hemochromatosis. *N. Engl. J. Med.* **294,** 302.

18. Feller, E.R., Pont, A., Wands, J.R., Carter, A.C., Foster, G., Kourides, I.A. & Isselbacher, K.J. (1977): Familial hemochromatosis. *N. Engl. J. Med.* **296,** 1422–1426.

19. Grace, N.D. & Powell, L.W. (1974): Iron storage disorders of the liver. *Gastroenterology* **64,** 1257–1283.

20. Powell, L.W., Halliday, J.W. & Cowlishaw, J.L. (1978): The relationship between serum ferritin and total body iron stores in idiopathic haemochromatosis. *Gut* **19,** 538–542.

21. Chapman, R.W.G., Williams, G., Bydder, G., Dick, R., Sherlock, S. & Kreel, L. (1980): Computed tomography for determining liver iron content in primary haemochromatosis. *BMJ* **1,** 440–442.

22. Gollan, J. (1983): Diagnosis of hemochromatosis. *Gastroenterology* **84,** 418–431.

23. Howard, J.M., Ghent, C.N., Carey, L.S., Flanagan, P.R. & Valbert, L.S. (1983): Diagnostic efficacy of hepatic computed tomography in the detection of body iron overload. *Gastroenterology* **84,** 209–215.

24. Brittenham, G.M., Farrell, D.E., Harris, J.W., Feldman, E.S., Danish, E.H., Muir, W.A., Tripp, J.H. & Bellon, E.M. (1982): Magnetic-susceptibility measurement of human iron stores. *N. Engl. J. Med.* **307,** 1671–1675.

25. Bassett, M.L., Halliday, J.W. & Powell, L.W. (1979): Early detection of idiopathic haemochromatosis: relative value of serum ferritin and HLA typing. *Lancet* **ii,** 4–7.

26. Powell, L.W., Halliday, J.W. & Fletcher, L.M. (1994): Distinction between haemochromatosis and alcoholic siderosis. In *Alcoholic Liver Disease*, 2 Edn. ed. Hall, P. *Edward Arnold*, Sevenoaks. pp. 199–216.

27. Searle, J., Kerr, J.F.R., Halliday, J.W. & Powell, L.W. (1994): Iron storage disease. In: *Pathology of the liver* 3rd edn., eds. R.N.M. MacSween, P.P. Anthony, P.J. Scheuer, B.C. Portmann & A.D. Burt, pp. 219–241. London: Churchill Livingstone.

28. Klausner, R.D. (1988): From receptors to genes – insights from molecular iron metabolism. *Clin. Res.* **36,** 494– 500.

29. Bothwell, T.H. (1972): Iron deficiency. *Med. J. Aust.* **2,** 433–438.

30. Teichmann, R. & Stremmel, W. (1990): Iron uptake by human upper small intestine microvillous membrane vesicles. Indication for a facilitated transport mechanism mediated by a membrane iron-binding protein. *J. Clin. Invest.* **86,** 2145.

31. Conrad, M.E., Umbreit, J.N., Moore, E.G., Peterson, R.D.A. & Jones, M.B.A. (1990): A newly identified iron binding protein in duodenal mucosa of rats. *J. Biol. Chem.* **265,** 5273–5279.

32. Stremmel, W., Arvailer, D., Voerbuchep, M., Teichmann, R., Diede, H.E. & Strohmeyer, G. (1991): The membrane iron binding protein is enriched in the liver of patients with primary hemochromatosis. *Hepatology* **14,** 142A.

33. McLaren, G.D., Nathanson, M.H., Jacobs, A., Trevett, D. & Thomson, W. (1991): Regulation of intestinal iron absorption and mucosal iron kinetics in hereditary hemochromatosis. *J. Lab. Clin. Med.* **117,** 390–401.

34. Kuhn, L.C. (1991): mRNA-protein interactions regulate critical pathways in cellular iron metabolism. *Br. J. Haematol.* **79,** 1–5.

35. Hentze, M.W., Caughman, S.W., Casey, J.W., Koeller, D.M., Rouault, T.A., Harford, J.B. & Klausner, R.D. (1988): A model for the structure and functions of iron-responsive elements. *Gene* **72,** 201–208.

36. Hentze, M.W., Seuanez, H.N., O'Brien, S.J., Harford, J.B. & Klausner, R.D. (1989): Chromosomal localization of nucleic acid-binding proteins by affinity mapping: assignment of the IRE-binding protein gene to human chromosome 9. *Nucleic Acids Res.* **17,** 6103–6108.

37. Hentze, M.W., Rouault, T.A., Harford, J.B. & Klausner, R.D. (1989): Oxidation-reduction and the molecular mechanism of a regulatory RNA-protein interaction. *Science* **244,** 357–359.

38. Whittaker, P., Skikne, B.S., Covell, A.M., Flowers, C., Cooke, A. & Lynch, S.L. (1989): Duodenal iron proteins in idiopathic hemochromatosis. *J. Clin. Invest.* **83,** 261–267.

39. Fracanzani, A.L., Fargion, S., Romeno, R., Piperno, A., Arosio, P. & Fiorelli, G. (1989): Immunohistochemical evidence for a lack of ferritin in duodenal absorptive epithelial cells in idiopathic hemochromatosis. *Gastroenterology* **96,** 1071–1078.

40. Pietrangelo, A., Rocchi, E., Rigo, G., Gerrari, A.L., Perini, M., Ventura, E. & Cairo, G. (1992): Regulation of transferrin, transferrin receptor and ferritin gene expression in the duodenum of normal anemic and siderotic subjects. *Gastroenterology* **102,** 802–809.

41. Pietrangelo, A., Casalgrandi, G., Quaglino, D., Gualdi, R., Conte, D., Milani, S., Montosi, G., Cesarini, L., Ventura, E. & Cairo, G. (1995: Duodenal ferritin synthesis in genetic hemochromatosis. *Gastroenterology* **108,** 208–217.

42. Banerjee, D., Falagan, O.R., Cluett, J. & Valberg, L.S. (1986): Transferrin receptors in the human gastrointestinal tract. *Gastroenterology* **91,** 861–869.

43. Anderson G.J., Powell L.W. & Halliday J.W. (1990): Transferrin receptor distribution and regulation in the rat small intestine. Effect of iron stores and erythropoiesis. *Gastroenterology* **98,** 576–585.

44. Anderson, G.J., Walsh, M.D., Powell, L.W. & Halliday, J.W. (1991): Intestinal transferrin receptors and iron absorption in the neonatal rat. *Brit. J. Haematol.* **77,** 229–236.

45. Srai, S.K.S., Epstein, O., Denham, E.S. & McIntyre, N. (1984): The ontogeny of iron absorption and its possible relationship to pathogenesis of haemochromatosis. *Hepatology* **4,** 1033.

46. Srai, S.K.S., Denham, E. & Epstein, O. (1987): Development changes in the villous uptake of iron and enterocyte iron binding proteins in the guinea pig duodenum. *Gut* **28,** A1333.

47. Summers, K.M., Tam, K.S., Bartley, P.B., Drysdale, J., Zoghbi, H.Y., Halliday, J.W. & Powell, L.W. (1991): Fine mapping of a chomosome 6 ferritin heavy chain gene: Relevance to haemochromatosis. *Hum. Genet.* **88,** 175–178.

48. Cook, J.D., Barry, W.E. & Hershko, C. (1973): Iron kinetics with emphasis on iron overload. *Am. J. Pathol.* **72,** 337–343.

49. Batey, R.G., Pettit, J.E., Nicholas, A.W., Sherlock, S. & Hoffbrand, A.V. (1978): Hepatic iron clearance from serum in treated hemochromatosis. *Gastroenterology* **75,** 856–859.

50. Adams, P.C., Reece, A.S., Powell, L.W. & Halliday, J.W. (1989): Hepatic iron in the control of iron absorption in a rat liver transplantation model. *Transplantation* **48,** 19–21.

51. Adams, P.C., Zhong, R., Haist, J., Flanagan, P.R. & Grant, D.R. (1991): Mucosal iron in the control of iron absorption in a rat transplantation model. *Gastroenterology* **100,** 370–374.

52. Powell, L.W. (1992): Does transplantation of the liver cure genetic hemochromatosis? *J Hepatol* **16**: 259–261

53. Sciot, R., Paterson, A.C., Van Den Oord, J.J. & Desmet, V.J. (1987): Lack of hepatic transferrin receptor expression in hemochromatosis. *Hepatology* **7,** 831–837.

54. Brissot, P., Wright, T.L., Ma, W.L. & Weisiger, R.A. (1985): Efficient clearance of non-transferrin bound iron by rat liver. *J. Clin. Invest.* **76,** 1463–1470.

55. Wright, T., Brissot, P., Ma, W.L. & Weisiger, R.A. (1986): Characterization of non-transferrin-bound iron clearance by rat liver. *J. Biol. Chem.* **261,** 10909–10914.

56. Wright, T., Fitz, J.G. & Weisiger, R.A. (1988): Non-transferrin-bound iron uptake by rat liver. *J. Biol. Chem.* **263,** 1842–1847.

57. MacDonald, R.A. (1964): *Hemochromatosis and hemosiderosis.* Illinois: Charles C. Thomas.

58. Wright, T.L. & Lake, J.R. (1990): Mechanisms of transport of non-transferrin-bound iron in basolateral and canalicular rat liver plasma membrane vesicles. *Hepatology* **12,** 398–504.

59. Mercer, J.F.B., Livingston, J., Hall, B., Paynter, J.A., Begy, C., Chadrasekharappa, S., Lockhart, P., Grimes, A., Bhave, M., Siemieniak, D. & Glover, T.W. (1993): Isolation of a partial candidate gene for Menkes disease by positional cloning. *Nature. Genet.* **3,** 20–25.

60. Fillet, G., Beguin, Y. & Bakdelli, L. (1989): Model reticuloendothelial iron metabolism in humans: Abnormal behaviour in idiopathic hemochromatosis and in inflammation. *Blood* **74,** 844–851.

61. Simon, M., Pawlotsky, Y., Bourel, M., Fauchet, R. & Genetet, B. (1975): Hémochromatose idiopathique: Maladie associée à l'antigène tissulaire HL-A3. *Nouv. Presse. Med.* **4,** 1432.

62. Bassett, M.L., Doran, T.J., Halliday, J.W., Bashir, H.V. & Powell, L.W. (1982): Idiopathic hemochromatosis: Demonstration of homozygous-heterozygous mating by HLA typing of families. *Hum. Genet.* **1,** 120–126.

63. Simon, M., Alexandre, J.L., Fauchet, R., Genetet, B. & Bourel, M. (1980): The genetics of haemochromatosis. *Prog. Med. Genet.* **4,** 135–168.

64. Simon, M., Le Mignon, L., Fauchet, R., Yaouanq, J., David, V., Edan, G. & Bourel, M. (1987): A study of 609 haplotypes marking for the hemochromatosis gene: (1) mapping of the gene near the *HLA-A* locus and characters required to define a heterozygous population and (2) hypothesis concerning the underlying cause of hemochromatosis-HLA association. *Am. J. Hum. Genet.* **41,** 89–105.

65. Jazwinska, E.C., Lee, S.C., Webb, S.I., Halliday, J.W. & Powell, L.W. (1993): Localization of the hemochromatosis gene close to D6S105. *Am. J. Hum. Genet.* **53,** 347–352.

66. Jazwinska, E.C., Pyper, W.R., Burt, M.J., Francis, J.L., Goldwurm, S., Webb, S.I., Lee, S.C., Halliday, J.W. & Powell, L.W. (1995): Haplotype analysis in Australian hemochromatosis patients: Evidence for a predominant ancestral haplotype exclusively associated with hemochromatosis. *Am. J. Hum. Genet.* **56,** 428–433.

67. Crawford, D.H.G., Halliday, J.W., Summers, K.M., Bourke, M.J. & Powell, L.W. (1993): Concordance of iron storage in siblings with genetic hemochromatosis: Evidence for a predominantly genetic effect on iron storage. *Hepatology* **17,** 833–837.

68. Crawford, D.H.G., Powell, L.W., Leggett, B.A., Francis, J.S., Fletcher, L.M., Webb, S.I., Halliday, J.W. & Jazwinska, E.C. (1995): Evidence that the ancestral haplotype in Australian hemochromatosis patients may be associated with a common mutation in the gene. *Am. J. Hum. Genet.* **57**, 362–367.

69. Williams, R., Smith, P.M., Spicer, E.J., Barry, M. & Sherlock, S. (1969): Venesection therapy in idiopathic haemochromatosis. *Q. J. Med.* **38,** 1–16.

70. Bassett, M.L., Halliday, J.W., Ferris, R.A. & Powell, L.W. (1984): Hemochromatosis: predictive accuracy of biochemical screening tests. *Gastroenterology* **87,** 628–633.

71. Niederau, C., Fischer, R., Sonnenberg, A., Stremmel, W., Trampish, H.J. & Strohmeyer, G. (1985): Survival and causes of death in cirrhotic and in noncirrhotic patients with primary hemochromatosis. *N. Engl. J. Med.* **313,** 1256–1262.

Iron Nutrition in Health and Disease, edited by Leif Hallberg and Nils-Georg Asp

Chapter 25

Genetics of haemochromatosis

M. Worwood[1], R. Raha-Chowdhury[1] and K.J.H. Robson[2]

[1]*Department of Haematology, University of Wales College of Medicine, Cardiff CF4 4XN,* [2]*MRC Molecular Haematology Unit, Institute of Molecular Medicine, John Radcliffe Hospital, Headington, Oxford OX3 9DU , UK*

Summary

Haemochromatosis is a disorder in which increased iron absorption leads to iron accumulation in the tissues and eventually to tissue damage. It is the most common autosomal recessive inherited disorder in parts of Northern Europe. In 1975 Simon and colleagues discovered the association between HLA-A3 and haemochromatosis. This led to the localization of the gene to chromosome 6 (6p21.3) and subsequent linkage analysis localized the gene to within 1 cM of HLA-A. With the development of the human genome project more markers for the region of chromosome 6 just telomeric to the HLA class 1 region have become available. New methods of high resolution linkage disequilibrium analysis have also been developed. These studies indicate that haemochromatosis appears to have originated from a founder mutation which has multiplied through successive generations. This mutation is associated with a haplotype which is common on haemochromatosis chromosomes from the UK, Sweden and Australia and which is rare in the general population. High resolution linkage disequilibrium analysis suggests that the gene is likely to be located telomeric to the genetic marker D6S105. This marker is located at least 2 cM from HLA-A towards the telomere. This work is not only contributing to the localization of the haemochromatosis gene but may indicate the number of mutations causing haemochromatosis and permit further speculation about spread of the disorder since the first mutation causing the biochemical abnormality occurred.

Introduction

Hereditary haemochromatosis is an inherited, metabolic abnormality in which increased absorption of iron causes gradual accumulation of iron in the tissues and eventually leads to tissue damage (see previous chapter). Men may develop significant iron overload at any time in adult life but in women iron overload is not usually seen until the menopause as the iron losses associated with menstruation and childbirth often compensate for the enhanced iron absorption. The gene causing the disorder has not yet been identified, neither is the primary biochemical abnormality known. In 1935 Sheldon[1] reviewed more than 300 published cases and made many proposals about the nature of the disorder including the suggestion that it was an inherited defect. In 1955, Finch and Finch[2] reviewed another 787 cases. Although the idea of haemochromatosis as an inherited disorder has received continuous support, MacDonald[3] described haemochromatosis as 'two conditions which when they occur together make up the disease but which are not causally related: iron excess and cirrhosis'.

In 1974, Saddi and Feingold[4] proposed a recessive mode of inheritance for the disorder. Two developments then led to the renewed interest in the condition and its genetic background. First, the serum ferritin assay was introduced by Addison *et al.*[5] and provided, for the first time, a convenient assay relating to storage iron levels. In practice it has not fulfilled expectations that it would facilitate early diagnosis but provides a valuable indicator of the degree of iron overload. Second, Simon *et al.*[6] described an association between the HLA antigens A3 and B14 and haemochromatosis which opened the door to genetic investigation.

Frequency of haemochromatosis

The disorder was considered to be relatively rare. For example, Finch and Finch[2] estimated the incidence to be approximately 1 in 10,000 (0.01 per cent). However, several autopsy studies involving from 8800 to 38,000 cases showed disease frequencies from 1 in 1000 (0.1 per cent) to 2 per 1000[7]. In the last few years there have been a number of large surveys in which the diagnosis has been made by a combination of biochemical screening (transferrin saturation and serum ferritin concentration) and the determination of liver iron concentration[8] (see Chapter 24). The results show a considerable variation in prevalence ranging from 0.05 per cent in central and southern Finland to over 1 per cent in north-eastern Quebec with prevalences of over 0.3 per cent in both Queensland and Utah. Of course the determined prevalence will depend on the method of detection. The early studies quoted by Finch and Finch[2] included only those presenting with clinical symptoms resulting from major iron overload, whereas both autopsy studies and biochemical screening will detect people with a more minor degree of iron accumulation who have not yet developed clinical symptoms.

However, many medical practitioners regard haemochromatosis as rare and there is a discrepancy between the number of patients with haemochromatosis and the expected number of homozygotes based on population screening. Many subjects may not develop a sufficient degree of iron overload to cause tissue damage. Whether environmental factors are responsible or there are several different mutations must await the identification of the gene.

Although there is good evidence to suggest that haemochromatosis is one of the most common inherited disorders in European populations there is little information about the frequency of iron overload in much of Asia, Africa or South America. Iron overload may also be found in patients with disorders of globin or haem synthesis. An example of a non-genetic form of iron overload has been the South African 'Bantu siderosis'[9] caused by the consumption of large quantities of beer brewed in iron pots. However, a recent study of Gordeuk *et al.*[10] has shown that there may be a genetic component although this does not appear to be an HLA-linked disorder.

It has been proposed that genetic haemochromatosis may have a selective advantage[11] in protecting against iron deficiency anaemia. Heterozygotes would suffer no ill-effects and homozygotes would not succumb until after their reproductive life.

Associations with HLA antigens

The HLA association led directly to the mapping of the haemochromatosis gene to the short arm of chromosome 6 (within 1 cM of HLA-A), confirmed the recessive nature of its inheritance and made it possible to trace the gene within the family once a diagnosis of haemochromatosis was made in a patient. The HLA haplotypes linked to haemochromatosis were shown to vary from family to family but were consistent within one family. These early studies have been reviewed by Simon *et al.*[12] and Edwards *et al.*[13].

Simon *et al.*[14] established clearly that the haemochromatosis gene was linked with HLA-A and that HLA-B alleles such as B7 and B14 were in linkage disequilibrium with HLA-A3. In Brittany, the most frequent haplotypes were A3,B7 and A3,B14 but other haplotypes are more common in other parts of Europe. Simon and colleagues[14] proposed that the haemochromatosis mutation was a 'rare if not unique event' which may have occurred in a chromosome carrying the A3,B7 haplotype (the 'ancestral' haplotype). They suggested that subsequent recombinations involving both B and (more rarely) A loci and population movements have produced the variable haplotype associations which have been described.

Recombinations involving the haemochromatosis gene and HLA class I genes

A number of recombinations involving haemochromatosis and HLA-A or HLA-B have been described[15–18]. They have not, however, resolved the debate about the haemochromatosis gene - centromeric or telomeric with respect to HLA-A.

Genotyping with probes for HLA class I genes

Southern blotting of HLA class I genes demonstrates the complexity of the gene family with up to 20 related genes[19]. Despite the difficulties of analysing often complex RFLP patterns, significant associations between HLA-A antigens and RFLPs with HLA class I probes have been demonstrated. However, the specific associations between genotypes and haemochromatosis which have been described reflect the well-known association between HLA-A3 and haemochromatosis[20–22].

Nature of the metabolic abnormality

The site of the abnormality

The intestinal mucosa, the liver, and phagocytic cells making up the reticuloendothelial system have been proposed as primary sites. Although there is evidence to support each possibility[23] the intestinal mucosa has attracted most support. Haemochromatosis is associated with anomalously low levels of ferritin in the absorptive epithelial cells but this may be secondary to enhanced iron absorption[24]. There is also evidence for an inappropriate expression of transferrin receptors on the basolateral, subnuclear region of villus epithelial cells in genetic haemochromatosis[25]. The receptor was expressed in untreated patients and normal subjects but not in patients with secondary iron overload. Thus there appeared to be a failure of down-regulation of the villus, enterocyte transferrin receptor which may be associated with a failure to restrict iron absorption. No such failure of regulation was found in the liver in patients with haemochromatosis. The function of ferritin in haem breakdown in macrophages has received much attention but no consistent abnormalities have been reported[26].

The search for candidate genes

Recent developments in gene mapping have made it possible to discount many candidate proteins as being the haemochromatosis gene (Table 1). There are two H ferritin gene sequences on the short arm of chromosome 6 but one (FTHPl) has now been shown to be centromeric to the glyoxylase locus[27]. Southern blotting of H ferritin genes has revealed polymorphisms but not specific associations with haemochromatosis[20,28,29]. No other iron binding or regulatory proteins have yet been located on chromosome 6.

Table 1 Chromosome location of genes coding for proteins of iron metabolism[8]

Name	Gene symbol	Location
Ferritin(H)	FTH1	11q13
	FTHL1-4	1p31-p22; 132.2-q42; 2q32-q33; 3q21-q23
	FTHL7,8	13q12; Xq26-q28
	10-16	5;8;9;14;17;6p;11q13
	FTHP1	6p21.3-p12
Ferritin (L)	FTL	19q13.3-q13.4
	FTLL1	20q12-qter
	FTLL2	Xp22.3-p21.2
Transferrin	TF	3q21
Transferrin receptor	TFRC	3q26.2-qter
Lactoferrin	LTF	3q21
Iron regulatory binding protein	IRP	9
Aconitase (soluble)	ACOI	9p22-q32
Haptoglobin	HP	16q22-q32
Haemopexin	HPX	11p15.5-15.4
δ-Aminolevulinate synthase 1	ALA-S1	3p21
δ-Aminolevulinate synthase 2 (erythroid specific)	ALA-S2	Xp11.21
Ferrochelatase	FECH	18q21.3
Haem oxygenase	HMOX1	22q12
Haem oxygenase (constitutive)	HMOX2	16p13.3

Recent advances in mapping the HLA class I region

In 1975 the only known genes in the HLA class I region were HLA-A, -B and -C. Since the initiation of the human genome mapping project there has been a rapid development of gene density in this region. Figure 1 shows a physical and genetic map for the region from HLA-B towards the telomere which includes HLA class I genes and other loci described in this review.

Linkage analysis - HFE and markers from 6p21.3 to 6pter

Two studies have been reported. Gasparini *et al.*[30] examined 25 families - a total of 136 subjects including 27 haemochromatosis patients. Individuals were classified under. seven liability classes depending on age and transferrin saturation. The marker loci included HLA-DQα, HLA-B, I–82, HLA-A, HLA-F, D6S105, D6S109 and D6S89. Data were analysed using MLINK, ILINK and LINKMAP programs. Pairwise linkage showed a maximum lod score of 6.27 for HFE versus HLA-B at a recombination fraction of 0.004. Multipoint linkage analysis gave the most likely position for the HFE locus as very close to I82. The authors also described a double recombination, one occurring between DQA and HLA-B and a second between HLA-A and HLA-F. They suggested that this places the limits for the region containing the HFE locus between DQA and HLA-F and supports the result of the linkage analysis. However they have since retracted this aspect of the paper[31].

Jazwinska *et al.*[32] used many of the same loci as markers - HLA-B, HLA-A, D6S105, D6S109, D6S89 and F13A - and examined 13 large pedigrees. No recombination was found between HFE and HLA-A or D6S105 and two-point analysis placed HFE within 1 cM of HLA-A and D6S105. A multipoint map (HLAB, HLA-A, D6S109) gave a gene location within 1 cM (proximal or telomeric) of HLA-A.

Allelic association studies

With the discovery of new, telomeric markers (Fig. 1) it has been found that D6S105 allele 8 (approximately 2 cM telomeric to HLA-A) is equally, or even more strongly associated with GH than HLA-A3[32,33]. By both Southern blotting[34] and PCR[35,36] it has been shown that alleles at HLA-F are in strong linkage disequilibrium with HFE. Alleles at D6S299, an informative marker approximately 4 cM distal to HLA-A, show no association with GH and this locus therefore represents a telomeric boundary for the HFE gene[34]. The microsatellite markers D6S258, D6S306, D6S461, D6S464[37] CS3 and CS5[38] also have alleles which are associated with haemochromatosis.

An analysis of linkage disequilibrium with markers (centromeric) D6S265, HLA-F, D6S306, D6S258, D6S306, CS3, D6S105, D6S464, CS5, D6S461, D6S299 (telomeric) has been completed for 130 chromosomes from unrelated patients with haemochromatosis and 180 control chromosomes[38]. We have also been able to establish haplotypes for 82 haemochromatosis chromosomes and 72 control chromosomes. Over 70 per cent of GH chromosomes carry a common, 'ancestral', haplotype 306–5, CS3–3 105–8, 464–9, CS5–4 which is found on only 6 per cent of control chromosomes. Some of these may carry the HFE gene since the gene frequency is 1 in 20 in the general population (it is difficult to detect heterozygotes by biochemical screening). A haplotype involving D6S265–1

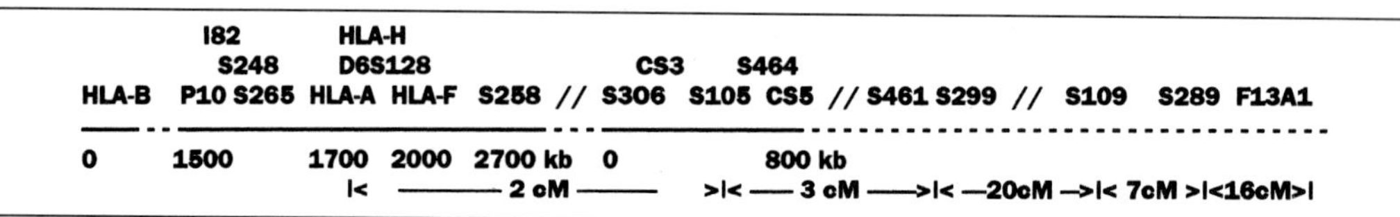

Fig. 1. Genetic and physical map of the HLA class I and more telomeric region of chromosome 6. Genetic loci discussed in the text are included. HLA-B, -A, -H and -F are HLA class 1 genes. P10, I82 and D6S128 were analysed by restriction fragment length polymorphisms. For other markers microsatellite sequences (dinucleotide repeats) have been analysed. Marker names have been abbreviated (i.e. D6S248 is written as S248). For further details see text and Ref. 47.

(HLA-A3) and D6S105–8 is an extension of the 'ancestral' haplotype described above and is present on up to 50 per cent of haemochromatosis chromosomes[38]. Thus HFE appears to have originated from a founder mutation which has multiplied through successive generations.

These allelic association data have now been analysed by a new likelihood method for the analysis of linkage disequilibrium[39]. Calculation of λ (the proportion of excess of allele *i* in chromosomes carrying the HFE gene) confirms that CS5 shows the maximum value, $\lambda = 0.74$ $p = 10^{-12}$) while the multipoint likelihood ratio analysis also gives a maximum value at CS5.

Hastbacka *et al.*[40] found that markers for the diastrophic dysplasia gene giving PeXcess values (comparable to λ) of this order lay within 180 kb of the gene. Our studies therefore indicate that the GH gene may lie within a few hundred kb of the marker CS5. However, although we have several close markers centromeric to CS5, we have no such markers close to CS5 toward the telomere (see Fig. 3). The next stage is therefore to find markers within 1000 kb of CS5 and towards the telomere in order to define the maximum value for λ and thus to provide a more precise location for the haemochromatosis gene.

A haemochromatosis-specific haplotype?

Haplotype analysis

Haplotypes involving HLA-A and -B (studies A3,B7) are associated with a high relative risk for haemochromatosis (see earlier) but are not specific for the disorder. Yaouanq *et al.*[41] has described a haplotype involving I82 allele 2 HLA-A3 and D6S128 allele 2 (D6S128 is a locus near HLA-H). However, this appears to be an HLA-A3 haplotype rather than a haemochromatosis-specific haplotype[42]. Homozygosity for both D6S265–1 and D6S105–8 is associated with a high relative risk for haemochromatosis of 214 (95 per cent CI = 26–1720). In this study[33] there were 42 patients and 376 controls and none of the controls possessed the homozygous genotype. Jazwinska *et al.*[36] have described a haplotype extending from D6S248 (within 30 kb of D6S265) to D6S105 and including D6S256–1 and D6S105–8 as being exclusively associated with haemochromatosis. This is the 'founder' haplotype described above and appears to be common in the UK[38], in Queensland[36] and in Sweden[43]. We have recently examined the frequency of the haplotype D6S265–1:D6S105–8 in 7820 blood donors from South Wales (Worwood *et al.*, submitted) and have concluded that chromosomes carrying this haplotype have an approximately 45 per cent risk of also carrying the gene for haemochromatosis.

Isolation of candidate genes for HFE

The first phase in any strategy for positional cloning of the HFE gene involves localizing the gene to a region which may then be dissected to reveal candidate genes. The region around HLA-A has been identified as a possible region. El Kahloun *et al.*[44] selected a yeast artificial chromosome (YAC B30) containing a 320 kb insert of genomic DNA including previously mapped genes from p10 to HLA-A and 6.7 (D6S128). This YAC was used to screen a cDNA library of human intestinal mucosa. Several cDNA clones were isolated which corresponded to new, non-HLA class I, structural genes. The authors have called these HCGI-VII, HCG standing for haemochromatosis candidate gene, as these genes are all within their selected region for the HFE gene. No sequence data are available for these genes. Both Wei *et al.*[45] and Goei *et al.*[46] have identified new genes from this region. Some of these may be identical to the seven novel genes found by El Kahloun *et al.*[44], but the number of genes already found indicates a gene density of one gene or pseudogene per 20 kb which is comparable with that in the HLA class II and III regions which were studied earlier.

What is the precise location of the HFE gene?

The studies described above locate the gene within a region extending from I82 to beyond D6S105. Some of the differences are easily explained. For example, Yaouanq *et al.*[41] did not include D6S105 in their list of markers so this analysis cannot be compared directly with that of Jazwinska *et al.*[32] or Worwood *et al.*[33]. Gasparini *et al.*[30] included D6S105 in their pedigree analysis but concluded that it was located about 3.5 cM from HFE. D6S105 has not been located on a physical map of the region so its distance from HLA-A or HLA-F in terms of kb is unknown. However, the gene order given in Fig. 1 has been verified by *in situ* hybridization of metaphase chromosomes[38].

A potentially useful marker for HFE should be HLA-F, located between HLA-A and D6S105. In one study the restriction enzyme selected has been uninformative[41] and Gasparini *et al.*[30] found no linkage disequilibrium between HLA-A and HLA-F despite their physical closeness (250 kbp). More recent analyses show that alleles at HLA-F are in strong linkage disequilibrium and haemochromatosis[35,36].

Genes identified in the appropriate region (see above) are all candidates for haemochromatosis once expression in the appropriate tissue has been demonstrated. Unfortunately there is still uncertainty that the intestinal mucosa is the site of the primary abnormality. The uncertainty about gene location, site of the primary abnormality and function (perhaps only a small change in a rate of iron transfer, for example) means that identification of the HFE gene may well depend on demonstration of a gene mutation which is common in haemochromatosis chromosomes but not in normal chromosomes.

Conclusion

Physical mapping, coupled with high resolution linkage disequilibrium analysis will determine a precise location for the gene causing haemochromatosis and permit a rapid search for the gene and for the causative mutations. At the same time knowledge of haplotypes involving close genetic markers will make it possible to compare haplotypes from different countries in order to determine the origin and migration patterns which have caused the present disease distribution. Furthermore as more specific haplotypes are described it becomes possible to assign a risk that any chromosome carried a haemochromatosis gene. This is clearly of value in providing patients with advice about the risk for their partner carrying the gene.

References

1. Sheldon, J.H. (1935): *Haemochromatosis.* London: Oxford University Press.

2. Finch, S.C. & Finch, C.A. (1955): Idiopathic hemochromatosis, an iron storage disease. A. Iron metabolism in hemochromatosis. *Medicine* **34,** 381–430.

3. MacDonald, R.A. (1964): *Hemochromatosis and Hemosiderosis.* Springfield, IL: Charles C. Thomas.

4. Saddi, R. & Feingold, J. (1974): Idiopathic haemochromatosis and diabetes mellitus. *Clin. Genet.* **5,** 242–247.

5. Addison, G.M., Beamish, M.R., Hales, C.N. *et al.* (1972): An immunoradiometric assay for ferritin in the serum of normal normal subjects and patients with iron deficiency and iron overload. *J. Clin. Pathol.* **25,** 326–329.

6. Simon, M., Bourel, M., Fauchet, R. & Genetet, B. (1976): Association of HLA-A3 and HLA-B14 antigens with idiopathic haemochromatosis. *Gut* **17,** 332–334.

7. Lindmark, B. & Eriksson, S. (1985): Regional differences in the idiopathic hemochromatosis gene frequency in Sweden. *Acta Med. Scand.* **218,** 299–304.

8. Worwood, M (1994): Genetics of Haemochromatosis. *Baill. Clin. Haematol.* **7,** 903–918.

9. Bothwell, T.H., Charlton, R.W., Cook, J.D. & Finch, C.A. (1977): Iron Metabolism in Man. Oxford: Blackwell Scientific Publications.

10. Gordeuk, V., Mukiibi, J., Hasstedt, S.J. *et al.* (1992): Iron overload in Africa. *New Engl. J. Med.* **326,** 95–100.

11. Motulksy, A.G. (1979): Genetics of hemochromatosis. *New Engl. J. Med.* **301,** 1291.

12. Simon, M., Alexandre, J.-L., Fauchet, R. *et al.* (1980): The genetics of hemochromatosis. In: *Progress in medical genetics*, New Series. Genetics of Gastrointestinal Disease, Vol. 4, eds. A.G. Steinberg, A.G. Bearn, A.G. Motulsky & G.B. Childs, pp. 135–168. Philadelphia: W.B. Saunders.

13. Edwards, C.Q., Skolnick, M.H. & Kushner, J.P. (1981): Hereditary hemochromatosis: Contributions of genetic analyses. *Prog. Hematol.* **12,** 43–71.

14. Simon, M., Le Mignon, L., Fauchet, R. *et al.* (1987): A study of 609 HLA haplotypes marking for the hemochromatosis gene: (l) mapping of the gene near the HLA-A locus and characters required to define a heterozygous population and (2) hypothesis concerning the underlying cause of hemochromatosis-HLA association. *Am. J. Hum. Genet.* **41,** 89–105.

15. Edwards C.Q., Griffen, L.M. & Dadone, M.M. (1986): Mapping the locus for hereditary hemochromatosis: localization between HLA-B and HLA-A. *Am. J. Hum. Genet.* **38,** 805–811.

16. David, V., Paul, P. & Simon, M. (1986): DNA polymorphism related to the idiopathic hemochromatosis gene: evidence in a recombinant family. *Hum. Genet.* **74,** 113–120.

17. Panajotopoulos, N., Piperno, A., Conte, D. *et al.* (1989): HLA typing in 67 Italian patients with idiopathic hemochromatosis and their relatives. *Tiss. Antig.* **33,** 431–436.

18. Powell, L.W., Summers, K.M., Board, P.G. *et al.* (1990)): Expression of haemochromatosis in homozygous subjects: implications for early diagnosis and prevention. *Gastroenterology* **98,** 1625–1632.

19. Geraghty, D.E., Koller, B.H., Hansen, J.A. & Orr, H.T. (1992): The HLA class I gene family includes at least six genes and twelve pseudogenes and gene fragments. *J. Immunol.* **149,** 1934–1946.

20. Cragg, S.J., Darke, C. & Worwood, M. (1988): HLA class I and H ferritin gene polymorphisms in normal subjects and patients with haemochromatosis. *Hum. Genet.* **80,** 63–68.

21. Hansen, J.L. & Kushner, J.P. (1989): The HLA class I locus: analysis of RFLPs in hereditary hemochromatosis. *Cytogenet. Cell. Genet.* **50,** 216–219.

22. Jouanolle, A.M., Yaouanq, J., Blayau, M. *et al.* (1990): HLA class I gene polymorphism in genetic hemochromatosis. *Hum. Genet.* **85,** 279–282.

23. Cox, T.M. (1990): Haemochromatosis. *Blood Reviews* **4,** 75–87.

24. Fracanzani, A.L., Fargion, S. & Romano, R. (1989): Immunohistochemical evidence for a lack of ferritin in duodenal absorptive epithelial cells in idiopathic hemochromatosis. *Gastroenterology* **96,** 1071–1078.

25. Lombard, M., Bomford, A.B., Poson, R.J. *et al.* (1990): Differential expression of transferrin receptor in duodenal mucosa in iron overload. Evidence for a site-specific defect in genetic hemochromatosis. *Gastroenterology* **98,** 976–984.

26. Raha-Chowdhury, R., Williams, B.J. & Worwood, M. (1993): Red cell destruction by human monocytes – changes in intracellular ferritin concentration and phenotype. *Europ. J. Haematol.* **50,** 26–31.

27. Summers, K.M., Tam, K.S., Bartley, P.B. *et al.* (1991): Fine mapping of a human chromosome 6 ferritin heavy chain pseudogene: relevance to haemochromatosis. *Hum. Genet.* **88,** 175–178.

28. Sampietro, M., Cairo, G., Piperno, A. *et al.* (1987): Analysis of the genes for transferrin, transferrin receptor as well as H and L subunits of ferritin in idiopathic haemochromatosis. *Ric. Clin. Labor.* **17,** 209–213.

29. David, V., Papadopoulos, P. & Yaouanq, J. (1989): Ferritin H gene polymorphism in idiopathic hemochromatosis. *Hum. Genet.* **81,** 123–126.

30. Gasparini, P., Borgato, L., Piperno, A. *et al.* (1993): Linkage analysis of 6p21 polymorphic markers and the hereditary hemochromatosis: localization of the gene centromeric to HLA-F. *Hum. Molec. Genet.* **2,** 571–576.

31. Gasparini, P. & Camaschella, C.: Personal Communication.

32. Jazwinska, E.C., Lee, S.C. & Webb, S.I. (1993): Localization of the hemochromatosis gene close to D6S105. *Am. J. Hum. Genet.* **53,** 347–352.

33. Worwood, M., Raha-Chowdhury, R., Dorak, M.T. *et al.* (1994): Alleles at D6S265 and D6S105 define a haemochromatosis-specific genotype. *Brit. J. Haematol.* **86,** 863–866.

34. Raha-Chowdhury, R., Bowen, D.J., Burnett, A.K. & Worwood, M. (1995): Allelic associations and homozygosity at loci from HLA-B to D6S299 in Genetic Haemochromatosis. *J. Med. Genet.* **32,** 446–452.

35. Raha-Chowdhury, R., Bowen, D.J. & Worwood, M. (1995): A new highly polymorphic marker in the 52 untranslated region of HLA-F shows strong allelic association with haemochromatosis. *Hum. Genet.* (in press).

36. Jazwinska, E.C., Pyper, W.R., Burt, M.J. *et al.* (1995): Haplotype analysis in Australian hemochromatosis patients: evidence for a predominant ancestral haplotype exclusively associated with hemochromatosis. *Am. J. Hum. Genet.* **56,** 428–433.

37. Gyapay, G., Morissette, J. & Vignal, A. (1994): The 1993–94 Genethon human genetic linkage map. *Nature Genet.* **7,** 246–249.

38. Raha-Chowdhury, R., Bowen, D.J., Stone, C. *et al.*. (1995): New Polymorphic microsatellite markers place the haemochromatosis gene telomeric to D6S105. *Hum. Mol. Genet.* (in press).

39. Terwilliger, J.D. (1995): A powerful likelihood method for the analysis of linkage disequilibrium between trait loci and one or more polymorphic marker loci. *Am. J. Human. Genet.* **56,** 777–787.

40. Hastbacka, J., de la Chapelle, A., Mahtani, M.M. *et al.* (1994): The diastrophic hysplasia gene encodes a novel sulphate transporter: positional cloning by fine-structure linkage disequilibrium mapping. *Cell* **78,** 1073–1087.

41. Yaouanq, J., Perichon, M., Chorney, M. *et al.* (1994): Anonymous marker loci within 400 kb of HLA-A generate haplotypes in linkage disequilibrium with the hemochromatosis gene (HFE). *Am. J. Hum. Genet.* **54,** 252–263.

42. Worwood, M., Dorak, M.T. & Raha-Chowdhury, R. (1994): Haplotypes in linkage disequilibrium with the hemochromatosis gene. (Letter) *Am. J. Hum. Genet.* **55,** 585–586.

43. Raha-Chowdhury, R., Olsson, K.S. & Worwood, M. (1995): Haplotype analysis with genetic markers within and telomeric to the HLA class I region in Swedish patients with haemochromatosis. Presentated at the Fifth Conference of the International Association for the study of disorders of Iron Metabolism, Boston 11–13 April.

44. El Kahloun, A., Chauvel, B. & Mauvieux, V. (1993): Localization of seven new genes around th HLA-A locus. *Hum. Molec. Genet.* **2,** 55–60.

45. Wei, H., Fan, W.-F., Xu, H. *et al.* (1993): Genes in one megabase of the HLA class I region. *Proc. Nat. Acad. Sci. USA* **90,** 11870–11874.

46. Goei, V.L., Parimoo, S., Capossela *et al.* (1994): Isolation of novel non-HLA gene fragments from the hemochromatosis region (6p21.3) by cDNA hybridization selection. *Am. J. Hum. Genet.* **54,** 244–251.

47. Volz, A., Boyle, J.M., Cann, H.M., Cottingham, R.W., Orr, H.T. & Ziegler, A. (1994): Report of the Second International Workshop on Human Chromosome 6. *Genomics* **21,** 464–472.

Iron Nutrition in Health and Disease, edited by Leif Hallberg and Nils-Georg Asp
©1996 John Libbey & Company Ltd., pp. 273–277

Chapter 26

Prevalence of haemochromatosis in Scandinavia

K. Sigvard Olsson

Department of Medicine, Mölndal Hospital, S–431 80 Mölndal, Sweden

Summary

Idiopathic or genetic hemochromatosis has been considered rare in Scandinavia, where iron deficiency was common in the past. Some studies have shown possible regional differences with a low figure in the south of Sweden. However, several studies from urban and rural regions of the three Scandinavian countries show a prevalence exceeding 0.33 per cent. This figure (g^2), means a gene frequency (g) of 5.7 per cent and a heterozygote frequency ($2 \times g$) of 11.4 per cent. Such high figures mean that the gene coding for genetic hemochromatosis is one of our most common mutant genes. The high prevalence might be a result of selective advantage of iron loading genes in iron poor areas.

Idiopathic or genetic haemochromatosis (GH) has been considered rare in Scandinavia. When Sheldon published his monograph in 1935, our three countries contributed with only five cases. Until 1955 18 additional cases had been published, 11 from Denmark[1] and seven from Norway[2], in nine reports. Finch and Finch concluded in 1955, that the incidence of GH was quite low in the Scandinavian countries and in England, where iron deficiency was common[3]. At the same time contrastingly high numbers were seen among former Europeans, who had left for Minnesota[4] or Australia, where Althausen *et al.* (in 1951) reported 23 patients from one single hospital[5]. The first prevalence study in Scandinavia was performed by Vogt after seeing three cases of GH in 1941. He reviewed 3518 autopsies from Oslo, found three cases and considered the frequency of GH in Norway the same as in Anglo-Saxon countries[2]. At this time prevalence figures were based only on clinically advanced cases representing the end stage of the disease.

The advent of laboratory routines including serum iron and transferrin saturation (TS) together with serum ferritin (SF) as a simple measure of iron storage, formed the basis for screening studies of families and populations from the mid-1970s. The discovery 1975 by Simon *et al.* that the gene coding for GH was HLA-related, further strengthened the possibility of early identification of homozygotic carriers of the GH genes in family studies[6].

Our own interest started in 1975 when a surprisingly high number of patients with GH was found at the county hospital in Östersund, Sweden, mainly because serum iron and TS had been included in the routine laboratory profile. The hospital is located in a sparsely populated area, known in the past for a high incidence of iron deficiency. A number of screening studies

Table 1. Prevalence of haemochromatosis in Scandanavia 1978-1989

Study size	No. found	%	Category: Location	Reference
197	4	2	men 30-39 y: Östersund, central Sweden	7
623	3	0.5	men 30-39 y, Östersund, central Sweden	8
4100	3	0.07	hosp. patients, Östersund, central Sweden	8
3300	8	0.24	Outpatients, Östersund, central Sweden	9
1310	3	0.23	blood donors, Östersund, central Sweden	9
68	1	1.4	men 31-40 y; Tröndelag, Norway	10
941	0	0	men 55 y; Malmö, Sweden	11
8834	9	0.10	autopsies; Malmö, Sweden	11
1660	0	0	men 50 y; Göteborg, Sweden	12
11920	9	0.08	hosp. patients; Stockholm, Sweden	12

was started in rural and urban Scandinavian areas and is summarized in Table 1.

Two studies[7,10] were from small rural districts and the results were not considered representative. Rather, they reflected local accumulations of the GH gene. Neither were the prevalence figures from Jämtland[8,9] considered representative for the Swedish population, because screening studies from the main urban areas of Sweden showed much lower values[11,12]. It was concluded that the average prevalence of GH in Scandinavia and in caucasian populations would be about 0.1 per cent instead of 0.4 per cent[12].

Possible explanations for divergent results

The low numbers found among hospital patients might seem paradoxical.

However, as inflammatory conditions, prevalent in this category, rapidly induce a fall in serum iron concentration in GH patients as well (Fig. 1), these individuals remain undetected in studies using transferrin saturation (TS) as the screening method.

The two screening studies of representative samples of middle-aged men from Göteborg and Malmö failed to detect one single case of GH.

These results might indicate regional differences of the prevalence of GH.

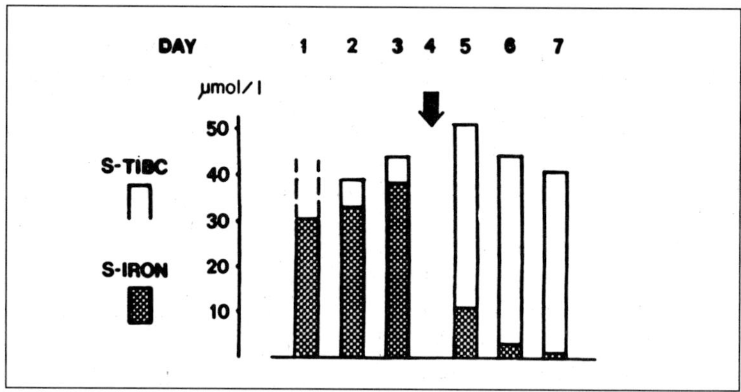

Fig. 1. Changes in serum iron and transferrin saturation in a man with haemochromatosis suffering from a myocardial infarction (arrow) on his 4th day in hospital.

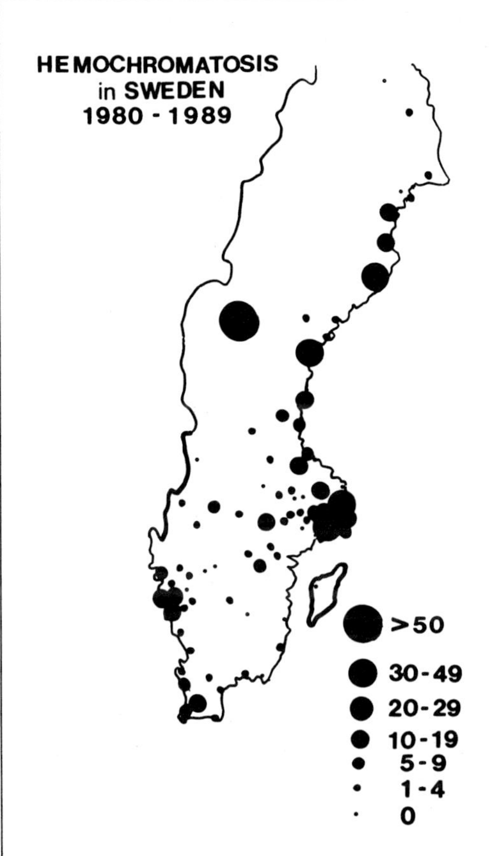

Fig. 2. Distribution of haemochromatosis detected at hospitals in Sweden between 1980 and 1989.

Are there regional differences of the prevalence of GH?

Even though hospital reports of GH patients might reflect a variable local interest for the disorder, rather than its prevalence, in 1991 we performed a study to get information about the geographical distribution of GH in Sweden. A questionaire asking for sex, age, TS, SF, liver tests of patients with GH diagnosed between 1980 and 1989 was sent to 91 departments of medicine at 88 hospitals in Sweden. Of 85 responses, there were 15 hospitals reporting no detected patients. There seemed to be a geographical difference of the distribution of the 503 (376 male, 127 female) reported patients (Fig. 2). Skåne, in the south of Sweden, with a population of 1.1 million, reported only 32 patients, as compared to 222 from the 4 northern counties (population 1.2 million). The county of Stockholm (population 1.6 million) fell between with 122 patients. These findings, together with the low prevalence reported from Malmö, might indicate a lower prevalence of iron loading genes in the south of Sweden.

In recent years there has been an increased interest to detect and treat GH individuals as early as possible. Screening studies mainly of blood donors from different parts of Scandinavia have been performed. (Table 2).

Preliminary results of screening for iron overload among 1810 blood donors of Göteborg, showed 67 GH subjects or 0.39 per cent[13].

Discussion

There is a risk that prevalence studies of rare diseases might be biased, because they are initiated at local hospitals in which an accumulation of the disease has been seen. This is perhaps unavoidable. However, in districts such as Fyn, Denmark, where GH has been considered rare (9 cases in 12 years from a population of 450.000), screening studies have also been made. In their study Wiggers *et al.* detected 9 GH individuals among 2417 male blood donors[14]. This study, together with the recent studies from Oslo and Göteborg, indicate that urban Scandinavian areas might present prevalence figures of GH, well in agreement with those from other caucasian populations[18]. It should be observed that the cut-off point of TS at the initial screening has been reduced

Table 2. Prevalence of haemochromatosis in Scandinavia 1990–1995

Study size	No found	%	Category; Location	Reference
2417	9	0.37	Male blood donors; Fyn, Denmark	14
1887	7	0.37	Random sample; Iceland	15
3975	17	0.43	18-year-old men: central Sweden	16
3500	12	0.34	Blood donors; Oslo, Norway	17

from 60–70 per cent in the early screenings to 50 per cent in recent studies.

The discrepancy between the few clinically detected GH patients in an area such as Fyn, and the relatively high numbers of GH individuals found at screenings might seem strange. Certainly there are GH patients who still go undetected; however, most GH individuals detected at screenings of families and populations have no clinical evidence of disease[18]. In other words, not all homozygotic carriers of iron loading genes will develop clinical disease. Therefore the cost-effectivenes of early screenings is difficult to determine[19,20].

Do these observations mean that screening is not needed?

Screening for GH of the general population in Scandinavia does not seem to be indicated, especially since all three countries have stopped the iron fortification of their food. However, screening studies are recommended first of all in GH families, but also in blood donors. The Scandinavian countries and Canada are favourable in this respect, because the blood banks accept the blood from healthy GH donors[20].

It is tempting to speculate about the causes of the probable regional difference of GH in Sweden with higher numbers found in the northern provinces. It could be an effect of increased awareness of the disorder in the north (because of data presented at regional meetings?). It could also be a result of genetic advantage of iron-loading genes in the iron-poor northern provinces. Such geographical differences in iron nutrition in Sweden were demonstrated by Odin in 1934[21] and discussed by Lundholm in 1939[22].

Conclusions

Screening studies of genetic haemochromatosis in Scandinavia have shown low figures in the south of Sweden. However, several studies from other urban and rural regions of the three Scandinavian countries show a prevalence exceeding 0.33 per cent. This figure (g^2), means a gene frequency (g) of 5.7 per cent or a heterozygote frequency ($2 \times g$) of 11.4 per cent. The gene coding for hereditary haemochromatosis is one of our most common mutant genes in Scandinavia. The high prevalence might be a result of selective advantage of iron loading genes in iron-poor areas.

References:

1. Christensen, R. (1955): Haemochromatosis. *Ugeskr. Laeger.* **117,** 445–451.
2. Vogt, J.H. (1944): Hemochromatosis. *Acta Path. Microbiol. Scand.* **21,** 461–471.
3. Finch, S.C. & Finch, C.A. (1955): Idiopathic Hemochromatosis, an iron storage disease. *Medicine* **34,** 381–430.
4. Butt, H.R. & Wilder, R.M. (1938): Hemochromatosis. Report of 30 cases in which the diagnosis was made during life. *Arch. Path.* **26,** 262–273.
5. Althausen, T.L., Doig, R.K., Weiden, S., *et al.* (1951): Hemochromatosis; investigation of 23 cases. *Arch. Int. Med.* **88,** 553–570.
6. Simon, M., Pawlotsky, Y., Bourel, M., Fauchet, R. & Genetet, B. (1975): Hémochromatose idiopathique: maladie associée à l'antigène tissulaire HL-A3? *Nouv. Presse Med.* **4,** 1432.
7. Olsson, K.S., Heedman, P.A. & Staugård, F. (1978): Preclinical hemochromatosis in a population on a high-iron-fortified diet. *JAMA* **239,** 1999–2000.
8. Olsson, K.S., Ritter, B., Rosén, U., Heedman, P.A. & Staugård, F. (1983): Prevalence of iron overload in Central Sweden. *Acta Med. Scand.* **213,** 145–150.
9. Olsson, K.S., Eriksson, K., Ritter, B. & Heedman, P.A. (1984): Screening for iron overload using transferrin saturation. *Acta Med. Scand.* **215,** 105–112.

10. Pedersen, K., Fölling, I., Lamvik, J. *et al.* (1985): Hereditär hemokromatose. *Tidsskr. Nor. Laegeforen.* **22,** 1385–1388.

11. Lindmark, B. & Eriksson, S. (1985): Regional differences in the idiopathic hemochromatosis gene frequency in Sweden. *Acta Med. Scand.* **218,** 299–304.

12. Hallberg, L., Björn-Rasmussen, E. & Jungner, I. (1989): Prevalence of hereditary haemochromatosis in two Swedish urban areas. *J. Intern. Med.* **225,** 249–255.

13. Olson, K.S. & Konar, R.M. Prevelance of iron overload among blood donors in Göteborg, Sweden. (1995) *Abstract Clin. Lab. Haem.* **17**, 372–373.

14. Wiggers, P., Dalhöj, J., Kiaer, H. *et al.* (1991): Screening for haemochromatosis: prevalence among Danish blood donors. *J. Intern. Med.* **230,** 265–270.

15. Jonsson, J.J., Johannesson, G.M., Sigfusson, N. *et al.* (1991): Prevalence of iron deficiency and iron overload in the adult Icelandic population. *J. Clin. Epidemiol.* **44,** 1289–1297.

16. Olsson, K.S., Marsell, R., Ritter, B. *et al.* (1995): Iron deficiency and iron overload in Swedish male adolescents. *J. Intern. Med.* **237,** 187–194.

17. Bell, H., Thordal, C., Raknerud, N. *et al.*. (1995): Prevalence of hemochromatosis in Norwegian healthy blood donors. Abstract volume. 5th Conference Int Ass for the Study of Disorders of Iron Metab. p. 95, Boston.

18. Edwards, C.Q. & Kushner, J.P. (1993): Screening for hemochromatosis. *N. Engl. J. Med.* **328,** 1616–1620.

19. Adams, P.C., Gregor, J.C., Kertesz, A.E. & Valberg, L.S. (1995): Screening blood donors for hereditary hemochromatosis: decision analysis model based on a 30-Year database. *Gastroenterology* **109,** 177–188.

20. Kushner, J.P. (1995): Screening for hemochromatosis. Editorial. *Gastroenterology* **109,** 316–317.

21. Odin, M. (1934): *En socialhygienisk undersökning i Västerbottens och Norrbottens län 1929–1931.* Lund: Håkan Olssons Boktryckeri.

22. Lundholm, I. (1939): Hereditary hypochromic anemia. *Acta Med. Scand.* Suppl 102.

Iron Nutrition in Health and Disease, edited by Leif Hallberg and Nils-Georg Asp

Chapter 27

Excess iron and risk of cancer

Richard G. Stevens

Pacific Northwest Laboratory, Richland, WA 99352, USA

Summary

Excess body iron may increase cancer risk by feeding existing transformed cells and/or by helping to create new transformed cells through oxidative stress. There is evidence bearing on this hypothesis from three sources: 1) cellular and subcellular, 2) animal, and 3) epidemiology studies. Whereas cellular studies clearly show that iron can damage DNA and animal studies have shown that iron can induce cancer, the epidemiological evidence is limited and mixed. At the extreme, haemochromatosis confers a hundred-fold increased risk of liver cancer. The question is whether, and to what extent moderate elevation of body iron increases risk of cancer in general, and if so, what cancer sites are most vulnerable. The mixed results from the epidemiological studies may reflect no real excess risk from iron, or may reflect an inadequate assessment of body iron, and therefore an inaccurate body iron determination.

Body iron in excess of that necessary to avoid anaemia offers no health benefit, and there is evidence that it may be a detriment. Therefore, an important question is whether a moderate elevation in body iron level leads to increased risk of cancer, and, if so, what cancer sites are most affected.

Introduction

Is iron good? Of course. It is necessary for life. Can iron be bad? Perhaps, in excess where it is not needed.

Just as iron is a nutritional requirement for humans, it is a nutritional requirement for human pathogens and transformed cells. Iron can also act as a potent pro-oxidant under some physiological circumstances. On this basis, excess iron may increase cancer risk by feeding existing transformed cells and/or by helping to create new transformed cells. The campaign against iron deficiency anaemia in under-nourished societies beginning early this century has obscured the potential harm that excess iron may cause in well-nourished societies. The issue is important because the Western diet includes high amounts of available iron[1], and this diet has been spreading throughout the world.

Although non-haem iron is effectively blocked from uptake in a normal iron replete person, haem iron is less well blocked. In addition, certain genetic polymorphisms allow some people to absorb iron more readily than others. In particular, hereditary haemochromatosis may be far more common than previously suspected[2]. People diagnosed with haemochromatosis are at greatly increased risk of cancer and heart attack[3,4]. The haemochromatosis gene product is unknown but it apparently affects uptake of iron from the gut, perhaps coding for an iron transport protein in the intestinal wall. Kravitz *et al.*[5] reported a transferrin saturation of 93 per cent and 83.7 per cent in male and female haemochromatosis homozygotes respectively, compared to only 32.8 per cent and 30.2 per cent in homozygous normal males and females. Obligate heterozygotes had intermediate transferrin saturations of 42.6 per cent and 40.1 per cent, respectively. Since the gene frequency of the abnormal haemochromatosis allele has been estimated to be 0.067 from a study of blood donors in Utah[2], it is estimated that approximately 12–14 per cent of the population may be heterozygotes. Therefore a large segment of the population may be at genetically determined increased risk of cancer due to chronically higher body iron stores (as reflected in higher transferrin saturation) resulting from the haemochromatosis gene (in either the homozygous or heterozygous state). There may well be other iron overload genetic polymorphisms as well[6].

The definitions of 'high body iron level' that are relevant to the two proposed mechanisms whereby iron might increase cancer risk[7,8] are: (1) high iron content of blood and interstitial fluid in a form that can be utilized by cancer cells (e.g. high transferrin saturation)[9], and (2) high intracellular iron content, particularly that iron associated with DNA, with ferritin, and with non-specific iron complexes that could participate in pro-oxidant reactions[10].

Cellular and subcellular evidence

The very quality that makes iron an effective energy transfer engine, its redox cycling capability, also makes it dangerous to cells and tissues. Complex biological systems have developed to utilize iron efficiently when it is needed, and to sequester it otherwise. These systems are not perfect.

Iron's potential for oxidative damage has been amply demonstrated in many cellular and subcellular systems. Added to a preparation of DNA and hydrogen peroxide, iron greatly increases strand breakage of the DNA[13]. In cellular systems, excess iron can increase chromosome damage[14] and can increase susceptibility of cells to damage by toxic chemicals and by ionizing radiation[15,16]. The deletarious biological effects of asbestos may be directly related to its iron content[17]. In particular, there is also evidence that the DNA oxidation by crocidolite asbestos and the silicate's mutagenicity in *Samonella typhimurium* (TA 102) involves iron in the fibre[18].

Animal evidence

There is a growing literature on the role of iron in carcinogenesis. For example, iron has been implicated in leukaemia in mice[19] and in cancers of colon in mice[20,21], breast in rats[22] and mice[23], lung in mice[24], and liver in mice[25]. Several of these studies have been of transplantation of tumour cells, and the subsequent differences in growth in iron deficient, iron replete, and iron overloaded animals. Such an experimental model is based directly upon Weinberg's[9] idea that iron is a limiting nutrient to cancer cells. Other experiments have examined whether iron augments the effects of a known carcinogen, and these test the idea that iron may act as a sensitizer to damage from prooxidant xenobiotics.

Human evidence

Liver cancer death is elevated several hundredfold among those diagnosed with hereditary haemochromatosis[3,4]. Whether other cancer sites are also elevated at more modest two- and threefold risks cannot be determined with the small numbers of haemochromatitics available for study. In the population at large, however, a limited number of epidemiological studies have reported associations of body iron level and risk of cancer in general. In these studies, iron level has been inferred from one or more of the following: serum ferritin, serum transferrin, total iron-binding capacity, and serum transferrin saturation.

Whether, and to what extent, elevated body iron increases cancer risk in general has been investigated in only a few studies. To obtain information on a large enough popuation to have meaningful results, surrogates for iron level have been used. In general, among healthy individuals, when body iron stores are high, transferrin saturation and serum ferritin are high, and TIBC and serum transferrin are low. These assumed relationships form the basis for the studies done to date.

Four studies have been consistent with the hypothesis that high body iron stores increase the risk of cancer, or general mortality, in men[26–28] or in women[29]. One study from Finland that was first presented in abbreviated form found no relationship between transferrin saturation and total cancer risk[30]. However, stomach cancer is a leading cause of cancer death in Finnish men, and after it is analyzed separately there is some support for increased risk of some cancer sites in those with high transferrin saturation or low TIBC in their study population[31]. In particular, relative risk of colon cancer was 3.04 among men and women with transferrin saturation greater than 60 per cent at baseline compared to those with transferrin saturation lower than 60 per cent. In the original report on the NHANES[28], for cancer of colon, risk in each quartile of transferrin saturation relative to a baseline of 1.0 for those under 22.8 per cent, increased to 1.76 in those 22.9–29.1 per cent, to 3.11 in those 29.2–36.7 per cent, and to 4.69 in those greater than 36.7 per cent. This striking result was consistent with the prediction of Graf and Eaton[32] who speculated that dietary phytate consumption would reduce risk of colon cancer by virtue of binding iron. The result was based on only 12 cases, however, and only provides the basis for investigating this relationship further in other population samples. Nelson *et al.*[33] reported risk of colonic adenoma was related to serum ferritin in a case-control study of 145 subjects with adenoma, 29 with colon cancer, and 159 controls who had undergone colonoscopy between 1984 and 1987 at Walter Reed Army Medical Center. The odds ratio associated with serum ferritin greater than 83 ng/ml versus lower values was ~2.3 for adenomas, whereas for colon cancer it was not significantly greater than 1.0. Because the ferritin assessment was done after diagnosis, the authors state that their adenoma result is more reliable than the cancer result because bleeding may have lowered body iron in those subjects with cancer.

An update of the NHANES study with four more years of follow-up has yielded further insight into the association of body iron and risk of cancer[34]. The data were examined with three goals: (1) hypothesis testing, (2) internal consistency, and (3) dose-response. For hypothesis testing, among 379 men who developed cancer over the study period (1971–1988), the mean transferrin saturation at enrollment was 32.1 per cent, whereas among 2908 who remained cancer free it was 30.7 per cent ($P = 0.015$); the difference for mortality was 32.3 per cent among 233 deaths versus 30.8 per cent among 3054 men not dying of cancer ($P = 0.025$). The mean differences among women were not significant. For internal consistency, the mean differences in TIBC and serum iron among men were consistent with the findings for transferrin saturation, and all three differences were stable over time when examined by years since the blood test.

For dose response, men and women were divided into five groups on the basis of baseline transferrin saturation: 0–30 per cent, 30– 40 per cent, 40–50 per cent, 50–60 per cent, and 60 per cent and higher. Nineteen per cent of men had a baseline transferrin saturation above 40 per cent (the last three groups), whereas only 10 percent of women had transferrin saturation above 40 per cent. Risk in each category was calculated relative to the lowest category by the Mantel-Haenszel procedure adapted to cohort studies using the computer software MOX[35]. Analyses were stratified on age (one year intervals), smoking and sex. For men and women combined, risk in each group relative to the first was 1.0, 0.95, 1.16, 1.31 and 1.81 (p for trend 0.012); for mortality the relative risks were 1.0, 0.96, 1.22, 1.29 and 1.73 (p for trend 0.049).

Merk *et al.*[36] found significantly reduced risk of cancer (all sites combined) in blood donors in Sweden. The authors discuss several possible explanations for their findings including a 'healthy donor' effect in which blood donors are a self-selected group with a generally healthy life style. The authors also point out, however, that their results are consistent with a protective effect of blood donation by virtue of lowering body iron level. This effect may have been particularly apparent in Sweden because the general population is heavily supplemented with iron both voluntarily and involuntarily[37,38]. on the other hand, a recent study from the Kaiser Permanente Health Plan has shown no relationships at all of transferrin saturation with cancer risk[39].

Conclusion and future studies

Future studies of the possible deleterious effects of excess body iron in cancer risk should include continued research on measures of body iron status. In order to conduct meaningful studies of disease risk, reliable exposure metrics are needed. Serum ferritin is believed to be well related to body iron in healthy people, but can also be elevated in inflammation unrelated to body iron. Transferrin saturation reflects a relevant iron measure, that of iron potentially available to cancer cells, but is thought to be highly variable in the middle range. New measures such as serum transferrin receptor[40] could be used in conjunction with other measures in future studies.

Other future avenues for research include interactions of the nutritional pro-oxidant iron with nutritional antioxidants, and the genetic polymorphisms of free radical scavenging systems. A difficult study, but potentially informative, would be a study of cancer risk in haemochromatosis heterozygotes. Without a blood test for heterozygous status, such a study is severly limited in size because subjects must be identified by pedigree analysis. Excess body iron may act as a sensitizer to ionizing radiation and toxic chemicals. And finally, the possible role of iron in prognosis after cancer diagnosis deserves attention[41].

Body iron in excess of that necessary to avoid anaemia offers no health benefit, and there is evidence that it may be a detriment. Therefore, an important question is whether a moderate elevation in body iron level leads to increased risk of cancer and, if so, what cancer sites are most affected.

References

1. Cook, J.D. (1990): Adaptation in iron metabolism. *Am. J. Clin. Nutr.* **51,** 301–38.
2. Edwards, C.Q., Griffen, L.M., Goldgar, D. *et al.* (1988): Prevalence of hemochromatosis among 11,065 presumably healthy blood donors. *N. Engl. J. Med.* **318,** 1355–1362.
3. Bradbear, R.A., Bain, C., Siskind, V., Schofield, F.D., Webb, S., Axelsen, E.M., Halliday, J.W., Bassett, M.L. & Powell, L.W. (1985): Cohort study of internal malignancy in genetic hemochromatosis and other chronic nonalcoholic liver diseases. *J. Natl. Cancer Inst.* **75,** 81–85.
4. Niederau, C., Fischer, R., Sonnenberg, A. *et al.* (1985): Survival and causes of death in cirrhotic and noncirrhotic patients with primary hemochromatosis. *N. Eng. J. Med.* **313,** 1256–1262.
5. Kravitz, K., Skolnick, M., Cannings, C. *et al.* (1979): Genetic linkage between hereditary hemochromatosis and HLA. *Am. J. Hum. Genet.* **31,** 601–619.
6. Gordeuk, V., Mukiibi, J., Hasstedt, S.J., Samowitz, W., Corwin, C.Q., West, G., Ndambire, S., Emmanual, J., Nkanza, N., Chapanduka, Z., Randall, M., Boone, P., Romano, P., Martell, R.W., Yamashita, T., Effler, P. & Brittenham, G. (1992): Iron overload in Africa. *New Engl. J. Med.* **326,** 95–100.
7. Stevens, R.G. & Kalkwarf, D.R. (1990): Iron, radiation, and cancer. *Environ. Health Perspec.* **87,** 291–300.
8. Stevens, R.G. (1992): Iron and Cancer. In: *Iron and human disease*, ed. R. Lauffer, pp. 333–347. Boca Raton, Florida: CRC Press.
9. Weinberg, E.D. (1984): Iron withholding: a defense against infection and neoplasia. *Physiological Reviews* **64,** 65–102.
10. Halliwell, B. & Gutteridge, J.M.C. (1990): Role of free radicals and catalytic metal ions in human disease: an overview. *Method. Enzymol.* **186,** 1–185.
11. Imlay, J.A. & Linn, S. (1988): DNA damage and oxygen radical toxicity. *Science* **240,** 1302–1309.
12. Loeb, L.A., James, E.A., Waltersdorph, A.M. & Klebanoff, S.J. (1988): Mutagenesis by autoxidation of iron with isolated DNA. *Proc. Natl. Acad. Sci.* **85,** 3918–3922.

13. Blakely, W.F., Fuciarelli, A.F., Wegher, B.J. & Dizdaroglu, M. (1990): Hydrogen peroxide-induced base damage in deoxyribonucleic acid. *Radiat. Res.* **121,** 338–343.

14. Whiting, R.F., Wei, L. & Stich, H.F. (1981): Chromosome-damaging activity of ferritin and its relation to chelation and reduction of iron. *Cancer Res.* **41,** 1628–1636.

15. Balla, G., Vercellotti, G.M., Eaton, J.W. & Jacob, H.S. (1990): Iron loading of endothelial cells augments oxidant damage. *J. Lab. Clin. Med.* **116,** 546–554.

16. Nelson, J.M. & Stevens, R.G. (1992): Ferritin-iron increases killing of Chinese hamster ovary cells by X irradiation. *Cell. Proliferation* **25,** 579–585.

17. Lund, L.G. & Aust, A.E. (1991): Iron-catalyzed reactions may be responsible for the biochemical and biological effects of asbestos. *BioFactors* **3,** 83–89.

18. Faux, S.P., Howden, P.J. & Levy, L.S. (1994): Iron-dependent formation of 8–hydroxydeoxyguanosine in isolated DNA and mutagenticity in Salmonella typhimurium TA102 induced by crocidolite. *Carcinogenesis* **15,** 1749–1751.

19. Bergeron, R.J., Streiff, R.R. & Elliott, G.T. (1985): Influence of iron on in vivo proliferation and lethality of L1210 cells. *J. Nutr.* **115,** 369–374.

20. Siegers, C.P., Bumann, D., Baretton, G. & Younes, M. (1988): Dietary iron enhances the tumor rate in dimethylhydrazine-induced colon carcinogenesis in mice. *Cancer Lett.* **41,** 251–256.

21. Siegers, C.P., Bumann, D., Trepkau, H.D., Schadwinkel, B. & Baretton, G. (1992): Influence of dietary iron overload on cell proliferation and intestinal tumorigenesis in mice. *Cancer Lett.* **65,** 245–249.

22. Thompson, H.J., Kennedy, K., Witt, M. & Juzefyk, J. (1991): Effect of dietary iron deficiency or excess on the induction of mammary carcinogenesis by 1-methyl-1-nitrosourea. *Carcinogenesis* **12,** 111–114.

23. Hann, H.W., Stahlhut, M.W. & Menduke, H. (1991): Iron enhances tumor growth: observation on spontaneous mammary tumors in mice. *Cancer* **68,** 2407–2410.

24. Yano, T., Obata, Y., Ishikawa, G. & Ichikawa, T. (1994): Enhancing effect of high dietary iron on lung tumorigenesis in mice. *Cancer Lett.* **76,** 57–62.

25. Smith, A.G., Francis, J.E. & Carthew, P. (1990): Iron as a synergist for hepatocellular carcinoma by polychlorinated biphenyls in AH-responsive C57BL/10ScSn mice. *Carcinogenesis* **11,** 437–444.

26. Stevens, R.G., Kuvibidila, S., Kapps, M., Friedlaender, J.S. & Blumberg, B.S. (1983): Iron-binding proteins, hepatitis B virus, and mortality in the Solomon Islands. *Am. J. Epidemiol.* **118,** 550–561.

27. Stevens, R.G., Beasley, R.P. & Blumberg, B.S. (1986): Iron-binding proteins and risk of cancer in Taiwan. *J. Natl. Cancer Inst.* **76,** 605–610.

28. Stevens, R.G., Jones, D.Y., Micozzi, M.S. & Taylor, P.R. (1988): Body iron stores and the risk of cancer. *N. Engl. J. Med.* **319,** 1047–1052.

29. Selby, J.V. & Friedman, G.D. (1988): Epidemiological evidence of an association of body iron stores and risk of cancer. *Int. J. Cancer* **41,** 677–682.

30. Takkunen, H., Reunanen, A., Knekt, P. & Aromaa, A. (1989): Body iron stores and the risk of cancer. *N. Engl. J. Med.* (letter) **320,** 1013–1014.

31. Knekt, P., Reunanen, A., Takkunen, H., Aromaa, A. & Hakulinen, T. (1994): Body iron stores and the risk of cancer. *Int. J. Cancer.* **56,** 379–382.

32. Graf, E. & Eaton, J.W. (1985): Dietary suppression of colonic cancer: fiber or phytate? *Cancer* **56,** 717–718.

33. Nelson, R.L., Davis, F.G., Sutter, E., Sobin, L.H., Kikendall, J.W. & Bowen, P. (1994): Body iron stores and risk of colonic neoplasia. *J. Natl. Cancer Inst.* **86,** 455–460.

34. Stevens, R.G., Graubard, B.I., Micozzi, M.S., Neriishi, K. & Blumberg, B.S. (1994): Moderate elevation of body iron level and increased risk of cancer occurrence and death. *Int. J. Cancer* **56,** 364–369.

35. Gilbert, E.S. & Buchanan, J.A. (1984): An alternative approach to analyzing occupational mortality data. *J. Occup. Med.* **26,** 822–828.

36. Merk, K., Mattsson, B., Mattsson, A., Holm, G., Gullbring, B. & Björkholm, M. (1990): The incidence of cancer among blood donors. *Int. J. Epidemol.* **19,** 505–509.

37. Olsson, K.S., Heedman, P.A. & Staugard, F. (1978): Preclincal hemochromatosis in a population on a high-iron-fortified diet. *JAMA* **239,** 1999–2000.

38. Reizenstein, P. (1990): Inducers and scavengers of free radicals in food. *Med. Oncol. & Tumor Pharmacother.* **7,** 67–68.

39. Herrington, L.J., Friedman, G.D., Baer, D., Selby, J.V. (1995): Transferrin saturation and risk of cancer. *Am J Epidemiol*, **142**, 692–698

40. Skikne, B.S., Flowers., C.H. & Cook, J.D. (1990): Serum transferrin receptor: a quantitative measure of tissue iron deficiency. *Blood* **75,** 1870–1876.

41. Cazzola, M., Bergamaschi, G., Dezza, L. & Arosio, P. (1990): Manipulations of cellular iron metabolism for modulating normal and malignant cell proliferation: achievements and prospects. *Blood* **75,** 1903–1919.

Iron Nutrition in Health and Disease, edited by Leif Hallberg and Nils-Georg Asp
©1996 John Libbey & Company Ltd., pp. 285–292

Chapter 28

Experimental studies on the role of iron in liver tumour development

Lennart C. Eriksson and Per Stål

Division of Pathology, Department of Immunology, Microbiology, Pathology and Infectious Diseases, Karolinska Institutet, Huddinge University Hospital, S-141 86 Huddinge, Sweden

Summary

The inability of liver tumour cells to accumulate iron in a situation of iron excess is seen in the preneoplastic stage, following initiation and is evident throughout the process of liver tumour development. It has even been used as a marker to identify and quantitate premalignant lesions, i.e. liver foci and liver nodules. Those lesions are also iron deficient compared to normal liver cells, as reflected by low levels of intracellular iron, haem and haem-containing enzymes. The rate of iron uptake in cells from liver nodules is decreased as compared to normal hepatocytes, in spite of an increased number of transferrin receptors on the cell surface. The affinity of the receptor to diferric transferrin is not altered. A possible explanation to the reduced receptor-mediated iron uptake is the decreased endosomal acidification and receptor-ligand dissociation found in those cells.

Iron is involved in many cellular processes, making it difficult to predict consequences of cellular iron deficiency and increased iron exposure on tumour development. The role of iron in oxidative stress reactions would indicate an increased risk for DNA damage and mutations in a situation of iron excess. Reduced iron content can contribute to the increased resistance to lipid peroxidation and cytotoxicity seen in cells of pre-neoplastic and pre-malignant liver lesions. The role of iron as a growth factor, however, can explain why those cells show increased growth response *in vivo* as well as *in vitro*. Genetic haemochromatosis is a common hereditary disorder associated with an increased risk of liver tumour development. In an animal model for studies of haemochromatosis using dietary carbonyl iron, the effect of iron in the initiation and promotion steps of hepatocarcinogenesis were tested. Iron at concentrations not associated with liver cirrhosis could not be shown to initiate or promote tumour formation via mechanisms involving genotoxic or mitogenic influences. The effect of long-term iron exposure, alone or in combination with other toxic compounds, during tumour progression is under evaluation. These results indicate that liver tumour development as a consequence of iron exposure is dependent on the development of liver cirrhosis.

The role of iron in tumour development is intriguing and controversial. Theoretical implications suggest roles for iron as a genotoxic, cytotoxic and mitogenic substance, with a putative carcinogenic potential. However, its influences on the carcinogenic process is not obvious and remains to be proven.

Introduction

It was soon recognized in experimental liver tumour models that preneoplastic and premalignant liver lesions did not accumulate iron in a situation of iron excess[1]. Human adenomas and hepatomas are also low in intracellular iron[2,3] and the role of iron deficient foci in the development of liver cancer in patients with haemochromatosis has recently been recognized[4].

Low iron content and iron uptake in liver tumour pre-stages and hepatocellular carcinoma

The inability of liver tumour cells to accumulate iron in a situation of iron excess is seen as early as the pre-neoplastic stage, following initiation and is evident throughout the process of liver tumour development[1,3]. It has been used as a marker to identify and quantitate premalignant lesions, such as liver foci and liver nodules. It was subsequently observed that many iron-containing and iron-dependent enzymes and processes were depressed in those lesions compared to normal or surrounding tissue. Reduced levels of haem-containing enzymes such as cytochrome P–450, cytochrome b_5, tryptophane 2,3–dioxygenase and catalase, as well as cellular haem, haem-binding protein and total cellular iron have been demonstrated in liver nodules[5]. Roomi *et al.*[6] and Stout and Becker[7] noticed an increased activity of haem oxygenase, a haem degrading activity, and a decrease in haem synthetizing activity, expressed as the activity of 5–aminolevulinic acid synthetase (ALA synthetase). In spite of reduced ALA synthetase and reduced iron uptake, haem synthesis in hepatic carcinomas appears to be normal[8].

The rate of iron uptake in cells from liver nodules is slower than in normal hepatocytes in spite of the fact that the number of transferrin receptors on the cell surface is greatly increased in those cells[9]. The affinity of the receptor to diferric transferrin is not altered. The number of membrane-bound diferric transferrin binding sites in homogenates is 20–60–fold higher in liver nodules than in normal liver, as compared to an eightfold relative increase in the organelles enriched in receptor sites, the plasma membrane and the endosomes. A possible explanation for the reduced receptor mediated iron uptake in liver nodules is a marked deficiency in endosomal acidification and receptor-ligand dissociation found in those cells[10]. Using a method which determines ATP-dependent acridine orange quenching in the presence of specific inhibitors for non-vacuolar activities (oligomycin, oubain, ortovanadate) the rate of acidification in a subcellular membrane fraction enriched in endosomal marker enzymes was reduced in liver nodules to less than 25 per cent of the normal activity. Rissler and Eriksson[11] showed a reduced rate of labelled diferric transferrin endocytosis in isolated hepatocytes from liver nodules, leaving a high proportion of the ligand on the cell surface. In addition, restoration of cell surface ligand binding capacity was slower than for normal cells. The available data suggest that, although binding of diferric transferrin to the receptor is high on the cell surface, dissociation of iron from the binding molecule is not taking place in the endosomes due to insufficient vacuolar acidification, which limits the uptake of iron into the cytoplasmic compartment (Fig. 1).

The role of iron in tumour development

Iron is involved in many cellular processes and it is hard to predict consequences of cellular iron deficiency, increased transferrin receptor expression and increased iron exposure on tumor development. Based on the knowledge of the sequential carcinogenic process several hypotheses can be formulated and investigated.

Iron toxicity

Genotoxic effects of iron on DNA have been demonstrated *in vitro*[12]. These effects may be mediated through an increased production of hydroxyl radicals via the iron-induced Fenton reaction[13,14]. Hydroxyl radicals react with DNA to produce single-strand nicks or oxidative damage, such as formation of 8–oxo–2′-deoxyguanosine. Iron may also participate in initation of lipid peroxidation via formation of hydroxyl radicals through the Fenton reaction or the Haber-Weiss reaction[15]. Lipid peroxidation of polyunsaturated fatty acid moieties in membrane phospholipids is most probably involved in iron-induced membrane damage, with severe functional implications for the cell, including cell death at heavy iron overload.

Iron as a growth factor

Transferrin is an essential growth factor in many cell systems[16]. Inhibition of transferrin binding to the receptor using antibodies against transferrin binding epitopes on the transferrin receptor inhibits growth[17]. The regulation of transferrin receptor expression is also affected by the growth status of the cell. The number of receptors on the cell surface is higher on proliferating cells[18], at least partly depending on receptor relocalization[19]. The intracellular iron requirement for iron-containing enzymes, including cytochromes and ribonucleotide reductase, necessary for cell proliferation, has been the rationale to explain increased receptor expression and transferrin dependence. The discovery that ferricyanide could replace diferric transferrin in melanoma cell cultures[20] showed that provision of nutritional iron was not the growth-limiting factor. Crane *et al.*[21] formulated the transplasma-membrane redox concept and showed that diferric transferrin is also an important electron acceptor for NADH oxidoreductases. In a review by Löw *et al.*[22], the properties and functions of plasma membrane oxidoreductases were described. Thorstensen and Romslo[23] have also summarized the role of transferrin for cellular growth.

Cell surface redox activity is associated with alkalinization of the cellular cytosol via proton extrusion through the Na^+/H^+ antiport[24–26] and restoration of intracellular NAD:NADH ratio[27]. Cellular control of pH and NAD stores[28] are important and rate limiting for growth. Transplasma membrane redox with electron transport to extracellular electron accepting substrates

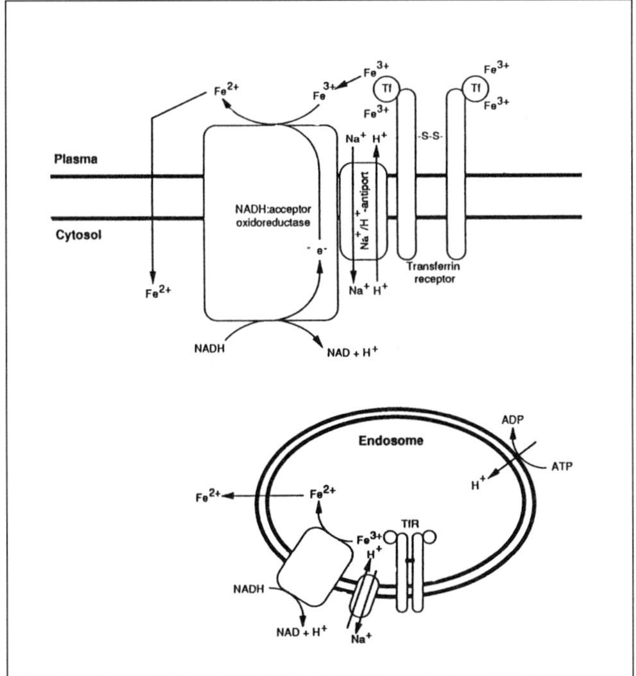

Fig. 1. Schematic presentation of cell surface binding and reduction of iron at the plama membrane and the release of iron from endosomes. Tf = transferrin, TfR = transferrin receptor. NADH-acceptor oxidoreductases reduce the iron at the cell surface and probably also in the endosome after iron has been released from transferrin in the acidic environment.

with appropiate reduction potential is important for themaintenance of growth-permitting homeostasis in the cell. The most abundant extracellular physiological substrate for plasma membrane redox reactions is diferric transferrin[28]. In fact, more ferric iron is used for redox purposes than for iron uptake and intracellular use[22]. Stimulation of transmembrane electron transfer by addition of diferric transferrin stimulates growth of many animal cells[28]. The influence of plasma membrane redox on growth regulation is emphasized by investigations showing that growth inhibitors, such as adriamycin and bleomycin, are also potent inhibitors of the redox system[29,30].

The stimulating effect of iron on cellular growth is thus dependent on the ability of the cell to position diferric transferrin in close association with the electron transport system. This ability is correlated to the number of diferric transferrin receptor sites on the cell surface. NADH diferric transferrin reductase is only one of several transplasma membrane oxidoreductase activities. Others are NADH oxygen oxidoreductase, NADH semidehydroascorbate reductase and NADPH thioredoxin reductase, all utilizing extracellular electron acceptors. Ferricyanide may act as an impermeable artificial acceptor for all these activities[22]. It was recently shown that proliferation of normal liver cells *in vitro*, on a growth permitting collagen type I biomatrix, was augmented by diferric transferrin[31,32]. This response was dose dependent in the range 0.1–30 M. Equimolar concentrations of ferricyanide could replace diferric transferrin. These data support previous findings from studies of other cell systems on the growth regulatory effect of available electron acceptors for cell surface redox reactions[28]. Isolated nodular cells showed a higher than normal spontaneous growth rate with a labelling index of 20 per cent, compared to the normal 10 per cent, and expressed an increased response to the growth-promoting activity of extracellular electron acceptors[32]. Thus the nodular cells contain an excess of constitutive diferric transferrin bound to the receptor, in close proximity to the reductase, due to their high surface transferrin receptor expression. This alteration would result in an activated plasma membrane redox activity, and to redox conditions that will not be rate limiting for cell proliferation.

These results, demonstrating mitogenic properties of iron compounds on normal hepatocytes and preneoplastic nodular cells *in vitro*, are supported by recent findings using an *in vivo* animal model of iron overload[33]. In this study, 9 weeks of treatment with dietary carbonyl iron resulted in a significantly increased number of S-phase nuclei (5′-bromodeoxyuridine incorporation in iron loaded livers), as compared with controls. Furthermore, the relative liver weights of iron-loaded livers were increased. However, it is not known whether or not liver

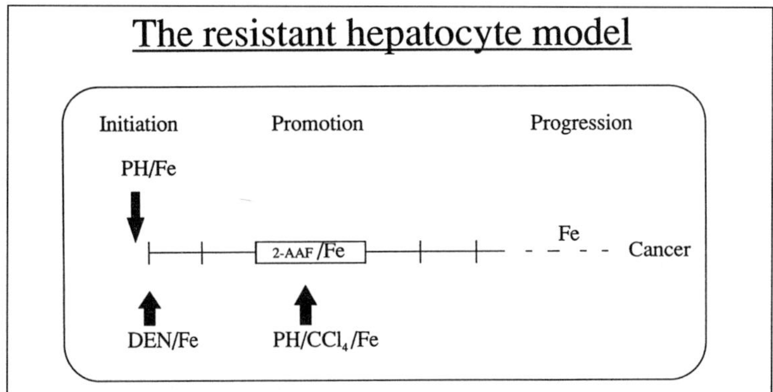

Fig. 2. Schematic representation of the Solt and Farber model for experimental hepatocarcinogenesis: PH = 2/3 partial hepatectomy, DEN = diethylnitrosamine 10 mg/kg, 2-AAF = 2-acetylaminofluorene in the diet (2 per cent), CCl_4 = carbon tetrachloride. Fe indicates where iron can replace a genotoxic or mitogenic component of the protocol.

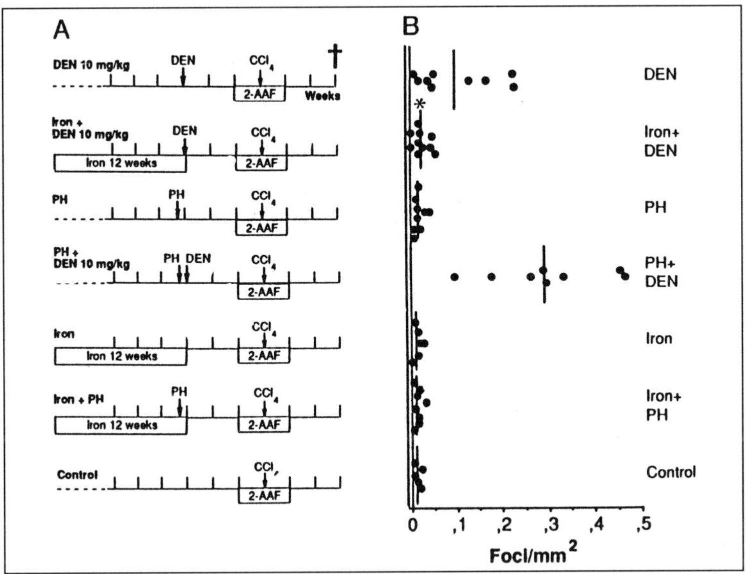

*Fig. 3(a) Schematic presentation of experiments on the role of iron in initiation. As indicated, 12 weeks of 2.5 per cent dietary iron exposure either replaced the genotoxic effect of DEN or the mitogenic effect of PH in different treatment combinations. (b) Number of glutathione-S transferase positive foci/mm^2. Each black dot represents one animal. * =$P < 0.05$ compared with animals treated with DEN 10 mg/kg.*

nodular cells, having enhanced proliferative response to exposure of iron compounds *in vitro*, would also exert accelerated growth following iron treatment *in vivo*.

Iron in experimental hepatocarcinogenesis

Using experimental animal models the genotoxic and/or mitogenic effects of excess iron can be sequentially studied in the different steps of the carcinogenic process (initiation, promotion and progression). In Fig. 2 the resistant hepatocyte model outlined by Solt and Farber is shown[34]. It indicates where iron, by replacing a genotoxic or mitogenic treatment, can be evaluated as an initiator, promoter or a compound that acts during progression. Hypothetically, iron can cause oxidative DNA damage and participate in initiation as a genotoxic compound, or by increasing cell replication enhance the fixation of DNA lesions and thus facilitate mutation of DNA. In the promotion phase, iron may act as a mitogen that preferentially stimulates initiated cells expressing an abundance of transferrin receptor molecules. During the progression phase, iron might selectively stimulate neoplastic growth, affect the frequency of neoplastic cell apoptosis, or act as a toxic compound that by itself or in combination with other noxious substances cause cell damage and cell death. A loss of liver cell mass may activate a regenerative response in the host. It is known that neoplastic liver lesions readily respond to regenerative growth stimulation, and in fact are more sensitive to such a stimulation than are normal liver cells. Over a prolonged period of time, subsequent genetic alterations followed by selection of cells with growth advantage create stepwise alterations in the cell populations and progression towards the malignant phenotype. Iron can participate in this process by its genotoxic effects, increasing the frequency of mutations taking place, accelerating the development of malignancy.

In an initiation/promotion protocol for experimental hepatocarcinogenesis described by Solt and Farber[34] the role of iron was tested according to the hypotheses outlined above. This animal model permits quantitative evaluation of the initiation event as well as evaluation of the power of the promoter regimen by morphometric analysis of the number and size of pre-neoplastic and neoplastic lesions. Iron is delivered as 3 per cent carbonyl iron in the diet for 12–21 weeks. Iron in this model, not resulting in cirrhosis, could not cause initiation or promotion by itself[33]. The results from the initiation experiments are shown in Fig. 3. Iron in combination with a complete initiation/promotion protocol decreased the number and the volume of pre-neoplastic lesions. Interference of iron with the regenerative growth promoter in the experimental situation is the most probable explanation for these unexpected findings. Thus, the effects of iron in this case should not be interpreted as an anticarcinogenic effect of iron.

The effect of long-term iron exposure, alone or in combination with other toxic compounds, during tumour progression is under evaluation. Taken together, these results indicate that liver tumour development, as a consequence of iron exposure, is dependent on the development of iron-induced liver cirrhosis[35], and that moderate iron overload, as seen in the carbonyl-iron model, does not exert significant initiating or tumour-promoting effects in the early phases of hepatocarcinogenesis.

The role of iron in tumour development is intriguing and controversial. Theoretical implications suggest roles for iron as a genotoxic, cytotoxic and mitogenic substance, with a putative carcinogenic potential. However, its influences on the carcinogenic process *in vivo* are not obvious and remain to be proved.

Acknowledgement

This work was supported by the Swedish Cancer Society.

References

1. Williams, G.M. & Yamamoto, R.S. (1972): Absence of stainable iron from preneoplastic and neoplastic lesions in rat liver with 8–hydroxyquinoline–induced siderosis. *J. Natl. Cancer Inst.* **49,** 685–692.

2. Deugnier, Y.M., Guyander, G., Crantock, L., Lopez, J.M., Yaouanq, J., Jouanolle, H., Campion, J.P., Launois, B., Halliday, J.W., Powell, L.W. & Brissot, P. (1993): Primary liver cancer in genetic hemochromatosis: A clinical, pathological and pathogenetic study of 54 cases. *Gastroenterology* **104,** 228–234.

3. Terada, T. & Nakanuma, Y. (1989): Iron-negative foci in siderotic macroregenerative nodules in human cirrhotic liver. A marker for incipient neoplastic lesions. *Arch. Pathol. Lab. Med.* **113,** 916–920.

4. Deugnier, Y.M., Charalambous, P., Le Quelleuc, D.L., Turlin, B., Searle, J., Brissot, P., Powell, L.W. & Halliday, J.W. (1993): Preneoplastic significans of hepatic iron-free foci in genetic hemochromatosis: a study of 185 patients. *Hepatology* **18,** 1363–1369.

5. Farber, E., Chen, Z.-Y., Harris, L., Lee, G., Rinaudo, J.S., Roomi, W.M., Rotstein, J. & Semple, E. (1989): The biochemical-molecular pathology of the stepwise development of liver cancer: new insights and problems. In: *Liver cell carcinoma,* eds. P. Bannasch, D. Keppler & G. Weber, pp. 273–291.

6. Roomi, M.W., Ho, R.K., Sarma, D.S.R. & Farber, E.A. (1985): A common biochemical pattern in preneoplastic hepatocyte nodules generated in four different models in the rat. *Cancer Res.* **45,** 564–571.

7. Stout, D.L. & Becker, F.F. (1987): Heme enzyme patterns in rat liver nodules and tumors. *Cancer Res.* **47,** 963–966.

8. Stout, D.L. & Becker, F.F. Normal heme synthesis in hepatic cancers despite reduced 5–aminolevulinic acid synthetase activity and iron uptake. *Cancer Res.* **29,** 19.

9. Eriksson, L.C., Torndal, U.-B. & Andersson, G.N. (1986): The transferrin receptor in hepatocyte nodules: binding properties, subcellular distribution and endocytosis. *Carcinogenesis* **7,** 1467–1474.

10. Andersson, G.N., Torndal, U.-B. & Eriksson, L.C. (1989): Decreased vacuolar acidification capacity in drug-resistant rat liver preneoplastic nodules. *Cancer Res.* **49,** 3765–3769.

11. Rissler, P. & Eriksson, L.C. (1990): Kinetics of transferrin endo- and exocytosis in normal and preneoplastic liver cells. *J. Cancer Res. Clin. Oncol.* **116,** 228.

12. Loeb, L.A., James, E.A., Waltersdorph, A.M. & Klebanoff, S.J. (1988): Mutagenesis by the autooxidation of iron with isolated DNA. *Proc. Natl. Acad. Sci. USA* **85,** 3918–3922.

13. Imlay, J.A., Chin, S.M. & Linn, S. (1988): Toxic DNA damage by hydrogen peroxide through the Fenton reaction *in vivo* and *in vitro. Science* **240,** 640–642.

14. Pryor, W.A. (1988): Why is the hydroxyl radical the only radical that comonly adds to DNA? Hypothesis: It has a rare combination of electrophilicity, high thermochemical reactivity and a mode of production that can occur near DNA. *Free Rad. Biol. Med.* **4,** 219–223.

15. Halliwell, B. & Gutteridge, J.M.C. (1984): Oxygen toxicity, oxygen radicals, transition metals and disease. *Biochem. J.* **219,** 1–14.

16. Barnes, D. & Sato, G. (1980): Serum-free culture, a unifying approach. *Cell* **22,** 649.

17. Trowbridge, I.S., Newman, R.A., Domingo, D.L. & Sauvage, C. (1984): Transferrinreceptors: structure and function. *Biochem. Pharmacol.* **6,** 925.

18. Arosio, P., Cairo, G. & Levi, S. (1989): Iron in immunity. In: *Cancer and inflammation*, eds. M. De Sousa & J.M. Brock, p. 55. Chichester: J. Wiley and Sons.

19. Hirose-Kumagai, A. & Akamatsu, N. (1989): Change in transferrin receptor distribution in regenerating rat liver. *Biochem. Biophys. Res. Commun.* **164,** 1105.

20. Ellem, K.A.O. & Kay, G.F. (1983): Ferricyanide can replace pyruvate to stimulate growth and attachment of serum restricted human melanoma cells. *Biochem. Biophys. Res. Commun.* **112,** 183.

21. Crane, F.L., Sun, I.L., Clark, M.G., Grebing, C. & Löw, H. (1985): Transplasma-membrane redox systems in growth and development. *Biochim. Biophys. Acta* **811,** 233.

22. Löw, H.E., Crane, F.L., Morré, D.J. & Sun, I.L. (1990): Oxidoreductase enzymes in the plasma membrane. In: *Oxidoreduction at the plasma membrane. Relation to growth and transport*, Vol. 1, eds. F.L. Crane, D.J. Morré & H.E. Löw, pp. 29. Boca Raton: CRC Press.

23. Thorstensen, K. & Romslo, I. (1990): The role of transferrin in the mechanism of cellular iron uptake. *Biochem. J.* **271,** 1–10.

24. Sun, I.L., Garcia-Canero, R., Liu, W., Toole-Simms, W., Crane, F. L., Morré, D.J. & Löw, H. (1987): Diferric transferrin reduction stimulates the Na^+/H^+ antiport of HeLa cells. *Biochem. Biophys. Res. Commun.* **145,** 467.

25. Sun, I.L., Toole-Simms, W., Crane, F.L., Morré, D.J., Löw, H. & Chou J.Y. (1988): Reduction of diferic transferrin by SV40 transformed pineal cells stimulates Na^+/H^+ antiport activity. *Biochim. Biophys. Acta* **938,** 17.

26. Hesketh, T.R., Morre, J.P., Morris, J.D.H., Taylor, M.V., Rogers, J., Smith, G.A. & Metcalf, J.C. (1985): A common sequence of calcium and pH signals in the mitogenic stimulation of eucaryotic cells. *Nature* **317,** 481.

27. Navas, P., Sun, I.L., Morré, D.J. & Crane, F.L. (1988): Relationship between $NAD^+/NADH$ levels and animal cell growth. In: *Plasma membrane oxidoreductases in control of animal and plant growth*, eds. F.L. Crane, D.J. Morré & H. Löw, p. 339. New York: Plenum Press.

28. Sun, I.L., Toole-Simms, W., Crane, F.L., Golub, E.S., de Pagán, T. D., Morré, D.J. & Löw, H. (1987): Retinoic acid inhibition of transplasmalemma diferric transferrin reductase. *Biochem. Biophys. Res. Commun.* **146,** 976.

29. Sun, I.L. & Crane, F.L. (1988): Control of transplasma membrane diferric transferrin reductase by antitumor drugs. In: *Plasma membrane oxidoreductases in control of animal and plant growth*, eds. F.L. Crane, D.J. Morré & H. Löw, p. 181. New York: Plenum Press.

30. Löw, H. & Crane, F.L. (1978): Redox function in plasma membranes. *Biochim. Biophys. Acta* **515,** 141.

31. Eriksson, L.C., Wollenberg, G.K., Quinn, B.A. & Hayes, M.A. (1989): Diferric transferrin stimulates hepatocyte proliferation in primary cultures. *Proc. Amer. Assoc. Cancer Res.* **30,** 67.

32. Nilsson, H. & Eriksson, L.C. (1994): Growth factor induced mitogenic effects and inositol phosphate responses in primary hepatocyte cultures from normal rat liver and rat liver nodules. *Carcinogenesis* **15,** 1821–1826.

33. Stål, P., Hultcrantz, R., Möller, L. & Eriksson, L.C. (1995): The effect of dietary iron on initiation and promotion in chemical hepatocarcinogenesis. *Hepatology* **21,** 521–528.

34. Solt, D.B. & Farber, E. (1976): New principle for the analyses of chemical carcinogenesis. *Nature* **263,** 702–703.

35. Stål, P. (1995): Role of iron overload in liver cell damage and hepatocarcinogenesis. Thesis.

Iron Nutrition in Health and Disease, edited by Leif Hallberg and Nils-Georg Asp
©1996 John Libbey & Company Ltd., pp. 293–301

Chapter 29

Body iron stores, lipid peroxidation and coronary heart disease

Jukka T. Salonen

Research Institute of Public Health, University of Kuopio, P.O. Box 1627, 70211 Kuopio, Finland

Summary

There is evidence from both basic research and epiemiology that supports the role of lipid peroxidation in atherogenesis and coronary disease. Redox-active forms of transition metals such as iron catalyse free radical production and can thus promote the oxidation of lipids.

In our prospective population study, both high dietary iron intake and elevated serum ferritin ≥ 200 µg/l, an indicator of elevated body iron stores, were associated with increased risk of myocardial infarct (MI) in almost 2000 men from Easter Finland. Our finding was repeated in a prospective population study from Canada and in the US Health Professionals Study in 45, 720 men, in which dietary intake of haem iron was significantly associated with an increased risk of infarct. Also negative studies have been published, but these all suffer from uninformative and unrealisble measurements of iron stores. In our small clionical trials, iron depletion by venosections reduced, and iron loading with ferrous sulphate increased, the osidation susceptibility of the atherogenic lipoproteins in men.

Our data suggest that a high dietary intake of iron or an enhaned iron absorption and the consequent accumalation of iron in the body may be associated with an excess risk of MI in eastern Finnish men and this increased risk could be due to the promotion of lipid peroxidation. Our findings need to be confirmed in further prospective population studies with proper measurements of iron stores, or, preferably, with DNA-tests of haemochromatosis. Eventually, clinical trials are needed either to verify or refute the hypotheses concerning the role of iron in atherosclerosis and cardiovascular diseases.

Iron, oxidative stress and lipid peroxidation

The role of iron in free radical reactions such as lipid peroxidation has been reviewed by several authors[1–6]. The ability of iron chelates or complexes to catalyse the formation of reactive oxygen species and stimulate lipid peroxidation *in vitro* has been demonstrated conclusively[1–6]. There is evidence suggesting that chelated iron acts as a catalyst for the Fenton reaction, facilitating the conversion of superoxide anion and hydrogen peroxide to hydroxyl radical, a species frequently proposed to initiate lipid peroxidation[1,2,6]. Agil *et al.* showed recently that the coincubation of human plasma with ferrous iron and hydrogen peroxide resulted in almost threefold increase of lipid peroxides, possibly by a Fenton reaction mechanism[7]. There are, however, also studies suggesting that the formation of hydroxyl radicals from ferrous peroxide does not fit into the Fenton reaction system[8].

There is less evidence of a role of iron in oxidative stress *in vivo*. To be able to promote free radical production in the human body, iron needs to be liberated from large binding proteins such as haemoglobin, transferrin or ferritin. It is thought that oxidative stress itself can provide the iron necessary for formation of reactive oxygen species[1,6]. For example, superoxide radical can mobilize iron from ferritin[9]. In iron overload lipid peroxidation has been detected in red blood cells[10, 11]. We observed in 60 eastern Finnish men a positive association between blood haemoglobin concentration and titre of autoantibodies against malondialdehyde (MDA) modified low density lipoprotein (LDL) (r = 0.27, P < 0.05), suggestive of a role of haem iron or the haemoglobin itself in lipid peroxidation *in vivo* in men[12].

Clinical evidence from randomized trials is even more scarce. We carried out a randomized double-masked trial of the effects of supplementation of men with low iron stores with either ferrous sulfate or iron polymaltose complex (IPC) on the oxidation susceptibility of atherogenic lipoproteins[13]. The design of the study comprised three parallel randomized groups, each receiving either 180 mg of iron as ferrous sulfate, 200 mg of iron as non-ionic iron polymaltose complex (IPC) or placebo for 6 months. The subjects were men aged 45–64 years with serum ferritin < 30 μg/l. IPC is an iron preparation which is absorbed very slowly in the whole intestine. Susceptibility of the combined fraction of very low density lipoprotein (VLDL) and LDL to oxidation was measured after induction with copper, or haemin and hydrogen peroxide[3,14,15].

Out of 48 randomized male subjects, 45 completed the 6 month measurements. Even though serum ferritin concentration increased more (2.2-fold) in the ferrous sulfate group than in the IPC group (1.3-fold), blood haemoglobin concentration increased more in the latter (by 2.2 per cent) than in the former (1.0 per cent) group (Table 1).

Of the main antioxidative vitamins, plasma ascorbate concentration increased similarly (between 34 per cent and 60 per cent) in all three groups because of the small vitamin C supplement (50 mg daily).

The main finding of the study was an increase of the susceptibility of VLDL + LDL to copper-induced oxidation in the ferrous sulfate group (Table 1). The maximal velocity of oxidation was increased by 8.3 per cent (95 per cent confidence interval (CI), 3.2 per cent, 12.4 per cent) in the ferrous sulfate group, remained almost unchanged in the placebo group and decreased by 5.7 per cent (95 per cent CI, –12.5 per cent, 0.6 per cent) in the IPC group. Thus the oxidation rate in the ferrous sulfate group was increased by 8.8 per cent (95 per cent CI, 2.4 per cent, 15.3 per cent, P = 0.009) compared to placebo and by 12.8 per cent (95 per cent CI, 5.0 per cent, 20.7 per cent, P = 0.009) compared to the IPC group. There were similar trends in the haemin-hydrogen peroxide-induced oxidation. The amount of conjugated dienes (a lipid peroxidation product) produced increased by 2.0 per cent in the ferrous sulfate group and decreased by 10.3 per cent in the IPC and by 4.5 per cent in the placebo group (P = 0.001 for heterogeneity, table). The net effect of the ferrous sulfate was an increase of 6.6 per cent (95 per cent CI, 0.7 per cent, 12.5 per cent, P = 0.028) compared to placebo and 13.8 per cent (95 per cent CI, 5.3 per cent, 22.3 per cent, P = 0.003) compared to IPC.

In our study, the conventional ferrous sulfate supplement increased lipid peroxidation. Ferrous sulfate is absorbed rapidly in the upper intestine. IPC is absorbed very slowly, and thus avoids rapid increases in serum iron. Both supplements were well tolerated and caused less gastrointestinal symptoms than regular ferrous sulfate preparations. We did not observe secular changes in either main plasma antioxidants or serum fatty acids that could have caused the observed treatment effects in the oxidation susceptibility of lipoproteins. On the contrary, changes in these determinants of lipid peroxidation, if anything, attenuated the observed treatment effects.

We carried out another study in which we tested the effect of reduction of body iron stores by venesections (blood letting) on the susceptibility to oxidation of atherogenic serum lipoproteins[15]. This was a randomized controlled cross-over trial in 14 regularly smoking men with elevated serum ferritin concentration. The study design comprised two 14-week study periods, with a 14 week wash-out period inbetween, with either blood donations or control. During the intervention periods, the subjects donated 450 mg (500 ml) of blood three times in 14 weeks. Oxidation resistance of VLDL + LDL was measured after inducing oxidation with haemin and H_2O_2.

Serum ferritin concentration was reduced by 44 per cent (95 per cent confidence interval (CI) 8–82 per cent, P = 0.021) during the venesection periods, the maximal oxidation velocity was decreased by 20 per cent (95 per cent CI 3–30 per cent, P = 0.032), and the lag time to start of oxidation lengthened (oxidation resistance increased) by 33 per cent (95 per cent CI 1–64 per cent, P = 0.036; Table 2). These observations indicate that the reduction of body iron stores by venesection can increase the oxidation resistance of serum VLDL + LDL in regularly smoking men.

Oxidative stress and atherogenesis

Atherosclerosis is a degenerative process in the arteries which is characterized in its early phase by endothelial cell injury, the accumulation of lipid and proliferation of smooth muscle cells and consequent thickening of the arterial wall. These and other pathophysiologic phenomena

Table 1. Mean baseline values and 6 month changes (SEM) of iron status indices, plasma ascorbate, serum lipids, and measurements of oxidation susceptibility of VLDL and LDL in 45 iron depleted male subjects

	Ferrous sulfate (n = 15)		**Iron polymaltose complex (n = 15)**		**Placebo (n = 15)**		**P-value for hetero-geneity of change from ANOVA**	**P-value for comparisons of changes between groups from Duncan multiple range test**		
	Before	Change	Before	Change	Before	Change		$FeSO_4$ vs. IPC	$FeSO_4$ vs. placebo	IPC vs. placebo
Blood haemoglobin (g/l)	145.3	1.5 (1.5	144.9	3.3 (2.2)	144.1	–3.6 (1.2)	0.0181	NS	< 0.05	< 0.05
Serum ferritin (µg/l)	21.5	46.8 (8.5)	20.5	27.4 (4.3)	19.5	5.0 (3.4)	< 0.0001	<0.05	< 0.05	< 0.05
Erythrocyte ferritin (µg/cell)	15.9	5.8 (2.2)	16.9	4.6 (2.4)	17.7	–2.9 (1.7)	0.0118	NS	< 0.05	< 0.05
Plasma ascorbate (µmol/l)	42.5	19.7 (5.6)	50.5	16.9 (5.6)	46.8	28.0 (5.6)	0.3614	NS	NS	NS
Serum LDL cholestrol (mmol/l)	3.72	0.35 (0.24)	3.80	–0.04 (0.17)	4.01	–0.40 (0.11)	0.0188	NS	< 0.05	NS
Serum HDL cholestrol (mmol/l)	1.08	0.01 (0.05)	1.13	0.00 (0.02)	1.12	0.05 (0.03)	0.6852	NS	NS	NS
Maximal oxidation velocity (slope) (mabs/min)										
copper induction	9.51	0.79 (0.24)	10.57	–0.60 (0.34)	10.24	–0.09 (0.20)	0.0025	< 0.05	<0.05	NS
haemin + H_2O_2 induction	0.72	–0.00 (0.06)	0.91	–0.16 (0.04)	0.83	–0.09 (0.05)	0.0675	< 0.05	NS	NS
Lag time to oxidation (min)										
copper induction	83.0	–3.3 (2.2)	87.3	–4.0 (3.0)	84.3	–4.3 (3.0)	NS	NS	NS	NS
haemin + H_2O_2 induction	125.3	20.3 (15.8)	100.8	55.7 (11.9)	94.4	36.0 (8.4)	0.1415	NS	NS	NS
Amount of oxidation after copper induction (maximal absorbance for conjugated dienes)	0.544	0.011 (0.014)	0.614	–0.063 (0.017)	0.577	–0.026 (0.006)	0.0012	< 0.05	NS	NS

in atherogenesis are assumed to be influenced by free radicals and oxidized lipids[12,16–18].

LDL particles contain polyunsaturated fatty acids and cholesterol that can be oxidized by oxidative free radicals. Oxidative and other chemical modifications of LDL make it immunogenic and are thought to increase its atherogenicity[18]. The oxidative modification of LDL in the human arterial wall is influenced by the availability of antioxidative mechanisms as well as the presence of transition metals such as iron, which act as catalysts of oxidation.

Autoantibodies to epitopes of oxidized LDL (Ox-LDL) have been shown in humans. To determine whether these antibodies are related to atherosclerotic progression, we compared the ratio of serum titre of autoantibodies to MDA-modified LDL to that for native LDL in baseline sera of 30 eastern Finnish men with accelerated 2-year progression of carotid atherosclerosis and 30 age-matched controls without progression[12]. IgG antibody titre was determined by solid phase RIA. To ensure the specificity of the measure, the ratio of antibody titres binding to MDA-LDL to binding to native LDL was used. Cases had significantly higher titre to MDA-LDL (2.67 versus 2.06, $P = 0.003$). In a multivariate logistic model, the difference in antibody titre remained significant ($P = 0.031$). Thus, the titre of auto-antibodies to MDA-LDL was an independent predictor of the progression of carotid atherosclerosis in a prospective study in Finnish men. This was the first epidemiologic study to show a role of oxidatively modified LDL in atherogenesis. Our finding has subsequently been repeated in a number of studies[19–21] (Table 3). No negative studies have been published.

Iron and atherosclerosis

In cholesterol-fed rabbits, iron overload has augmented the development of atherosclerotic lesions[22,23]. Araujo *et al.* administered 1.5 g of

Table 2. Mean (SE) baseline values and changes of indicators of iron status, possible confounding factors and the oxidation susceptibility of lipoproteins before and during blood letting and control in 14 male smokers

Parameter[a]	Venesection		Control		*P* for difference between periods[b]
	Before	Change	Before	Change	
Blood haemogolobin (g/l)	160.8 (2.1)	–9.1 (2.1)	159.9 (2.9)	–1.5 (2.0)	0.064
Blood haematocrit	0.47 (0.01)	–0.04 (0.01)	0.47 (0.01)	–0.02 (0.01)	0.066
Serum ferritin (μg/l)	209 (37)	135 (27)	171 (45)	–52 (23)	0.021
Body weight (kg)	89.6 (4.3)	–1.0 (0.05)	88.4 (4.3)	0.9 (0.3)	0.018
Smoking (cigarettes/day)	24.9 (2.2)	–0.4 (1.0)	26.1 (2.8)	–2.1 (1.2)	0.082
Serum albumin (g/l)	42.4 (0.9)	–0.36 (0.84)	42.7 (0.9)	–1.14 (0.58)	0.444
Serum haemopexin (g/l)	0.90 (0.07)	0.00 (0.07)	0.88 (0.07)	0.03 (0.07)	0.803
VDL/LDL oxidation suscptibility					
Maximal slope (mAbs/min)	0.888 (0.075)	0.762 (0.092)	0.762 (0.092)	0.081 (0.045)	0.032
Maximal slope cigarettes	0.041 (0.007)	0.039 (0.010)	0.039 (0.010)	0.004 (0.002)	0.018
Lag to start (min)	146 (17)	187 (31)	187 (31)	–7 (19)	0.036
Lag/cigarette	6.28 (0.83)	7.82 (1.15)	7.82 (1.15)	0.19 (0.84)	0.044
Serum TBARS (μmol/l)	0.88 (0.085)	0.79 (0.089)	0.79 (0.089)	–0.08 (0.076)	0.344
Serum TBARS/cigarette	0.038 (0.004)	0.033 (0.004)	0.033 (0.004)	0.005 (0.004)	0.058

[a]VLDL denotes very low density lipoprotein; LDL, low density lipoprotein; TBARS, thiobarbituric acid-reactive substances. [b] Based on paired *t*-tests comparing changes in venecetion and control periods ($n = 14$ pairs).

Table 3. Studies showing an association between antibodies against oxidized LDL and atherosclerosis or CHD

Study	Reference	Study design and sample size	Ox-LDL titre 9 (ratio)
KIHD 2 year follow-up	12	Nested case-control, 30 men with fast atherogenesis and 30 controls	2.67 *vs*. 2.06, P=0.003
KAPS 1 year follow-up	19	ohort, 212 men	IMT incr. 0 *vs*. 0.13 mm/year, $P < 0.001$
Italian	20	Cross-sectional, 94 patients and 42 controls	2.39 *vs*. 2.04, $P < 0.01$
Helsinki heart study	21	Nested case-control, 135 men with AMI and 135 controls	0.412 *vs*. 0.356 $P = 0.002$

iron dextran in 30 doses to eight hypercholesterolaemic and six normocholesterolemic New Zealand White rabbits[22]. There were hypercholesterolemic ($n = 6$) and normocholesterolemic ($n = 6$) untreated control groups. The lesion area was 18.5 per cent in the iron-overloaded group, as compared 5.7 per cent in the cholesterol-fed group ($P = 0.03$ for difference). There were no lesions in rabbits on normal diet. Thiobarbituric acid-reactive substances (TBARS) were higher in iron-overloaded than cholesterol-fed group in liver, spleen and aorta. Similar results were reported by Weiner *et al.*[23]. In nine New Zealand rabbits, 19.2 per cent ($P = 0.04$) of aorta was occupied by plaques in iron and cholesterol fed rabbits versus 7.6 per cent in the cholesterol-fed and 0.0 per cent in normal diet groups.

There are few studies of the role of body iron stores directly affecting atherosclerosis in humans. An Austrian group reported an association between serum ferritin concentration and the severity of carotid atherosclerosis in a cross-sectional study in 847 men and women aged 40–79[24]. They also observed a synergism between high ferritin and high serum cholesterol. In another cross-sectional population study, however, no association was found between serum ferritin concentration and carotid atherosclerosis[25].

In a cross-sectional autopsy study in 41 cases of iron overload and 82 matched controls, there was less advanced coronary disease in the cases than the controls[26]. This finding has been thought to be explained by a selection bias[27]. It has also been speculated that the reportedly lower prevalence of atherosclerosis in haemochromatosis patients could be due to reduced cholesterol synthesis in the liver[28].

Iron and coronary heart disease

We investigated the association of serum ferritin concentration and dietary iron intake with the risk of acute myocardial infarction in 1931 randomly selected men aged 42, 48, 54 or 60 years who had no symptomatic coronary heart disease at entry, examined in the Kuopio Ischaemic Heart Disease Risk Factor Study (KIHD) in 1984–1989[29]. In a multivariate model adjusting for the major coronary risk factors, serum ferritin ≥ 200 μg/l was associated with a 2.2–fold (95 per cent confidence interval 1.2–4.0, P<0.01) risk of acute myocardial infarction. This association was stronger in men with serum low density lipoprotein cholesterol concentration ≥5.0 mmol/l (193 mg/dl) than in others. In another model, a high dietary intake of iron was associated with an increased risk. We have hypothesized that these associations could be explained by the catalytic effect of iron on lipid peroxidation[5].

The original finding was repeated later in a more thorough statistical analysis that was based on 2 years longer follow-up time[30]. The results were virtually identical. Other nutrients and inflammation as possible confounders of the observed association were ruled out. Our data suggest that high stored iron level is a risk factor for acute myocardial infarction in men with no prevalent CHD.

The publication of our findings created a lot of interest about the role of body iron stores as a possible new risk factor for CHD. The associ-

Table 4. Prospective population studies concerning body iron stores and the risk of CHD

Study	Reference	Sample size	Events	Measurement	Result: relative risk
KIHD 3 year follow-up	Salonen *et al.* *Circulation* 1992; **86**: 803	1931 M aged 42–60 with no clinical CHD	51 AMIs	Serum ferritin > 200 μg/l	2.2 (95% CI 1.2, 4.0)
Canadian	Morrison *et al.* *Epidemiology* 1994; **5**; 243	9920 M+F aged 35–79	224 fatal MIs	Serum iron > 175 μg/l	2.2 (1.01, 4.7) for M, 5.5 (1.7, 18.1) for F
Icelandic	Magnusson *et al.* *Circulation* 1994; **89**: 102	2036 M+ F aged 25–74	81 AMIs	Serum ferritin, TIBC	TIBC had an inverse association (*P*=0.002), results for ferritin equivocal
NHANES	Sempos *et al.* *NEJM* 1994; **330**: 1119	3713 M+F aged 45–74	350 MIs, 842 CHD, 293 CHD deaths	Transferrin saturation	No consistent association
Finnish Mobile Clinic	Reunanen *et al.*, *J Int Med*, 1995; **238**, in press	6086 M, 6102 F aged 45–64	In M 739, in F 245 CHD deaths	Transferrin saturation	In M, no association in F, U-shaped relationship
US Health Professionals	Ascherio *et al.* *Circulation* 1994; **89**: 969	44933 M aged 40–75 with no self-reported CVD	249 non-fatal AMIs, 137 CHD deaths	Dietary haem iron by food frequency questionnaire	1.42 (1.02, 1.98) in top 20% of haem iron intake
Kaiser Permanente	Baer *et al.* *Circulation* 1994; **331**: 1159	46932 M+F aged ≥ 30	969 men and 871 had AMI-related hospitalisation	Transferrin saturation	1.3 (1.0, 1.8), P = 0.084 for TS ≥ 62%
KIHD 5 year follow-up	Salaonen *et al.* *NEJM* 1994; **331:** 1159	1931 M aged 42–60 with no clinical CHD	83 AMIs	Serum ferritin > 200 μg/l	2.0 (95% CI 1.2, 3.1, P = 0.004)
Seven countries, Dutch cohort	Van Asperen *et al.* *Int J Epidemiol* 1995; **24**: 665	260 M+F aged 64–87, 22% had CHD history	50 CHD deaths	Transferrin saturation	0.4 for M, 1.4 for F. not significant

ation between body iron stores and the risk of CHD has now been examined in at least in eight prospective studies (Table 4). In a prospective population study from Canada, Morrison *et al.* reported an association between serum iron and the risk of fatal AMI in 9920 men and women[31]. Also in this Canadian cohort, high serum iron and high serum cholesterol had a synergistic relation with CHD. Only our and the Canadian study have observed an unequivocal direct relationship. In the study from Iceland, 'in a univariate analysis, log(ferritin) had a positive correlation with myocardial infarction (relative risk 1.6, P<0.001), but after taking sex and age into account, it lost all predictive power (RR 1.0, $P = 0.78$)'[32]. In this study, low iron-binding capacity was associated with increased risk of AMI[32].

Our finding concerning the role of dietary iron intake was confirmed in the US Health Professionals Study in 45,720 men aged 40–75 with no self-reported history of cardiovascular disease[33]. In this large prospective study, dietary intake of haem iron (but not that of total iron) had a consistent and statistically significant association with an increased risk of myocardial infarction.

Unfortunately in most old epidemiologic follow-up studies serum transferrin saturation has been used to estimate body iron stores (Table 4). This measurement has a large analytical variability and is lowered in inflammation and probably also in chronic atherosclerosis and CHD. Most studies also suffered from the lack of sufficient range in transferrin saturation within the study populations. In addition, serum transferrin saturation is confounded by prevalent diseases. In any of the published studies in which no association was observed between transferrin saturation and CHD, neither clinical examination nor exercise test was performed to assess prevalent CHD. Consequently, these study populations are mixes of both previously healthy persons (as in our study) and persons with either occult or clinical CHD. It is possible and may be even probable that in persons with angina pectoris or myocardial infarction, the sufficiency of iron stores becomes more important than the disadvantageous effects of excessive iron stores.

Conclusions

Iron is a powerful catalyst of free radical formation and lipid peroxidation *in vitro*. Taken together, our iron supplementation and iron depletion trials provide evidence for the role of iron in lipid peroxidation in humans. The susceptibility of human lipoproteins to oxidation appeared to be influenced by the availability of different types of iron within the physiological range of iron status. Our findings have important implications regarding the treatment of iron deficiency anaemia. They indicate that a rapid correction of iron stores by supplementing with ferrous sulfate, at least in combination with ascorbate, may have undesirable health effects and suggest that if iron supplementation is necessary, non-ionic iron polymaltose products may be preferable to ferrous sulfate. Before any clinical recommendations are given, however, our findings need to be repeated in larger clinical trials. Two animal experiments have suggested that iron over-loading promotes the progression of atherosclerosis in cholesterol-fed rabbits.

Epidemiologic evidence concerning the role of iron stores in coronary heart disease is inconsistent although suggestive of a relationship, as all negative studies are undermined by large measurement variability that probably explains the lack of observed association.

More clinical trials concerning the effects of iron depletion and iron supplementation on lipid peroxidation in humans are warranted, and eventually a trial of the effect of iron depletion on atherosclerotic progression or coronary events is necessary to conclusively verify of refute the theory concerning the role of excess iron in atherogenesis and coronary heart disease.

Acknowledgements

I would like to thank the faculty and staff of the Research Institute of Public Health, University of Kuopio, for their contributions to the studies cited.

References

1. Gutteridge, J.M.C. & Halliwell, B. (1989): Iron toxicity and oxygen radicals. *Balliere's Clinical Haematology* **2,** 195–256.

2. Halliwell, B. & Gutteridge, J.M.C. (1990): Role of free radicals and catalytic metal ions in human disease: an overview. *Method. Enzymol.* **186**, 1–85.

3. Balla, G., Jacob, H.S., Eaton, J.W., Belcher, J.D. & Vercellotti, G.M. (1991): Hemin: a possible physiological mediator of low density lipoprotein oxidation and endothelial injury. *Arterioscler. Thromb.* **11,** 1700–1711.

4. Ryan, T.P. & Aust, S.D. (1992): The role of iron in oxygen-mediated toxicities. *Crit. Rev. Toxicol.* **22,** 119–141.

5. Salonen, J.T. (1993): The role of iron as a cardiovascular risk factor. *Curr. Opinion Lipidol.* **4,** 277–282.

6. Stohs, S.J. & Bagghi, D. (1995): Oxidative mechanisms in the toxicity of metal ions. *Free Rad. Biol. Med.* **18,** 321–336.

7. Agil, A., Fuller, C.J. & Jialal, I. (1995): Susceptibility of plasma to ferrous iron/hydrogen peroxide-mediated oxidation: demonstration of a possible Fenton reaction. *Clin. Chem.* **41,** 220–225.

8. Luzzatto, E., Cohen, H., Stockheim, C., Wieghardt, K. & Meyerstein, D. (1995): Reactions of low valent transition metal complexes with hydrogen peroxide. Are they 'Fenton-like' or not? 4. the case of Fe(II)L, L = EDTA, HEDTA and TMCA. *Free Rad. Res.* **23,** 453–463.

9. Carlin, G. & Djursater, R. (1984): Xanthine oxidase induced depolymerization of hyaluronic acid in the presence of ferritin. *FEBS Lett.* **177,** 27–30.

10. Rice-Evans, C.A. & Baysal, E. (1987): Iron-mediated oxidative stress in erythrocytes. *Biochem. J.* **244,** 191–196.

11. Herhsko, C. (1989): Mechanism of iron toxicity and its possible role in red cell membrane damage. *Semin. Hematol.* **26,** 277–285.

12. Salonen, J.T., Ylä-Herttuala, S., Yamamoto, R., Butler, S., Korpela, H., Salonen, R., Nyyssönen, K., Palinski, W. & Witztum, J.L. (1992): Autoantibody against oxidized LDL and progression of carotid atherosclerosis. *Lancet* **339,** 883–887.

13. Salonen, J.T., Nyyssönen. K., Porkkala-Sarataho, E., Tuomainen, T.-P., Geisser, P. & Salonen, R. Oral supplementation with ferrous sulfate but not with non-ionic iron polymaltose complex increases the susceptibility of plasma lipoproteins to oxidation (unpublished).

14. Nyyssönen, K., Porkkala, E., Salonen, R., Korpela, H. & Salonen, J.T. (1994): Increase in oxidation resistance of atherogenic serum lipoproteins following antioxidant supplementation: a randomized double-blind placebo-controlled trial. *Eur. J. Clin. Nutr.* **48,** 633–642.

15. Salonen, J.T., Korpela, H., Nyyssönen, K., Porkkala, E., Tuomainen, T.-P., Belcher, J.D., Jacobs, D.R. Jr. & Salonen, R. (1995): Lowering of body iron stores by blood letting and oxidation resistance of serum lipoproteins: a randomized cross-over trial in smoking men. *J. Int. Med.* **237,** 161–168.

16. Halliwell, B. (1994): Free radicals, antioxidants, and human disease: curiosity, cause, or consequence? *Lancet* **344,** 721–724.

17. Steinberg, D. & Workshop Participants. (1992): Antioxidants in the prevention of human atherosclerosis. *Circulation* **85,** 2337–2344.

18. Witztum, J.L. (1994): The oxidation hypothesis of atherosclerosis. *Lancet* **344,** 793–795.

19. Salonen, J.T., Tatzber, F., Salonen, R., Nyyssönen, K., Korpela, H., Ehnholm, C. & Esterbauer, H. (1992): Autoantibodies against oxidized LDL associated with accelerated atherosclerosis progression in hypercholesterolemic men. *Eur. Heart J.* **13,** 391.

20. Maggi, E., Chiesa, R., Melissano, G., Castellano, R., Astore, D., Grossi, A., Finardi, G. & Bellomo, G. (1994): LDL oxidation in patients with severe carotid atherosclerosis. A study of *in vitro* and *in vivo* oxidation markers. *Arterioscler. Thromb.* **14,** 1892–1899.

21. Puurunen, M., Mänttari, M., Manninen, V., Tenkanen, L., Alfthan, G., Ehnholm, C., Vaarala. O., Aho, K. & Palosuo, T. (1994): Antibody against oxidized low-density lipoprotein predicting myocardial infarction. *Arch. Intern. Med.* **154,** 2605–2609.

22. Araujo, J.A, Romano, E.L., Brito, B.E., Parthe, V., Romano, M., Bracho, M., Montano, R.F. & Cardier, J. (1995): Iron overload augments the development of atherosclerotic lesions in rabbits. *Arterioscler. Thromb. Vasc. Biol.* **15,** 1172–1180.

23. Weiner, M.A., Paige, S.B. & Bailey, S.R. (1994): Antioxidant therapy decreases atherosclerotic plaque burden in an iron loaded animal model. *Eur. Heart J.* **15,** 425.

24. Kiechl, S., Aichner, F., Gerstenbrand, F., Egger, G., Mair, A., Rungger, G., Spögler, F., Jarosch, E., Oberhollenzer, F. & Willeit, J. (1994): Body iron stores and presence of carotid atherosclerosis. Results from the Bruneck Study. *Arterioscler. Thromb.* **14,** 1625–1630.

25. Moore, M., Folsom, A.R., Barnes, R.W. & Eckfeldt, J.H. (1995): No association between serum ferritin and asymptomatic carotid atherosclerosis. The Atherosclerosis Risk in Communities (ARIC) Study. *Am. J. Epidemiol.* **141,** 719–723.

26. Miller, M. & Hutchins, G.M. (1994): Hemochromatosis, multiorgan hemosiderosis, and coronary artery disease. *JAMA* **272,** 231–233.

27. Sullivan, J.L. (1995): Hemochromatosis and coronary artery disease (letter). *JAMA* **273,** 25–26.

28. Herbert, V. (1994): Iron worsens high-cholesterol-related coronary artery disease. *Am. J. Clin. Nutr.* **60,** 299–302.

29. Salonen, J.T., Nyyssönen, K., Korpela, H., Tuomilehto, J., Seppänen, R. & Salonen, R. (1992): High stored iron levels are associated with excess risk of myocardial infarction in eastern Finnish men. *Circulation* **86,** 803–811.

30. Salonen, J.T., Nyyssönen, K. & Salonen, R. (1994): Body iron stores and the risk of coronary heart disease. *N. Engl. J. Med.* **331,** 1159.

31. Morrison, H.I., Semenciw, R.M., Mao, Y. & Wigle, D.T. (1994): Serum iron and risk of fatal acute myocardial infarction. *Epidemiology* **5,** 243–246.

32. Magnusson, M.K., Sigfusson, N., Sigvaldason, H., Johannesson, G.M., Magnusson, S. & Thorgeirsson, G. (1994): Low iron-binding capacity as a risk factor for myocardial infarction. *Circulation* **89,** 102–108.

33. Ascherio, A., Willet, W.C., Rimm, E.B., Giovannucci, E. & Stampfer, M.J. Dietary iron intake and risk of coronary heart disease. *Circulation* **89,** 969–974.

Iron Nutrition in Health and Disease, edited by Leif Hallberg and Nils-Georg Asp
©1996 John Libbey & Company Ltd., pp. 303–311

Chapter 30

Epidemiological studies relating iron status to coronary heart disease and cancer

Alberto Ascherio and Walter C. Willett

Department of Nutrition and Department of Epidemiology, Harvard School of Public Health, and Channing Laboratory, Department of Medicine, Harvard Medical School and Brigham and Women's Hospital, Boston, MA USA

Summary

The observation that iron overload increases myocardial damage caused by anoxia and reperfusion in animal experiments, and it s potential role in lipoprotein oxidation, have renewed interest in the hypothesis that high body iron may be a risk factor for coronary heart disease (CHD). The ability of iron to catalyse the production of free radicals, which may increase oxidative stress and damage DNA, has also raised concern about the possibility that excess body iron may increase the risk of cancer. However, the results of epidemiological studies have been conflicting, and do not provide convincing evidence of an adverse effect of iron. One of the complexities in interpreting the results of these studies is the use of different measures of iron status. Transferrin saturation is poorly correlated with iron stores, except when they are fully depleted or overloaded. Serum ferritin in healthy individuals is a better indicator if iron stores, but it increases in several inflammatory states which may precede the clinical diagnosis of cancer or CHD. Some of the published studies may have failed to detect an association because of inadequate assessment of iron status or small number of cases. For this reason, and because of their substantial public health implications, stronger evidence is needed to reject the hypothesis that iron status adversely affects the risk of CHD or cancer.

Iron and coronary heart disease

In 1981 Sullivan proposed that premenopausal women are protected from coronary heart disease (CHD) because of their low levels of stored iron[1]. In support of this hypothesis, he cited the increased risk of CHD among women with hysterectomy but no oophorectomy in the Framingham study, the cardiomyopathy associated with iron overload, and the low incidence of CHD among men and women in developing countries, who are likely to have low iron stores. However, the subsequent observation that women taking postmenopausal estrogens (with or without hysterectomy) have a risk of CHD similar to that of premenopausal women, suggested that reduced estrogens rather than excess iron largely account for the increased risk after menopause[2].

The hypothesis that high iron stores increase the risk of CHD was renewed by the results of animal experiments indicating that iron overload increases, whereas the iron chelator desferrioxamine decreases, myocardial damage caused by anoxia and reperfusion. These effects have been

Table 1. Epidemiological studies on iron status and risk of acute myocardial infarction (AMI) or fatal coronary heart disease (CHD)

Study	Population (Cases)				Length of follow-up (years)	Type of Outocome	Measures of iron status	Association with risk
	Men		Women					
Salonen *et al.*[5]	1,931	(46)	–	–	3	AMI	ferritin, iron intake	+ +
Stampfer *et al.*[7]		(238)	–	–		AMI	ferritin	0
Magnusson *et al.*[8]	990	(53)	1,046	(18)	8.5	AMI	ferritin, Serum iron TIBC	0 0 –
Morrison *et al.*[9]	≈4,238	(141)	≈5,682	(83)	≈15	Fatal CHD	serum iron iron intake[c]	0[a] + ≥ 175 µg/l 0
Sempos *et al.*[11]	2,022	(189)	2,496	(161)	15[b]	AMI	Transferrin saturation, iron intake[c]	0 0
Ascherio *et al.*[17]	44,933	(386)	–	–	3.5	AMI	iron intake haem iron intake	0 +
Baer *et al.*[16]	15,167	(969)	31,765	(871)	14	AMI	Transferrin saturation	0

[a] Result not in original article.
[b] First 5 years excluded.
[c] Single 24-hour recall.

attributed to the ability of free iron to catalyse the formation of highly reactive radicals from superoxide and hydrogen peroxide, which are generated after restoration of blood flow to ischaemic myocardium and contribute to myocardial damage[3]. The free iron required for this reaction may be released from ferritin after being reduced to the ferrous state by the superoxide radicals generated during reperfusion of ischaemic tissue[4]. Whether similar reactions may occur in the absence of ischaemia is still unsettled; a role for iron in promoting LDL oxidation and atherosclerosis has been proposed, but evidence is sparse[5]. Evidence from several epidemiological studies has only recently been published, and is summarized in Table 1.

In 1992, Salonen reported from a prospective study in Finland a twofold increase in acute myocardial infarction among men with serum ferritin levels above 200 µg/l (25 per cent of the cohort) compared to those below this level[6]. The study included 1931 men without symptomatic CHD who were examined in eastern Finland between 1984 and 1989 and followed for an average of 3 years. During the follow-up, 51 men experienced an acute myocardial infarction. The association between ferritin and risk of myocardial infarction was not explained by other risk factors. However, conflicting findings were later reported from two other investigations that also used serum ferritin as a marker of body iron stores. In a preliminary analysis among US male physicians, based on 238 cases, Stampfer and colleagues reported no significant association between serum ferritin levels and risk of myocardial infarction[7]. In a cohort study among 2036 Icelandic men and women followed for an average of 8.5 years, no association was found between serum ferritin or serum iron and risk of myocardial infarction (81 cases)[8]. In the latter investigation, however, serum total iron-binding capacity was inversely related to risk of myocardial infarction. Since it is well established that serum ferritin is a more reliable indicator of total iron stores than the total iron-binding capacity, these results suggest that iron stores *per se* are not an important determinant of CHD.

In the other published studies serum ferritin had not been measured, and investigators had to rely on less reliable indicators of iron status. In a Canadian cohort with a follow-up of 17 years, an increased risk of fatal myocardial infarction (224 cases) was found among men and women with abnormally high serum iron concentrations presumed to represent iron overload[9]. The risk of fatal acute myocardial infarction among individuals with baseline serum iron concentrations of 175 µg/dl or above (representing 2.8 per cent of men and 0.8 per cent of women in the cohort) was twice for men and five times for women that of participants with serum iron below 120 µg/dl. No association between serum iron and risk of fatal AMI was observed at concentrations below 175 µg/dl. Since serum iron concentrations above 175 µg/dl are likely to occur in individuals who are genetically predisposed, whether the genotype, such as the haemochromatosis gene or other genes covarying with it, or the accumulated iron are increasing the risk of fatal AMI cannot be established from these data[10].

The association between serum transferrin saturation and risk of CHD has been examined among men and women participating in the National Health and Nutrition Examination Survey I (NHANES)[11]. The study population included 4518 subjects 45–74 years of age, recruited from 1971 to 1974, and free of CHD at baseline, who were followed for an average of 14.6 years. All deaths or incident events within the first 5 years of follow-up were excluded to minimize the effects of pre-existing disease on serum transferrin saturation. The relative risk for the highest quintile of transferrin saturation compared to the lowest was 0.72 (95 per cent CI 0.51–1.00) for men, and 0.85 (95 per cent CI 0.60–1.21) for women. However these results are not incompatible with an association between body iron stores and risk of CHD, because, as recognized by Sempos *et al.*, transferrin saturation is an indicator of circulating iron available to tissues, but is poorly correlated with body iron stores except when they are fully depleted or overloaded[12,13]. In addition, there is substantial diurnal and day-to-day variation in individual serum transferrin saturation values. In contrast with transferrin saturation, serum ferritin levels reflect iron stores over the wide normal range as well as at the extremes, and are more stable[14]. An association of CHD incidence with the more extreme levels of transferrin saturation among women, but not among men, was reported in a previous analyses of the same data[15]; women in the top tail of the distribution of transferrin saturation (-> 60 saturated) had a relative risk of 2.6 (95 per cent confidence interval: 0.7, 9.2) compared with women with low transferrin saturation (< 15 per cent saturated); the comparable relative risk for men was 0.8. Similar analyses have been conducted among 46,932 participants in the Kaiser-Permanente Multiphasic Health Clinic who had their serum transferrin saturation measured between 1969 and 1971 and were followed for a mean of 14 years, starting 2 years after the blood collection. During the follow-up, 969 men and 871 women were admitted to a hospital for acute myocardial infarction[16]. Transferrin saturation was categorized as low (≤ 10 per cent), normal (11 per cent to 61 per cent), or elevated (≥ 62 per cent). The low transferrin saturation category, comprising 1.8 per cent of the study population, included a substantial proportion of individuals with anaemia (28 per cent of the men, and 46 per cent of the women) and microcytosis (36 per cent overall); the elevated transferrin saturation category comprised 2.3 per cent of the study population and it was likely to include most individuals with iron overload. The relative risks of myocardial infarction for the low compared to the normal category of transferrin saturation were 0.8 among men (95 per cent 6 CI 0.3–2.6), and 1.2 among women (95 per cent CI 0.7–2.1). Comparable figures for men and women with elevated transferrin saturation were 1.3 (95 per cent CI 0.9–2.0) and 1.3 (0.8–2.4), respectively. The authors reported that the results for transferrin saturation were unchanged after excluding individuals who reported an acute myocardial infarction before the collection of the blood sample, or those with transferrin saturation ≤10 per cent and total iron-binding capacity below 250 µg/l (because they were more likely to have anaemia of chronic disease rather than iron deficiency). However, these exclusions, although appropriate, must have widened the confidence intervals of the relative risks, adding to the uncertainty of the conclusions that can be derived from this study. Other limitations of this study are the use of hospital admissions rather than incident events as endpoints (patients who died of myocardial infarction before being admitted to the hospital were not included among the cases), and the inclusion of individuals with diseases or conditions which may be associated with both transferrin saturation (in some cases indirectly, for example if they contraindicate blood donations) and risk of acute myocardial infarction, such as severe atherosclerosis or post coronary bypass surgery status, and use of aspirin or anticoagulants, among others.

A primary reason for interest in the relation of iron stores with risk of CHD is the possibility that higher *intake* of iron may increase risk; this has been addressed directly in several studies. In the Finnish cohort, dietary iron – assessed by 4 day food recording – was positively associated with risk of myocardial infarction; risk increased 5 per cent for each mg of iron daily[6]. A lack of association was reported in the Canadian cohort, and also in the report by Sempos and colleagues. However, in both studies iron intake was estimated with a single 24 h recall which, as recognized by the authors, is a poor indicator of individual long-term intakes[9,11]. In a large cohort study among US men in which diet was assessed using a semiquantitative food frequency questionnaire, we found no association between intake of non-haem iron (from foods and supplements) and risk of CHD or myocardial infarction. However, haem iron (mainly from red meat) was directly related to risk of myocardial infarction[17]. Since Finnish men have a high meat intake, total iron intake may reflect haem iron and meat intake to a greater degree in the Finnish cohort, whereas it reflects largely non-meat sources and supplements in the US. Although confounding by other factors cannot be totally excluded at this time, the distinction of dietary iron from haem and non-haem sources is important, because absorption of the latter is better regulated according to body needs. Even if iron stores were to adversely affect coronary risk, intake of non-haem iron would be unlikely to increase the risk of CHD among individuals with normal iron metabolism, because absorption of non-haem iron is minimal if iron stores are repleted. Concern remains that the small fraction of persons homozygous for haemochromatosis (about 1 in 300) might experience elevated risk of CHD due to iron intake within the range of US diets. The available studies do not exclude such an effect in a small subgroup.

Iron and cancer

In 1984 Weinberg proposed that withholding of iron - an essential growth factor for cancer cells - is an important defense mechanism of the human body against neoplasia, and suggested that iron supplementation may increase the risk of cancer[18]. The recognition that iron can catalyse the production of oxygen radicals (Halliwell 1986[32]), which have been implicated in several steps of carcinogenesis[19], has further strengthened the biological plausibility for its role as a potential risk factor for cancer. Some support to this hypothesis has been provided by laboratory[20] and animal experiments[21–23]. In this presentation, we will review the evidence from epidemiological studies addressing the relationship of iron status or iron intake with risk of cancer (Table 2).

In 1986 Stevens *et al.* reported a positive association between baseline serum ferritin and risk of death from cancer or development of primary hepatocellular carcinoma (PHC) in a prospective study of Chinese male government workers in Taiwan[24]. The study population comprised 21,513 men (including 3454 HBV carriers) who were enrolled between 1975 and 1978 and were followed until 1983. The study was originally designed to examine the association between HBV and PHC, and information on other cancers was only available for men who died during the follow-up period. There was no significant difference in mean serum ferritin between 122 men who died of cancer other than PHC (149.1 µg/ml) and their controls (142.1 µg/ml), whereas serum ferritin was significantly higher among the 70 men who developed PHC

Table 2. Epidemiological studies on iron status and risk of cancer

Study	Population		Length of follow-up (years)	Measures of iron status	Association with risk		
	Men	Women			All cancers	Specific Sites	
Stevens *et al.*[24]	21,513	–	8	ferritin	0 ($n = 122$) (excluding PHC)	PHC ($n = 70$)	+
				serum transferrin	–	PHC	0
Selby *et al.*[25]	80,007	94,500	8 (first 2 years ignored)	use of iron supplements	0 ($n = 6{,}842$) (excluding lung)	lung ($n = 120$) ($n = 99$)	– women 0 men
	14,333	29,219	– (first 2 years ignored)	TIBC	0 ($n = 1{,}750$) (excluding lung)	lung	– women 0 men
Stevens *et al.* [29]	3,287	5,269	14 (first 4 years ignored)	transferrin saturation	+ men ($n = 379$) 0 women ($n = 340$)	esophagus ($n = 9$) bladder ($n = 17$) other urinary ($n = 12$)	+ men + men – men
				TIBC	– men 0 women	esophagus	– men
				iron intake	0		
						colon ($n = 25$)	+ men
Knekt[30]	18,813	22,463	14	transferrin saturation	0	stomach ($n = 120$)	– men
				TIBC	0	lung, stomach ($n = 416$)	– men + men
				serum iron	0	rectum ($n = 40$) stomach	+ women – men

(121.4 µg/ml) than among their controls (99.5 µg/ml, $P < 0.05$).

The mean increase in ferritin compared to the controls was higher among the 10 cases of PHC that occurred within the first year from the serum collection (60 µg/ml) than among the cases that occurred at least two years later (16.4 µg/ml), suggesting that pre-existing PHC increased the serum ferritin levels among the cases. In the same population, a significant inverse association was found between serum transferrin and risk of death from cancer (excluding PHC), but not between serum transferrin and risk of PHC. The correlation between serum transferrin and iron status, however, is poor, and the reported association could also be due to an effect of undiagnosed cancer on serum protein levels. Thus, the overall results of this study do not support an association between iron status and risk of cancer. However, noting that the coefficients for serum ferritin in proportional hazard models with PHC or other cancers as outcomes were not statistically different from each other, the authors fitted a model assuming that the two coefficients were equal. The model, which included also two coefficients (one for each outcome) for transferrin, was found to make a significant improvement over the null model (i.e. with all coefficients zero), and was used to support the conclusion that iron status is related to risk of cancer at any site. However the significance of the model was due to the positive association of ferritin with risk of PHC, and to the inverse association of transferrin with risk of other cancer, which, as explained above, are both unlikely to be causal. On the other hand, it is worth noting that the inclusion of 24 stomach cancer may have attenuated a possible positive association between serum ferritin and cancer at other sites, since stomach cancer has been associated with lower ferritin levels 5 or more years before the diagnosis (Akiba 1991[31]), perhaps due to hypochlorhydria (frequently associated with athrophic gastritis, a condition related to stomach cancer) or bleeding from early undetected lesions.

The association between recent iron use or anaemia and risk of cancer was examined in a cohort of 174,507 persons who had been examined between 1964 and 1973 at the Kaiser Permanente Medical Center in California[25]. The first 2 years of follow-up after enrollment in the study were ignored, to reduce the possibility that undetected cancer at baseline lead to iron use or anaemia. The average follow-up was 8.3 years (range 2.1–16 years). The age- and smoking-adjusted risk of lung cancer was lower among women with history of recent use of iron supplements compared to those without such history (relative risk 0.60, 95 per cent CI 0.37–0.97), and among women with anaemia compared to those without anaemia (relative risk 0.61, 95 per cent CI 0.38–0.98). No significant associations were found with cancer at other sites or among men. Since women with recent use of iron had lower haemoglobin levels and higher total iron-binding capacity than non-users, even after taking the iron medication, the authors concluded that the inverse association observed was probably due to a protective effect of iron deficiency. They acknowledged, however, the possibility that the observed associations were due to residual confounding by smoking, that was inversely related to use of iron in women, and directly related to haemoglobin levels in both sexes. A subgroup of 43,552 members was enrolled during a period in which total iron-binding capacity was part of the check-up. Among women in this group, there was an inverse association between total iron-binding capacity and risk of lung cancer; the relative risk for the highest quartile compared to the lowest was 0.41 (95 per cent CI 0.23–0.73). As for iron supplement use, no significant associations were found for other cancers or among men. Since total iron-binding capacity was unrelated to smoking, this result is less likely to reflect residual confounding from this variable. However, as previously discussed, total iron- binding capacity is reduced by chronic infection and malignancy, and the possibility cannot be excluded that preclinical cancer caused the lower levels observed among cases. To address this possibility, it would have been useful to present analyses stratified by different periods of follow-up.

A group including two authors of the Taiwan study, reported a positive association between serum transferrin saturation and risk of cancer, and an inverse association between total iron-binding capacity and risk of cancer, among men and women in the National Health and Nutrition Examination Survey I (NHANES)[26]. The study population comprised 14,384 adults 25–74 years of age, recruited from 1971 and 1975, who did not have cancer at the time of the initial interview. Of these subjects, 13,292 were traced and reinterviewed between 1981 and 1984. Because preclinical cancer may affect serum transferrin saturation and total iron-binding capacity, analyses were restricted to individuals who remained cancer free and alive for at least 4 years after the blood was drawn. In this group, baseline total iron-binding capacity was available for 3355 men and 5367 women, who developed 242 cases and 203 cases of cancer, respectively, during the follow-up. The follow-up of this population has been later extended to 1988, and the analyses have been replicated with 379 cancer cases (including 233 cancer deaths) among men, and 340 cancer cases (including 174 cancer deaths) among women (Stevens 1994[29]). For the following review, we have been referring to the latest publication, unless otherwise specified. Since serum ferritin was not measured in the NHANES study, analyses were performed using serum transferrin saturation and total iron-binding capacity as surrogate markers of iron status. It is noteworthy that the *P* values reported in these articles are one-tailed; the two-tailed *P* values would be approximately twice the reported values, and often would fail to reach the standard significance level. The mean transferrin saturation was 32.1 per cent among men who developed cancer, and 30.7 per cent among those who remained cancer free (one-tailed $P = 0.015$). The comparable figures among women were 28.2 per cent and 27.3 per cent (one-tailed $P = 0.09$). Men, but not women, who developed cancer also had a lower total iron- binding capacity than men who remained cancer free (346.0 g/dl versus 350.9

g/dl, one-tailed P = 0.035). When men and women were divided into five categories according to their level of transferrin saturation, those with the highest levels of saturation also had the highest risk of cancer. Compared to men and women with transferrin saturation below 30 per cent (a category which included 52 per cent of all men and 66 per cent of all women), those with transferrin saturation between 50 and 60 per cent (a category which included 4 per cent of men and 2 per cent of women) had a relative risk of 1.38 (90 per cent CI 1.00–1.99) and those with transferrin saturation of 60 per cent or more (a category which included 2 per cent of all men and 1 per cent of all women) had a relative risk of 1.81 (90 per cent CI 1.21–2.71). Thus, levels of transferrin saturation often suggestive of haemochromatosis and iron overload were associated with an increased risk of cancer. The comparison of mean values of biochemical variables by cancer site among men showed significantly higher transferrin saturation among cases of esophageal (43.7 per cent, n = 9) and bladder (38.1 per cent, n = 17) cancer compared to controls (30.7 per cent, n = 2908). The mean transferrin saturations among men with cancer of other sites were 33.0 per cent for colon (n = 25), 34.7 per cent for rectum (n = 14), 31.9 per cent for lung (n = 75), and 26.0 per cent for stomach (n = 10). Although transferrin saturation is a poor indicator of body iron stores[12,13] when these are within the normal range, high levels of transferrin saturation (60 per cent) are suggestive of iron overload and are frequently associated with abnormal iron metabolism. Thus this study does provide some indirect evidence that iron overload is associated with an increased risk of cancer, although whether this is due to the effect of iron itself rather then genetic predisposition remains unsettled.

Further evidence on the association between iron overload and risk of cancer has been provided by a large prospective investigation conducted in Finland[27]. The population included in the analyses comprised 41,276 persons (18,813 men and 22,463 women) aged 20–74 years and who never had cancer, recruited by a mobile health clinic throughout the country during the period 1966–1972. Information on subsequent cancer incidence was obtained through the Finnish Cancer Registry. During a mean follow-up of 14 years, 2469 cases of cancer were registered. No significant differences in mean levels of serum iron, total iron-binding capacity, or transferrin saturation, were found between individuals who developed cancer and subjects who remained cancer free. Some significant associations were found for cancer at single sites. The incidence of stomach cancer was inversely related with transferrin saturation and serum iron, and positively associated with total iron-binding capacity among men. The incidence of lung cancer was inversely associated with total iron-binding capacity among men, whereas the incidence of rectal cancer was positively associated with total iron-binding capacity among women. Also, the relative risk of all cancers combined did not vary significantly between quartiles of transferrin saturation. However, an increased risk of cancer was observed among men and women with transferrin saturation above 60 per cent (a category comprising 3 per cent of the total population). After adjustment for age and smoking, the relative risk of cancer at any site for men and women with transferrin saturation above 60 per cent was 1.39 (95 per cent CI 1.08–1.79) for men and 1.48 (95 per cent CI 0.99–2.20) for women as compared to subjects with lower saturation levels. The strongest association was found with colon cancer. The relative risk for men and women combined was 3.04 (95 per cent CI 1.64–5.62), and persisted after adjustment for several potential confounders and after exclusion of cases occurring during the first 5 years of follow-up. Thus, these findings do not imply that there is an association between iron status and risk of cancer among individuals with normal iron metabolism, but they are consistent with the hypothesis that excessive iron stores may increase the risk of cancer, particularly of the large intestine.

Because of the homeostatic control over iron absorption, intake of iron is not correlated with iron stores in most populations, and therefore studies of dietary iron do not provide much information on the association of iron status with cancer risk. It is possible that iron intake is itself a risk factor for cancer; however, the effect of dietary iron, if any, is likely to be modified by the iron status that regulates the amount of iron absorbed. In the NHANES study, there was no association between iron intake and risk of cancer[26]. However, iron intake was estimated with a single 24 h recall, which, as recognized by the authors, is a poor indicator of individual long-term intakes. Although a positive association between red meat intake and risk of colon cancer has been reported in several studies[28], it is far from clear whether this is due to iron itself or to other components of red meat.

Conclusion

Evidence linking iron status with risk of CHD or cancer is unconvincing, and does not justify changes in food fortification or medical practice, particularly because the benefits of assuring adequate iron intake during growth and development are well established. However, most published studies have included mainly men with normal iron stores and have included small number of CHD or cancer cases or have not adequately assessed iron status. Thus, they have had little capacity to detect an association of iron status with risk of CHD or cancer, particularly in the deficient or overload ranges of iron nutriture. Stronger evidence is needed before rejecting the hypothesis that greater iron stores increase the incidence of CHD or cancer.

References

1. Sullivan, J.L. (1981): Iron and the sex difference in heart disease risk. *Lancet* **1,** 1293–1294.

2. Stampfer, M.J., Colditz, G.A., Willett, W.C. *et al.* (1991): Postmenopausal estrogen therapy and cardiovascular disease. *N. Engl. J. Med.* **83,** 325:756–762.

3. McCord, J.M. (1991): Is iron sufficiently a risk factor in ischemic heart disease? *Circulation* **83,** 1112–1114.

4. Biemond, P., Swaak, A.J., Beindorff, C.M. & Koster, J.F. (1986): Superoxide-dependent and -independent mechanisms of iron mobilization from ferritin by xanthine oxidase. *Biochem. J.* **239,** 169–173.

5. Sullivan, J.L. (1992): Stored iron and ischemic heart disease: Empirical support for a new paradigm. *Circulation* **86,** 1036–1037.

6. Salonen, J.T., Nyyssonen, K., Korpela, H., Tuomilehto, J., Seppanen, R. & Salonen, R. (1992): High stores iron levels are associated with excess risk of myocardial infarction in Eastern Finnish men. *Circulation* **86,** 803–811.

7. Stampfer, M.J., Grodstein, F., Rosenberg, I., Willett, W.C. & Hennekens, C. (1993): A prospective study of plasma ferritin and risk of myocardial infarction in US physicians. *Circulation* **87,** 688 (abstract).

8. Magnusson, M.K., Sigfusson, N., Sigvaldson, H., Johannesson, G.M., Magnusson, S. & Thorgeirsson, G. (1994): Low iron-binding capacity as a risk factor for myocardial infarction. *Circulation* **89,** 102–108.

9. Morrison, H.I., Semenciw, R.M., Mao, Y. & Wigle, D.T. (1994): Serum iron and risk of fatal acute myocardial infarction. *Epidemiology* **5,** 243–246.

10. Ascherio, A. & Hunter, D. (1994): Iron and myocardial infarction (editorial). *Epidemiology.* **5,** 135–137.

11. Sempos, C.T., Looker, A.C., Gillum, R.F. & Makuc, D.M. (1994): Body iron stores and the risk of coronary heart disease. *N. Engl. J. Med.* **330,** 1119–1124.

12. Beaton, G.H., Corey, P.N. & Steele, C. (1989): Conceptual and methodological issues regarding the epidemiology of iron deficiency and their implications for studies of the functional consequences of iron deficiency. *Am. J. Clin. Nutr.* **50,** 575–588.

13. Cook, J.D., Finch, C.A. & Smith, N.J. (1976): Evaluation of the iron status of a population. *Blood* **48,** 449–455.

14. Cook, J.D., Lipschitz, D.A., Miles, L.E.M. & Finch, C.A. (1974): Serum ferritin as a measure of iron stores in normal subjects. *Am. J. Clin. Nutr.* **27,** 681–687.

15. Giles, W.H., Anda, R.F., Williamson, D.F., Yip, R. & Marks, J. (Letter) (1993): *Circulation* **87,** 2065–2066.

16. Baer, D.M., Tekawa, I.S. & Hurley, L.B. (1994): Iron stores are not associated with acute myocardial infarction. *Circulation* **89,** 2915–2918.

17. Ascherio, A., Willett, W.C., Rimm, E.B., Giovannucci, E.L. & Stampfer, M.J. (1994): Dietary iron intake and risk of coronary heart disease among men. *Circulation* **89,** 969–974.

18. Weinberg, E.D. (1984): Iron withholding: a defense against infection and neoplasia. *Physiol. Rev.* **64,** 65–102.

19. Cerutti, P.A. (1985): Prooxidant states and tumor promotion. *Science* **227,** 375–381.

20. Babbs, C.F. (1990): Free radicals and the etiology of colon cancer. *Free Biol. Med.* **8,** 191–200.

21. Siegers, C.P., Bumann, D., Baretton, G. & Younes, M. (1988): Dietary iron enhances the tumour rate in dimethylhydrazine-induced colon carcinogenesis in mice. *Cancer Lett.* **41,** 151–256.

22. Hann, H.W., Stahlhut, M.W. & Blumberg, B.S. (1988): Iron nutrition and tumor growth: decreased tumor growth in iron-deficient mice. *Canc. Res.* **48,** 4168–4170.

23. Nelson, R.L., Yoo, S.J., Tanure, J.C., Andrianpoulos, G. & Misumi, A. (1989): The effect of iron on experimental colorectal carcinogenesis. *Anticancer Res.* **9,** 1477–1482.

24. Stevens, R.G., Beasley, R.P. & Blumberg, B.S. (1986): Iron-building proteins and risk of cancer in Taiwan. *JNCI* **76,** 605–610.

25. Selby, J.V. & Friedman, G.D. (1988): Epidemiologic evidence of an association between body iron stores and risk of cancer. *Int. J. Cancer* **41,** 677–682.

26. Stevens, R.G., Jones, D.Y., Micozzi, M.S. & Taylor, P.R. (1988): Body iron stores and the risk of cancer. *N. Engl. J. Med.* **319,** 1047–1052.

27. Knekt, P., Reunanen, A., Jarvinen, R., Seppanen, R., Heliovaara, M. & Aromaa, A. (1994): Antioxidant vitamin intake and coronary mortality in a longitudinal population study. *Am. J. Epidemiol.* **139,** 1180–1189.

28. Giovannucci, E. & Willett, W.C. (1995): Dietary factors and risk of colon cancer. *Ann. Med.* **26,** 443–452.

29. Stevens, R.G., Graubard, B.I., Micozzi, M.S., Neriishi, K. & Blumberg, B.S. (1994): Moderate elevation of body iron level and increased risk of cancer occurence and death. *Int. J. Cancer.* **56,** 364–369

30. Knekt, P., Reunanen, A., Takkunen, H., Aramaa, A., Heliövarra, M. & Hakulinen, T. (1994): Body iron stores and risk of cancer. *Int. J. Cancer.* **56**, 379–382.

31. Akiba, S., Neriishi, K., Blot, W.J., Kabuto, M., Stevens, R.G., Kato, H. & Land, C.E. (1991): Serum ferritin and stomach cancer risk among a Japanese population. *Cancer.* **67**, 1707–1712

32. Halliwell, B. & Gutteridge, J.M.C. (1986): Oxygen free radicals and iron in relation to biology and medicine: some problems and concepts. *Bioch & Bioph* (No. 2). **246**, 501–514

Iron Nutrition in Health and Disease, edited by Leif Hallberg and Nils-Georg Asp
©1996 John Libbey & Company Ltd., pp. 313–324

Chapter 31

Breast feeding and formulas: the role of lactoferrin?

Bo Lönnerdal

Department of Nutrition, University of California, 3135 Meyer Hall, Davis, CA 95616 USA

Summary

Iron status of breast-fed infants is satisfactory for 6–9 months after birth. This is somewhat surprising considering the low concentration of iron in breast milk and suggests that iron utilization is exceptionally high in breast-fed infants. Infants fed milk formula without iron fortification frequently develop iron deficiency at this age, even though the iron level of such formula is higher than that of breast milk. Iron absorption studies as well as balance studies in infants suggest that iron absorption is higher from breast milk than from formula. The factor(s) responsible for the high absorption of iron from breast milk is not yet known. A possible candidate is lactoferrin, the major iron-binding protein in breast milk. This protein is present in high concentrations in breast milk, whereas the concentration in formula is low. Lactoferrin is resistant against proteolysis and significant proportions of intact lactoferrin can be found in the stool of breast-fed infants. Our *in vitro* studies show that conditions similar to those of the gastrointestinal tract of infants favour redistribution of iron from other ligands in breast milk to lactoferrin, so that a larger proportion of iron is bound to lactoferrin after limited digestion than originally in breast milk. Specific receptors for human lactoferrin have been found in intestinal brush border membranes from human infants. This receptor recognizes human lactoferrin but not bovine lactoferrin. There is little *in vivo* evidence for a direct role of human lactoferrin in iron absorption in infants. However, most clinical studies that do not show any effect of lactoferrin on iron status of infants have used bovine lactoferrin, which cannot bind to the intestinal receptor. Studies on human lactoferrin in animal models have not given support for lactoferrin in iron absorption either, although species differences may explain this. Recombinant human lactoferrin is now being produced. Long-term clinical studies of this lactoferrin added to formula are needed to evaluate better the role of lactoferrin in iron absorption.

Introduction

The iron requirement of infants has been estimated by several investigators. Usually, losses are determined by analysis of iron in the stool and urine (very small for infants) and, occasionally, estimates of skin losses. A provision for growth is then added to cover tissue expansion and red blood cell synthesis. For infants 0–6 months of age, this iron requirement has been estimated to 0.49 mg/day and between 6–12 months of age to 0.90 mg/day[1]. An inherent problem with this approach is that breast milk only provides a maximum of 0.2–0.3 mg/day during the first 6 months of age, i.e. even if all this iron would be absorbed (which is not likely), the iron provided from breast milk would not meet the requirements. A counter-argument commonly used is that most iron in red blood cells will be recycled during the first 3–4 months of age and that stored iron can be used to meet the need for iron. Still, the fact that exclusively breast-fed infants have satisfactory iron status at 6 months of age and in most cases up to 9 months[2] of age may argue for the iron requirements being overestimated, but also that iron in breast milk is exceptionally well utilized by the breast-fed infant.

Iron status of breast-fed and formula-fed infants

Even if current estimates of iron requirements of infants may be inflated, it is evident that breast-fed infants utilize iron from their diet very effectively. This has been shown by a variety of methods (see below) in several populations and settings. However, infants fed milk formula which has not been fortified with iron are frequently found to have iron deficiency or iron deficiency anaemia at 6 months of age[3,4]. The lower iron status of infants fed unfortified formula as compared to breast-fed infants also supports a high bioavailability of iron from breast milk, as the iron content of this formula is higher than that of breast milk. Such formulas previously contained about 0.7 mg of iron per litre, but recently the iron concentration has been increased to 1.0 mg/l, or higher. Cow's milk in itself only contains about 0.1–0.2 mg of iron per litre, but mineral salts and other components added to formula increase the iron level substantially. Thus, by choosing various raw materials, the iron level of unfortified formula can be raised without defining it as 'iron fortified' formula. This is not a moot point as earlier studies may have shown anaemia in infants fed 'unfortified' formula, whereas more recent studies using 'unfortified' formula may fail to do so.

Breast-fed infants have satisfactory iron status at 6 months of age as indicated by both haemoglobin (>105 g/l), MCV, transferrin saturation, and ferritin (>12 μg/l) values[2,5,6]. Infants fed iron fortified formula have also been shown to have excellent iron status at 6, 9 and 12 months of age[6–8]. The level of iron fortification needed to assure satisfactory iron status is, however, a matter of disagreement. Infant formula in the USA usually contains 12–14 mg of iron per litre, whereas formulas in Europe contain 6–7 mg/l. We have recently evaluated the capacity of milk formula with lower levels of iron fortification to provide adequate amounts of iron to healthy term infants exclusively fed formula up to 6 months of age[6,9]. Our first study showed that feeding a whey predominant formula with 4 mg of iron per litre resulted in satisfactory iron status at 6 months of age[6]. A subsequent study of the same formula with 2 mg of iron per litre showed similar results, i.e. serum ferritin concentrations of all infants were higher than 12 μg/l[9].

The observation that infants fed breast milk, which contains 0.2–0.4 mg of iron per litre[10], had better iron status at 6 months of age than infants fed formula with 0.7 mg of iron per litre can be used as indirect evidence to support the notion that iron bioavailability is considerably higher from breast milk than from milk formula. However, radioisotope studies also support a high bioavailability of breast milk iron. Garby and Sjolin[11] showed early that iron absorption is high in breast-fed infants and that absorption is highest during early infancy. Schultz and Smith[12] showed that iron absorption from cow's milk is substantially lower than from breast milk. By using the extrinsic tag method, Saarinen et al.[13] demonstrated that iron absorption from breast milk is around 50 per cent, whereas it is substantially lower (≈20 per cent) from milk formula. Although the method of extrinsic labelling may not be entirely valid for breast milk[14,15], there is no doubt that some component(s) of breast milk leads to high iron absorption, while some component of cow's milk (and formula) causes lower iron absorption[14]. Therefore, several studies have attempted to evaluate the relative influence of different constituents of breast milk and formula on iron absorption.

Differences in the composition of breast milk and formula

A major difference in iron-binding between breast milk and cow's milk formula is that the major part of iron in breast milk is found in the whey (soluble) fraction (65–81 per cent), whereas by far most of the iron in cow's milk is bound to casein (61–73 per cent)[16]. Since some cow's milk formulas are adapted, i.e. whey proteins are added to make the whey:casein ratio more similar to that of human milk (60:40), somewhat less iron is bound to casein in this type of formula as compared to conventional casein-predominant formula. However, the strong affinity of bovine (cow) casein to iron will always make casein the dominant iron-binding component of milk formula. Only small fractions of iron in cow's milk are bound to lipids (13–18 per cent) or are found in the whey fraction (9–15 per cent).

In the human milk whey fraction, most of the iron is bound to lactoferrin[10], a milk protein synthesized by the mammary gland. This protein is present in human milk at high concentrations[10], whereas cow's milk only contains a very low concentration of lactoferrin[17]. The remainder of the iron in human whey is associated with low molecular weight compounds, most likely citrate[14]. Another significant fraction of iron in breast milk is associated with the fat fraction (19–26 per cent), most probably in the form of iron-containing, membrane-bound enzymes[18]. Only a small fraction of iron in human milk is bound to casein (2–14 per cent). Thus, the considerable difference in iron- binding between human milk and cow's milk may be explained by the high concentration of lactoferrin in breast milk with a high affinity towards iron and its low concentration of casein as well as the high concentration of highly phosphorylated casein in cow's milk with high affinity towards iron and a very low concentration of lactoferrin.

Properties of lactoferrin

Lactoferrin was first isolated from milk in 1960[19]. It is similar to transferrin in that it has a molecular weight of 80 kDa and binds two atoms of ferric iron together with either bicarbonate or carbonate as anions[20]. However, they are different gene products and there is no cross-reactivity of one antibody towards the other protein. Lactoferrin has an affinity constant for iron which is several orders of magnitude higher than that of transferrin and lactoferrin maintains its iron-binding capacity at a lower pH than does transferrin. The lactoferrin molecule contains two lobes, which are similar but not identical, and the lobes are connected by an alpha-helical extended segment. Lactoferrin is a glycoprotein; it contains one glycan per lobe and the bi- or tri-antennar structure contains terminal fucose residues[21]. The protein is unusually resistant against proteolysis, particularly in its iron-saturated form[22].

Table 1. Suggested biological activities for lactoferrin

Enhancer/facilitator of iron absorption
Bactoeriostatic agent
Bactericidal agent
Phagocytic killing
Growth factor
Immunostimulatory factor
Transcription factor

Lactoferrin has been proposed to have several physiological functions (Table 1). It was originally suggested that apolactoferrin may have a bacteriostatic function by withholding iron from iron-demanding pathogens[23]. As lactoferrin in breast milk is only saturated with iron to about 14 per cent[10], this might be a mechanism to help breast-fed infants resist infection. More recently, it was shown that a fragment of lactoferrin, named lactoferricin[24], may exert a direct bactericidal effect on some bacteria. Although both these effects have been clearly demonstrated *in vitro*, there is scant evidence for these functions *in vivo*.

Since lactoferrin binds a substantial part of iron in breast milk, it was hypothesized that lactoferrin may promote iron absorption in breast-fed infants[14]. The finding of significant quantities of intact lactoferrin in the stool of breast-fed infants, even up to the age of 4 months[25], supported this idea. Although some digestion of lactoferrin certainly occurs, up to 10–14 per cent of all lactoferrin appears to escape digestion. When calculating the iron-binding capacity of this amount of lactoferrin on a molar basis, it is more than adequate to carry all iron in breast milk. The ability of lactoferrin to partially escape digestion may be explained by the relatively high gastric pH of breast-fed infants, the comparatively low activity of gastric and pancreatic proteases and, particularly, the resistance of this molecule towards proteolytic attack.

A stimulatory effect of lactoferrin on intestinal cell growth has been suggested[26,27]. However, these findings should be viewed with some caution as they were made in the rat, a species that does not have lactoferrin in its milk[17]. It is possible that lactoferrin has some mitogenic effect, but support for this in humans has not yet been obtained. Lactoferrin is also involved in immune function, particularly in phagocytic killing by macrophages and is believed to be synthesized by neutrophils[28,29]. Part of the involvement of lactoferrin in immune function may be explained by the stimulatory effect of lactoferrin on cytokine release by cells[30]. Finally, it is known that lactoferrin binds avidly to DNA[31] and very recent findings of highly specific binding of lactoferrin to DNA sequences in the nucleus suggest that lactoferrin may act as a transcription factor and thus regulate cellular events[32]. Further research is needed to evaluate this potential function of lactoferrin.

Lactoferrin receptors

The observation that lactoferrin is resistant towards proteolysis led to the suggestion of specific structures, or receptors, for lactoferrin in the small intestine. Such receptors may then facilitate the binding of lactoferrin to the mucosa and subsequently the delivery of iron to the intestinal cell. Studies by Cox *et al.*[33] showed that lactoferrin (and iron) bound to human adult intestinal tissue in a saturable and specific manner, supporting the notion of a lactoferrin receptor. Subsequent studies in the mouse demonstrated such a receptor and provided some biochemical data[34,35]. We first isolated the lactoferrin receptor from brush border membranes from infant rhesus monkey small intestine[36]. The receptor was found to be specific for human and rhesus lactoferrin, but did not bind bovine lactoferrin or human transferrin. Subsequent studies in the rhesus monkey showed that the receptor binds both iron- and manganese-saturated lactoferrin as well as apolactoferrin[37]. The receptor appears to be present at all ages, including the fetus, but the number of receptors per tissue weight appeared highest during infancy, i.e. the period when the intestine would be likely to be exposed to lactoferrin[36]. Studies in piglets showed no variation in receptor affinity or number of receptors during the infancy period and the receptor was present in similar quantities in all parts of the small intestine[38].

The receptor was subsequently purified from human fetal and infant small intestine by affinity chromatography on an immobilized lactoferrin column and was found to have a molecular weight around 115 kDa[39]. The lactoferrin receptor is highly specific for human lactoferrin, is glycosylated and has a subunit molecular weight of about 37 kDa. Deglycosylated lactoferrin binds to the receptor with similar affinity, suggesting that the glycans are not needed for receptor recognition. We have recently cloned the human lactoferrin receptor from a human small intestinal cDNA library and are presently sequencing the clone (unpublished data). Lactoferrin receptors have also been isolated from mouse small intestine[35] and human lymphocytes[40]. Although the size of the receptors are relatively similar, there appears to be differences between investigators regarding the existence of subunits. This may, however, be explained by differences in species and/or cell type studied.

Distribution of iron in breast milk and formula prior to and following digestion

The capacity of lactoferrin to resist digestion results in a fraction of lactoferrin remaining intact in the gastrointestinal tract. Although not all iron in breast milk is bound to lactoferrin initially, the conditions in the milk and the gastrointestinal tract are such that they may promote redistribution of iron from other ligands in the milk to lactoferrin. Human milk is a good source of citrate which is known to chelate iron and keep it in soluble form. At the gastric pH of breastfed infants, which is commonly around 4–5, iron remains bound to lactoferrin but becomes dissociated from citrate and, most likely, also from other minor ligands such as membrane proteins and casein.

The addition of pancreatic fluid to this partially digested mixture provides a high concentration of bicarbonate, which is known to facilitate iron binding by lactoferrin. Thus, when approaching the luminal uptake phase, a vast majority of iron in breast milk may be bound to lactoferrin. As shown in Table 2, a preliminary *in vitro* experiment in which breast milk was exposed to first pepsin at pH 4 and then addition of bicarbonate to pH 7 to mimic digestion in the gastrointestinal tract of infants supports this notion. Iron was followed by ^{59}Fe and incubation times of 15 and 30 min, respectively, were used at 37 °C. Lactoferrin was separated from the whey by affinity chromatography on heparin–Sepharose. It is evident that more iron was found associated to lactoferrin (or large fragments thereof) following digestion than initially. A simple calculation reveals that if human milk has a lactoferrin concentration of ≈ 1 mg/ml which corresponds to ~ 15 μM and 10 per cent remains undigested, the 1.5 μM of lactoferrin can bind 3 μM of iron – which is about the total iron concentration of breast milk! Thus, undigested lactoferrin has the potential of binding all the iron in breast milk in the upper small intestine, i.e. the site of absorption.

A major difference between breast milk and cow's milk or formula is that most iron in breast milk is soluble, whereas a substantial part of iron in cow's milk is associated with casein, which is present in the form of micelles. When the pH is lowered in the stomach, bovine casein has a tendency to precipitate and form a partially insoluble clot, which may resist digestion. In addition, partial digestion of casein may result in phosphopeptides which can bind iron and make it unavailable for absorption. A negative effect of bovine casein on iron absorption has been documented[41]. Human casein, however, is less phosphorylated, is present in much lower concentrations and is less prone to precipitate at lower pH. Thus, cow's milk casein may have a significant negative influence on iron absorption in infants, whereas human lactoferrin may enhance iron uptake.

Effect of bovine lactoferrin on iron absorption

Animal models

The potential effect of lactoferrin on iron absorption and/or iron status has been evaluated in several animal models. As bovine lactoferrin was the first lactoferrin source that was likely to be available in large quantities, most studies have used bovine lactoferrin.

Table 2. Iron distribution following in vitro digestion of ^{59}Fe-labelled human milk (percentage of total counts)

	Untreated	pH 4[a]	Pepsin[b]	Bicarbonate[c]
Whey	82	80	78	91
Fat	5	5	16	5
Pellet (casein)	13	16	7	5
Non-Lf[d]	24	31	32	33
Lf[e]	76	69	68	67

[a]Milk was adjusted to pH 4 with hydrochloric acid.
[b]Milk was incubated with pepsin at pH 4 and 37 °C for 30 min.
[c]Sodium bicarbonate was added to the milk so that the pH was adjusted to 7.0.
[d]Material passing heparin-Sepharose.
[e]Material binding to heparin-Sepharose (i.e. lactoferrin).

The effect of adding bovine lactoferrin to milk formula was evaluated in suckling piglets[42]. This animal model was chosen since sow milk has relatively high levels of lactoferrin and the newborn piglet has a high requirement for dietary iron. Piglets were fed a 'piglet formula' (based on the composition of sow milk) with iron added in the form of bovine lactoferrin or as ferrous sulfate. The formulas were radiolabelled with ^{59}Fe and the piglets were fed the formula in a fasting state. Radioisotope incorporation in red blood cells and plasma appearance were monitored following dosing. No significant differences were found in net iron uptake between the two forms of iron, although iron uptake into RBCs and plasma appeared somewhat more rapid from lactoferrin than from ferrous sulfate.

The mouse has also been used as an animal model for studying iron absorption from lactoferrin[43]. Iron status of mice fed a milk diet supplemented with iron as bovine lactoferrin was similar to that of mice fed iron as ferrous chloride when the mice had been depleted of iron prior to the supplementation. In contrast, milk supplemented with ferric chloride resulted in better iron status than lactoferrin-supplemented milk when iron status was satisfactory. This may suggest that the role of lactoferrin in iron absorption may depend on the iron status of the individual.

Although the rat does not have any lactoferrin in its milk, attempts have been made to use this species for evaluation of the effect of lactoferrin on iron absorption. When weanling rats were fed a diet with iron provided as lactoferrin, iron status was shown to be higher than in rats fed a diet with ferrous sulfate as the iron source[44]. This was somewhat surprising but a possible explanation was subsequently obtained when it was found that rat small intestine contains a transferrin receptor and that this receptor recognizes bovine lactoferrin[45]. Thus, the rat, which has transferrin as a major iron-binding protein in its milk, is able to utilize iron from bovine lactoferrin, whereas human lactoferrin did not bind to this receptor. It is therefore questionable if the rat is a good model for the human infant with regard to iron absorption and the role of lactoferrin.

Human studies

Iron absorption from infant formula supplemented with bovine lactoferrin was evaluated by Fairweather-Tait *et al.*[46]. Seven-day-old term infants were fed whey-predominant formula extrinsically labelled with a stable isotope, ^{58}Fe, during a 3 day balance period. The experimental formula contained 2.85 g of lactoferrin per litre, whereas the control formula contained no extra lactoferrin. Iron absorption was similar from the two formulas, 46 per cent versus 44 per cent, respectively. A drawback with the study was that the lactoferrin-supplemented formula contained 0.86 mg of iron per litre, while the control formula contained 0.4 mg/l. As iron absorption decreases with the amount of iron in a meal, it is not known whether iron absorption was higher from the lactoferrin-supplemented product, but reduced because of the higher iron concentration. Similar iron concentrations in the two products would have allowed such an evaluation.

Iron balance studies on formula fortified with bovine lactoferrin were performed by Schulz-Lell *et al.*[47]. Term infants, 3–17 weeks old, were used in this study and the balances were performed during 3 days. Whey-predominant formula with either 1 g of bovine lactoferrin per litre or no lactoferrin added were used, and the iron concentration of these products were 1.1 and 0.77 g/l, respectively. Iron retention from the lactoferrin-supplemented formula was 36 per cent and from the control formula 28 per cent; this difference was not significant. Iron retention from breast milk was found to be 47 per cent. Again, similar iron levels in the two products would have been preferable from a methodological point of view.

The long-term effects of feeding infant formula supplemented with bovine lactoferrin was evaluated by Chierici *et al.*[48]. Term infants were fed from birth to 5 months of age either whey-predominant formula supplemented with 0.1 or 1.0 g/l of lactoferrin or the same formula without lactoferrin added. The iron concentration of the three formulas were 0.73, 0.98 and 0.70 mg/l, respectively. Iron status as assessed by serum ferritin concentrations at 5 months of age was 18, 25 and 20 μg/l, respectively. Although the ferritin values were slightly higher for the group fed formula with the higher concentration of lactoferrin, it should be noted that the iron concentration of this product was also slightly higher. As the formula was fed exclusively for 5 months, it is feasible that the slightly higher iron concentration, and not lactoferrin *per se*, was the reason for the somewhat higher ferritin concentrations. Again, it is apparent that when the effect of lactoferrin is to be evaluated, the iron concentrations of the diets studied need to be closely matched in order to identify the role of lactoferrin on iron absorption or status.

Bovine lactoferrin has also been used to substitute part of the iron in infant formula. Term infants were exclusively fed whey-predominant formula from 6 weeks to 6 months of age[6]. The formula contained ferrous sulfate at 4 or 7 mg of iron per litre or bovine lactoferrin providing 1.4 mg of iron and ferrous sulfate providing 2.6 mg of iron per litre. At 6 months of age, infants in all groups had satisfactory haemoglobin values and no incidence of iron deficiency as judged by serum ferritin concentrations (< 12 μg/l). There were no significant differences between groups fed the two iron levels or between the groups fed lactoferrin-iron and ferrous sulfate versus ferrous sulfate alone.

It is possible that the lack of positive effect of lactoferrin on iron absorption and iron status found in these studies can be explained by the inability of bovine lactoferrin to bind to the intestinal lactoferrin receptor (see above). Instead of binding to the receptors, lactoferrin may be digested in the small intestine and iron released for absorption. In the high ascorbic environment created by the formula, this iron is likely to be in the ferrous form and consequently be absorbed to an extent similar to that of ferrous sulfate.

The effect of human lactoferrin on iron absorption

Animal studies

The newborn rhesus monkey is an excellent model for the human infant. Its nutrient requirements and the development of its gastrointestinal function are very similar to human infants. In addition, rhesus monkey milk has a composition which closely resembles that of human milk[49]. In fact, lactoferrin is the major iron-binding protein of rhesus milk and the isolated protein was found to be almost identical to human lactoferrin with regard to molecular weight, carbohydrate content, amino acid composition and *N*-terminal sequence[50]. Close similarity was demonstrated by the binding of the human lactoferrin antibody to rhesus lactoferrin. Similar to the human lactoferrin receptor, bovine lactoferrin was not found to bind to the rhesus lactoferrin receptor.

We therefore used the infant rhesus monkey to evaluate the effect of human lactoferrin as well as bovine lactoferrin on iron absorption[51]. Care was taken to assure proper labelling of all iron-binding ligands with an extrinsic tag of ^{59}Fe and that a realistic meal size was used. Fasted animals were then fed the radiolabelled meals consisting of human milk whey-predominant formula with without ferrous sulfate fortification or bovine or human lactoferrin. Iron (^{59}Fe) retention was monitored in a whole body counter. In order to correct for large interindividual variations in iron absorption, a reference dose of ^{55}Fe in a ferrous ascorbate solution was given to each animal. No significant differences in iron absorption were found between groups. It is possible that the bovine lactoferrin was ineffective because of its lack of binding to the lactoferrin receptor and that the human lactoferrin had been somewhat altered during the isolation procedure and therefore did not behave as when *in vivo*. Alternatively, human and bovine lactoferrin may not have a pronounced effect on iron absorption in this model.

Human studies

Obtaining large quantities of isolated human lactoferrin for clinical studies on human infants has been difficult. We therefore used an alternative approach to evaluate the effect of human lactoferrin on iron absorption in human infants[52]. In this study, term, healthy infants were given breast milk or breast milk without lactoferrin, and iron absorption was followed by using a stable isotope of iron (^{58}Fe) and iron incorporation into red blood cells. Lactoferrin was removed by first gently removing fat and casein from the breast milk by centrifugation and then separating the lactoferrin from the whey fraction by affinity chromatography on heparin-Sepharose. The lactoferrin-free whey was then added back to the fat and the casein and the fractions were then gently stirred to homogeneity. Intact breast milk and lactoferrin-free breast milk were then extrinsically labelled with the isotope. A period of 48 h of labelling was used to assure proper labelling (isotope exchange). All infants were exclusively breast-fed and each infant was fed their own mother's milk. Iron absorption was found to be slightly higher from the lactoferrin-free milk than from intact breast milk. However, caution must be used when evaluating these results. In order to feed sufficient quantities of the stable isotope to allow detection, relatively large volumes of milk were needed and, consequently, larger infants. Therefore, all infants except one were older than four months of age. We have found earlier that by this age most of the lactoferrin in breast milk is digested and it is therefore possible that the amount of intact lactoferrin that survived and reached the receptors was very small. It is interesting to note that in the only infant that was younger than four months, iron absorption was higher from intact breast milk than from the lactoferrin-free milk. Unfortunately, the total number of infants studied was low. It should also be cautioned that even if we attempted to remove the lactoferrin by gentle methods, the milk had been processed, possibly altering its properties and therefore, possibly, the effect on iron absorption. Finally, the role of homeostasis on iron absorption must be carefully considered. It is possible that long-term iron status has more pronounced effects on iron absorption (and erythrocyte incorporation of iron) than dietary components during a short-term study. However, evaluation of iron status at this age is very difficult. Thus, the relative importance of these two factors is complicated to assess with any degree of certainty.

Recombinant human lactoferrin

With the advent of the techniques of genetic engineering it has become possible to produce recombinant human lactoferrin. The cDNA for human lactoferrin was cloned and the gene has subsequently been inserted into yeast[53], baby hamster kidney (BHK) cells[54], *Aspergillus*[55] and cows[56]. The two latter systems are likely to produce large quantities of recombinant lactoferrin that may be used in infant formula manufacture. There are, however, still many hurdles to overcome before this will occur. The stability of the transgene in transgenic cows and the long time needed for each generation are some of the problems encountered with this approach. Expression levels and potential antigenic contaminants from the fungi are potential problems with the *Aspergillus* system. Approval from authorities to use the recombinant lactoferrin in infant diets may also be difficult to obtain, as noted in some European countries. Finally, the effect of heat treatment of the formula on the biological properties of the recombinant lactoferrin needs to be evaluated carefully. Although there are several apparent obstacles before recombinant lactoferrin can be produced in large scale and incorporated into infant formula, it is likely that the effect of human lactoferrin on iron absorption can be evaluated more carefully with the recombinant form. The slight concern that the recombinant form of lactoferrin will have a different glycan composition than native human lactoferrin is largely alleviated by the finding that the glycans are not required for receptor recognition[39].

Is there a role for lactoferrin in iron absorption?

It is apparent from the discussion above that there is little unequivocal evidence for improved iron absorption from neither human or bovine lactoferrin. There is, however, ample evidence for a lactoferrin receptor in the small intestine, which strongly suggests that lactoferrin is involved in iron delivery to the cell. Recent studies have shown that human lactoferrin facilitates the uptake of iron into human small intestinal cells in culture[57,58]. However, lactoferrin is digested inside the cell and the iron is released. Thus, other factors may determine the subsequent fate of this iron. There are also other biological advantages with lactoferrin as a vehicle for iron absorption. First, lactoferrin has the capacity to bind and deliver ferric iron, which is less prone to cause any oxidative damage. Second, iron bound to lactoferrin is less likely to cause any interaction with the absorption of other divalent cations. It has been shown previously that higher levels of iron may reduce copper absorption[59] and copper and selenium status[6]. Thus, presenting iron in the form of human lactoferrin may be a biologically 'safe' way to assure iron absorption in breast-fed infants and to minimize any negative effects of iron.

References

1. Stekel, A. (1984): Iron requirements in infancy and childhood. In: *Iron nutrition in infancy and childhood*, ed. A. Stekel, pp. 1–10. New York: Nestle Nutrition/Raven Press.

2. Siimes, M.A., Salmenperä, L. & Perheentupa, J. (1984): Exclusive breast-feeding for 9 months: risk of iron deficiency. *J. Pediatr.* **104,** 196–199.

3. Saarinen, U.M. & Siimes, M.A. (1977): Iron absorption from infant milk formula and the optimal level of iron supplementation. *Acta Paediatr. Scand.* **66,** 719–722.

4. Picciano, M.F. & Deering, R.H. (1980): The influence of feeding regimens on iron status during infancy. *Am. J. Clin. Nutr.* **33,** 746–753.

5. Duncan, B., Schifman, R.B., Corrigan, J.J. & Schaefer, C. (1985): Iron and the exclusively breast-fed infant from birth to 6 months. *J. Pediatr. Gastroenterol. Nutr.* **4,** 421–425.

6. Lönnerdal, B. & Hernell, O. (1994): Iron, zinc, copper and selenium status of breast-fed infants and infants fed trace element fortified milk-based infant formula. *Acta Paediatr.* **83,** 367– 373.

7. Fuchs, G.J., Farris, R.P., DeWier, M., Hutchinson, S.W., Warrier, R., Doucet, H. & Suskind, R.M. (1993): Iron status and intake of older infants fed formula *vs* cow milk with cereal. *Am. J. Clin. Nutr.* **58,** 343–348.

8. Bradley, C.K., Hillman, L., Pennridge Pediatric Associates, Sherman, A.R., Leedy, D., Caylor-Nickel Research Institute Inc. & Cordano, A. (1993): Evaluation of two iron-fortified, milk-based formulas during infancy. *Pediatrics* **91,** 908–914.

9. Hernell, O., Lönnerdal, B. (1996): Iron requirements and prevalence of iron deficiency in term infants during the first 6 months of life (this volume, Chapter 13).

10. Fransson, G.B. & Lonnerdal, B. (1980): Iron in human milk. *J. Pediatr.* **2,** 693–701.

11. Garby, L. & Sjolin, S. (1959): Absorption of labelled iron in infants less than three months old. *Acta Paediatr.* **48,** (suppl. 117) 24–28.

12. Schultz, J. & Smith, N.J. (1958): A quantitative study of food iron in infants and children. *J. Dis. Child* **95,** 109– 119.

13. Saarinen, U., Siimes, M. & Dallman, P. (1977): Iron absorption in infants: High bioavailability of breast-milk iron as indicated by the extrinsic tag method of iron absorption and by the concentration of serum ferritin. *J. Pediatr.* **91,** 36–39.

14. Lönnerdal, B. (1984): Iron in breast milk. In: *Iron nutrition in infancy and childhood*, ed. A. Stekel, Vol. 4, pp. 95–118. Nestlé Nutrition Workshop Series. New York: Raven Press.

15. Gislason, J., Jones, B., Lönnerdal, B. & Hambraeus, L. (1992): Iron absorption differs in piglets fed extrinsically and intrinsically ^{59}Fe-labelled sow's milk. *J. Nutr.* **122,** 1287–1292.

16. Fransson, G.B. & Lönnerdal B. (1983): Distribution of trace elements and minerals in human and cow's milk. *Pediatr. Res.* **17,** 912–915.

17. Masson, P.L. & Heremans, J.F. (1971): Lactoferrin in milk from different species. *Comp. Biochem. Physiol.* **39B,** 119–129.

18. Kunz, C. & Lönnerdal, B. (1992): Re-evaluation of the whey protein/casein ratio of human milk. *Acta Paediatr.* **81,** 107–112.

19. Johansson, B.G. (1960): Isolation of an iron-containing red protein from human milk. *Acta Chem. Scand.* **14,** 510–512.

20. Lönnerdal, B. & Iyer, S. (1995): Lactoferrin: molecular structure and biological function. *Ann. Rev. Nutr.* **15,** 93–110.

21. Spik, G., Coddville, B. & Montreuil, J. (1988): Comparative study of the primary structures of sero-, lacto- and ovotransferrin glycans from different species. *Biochimie* **70,** 1459–1469.

22. Brines, R.D. & Brock, J.H. (1983): The effect of trypsin and chymotrypsin on the in vitro antimicrobial and iron-binding properties of lactoferrin in human milk and bovine colostrum: unusual resistance of human lactoferrin to proteolytic digestion. *Biochim. Biophys. Acta* **759,** 229–35.

23. Bullen, J.J., Rogers, H.J. & Leigh, L. (1972): Iron-binding proteins in milk and resistance to Escherichia coli infection in infants. *Br. Med. J.* **1,** 69–65.

24. Tomita, M., Bellamy, W., Takase, M., Yamauchi, K., Wakabayashi, H. & Kawase, K. (1991): Potent antibacterial peptides generated by pepsin digestion of bovine lactoferrin. *J. Dairy Sci.* **74,** 4137–4142.

25. Davidson, L.A. & Lönnerdal, B. (1987): Persistence of human milk proteins in the breast-fed infant. *Acta Pediatr. Scand.* **76,** 733–740.

26. Nichols, B.L., McKee, K.S., Henry, J.F. & Putman, M. (1987): Human lactoferrin stimulates thymidine incorporation into DNA of rat crypt cells. *Pediatr. Res.* **21,** 563–567.

27. Nichols, N.L., McKee, K., Putman, M., Henry, J.F. & Nichols, V.N. (1989): Human lactoferrin supplementation of infant formulas increases thymidine incorporation into the DNA of rat crypt cells. *J. Pediatr. Gastroenterol. Nutr.* **8,** 102–109.

28. Birgens, H.S., Hansen, N.E., Karle, H. & Kristensen, L.O. (1983): Receptor binding of lactoferrin by human monocytes. *Br. J. Haematol.* **54,** 383–391.

29. Ellison, R.T. & Giehl, T.J. (1991): Killing of gram-negative bacteria by lactoferrin and lysozyme. *J. Clin. Invest.* **88,** 1080–1091.

30. Crouch, S.P.M., Slater, K.J. & Fletcher, J. (1992): Regulation of cytokine release from mononuclear cells by the iron-binding protein lactoferrin. *Blood* **80,** 235–240.

31. Hutchens, T.W., Henry, J.F., Yip, T.T., Hachey, D.I., Schanler, R.J., Motil, K.J. & Garza, C. (1991): Origin of intact lactoferrin and its DNA-binding fragments found in the urine of human-milk fed preterm infants. Evaluation of stable isotope enrichment. *Pediatr. Res.* **29,** 243–250.

32. He, J. & Furmanski, P. (1995): Sequence specificity and transcriptional activation in the binding of lactoferrin to DNA. *Nature* **373**, 721–727.

33. Cox, T.M., Mazurier, J., Spik, G., Montreuil, J. & Peters, T.J. (1979): Iron binding proteins and influx of iron across the duodenal brush-border. Evidence for specific lactotransferrin receptors in the human intestine. *Biochim. Biophys. Acta* **558,** 129–141.

34. Hu, W.L., Mazurier, J., Sawatzki. G., Montreuil, J. & Spik, G. (1988): Lactotransferrin receptor of mouse small intestinal brush border. *Biochem. J.* **248,** 435–441.

35. Hu, W.L., Mazurier, J., Montreuil, J. & Spik, G. (1990): Isolation and partial characterization of a lactotransferrin receptor from mouse intestinal brush border. *Biochemistry* **29,** 535–541.

36. Davidson, L.A. & Lönnerdal, B. (1988): Specific binding of lactoferrin to brush-border membrane: ontogeny and effect of glycan chain. *Am. J. Physiol.* **254,** G580–G585.

37. Davidson, L.A. & Lönnerdal, B. (1989): Fe-saturation and proteolysis of human lactoferrin: effect on brush-border receptor-mediated uptake of Fe and Mn. *Am. J. Physiol.* **257,** G930–G934.

38. Gislason, J., Iyer, S., Hutchens, T.W. & Lönnerdal, B. (1993): Lactoferrin receptors in piglet small intestine: binding kinetics, specificity, ontogeny and regional distribution. *J. Nutr. Biochem.* **4,** 528–533.

39. Kawakami, H. & Lönnerdal, B. (1991): Isolation and function of a receptor for human lactoferrin in human fetal intestinal brush-border membranes. *Am. J. Physiol.* **261,** G841–G846.

40. Mazurier, J., Legrand, D., Hu, W.L., Montreuil, J. & Spik, G. (1989): Expression of human lactotransferrin receptors in phytohemagglutinin-stimulated human peripheral blood lymphocytes. Isolation of the receptors by antiligand-affinity chromatography. *Eur. J. Biochem.* **179,** 481–487.

41. Hurrell, R.F., Lynch, S.R., Trinidad, T.P., Dassenko, S.A. & Cook, J.D. (1989): Iron absorption as influenced by bovine milk proteins. *Am. J .Clin. Nutr.* **49,** 546–552.

42. Fransson, G.B., Thoren-Tolling, K., Jones, B., Hambraeus, L. & Lönnerdal, B. (1983): Absorption of lactoferrin-iron in suckling pigs. *Nutr. Res.* **3,** 373–384.

43. Fransson, G.B., Keen, C.L. & Lönnerdal, B. (1983): Supplementation of milk with iron bound to lactoferrin using weanling mice: I. Effects on hematology and tissue iron. *J. Pediatr. Gastroenterol. Nutr.* **2,** 693–700.

44. Kawakami, H., Hiratsuka, M. & Dosako, S. (1988): Effects of iron-saturated lactoferrin on iron absorption. *Agric. Biol. Chem.* **52,** 903–908.

45. Kawakami, H., Dosako, S. & Lönnerdal, B. (1990): Iron uptake from transferrin and lactoferrin by rat intestinal brush-border membrane vesicles. *Am. J. Physiol.* G535–G541.

46. Fairweather-Tait, S.J., Balmer, S.E., Scott, P.H. & Ninski, M.J. (1987): Lactoferrin and iron absorption in newborn infants. *Pediatr. Res.* **22,** 651–654.

47. Schulz-Lell, G., Dörner, K., Oldigs, H.D., Sievers, E. & Schaub, J. (1991): Iron availability from an infant formula supplemented with bovine lactoferrin. *Acta Paediatr. Scand.* **80,** 155–158.

48. Chierici, R., Sawatzki, G., Tamisari, L., Volpato, S. & Vig,i V. (1992): Supplementation of an adapted formula with bovine lactoferrin. 2. Effects on serum iron, ferritin and zinc levels. *Acta Paediatr.* **81,** 475–479.

49. Lonnerdal, B., Keen, C.L., Glazier, C.E. & Anderson, J. (1984): A longitudinal study of rhesus monkeys (Macaca mulatta) milk composition: trace elements, minerals, protein, carbohydrate and fat. *Pediatr Res.* **18,** 911–914.

50. Davidson, L.A. & Lönnerdal, B. (1986): Isolation and characterization of monkey milk lactoferrin. *Pediatr. Res.* **20,** 197–201.

51. Davidson, L.A., Litov, R.E. & Lönnerdal, B. (1990): Iron retention from lactoferrin-supplemented fommulas in infant rhesus monkeys. *Pediatr. Res.* **27,** 176–180.

52. Davidsson, L., Kastenmayer, P., Yuen, M., Lönnerdal, B. & Hurrell, R.F. (1994): Influence of lactoferrin on iron absorption from human milk in infants. *Pediatr. Res.* **35,** 117–124.

53. Liang, Q. & Richardson, T. (1993): Expression and characterization of human lactoferrin in yeast Saccharomyces cerevisiae. *J. Agric. Food Chem.* **41,** 1800–1807.

54. Stowell, K.M., Rado, T.A., Funk, W.D. & Tweedie, J.W. (1991): Expression of cloned human lactoferrin in baby-hamster kidney cells. *Biochem. J.* **276,** 349–345.

55. Ward, P.P., May, G.S., Headon, D.R. & Conneely, O.M. (1992): An inducible expression system for the production of human lactoferrin in Aspergillus nidulans. *Gene* **122,** 219–223.

56. Krimpenfort, P. (1993): The production of human lactoferrin in the milk of transgenic animals. *Cancer Detection & Prevention* **17,** 301–305.

57. Iyer, S., Yuen, M. & Lönnerdal, B. (1993): Binding and uptake of human lactoferrin by its intestinal receptor studied in Caco-2 cells. *FASEB J.* **7,** A64. (Abstract)

58. Mikogami, T., Heyman, M., Spik, G. & Desjeux, J.F. (1994): Apical-to-basolateral transepithelial transport of human lactoferrin in the intestinal cell line HT-29CL. 19A. *Am. J. Physiol.* **267,** G308–G315.

59. Haschke, F., Ziegler, E.E., Edwards, B.B. & Fomon, S.J. (1986): Effect of iron fortification of infant formula on trace mineral absorption. *J. Pediatr. Gastroenterol. Nutr.* **5,** 768–773.

Iron Nutrition in Health and Disease, edited by Leif Hallberg and Nils-Georg Asp
©1996 John Libbey & Company Ltd., pp. 325–329

Chapter 32

Iron nutritional status during early childhood - the importance of weaning foods to combat iron deficiency

Ferdinand Haschke and Christoph Male

University of Vienna, 18–20 Währinger Gürtel, A - 1090 Vienna, Austria

Summary

Socioeconomic factors, low iron intake with food, delayed introduction of solids, and the early introduction of cow's milk are the main factors contributing to high prevalence of iron deficiency in most industrialized and developing countries. In most European countries, public health measures and food-fortification programmes still need to be improved. Metabolic and clinical studies have shown that iron fortified cereals and baby foods can be alternatives to iron fortified formulas to combat iron deficiency during late infancy.

Epidemiology of iron deficiency and anaemia

Epidemiological data

Data on prevalence of iron deficiency and anaemia related to iron deficiency have been summarized by WHO in 1985[4] (Table 1). Such data are important since even mild or moderate iron deficiency anaemia in the second 6 months of life and beyond infancy can be associated with delayed mental and motor development and the outcome after appropriate iron treatment is inconsistent[13,14,19]. It may be that relatively brief periods of iron deficiency during a vulnerable 'age window of risk' can result in long-lasting consequences for behavioural and mental developmental status even in a school population. If this is true, a public health shift from early detection and treatment to primary prevention of iron deficiency anaemia is appropriate for most countries in the world.

Table 1 Prevalence of iron deficiency (0–5) years

Region	No studies	Prevalence	Mean (range)
Africa	45	59	(15–93)
Latin America	35	34	(12–69)
East Asia	5	46	(15–80)
South Asia	43	51	(2–92)
Europe			
Northern	3	5	(0–11)
Western	2	6	(3–9)
Southern	1	34	
Eastern	–	34 (?)	

Source: WHO[4]

Surveys of anaemia world–wide for children between and 5 years of age indicate that[4] (Table 1) estimated prevalences in less developed countries are generally high. Since the agespan is rather wide, it is impossible to obtain specific information published on infants.

Few studies from European countries are included in the WHO report, but it seems rather evident that the estimated prevalences were lower in the 1970s and 1980s in Europe than in less developed countries. Recent data on the prevalence of iron deficiency and anaemia were collected between 1992 and 1994 as part of the Euro-Growth study. During this longitudinal study to evaluate the interactions between nutrition, health and growth, blood samples of 520 healthy infants from 11 European cities were collected at 12 months of age. Nine point eight per cent had haemoglobin values below 11 g/dl and 23.7 per cent had ferritin values below 12 ng/ml. Six per cent of the infants were anaemic and had signs of iron deficiency (low ferritin and/or low MCV). This indicates that public health measures and food-fortification programmes still need to be improved in most European countries.

Recent data from Canada and the USA are also available. Fullterm infants born between 1990 and 1992 were studied by Zlotkin *et al.*[22]. Their age at the time of blood sampling was between 8.5 and 15.5 months and infants with acute or chronic diseases were excluded. The laboratory results of 428 infants from four Canadian cities indicate that 8 per cent had haemoglobin levels below 11 g/dl. However, only 1.1 per cent of the infants studied had haemoglobin values below 10 g/dl. One out of three Canadian infants at that age range had depleted iron stores, if 10 ng/ml was considered as the adequate cut-off value. It is of interest that only 4.3 per cent of the infants had both low haemoglobin and ferritin values. Thus in more than 50 per cent of the infants with anaemia there was no biochemical proof of iron deficiency. During this conference Dallman *et al.* (1995) presented preliminary data from the NHANES III from the USA, where the prevalence of iron deficiency anaemia in children between 1 and 2 years of age is now as low as 3.5 per cent, substantially lower than in Canada and Europe.

Factors contributing to anaemia

Infection, genetic and socioeconomic factors, and low iron intake play important roles in the development of hypochromic anaemia during early childhood. Evidence suggests that the prevalence of iron deficiency anaemia in young British children varies greatly according to social circumstances and has been shown to approach 30 per cent in the most disadvantaged groups (Stevens 1991). Preliminary data from the NHANES III[1] indicate that iron intake in the US is higher than in Austria, a member country of the European Union (Table 2). This is probably related to the general use of iron fortified formulas and the higher iron-fortification level of infant formulas in the USA. Indeed, it seems that the prevalence of iron deficiency during late infancy is lower in the USA than in Europe.

Does prolonged exclusive breast-feeding contribute to poor iron-nutritional status? It is well established that iron concentration in breast-milk declines during the course of lactation[17]. Studies on exclusively breast-fed infants in different countries show that iron deficiency is virtually absent at 6 months of age but may become evident in a small percentage of infants at 9–12 months of age[10,11,16]. Another factor contributing to iron deficiency in industrialized and developing countries is the early introduction of cow's milk into the infants diet. Consumption of cow's milk as the liquid part of the infants diet results in low iron intake, can cause gastrointestinal blood loss, and negatively interacts with iron absorption because of the high protein and calcium concentrations in cow's milk[7,21]. Both the Canadian[23] and the Euro-Growth[16] studies confirm the negative influence of early introduction of cow's milk on iron nutritional status of older infants.

Table 2. Mean iron intake (g/day) between 2 and 24 months

Month	**NHANES III, USA 1988–91**	**Austria 1988**
< 11	15.5	4.8[a] 10.3[b]
12–24	9.5	7.4

[a]Non-fortified formula [b]Iron fortified formula

Weaning foods to combat iron deficiency

Cereals

There are several reasons for selecting iron fortified infant cereals as a vehicle to combat iron deficiency. Cereal products are relatively inexpensive and have a long shelf life. Moreover, they are distributed through infant feeding programmes in industrialized and developing countries. Although they have been on the market since the 1950s, their effectiveness in preventing iron deficiency is still under discussion. A major disadvantage of infant cereal as the main source of iron is that the amount consumed varies substantially from infant to infant.

Iron absorption from infant cereals

The first data in 4–6 month-old infants were published by Rios[17], who used iron–59 as an extrinsic label to calculate the absorption of fortification iron from rice cereal and infant formula in 4–6 month-old infants. Geometric mean absorption was 0.7 per cent for ferric orthophosphate, 1 per cent for sodium iron pyrophosphate, 2.7 per cent for ferrous sulfate, and 4 per cent for electrolytic iron powder. Absorption of electrolytic iron from cereal was about 4 per cent, which was similar to the percentage iron absorption from infant formulas fortified with ferrous sulfate. However, if added to dry infant cereals, ferrous sulfate would promote oxidative rancidity and the electrolytic iron powder studied[17] was of considerably smaller particle size than that used in commercial fortification of infant cereals. Ferrous fumarate has been suggested as an attractive iron preparation for cereal fortification[12]. The stable isotope technique[7] showed that mean erythrocyte incorporation of iron from rice-based cereal meals fortified with ferrous sulfate and ferrous fumarate in 4–6-month-old infants was 4.4 per cent and 4.0 per cent of intake, respectively. Recently it has been shown that the addition of ascorbic acid to a whole-wheat breakfast cereal test meal increases mean erythrocyte incorporation of iron from 3.1 to 7.5 per cent of intake[15].

Clinical data

The results of clinical studies on iron nutritional status of infants receiving iron fortified cereals are conflicting[20]. Comparisons between iron fortified rice cereal and unfortified rice cereal were made in infants who were exclusively breast-fed for more than 4 months, and with iron fortified formula in infants who were weaned to formula before 4 months of age. The infants were followed from 4 to 15 months of age. The cumulative percentages of infants excluded from the study until 15 months of age on the basis of a low haemoglobin value (<105 g/l) were 4 per cent, 8 per cent, and 24 per cent in the groups fed the fortified formula, fortified cereal, and non-fortified food, respectively. The authors concluded that iron fortified infant cereal can play a significant role in prevention of iron deficiency anaemia but iron fortified formulas presented a slight advantage. Fuchs *et al.*[8] prospectively studied infants from 4–6 to 12 months of age who were randomly assigned to receive whole cow's milk plus iron fortified cereal, one of two iron fortified follow-up formulas, or an iron fortified infant formula. By 12 months of age, mean serum ferritin (Fig. 1) and mean corpuscular volume of the erythrocytes were lower in the group fed cow's milk and the iron fortified cereal. Moreover, 29 per cent of the infants in that group had serum ferritin values below 12 ng/ml and 24 per cent MCV below 70 fl. In the three groups fed the iron fortified formulas, low ferritin values were found in 0–4 per cent only and low MCV in 0–7 per cent. It remains uncertain whether poor bioavailability of iron from cereal and/or feeding of cow's milk was the main factor contributing to poorer iron nutritional status than in the other groups at 12 months of age.

Other weaning foods

Commercially prepared baby foods fortified with ferrous sulfate and ascorbic acid are available in many European countries. If meat is also present, the iron in these foods is assumed to be of high bioavailability because meat and ascorbic acid[2,5] enhance the bioavailability of non-haem (i.e. fortification) iron. In a prospective study, healthy term infants received non-fortified formula and iron mainly from fortification iron in baby foods from 4 to 12 months of age[8]. Their mean iron intake was only 0.42–0.65 mg/kg/day between 274 and 365 days of age, which is substantially below the estimated requirements[7]. However, none of the infants had a

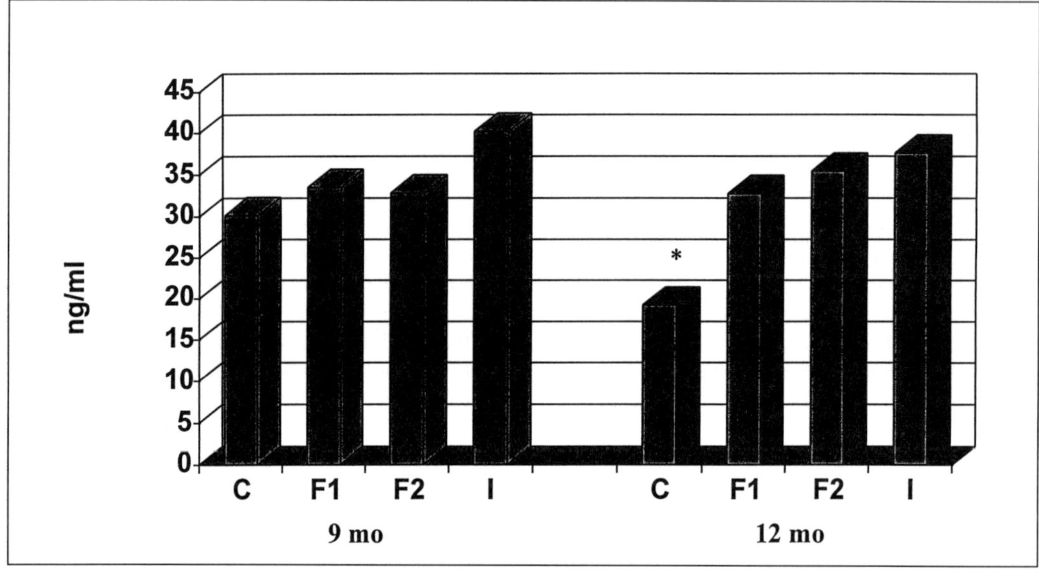

*Fig. 1. Serum ferritin of infants fed iron fortified cereal + cow's milk (C), iron fortified follow-up formulas (F1, F2), or iron fortified infant formula (I). * Indicates $p < 0.05$ compared to F1,F2, and I. (Data from Fuchs et al.,[8])*

haemoglobin value below 100 g/l and only 8 per cent had ferritin below 10 ng/ml at 12 months of age. This indicates that regular feeding of such baby foods may be a convenient and effective way of providing iron to infants who are breast-fed or receive cow's milk between 6 and 12 months of age.

References

1. Alaimo, K., McDowell, M.A., Briefel, R.R., Bischof, A.M., Caughman, C.R., Loria, C.M. & Johnson, C.L.: *Dietary intake of vitamins, minerals, and fiber of persons ages 2 months and over in the United States.* Third National and Nutrition Examination Survey, Phase 1 (1988–1991).
2. Cook, J.D. & Monsen, E.R. (1976): Food iron absorption.III Comparison of the effect of animal proteins on nonheme iron absorption. *Am. J. Clin. Nutr.* **29,** 859–867.
3. Dallman, P.R., Looker, A.C., Carroll, M. & Johnson, C.L. (1996): Influence of age on laboratory criteria for the diagnosis of iron deficiency and iron deficiency anemia in infants and children (this volume, Chapter 6).
4. DeMaeyer, E. & Adiels-Tegman, M. The prevalence of anemia in the world. *World Health Stat. Q.* **38,** 302–316.
5. Derman, D.P., Bothwell, T.H. & MacPhail, A.P. (1980): Importance of ascorbic acid in the absorption of iron from infant foods. *Scand. J. Hematol.* **25,** 193–201.
6. Fairweather-Tait, S., Fox, T., Wharf, G. & Eagles, J. (1995): The bioavailability of iron in different weaning foods and the enhancing effect of a fruit drink containing ascorbic acid. *Pediatr. Res.* **37,** 389–394.
7. Fomon, S.J. (1993): *Nutrition of Normal Infants.* Mosby, St.Louis.

8. Fuchs, G.J., Farris, R.P., DeWier, M., Hutchinson, S.W., Warrier, R., Doucet, H. & Suskind, R.M. (1993): Iron intake of older infants fed formula *vs* cow milk with cereal. *Am. J. Clin. Nutr.* **58,** 343–348.

9. Haschke, F., Pietschnig, B., Vanura, H., Heil, M., Steffan, I., Hobiger, G., Schuster, E. & Camaya, Z. (1989): Iron intake and iron nutritional status of infants fed iron-fortified beikost with meat. *Am. J. Clin. Nutr.* **47,** 108–112.

10. Haschke, F., Vanura, H., Male, C., Owen, G., Pietschnig, B., Schuster, E., Krobath, E. & Huemer, C. (1993): Iron nutrition and growth of breast- and formula-fed infants during the first 9 months of life. *J. Pediatr. Gastroenterol. Nutr.* **16,** 151–156.

11. Hernell, O., Lundström, M., Persson, L.A. & Lönnerdal, B. (1996): Iron requirements and prevalence of iron deficiency during the first year of life in term infants (this volume, Chapter 12).

12. Hurrell, R.F., Furniss, D.E., Burri, J., Whittaker, P., Lynch, S.R. & Cook, J.D. (1989): Iron fortification of infant cereals: a proposal for the use of ferrous fumarate or ferrous succinate. *Am. J. Clin. Nutr.* **49,** 1274–1282.

13. Lozoff, B., Brittenham, G.M., Wolf, A.W., McClish, D.K., Kuhnert, P.M., Jimenez, E., Jimenez, R., Mora, L.A., Gomez, I. & Krauskoph, D. (1987): Iron deficiency and iron therapy effects on infant developmental test performance. *Pediatrics* **79,** 981–995.

14. Lozoff, B. (1994): Iron deficiency and infant development. *J. Pediatr.* **125,** 577–578.

15. Male, C., Barko, E., Freeman, V., Golser, A., Guerra, A., Haschke, F., van't Hof, M., Manrique, M., Persson, L., Radke, M., Salerno, C., Sanchez, E., Tojo, R. & Zachou, T. (1995): Iron status of European infants at 12 months of age. (abstract) 7th European Nutrition Conference, Vienna.

16. Pisacane, A., De Vizia, B., Valiante, A., Vaccaro, F., Russo, M., Grillo, G. & Giustardi, A. (1995): Iron status in breast-fed infants. *J. Pediatr.* **127,** 429–431.

17. Rios, E., Hunter, R.E., Cook, J.D., Smith, N.J. &., Finch, C.A. (1975): The absorption of iron as supplements in infant cereal and infant formulas. *Pediatrics* **55,** 686–693.

18. Siimes, M.A., Vuori, E. & Kuitunen, P. (1979): Breast milk iron - a declining concentration during the course of lactation. *Acta Paediatr. Scand.* **68,** 29–31.

19. Walter, T. (1993): Impact of iron deficiency on cognition in infancy and childhood. *Eur. J. Clin. Nutr.* **47,** 307–316.

20. Walter, T., Dallman, P.R., Pizarro, F., Velozo, L., Pena, G., Bartholomey, S.J., Hertrampf, E., Olivares, M., Letelier, A. & Arredondo, M. (1993): Effectiveness of iron-fortified infant cereal in prevention of iron deficiency anemia. *Pediatrics* **91,** 976– 982.

21. Ziegler, E.E., Fomon, S.J., Nelson, S.E., Rebouche, C.J., Edwards, B.B., Rogers, R.R. & Lehman, L.J. (1990): Cow milk feeding in infancy: further observations on blood loss from the gastrointestinal tract. *J. Pediatr.* **116,** 11–18.

22. Zlotkin, S.h., Marie, M.S., Kopelman, H. & Jones, A. (1995): The prevalence of iron depletion and iron-deficiency anemia in a randomly selected group of infants from four Canadian cities (unpublished).

Iron Nutrition in Health and Disease, edited by Leif Hallberg and Nils-Georg Asp
©1996 John Libbey & Company Ltd., pp. 331–339

Chapter 33

Strategies to prevent iron deficiency in adults

T.H. Bothwell

Department of Medicine, University of the Witwatersrand Medical School, 7 York Road, Parktown 2193, Johannesburg, South Africa

Summary

Although supplementation and fortification programmes have been the ones that have received most attention, there is a good deal of current interest in the possible role of dietary modifications on iron nutrition. In this context, the two main approaches that might be followed involve the increased consumption with meals of fruits and vegetables containing ascorbic acid and the decreased consumption of inhibitors, such as tea. In addition, a reduction in the phytate content of cereals by better milling techniques is another potential strategy. Although it is still not clear how these various approaches can be translated into realistic programmes to combat nutritional iron deficiency, it should be emphasized that food education may for some time be the main and even the only method available for improving iron nutrition in certain parts of the world.

Introduction

Iron deficiency anaemia remains a major problem in the world today and is particularly prevalent in developing countries. The groups that are particularly vulnerable are infants, young children and women during their reproductive times. Because of the high prevalence of iron deficiency anaemia and its attendant pathological sequelae, various strategies have been devised to prevent it, including iron supplementation and fortification. The strategies have varied from those targeted at vulnerable groups, such as infants, to broader based fortification programmes supplying increased amounts of dietary iron to the population at large. The current situation, insofar as infants are concerned, has already been reviewed at this symposium and the present discussion will therefore be confined to adults. In this discussion particular attention will be paid to areas of uncertainty and debate, since there are several recent reviews in which guidelines for the implementation of supplementation and fortification programmes have been laid down[1] and the relative advantages of different iron fortificants have been analysed[2–5]. Nevertheless, several questions relating to the efficacy and safety of the current fortification programmes in industrialized societies still remain, while the prevention of iron deficiency in developing countries using fortification strategies is an issue that remains largely unaddressed.

Current iron fortification policies

In general, fortification involves the addition of nutrients to foods in order to maintain or improve the quality of the diet. Such nutrients are usually added to cereals, such as milled wheat flour and corn meal, which tend to be processed centrally and consumed by a large proportion of the population. The degree to which fortification forms the basis of a nutritional intervention programme depends on how much of the nutrient is added. Insofar as iron is concerned, there are significant variations from country to country in the amounts of fortification iron that are used. For example, until recently wheat flour was fortified with 65 ppm in Sweden, as compared with 44 ppm in the USA and 16.5 ppm in the UK[6]. This last figure does not even raise the iron content of the flour to that of the native whole wheat prior to milling, whereas the Swedish fortification doubles it. Such considerations must be borne in mind when attempting to assess the overall effects of different fortification programmes.

Practical aspects of iron fortification

The amounts of fortification iron absorbed from a particular diet are dependent on three factors. These include the iron status of the individuals consuming the diet, the composition of the diet, and the relative bioavailability of the iron fortificant[4]. Iron status is important, in that more iron is absorbed when the body is iron deficient. However, the actual amounts absorbed are markedly influenced by the nature of the diet. There are two types of iron in the diet, haem iron (derived from haemoglobin and myoglobin) and non-haem iron (derived mainly from cereals, vegetables and fruit)[7,8]. Most forms of non-haem iron in a meal, whatever their origin, enter a common pool during digestion and are thus equally susceptible to a number of promoters and inhibitors of iron absorption. The major promoters of iron absorption are meat and ascorbic acid, whereas the major inhibitors are phytates and polyphenols. Iron fortificants, in their turn, are also affected by such factors, with their relative bioavailability also affected by the degree to which they enter the common pool of dietary non-haem iron.

Iron fortificants

Soluble iron fortificants, such as ferrous sulfate, enter the common pool of non-haem iron completely and are absorbed to the same degree as is the intrinsic non-haem iron in the diet[2–5]. Ferrous salts are therefore well absorbed when added to varied Western-type diets but are poorly bioavailable when added to the staple cereal diets consumed in many developing countries, since these diets contain large amounts of inhibitors of iron absorption. Ferrous sulfate and other soluble iron complexes can only be used as fortificants in certain defined situations, since they are chemically reactive and tend to produce undesirable organoleptic changes over time in the vehicles to which they are added[9]. As a result, several other fortificants, which are less soluble under the conditions prevailing in the upper gastrointestinal tract, are in common use. Although such inert compounds do not cause organoleptic changes when stored in a variety of vehicles, they tend to be less well absorbed[2–5]. Their relative bioavailability has been assessed on the basis of their physical characteristics (particle size, reactive surface areas, and solubility in acid), their capacity as compared with ferrous sulfate to restore the haemoglobin level in iron deficient rats, and the degree to which they exchange with the common pool of non-haem iron in the diet in human absorption studies. Reasonable agreement between these different methods has recently been reported in one study in which they were directly compared[10].

There are three type of elemental iron powders which have been used for iron fortification. Carbonyl iron has the smallest particle size and the greatest solubility in dilute hydrochloric acid, followed by electrolytic iron and then by H-reduced iron[11]. However, it has been difficult to translate such characteristics into meaningful bioavailability figures, since different methodologies have provided conflicting results[5,12]. As judged by haemoglobin regeneration in iron deficient rats, elemental iron powders are about half as bioavailable as ferrous sulfate, whereas human absorption studies using radioactively labelled powders have given widely differing results, which are probably attributable to the fact that some of the tested materials differed physically from the commercial compounds[5]. However, in two studies in which the characteristics of the tested material were similar to those of commercially available powders, very low figures for bioavailability were obtained[13,14]. Carbonyl iron was found to have a relative bioavailability which was between 5 and 20 per cent of that of ferrous sulfate[14] and similar low figures were obtained with electrolytic iron which had been made radioactive by neutron activation[15]. The bioavailability of ferric pyrophosphate and ferric orthophosphate, which are other compounds used to fortify cereals, has also been studied in humans. Ferric pyrophosphate was found to have a relative bioavailability of 39 per cent, whereas that of ferric orthophosphate varied from 10 to 31 per cent[5,12].

Vehicles for iron fortification

Bakery products and wheat flour have been fortified to varying levels with iron for several decades and represent the main vehicles for fortification in a number of countries. Ferric pyrophosphate and ferric orthophosphate are widely used in Europe as fortificants in cereals, whereas ferrous sulfate and elemental powders are used in the USA[5]. Ferrous sulfate is very satisfactory as a fortificant when added during the preparation of bread and bakery products, since it is absorbed as well as the intrinsic iron in the flour. It is, however, unsatisfactory in stored flour because of the organoleptic problems it and other soluble sources of iron produce[9]. It is for this reason that elemental iron powders are used in the USA in stored flour and cereal products. In Sweden, carbonyl iron has been the fortificant that has been used[14].

Impact of iron fortification

Fortification iron accounts for about 10 per cent of the dietary intake in the United Kingdom, 20 per cent in the United States and 40 per cent until recently in Sweden[5]. The high levels of fortification in Sweden can be ascribed to the fact that there has been a steady drop in the iron content of the diet over the years. This drop has been ascribed to a number of factors, including changes in eating habits, a marked reduction in the use of iron cooking utensils and increased removal of iron in milling procedures[15]. In assessing the effects of these various fortification programmes, particular attention has been paid to the changes that have occurred in the prevalence of iron deficiency anaemia in different countries. For example, the prevalence in Swedish women dropped from between 25 and 30 per cent in the 1960s to about 7 per cent in the mid-1970s[15]. An even lower prevalence was recorded in the USA in the NHANES II survey, with figures of 0.2 per cent in adult men and 2.6 per cent and 1.9 per cent in pre- and post-menopausal women, respectively[16]. What is more difficult to assess is the degree to which these improvements can be ascribed to iron fortification *per se*. In this context, the figures in Sweden take on particular relevance, since it is the country in which the levels of iron fortification were until recently the highest. Although iron fortification of wheat flour was thought initially to have played a significant role in reducing the prevalence of iron deficiency anaemia[15], it is difficult to reconcile these conclusions with the recently discovered low bioavailability of the fortificant, carbonyl iron[14]. Insofar as the USA is concerned, it is more difficult to make judgements. As discussed previously, there are still doubts as to the relative bioavailability of commercially used electrolytic powders, but the ferrous sulphate added in the preparation of bread and bakery products is a good source of bioavailable iron. It is, however, not clear what relative amounts of these two types of fortificant are consumed by the population.

Because of real doubts concerning the effectiveness of some current fortification programmes, attention needs to be directed to other factors that may have led over the past decades to a decline in the prevalence of iron deficiency anaemia. In this context, two potentially important ones are a reduction in menstrual blood losses due to increasing use of oral contraceptives and the widespread consumption of 'over the counter' preparations containing iron and vitamin supplements[15]. There are also other factors which stem from increased affluence, including smaller families and a wider selection of foods. Perhaps some insight into the relative effects of these various factors and of iron fortification on iron status will be obtained in Sweden over the coming years, since fortification of flour with iron was stopped at the beginning of 1995.

Safety of iron fortification

From the preceding discussion it is apparent that there are still doubts on the relative effectiveness of current fortification programmes in industrialized countries. This aspect has, however, received much less attention than questions relating to the safety of such programmes. It has been argued that attempts to reduce the prevalence of iron deficiency anaemia in women of fertile age expose iron replete subjects to excessive quantities of dietary iron[17]. At special potential risk are those with a tendency to absorb excessive quantities. In this context, subjects homozygous for the HLA-linked iron-loading gene that is associated with haemochromatosis, which occurs with a prevalence of up to 0.3 per cent in some Caucasoid populations, have received special attention[18]. From what is known of iron balance it seems likely that increasing the quantities of bioavailable iron in the diet would have two effects[17]. First, subjects destined to present clinically due to the pathological affects of excessive iron deposits would do so at younger ages than previously. Second, a proportion of asymptomatic homozygotes with only moderate iron overload would be expected to accumulate enough iron to develop clinical symptoms. Recently the debate has widened, with disturbing claims, based on epidemiological data, which suggest that subjects with only modestly raised iron stores are at greater risk of developing malignancy[19] and ischaemic heart disease[20]. Although the debate on this issue is still an open one, it does raise issues relating to the desirability of fortification programmes which supply increased amounts of iron not only to those who need it but also to those who do not. As a result, increasing attention needs to be focused on programmes that are targeted at the most vulnerable sectors of the population, namely infants, young children and pregnant mothers.

Iron fortification strategies for developing countries

There is a real need for effective fortification programmes in many developing countries, since iron deficiency anaemia remains a major problem[21]. Although several countries including Chile, Guyana, Kenya, Zambia and Nigeria require that iron be added to flour[5], logistic problems have largely prevented the development of fortification programmes in the majority. There are two main reasons for this. First, most potential vehicles are not centrally processed and, as a result, alternative ones have had to be used. These have included salt, sugar and condiments. The second problem relates to the predominantly cereal diets consumed by many of the poorer populations. The iron in the cereals, which make up a high proportion of these diets, is poorly absorbed for two reasons[7,8]. Cereals contain large amounts of phytates and polyphenols, which inhibit iron bioavailability, and the diet also contains inadequate amounts of promoters of iron absorption, such as ascorbic acid, meat and fish. If fortification iron is added to such a diet it is affected by the same ligands that inhibit the absorption of the intrinsic iron in the food and is therefore as poorly absorbed.

Several strategies have been developed to render fortification iron more bioavailable. One that has been reported to have been successful involved the use of a stable form of iron, iron orthophosphate, and a promoter of iron absorption, sodium hydrogen sulfate[22]. Perhaps the most promising of the approaches is one involving the use of the chelate iron EDTA as a fortificant. It has two major advantages. It is less affected by inhibitory ligands in the diet than are soluble ferrous salts[22] and it remains stable in the presence of several vehicles, including fish sauce[23], masala[24] and sugar[25]. The efficacy of iron EDTA as a fortificant has been demonstrated in three separate studies[23,23,25]. Particularly impressive were the results in a South African study which demonstrated an overall drop in the prevalence of anaemia in adult Indian women from 22 per cent to 5 per cent over a 2 year period[24]. Equally important was the fact that there was no significant rise in the levels of serum ferritin (and hence iron stores) in adult males. Curry powder was used as the vehicle in this targeted trial in order to ensure that the iron replete black population was not exposed to extra dietary iron. On the basis of all the current evidence, the International Nutritional Anaemia Consultative Group (INACG) has recently produced a monograph on FeNaEDTA which is intended for use by industry, donor agencies, governments, non-governmental organizations and research institutions[26]. In addition, the Joint (FAO/WHO) Expert Committee on Food Additives (JECFA) has granted provisional approval for NaFeEDTA to be used in food fortification programmes. The Codex Alimentarium Commission of the WHO and the Food Agriculture Organization (FAO) bases food standards on JECFA recommendations.

Iron supplementation

Iron requirements during pregnancy are greater than can be supplied by even an optimal diet and for these requirements to be satisfied the mother must enter pregnancy with adequate stores. It is because of such considerations that supplemental iron is widely used during pregnancy. The usual supplement is 30–100 mg daily and it is normally combined with 250–500 ng folate in a once daily formulation. The need for such routine supplementation has, however, been questioned, since data in a recent USA study indicate that iron deficiency anaemia only affects 2.6 per cent of pre-menopausal women[16]. At the same time, data derived from serum ferritin levels suggest that only 15 per cent of women in the USA and 10 per cent of women in Sweden have stores in the range of 300–500 mg, which is the amount required for a full expansion of the red cell mass in the latter part of pregnancy[16,27]. The debate therefore really centres around the issue as to whether such pregnancies are at increased risk. If supplementation is not to be applied routinely in pregnancy, then two prerequisites should be fulfilled. First, there should be prior knowledge of the iron status of the particular group or individual and, secondly, adequate monitoring should be available. If these prerequisites cannot be met then iron supplementation still seems warranted as a means of ensuring optimal iron nutrition in the latter part of pregnancy.

At a practical level, there are several problems associated with the application of effective supplementation programmes, especially in developing countries where the need is greatest. A major one is the lack of compliance attendant on long-term daily administration. In the case of iron, this is compounded by gastrointestinal side effects, especially with higher dosages. Current strategies that have been suggested for overcoming poor compliance include smaller once daily doses (30–60 mg)[28], twice weekly schedules[29], and the use of better tolerated iron preparations (e.g. a gastric delivery system in which the ferrous sulfate is incorporated into a slow release hydrocolloid matrix)[30]. Another strategy perhaps of equal importance for improving compliance is proper education on the importance of supplementation and advice on side effects[28]. At a more general level, prerequisites for effective supplementation programmes include adequate budgetary provisions, the establishment of reliable standards for the supply and storage of the supplements and appropriate training of health professionals. For such programmes to be successful they must not stand alone but must be integrated into the overall provision of primary health care.

Prevention of iron deficiency by diet

Programmes to prevent iron deficiency have focused mainly on iron fortification and supplementation. However, neither of these approaches precludes the use of other strategies to modify iron balance. In this context, the iron status of the body is determined by the degree to which iron absorption from the diet matches iron losses. Both sides of the equation can be modified. For example, menstrual losses can be lowered by oral contraceptive use, while blood loss from the gut can be reduced by combating hookworm infestation in areas where it is endemic. Similarly, iron balance can be influenced by improving iron absorption from the diet. It is this latter approach which is the subject of the present section.

As mentioned previously, the two major sources of dietary iron are haem iron and non-haem iron[7,8]. Haem iron, which is present in meat, poultry and fish, is highly bioavailable and there is epidemiological evidence that iron status correlates well with meat intake[31]. In contrast, the absorption of non-haem iron is variable, being dependent on the relative proportions of promoters and inhibitors of iron absorption present in the diet. The one major promoter is ascorbic acid. The second is meat. Not only is the haem iron in meat, poultry and fish well absorbed, but the meat itself promotes the absorption of non-haem iron[7]. Other promoters include fermented foods, such as sauerkraut and soy sauce[32,33]. The two major inhibitors are phytate, present in cereals, nuts and vegetables, and iron-binding phenolic compounds, which are found in tea, coffee, legumes, sorghum and some spices (e.g. oregano)[7,8,34], Other inhibitors include soy products[35] and calcium[36].

One obvious way to improve dietary iron bioavailability by dietary modification is to encourage increased consumption of meat. This is, however, not a practical option for two reasons. Not only is meat expensive but its increased consumption may have other deleterious effects. The alternative is to raise the relative proportion of promoters of non-haem iron absorption in the diet and to decrease the proportion of inhibitors. Within the context of a Western-type diet, possible approaches include such measures as the ingestion of orange juice with meals and the exclusion of tea. One recent strategy that was found to be effective was the reduction of the cheese and milk content of the main iron-containing meals[36,37]. However, the potential effectiveness of such manipulations in the context of the mixed and varied diets consumed in industrialized countries is probably much less than absorption studies involving single meals would suggest[38].

It is in developing countries, where diets are much less varied, that dietary measures have the greatest potential[28,34,39,40]. The intake of meat and fish is usually low and the intake of ascorbic acid is also often low. In contrast, the dietary contents of phytate and iron- building phenolic compounds are usually raised[34]. Although it is usually not feasible to increase the consumption of meat, strategies need to be developed to encourage increased production and consumption of fruit and vegetables containing reasonable amounts of ascorbic acid and to discourage the consumption of inhibitors of iron absorption, such as tea, with the major iron-containing meals. If, however, meaningful education programmes are to be mounted, more needs to be known of the major promoters and inhibitors of iron absorption in regional diets so that advice can be tailored to local needs. Coupled with such programmes is the need to introduce improved milling procedures in order to reduce further the phytate content of wheat and other cereals[34]. For food-based preventive programmes to be effective it is important that they be developed as part of more general nutritional education and that they remain firmly embedded within the primary health care delivery system.

References

1. International Nutritional Anemia Consultative Group (INACG) (1979): *Guidelines for the eradication of iron deficiency anemia.* A Report of the International Nutritional Anemia Consultative Group. pp. 1–29. Washington: Nutrition Foundation.

2. Cook, J.D. & Reusser, M.E. (1983): Iron fortification: an update. *Am. J. Clin. Nutr.* **38,** 648–659.

3. Hurrell, R.F. (1984): Bioavailability of different iron compounds used to fortify formulas and cereals: technological problems. In: *Iron nutrition in infancy and childhood*, ed. A Stekel, pp. 147–148. New York: Raven Press.

4. Hallberg, L. (1985): Factors influencing the efficacy of iron fortification and the selection of fortification vehicles. In: *Iron fortification of foods*, eds. F.M. Clydesdale & K.L. Weinerpp, pp. 7–28. New York: Academic Press.

5. Bothwell, T.H. & MacPhail, A.P. (1992): Prevention of iron deficiency by food fortification. In: *Nutritional anemias*, eds. S.J. Forman & S. Zlotzin, pp. 183–192. New York: Raven Press.

6. Barrett, F. & Ranum, P. (1985): Wheat and blended cereal foods. In: *Iron fortification of food*, eds. F.M. Clydesdale & K.L. Weiner. pp. 75–109. New York: Academic Press.

7. Hallberg, L. (1981): Bioavailability of dietary iron. *Annu. Rev. Nutr.* **1,** 123–147.

8. Baynes, R.D. & Bothwell, T.H. (1990): Iron deficiency. *Annu. Rev. Med.* **10,** 133–148.

9. Hurrell, R.F. (1985): Types of iron fortificants: non-elemental sources. In: *Iron fortification of foods*, eds. F.M. Clydesdale & K.L. Weiner, pp. 39–53. New York: Academic Press.

10. Forbes, A.L., Adams, C.E., Arnaud, M.J., Chichester, C.O., Cook, J.D., Harrison, B.N., Hurrell, R.F., Kahn, S.G., Morriss, E.R., Tanner, J.T. & Whittaker, P. (1989): Comparison of *in-vitro*, animal and clinical determinations of iron bioavailability. *Am. J. Clin. Nutr.* **49,** 225–238.

11. Patrick, J.Jr (1985): Types of iron fortificants: elemental sources. In: *Iron fortification of foods*, eds. F.M. Clydesdale & K.L. Weiner, pp. 31–38. New York: Academic Press.

12. Hurrell, R.J. (1985): Prospects of improving the iron fortification of foods. In: *Nutritional anemias*, eds. S.J. Foman & S. Zlotzin, pp. 193–201. New York: Raven Press.

13. Elwood, P.A. (1968): Radio-active studies of the absorption by human subjects of various iron preparations from bread. In: *Iron in flour*, Ministry of Health Reports on Public Health and Medicine. Subject no. 117, pp. 1–50. London: HMSO.

14. Hallberg, L., Brune, M. & Rossander, L. (1986): Low bioavailability of carbonyl iron in man: studies on iron fortification of wheat flour. *Am. J. Clin. Nutr.* **43,** 59–67.

15. Hallberg, L., Bengtsson, C. & Garby, L. (1979): An analysis of factors leading to a reduction in iron deficiency in Swedish women. *Bull. WHO* **57,** 147–954.

16. Cook, J.D., Skikne, B.S., Lynch, S.R. & Reusser, M.E. (1986): Estimates of iron sufficiency in the US population. *Blood* **68,** 726–731.

17. Bothwell, T.H. & Charlton, R.W. (1982): A general approach to the problems of iron deficiency and iron overload in the population at large. *Sem. Hematol.* **19,** 54–57.

18. Bothwell, T.H., Charlton, R.W. & Motulsky, A.G. (1995): Hemochromatosis. In: *The metabolic and molecular bases of inherited disease*, eds. C.R. Scriver, A.L. Beaudet, W.S. Sly & D. Valle, pp. 2237–2269. New York: McGraw Hill.

19. Stevens, R.G., Jones, D.Y., Micozzi, M.S. & Taylor, P.R. (1988): Body iron stores and the risk of cancer. *New Engl. J. Med.* **319,** 1047–1052.

20. Salonen, J.T., Nyssnen, K., Korpela, H., Tuomilehto, J., Seppnen, R. & Salonen, R. (1992): High stored iron levels are associated with excess risk of myocardial infarction in Eastern Finnish men. *Circulation* **86,** 803–811.

21. De Maeyer, E. & Adiels-Tegman, M. (1985): The prevalence of anaemia in the world. *World Health Stat. Q.* **38,** 302–316.

22. MacPhail, A.P., Charlton, R., Bothwell, T.H. & Bezwoda, W. (1985): Experimental fortificants. In: *Iron fortification of foods*, eds. F.M. Clydesdale & K.L. Weiner, pp. 7–28. New York: Academic Press.

23. Garby, L. & Areekul, S. (1974): Iron supplementation in Thai fish sauce. *Ann. Trop. Med. Parasitol.* **68,** 467–476.

24. Ballot, D.E., MacPhail, A.P., Bothwell, T.H., Gillooly, M. & Mayet, F. (1989): Fortification of curry powder with NaFe(III)EDTA in an iron-deficient population; report of a controlled iron-fortification trial. *Am. J. Clin. Nutr.* **49,** 162–169.

25. Viteri, F.E., Alvarez, E., Batres, R., Torun, B., Pineda, A., Mejia, L.A. & Sylvie, J. (1995): Fortification of sugar with iron sodium ethylenediamine tetraacetate (FeNaEDTA) improves iron status in semi rural Guatemalan populations. *Am. J. Clin. Nutr.* **61,** 1153–1163.

26. Lynch, S.R., Bothwell, T.H., Hurrell, R.H. & MacPhail, A.P. (1993): Iron EDTA for food fortification. A Report of the International Nutritional Anemia Consultative Group. pp. 1–54. Washington: Nutrition Foundation.

27. Hallberg, L. (1992): Iron balance in pregnancy and lactation. In: *Nutritional anemias*, eds. S.J. Foman & S. Zlotkin, pp. 13–25. New York: Raven Press.

28. Yip, R. (1994): Iron deficiency: contemporary scientific issues and international programmatic approaches. *J. Nutr.* **124,** 1479s–1490s.

29. Schultink, W., Gross, R., Gliwitzki, M., Karyadi, D. & Matulessi, P. (1995): Effect of daily *vs* twice weekly iron supplementation in Indonesian preschool children with low iron status. *Am. J. Clin. Nutr.* **61,** 111–115.

30. Simmons, W.K., Cook, J.D., Bingham, K.C., Thomas, M., Jackson, J., Jackson, M., Ahluwalia, N., Kahn, S.G. & Patterson, A.W. (1993): Evaluation of a gastric delivery system for iron supplementation in pregnancy. *Am. J. Clin. Nutr.* **58,** 622–626.

31. Takkunen, H. & Seppanen, R. (1975): Iron deficiency and dietary factors in Finland. *Am. J. Clin. Nutr.* **28,** 1141–1147.

32. Gillooly, M., Bothwell, T.H., Torrance, J.D., MacPhail, A.P., Derman, D.P., Bezwoda, W.R., Mills, W., Charlton, R.W. & Mayet, E. (1983): The effects of organic acids, phytates and polyphenols on the absorption of iron from vegetables. *Br. J. Nutr.* **49,** 331–342.

33. Baynes, R.D., Macfarlane, B.J., Bothwell, T.H., Siegenberg, D., Bezwoda, W.R., Schmidt, U., Lamparelli, R.D., Mayet, F. & MacPhail, A.P. (1990): The promotive effect of soy sauce on iron absorption in human subjects. *Eur. J. Clin. Nutr.* **44,** 419–424.

34. Hallberg, L., Rossander-Hultén, L. & Brune, M. (1992): Prevention of iron deficiency by diet. In: *Nutritional anemias*, eds. S.J. Foman & S. Zlotkin, pp. 168–178. New York: Raven Press.

35. Lynch, S.R., Dassenko, S.A., Cook, J.D., Juillerat, M.-A. & Hurrell, R.F. (1994): Inhibitory effect of a soybean-protein-related moiety on iron absorption in humans. *Am. J. Clin. Nutr.* **60,** 567–572.

36. Hallberg, L., Brune, M., Erlandsson, M., Sandberg, A.-S. & Rossander-Hultén, L. (1991): Calcium: effect of different amounts on nonheme- and heme-iron absorption in humans. *Am. J. Clin. Nutr.* **53,** 112–119.

37. Gleerup, A., Rossander-Hultén, L., Gromatkovski, E. & Hallberg, L. (1995): Iron absorption from the whole diet: comparison of the effect of two different distributions of daily calcium intake. *Am. J. Clin. Nutr.* **61,** 97–104.

38. Cook, J.D., Dassenko, S.A. & Lynch, S.R. (1991): Assessment of the role of nonheme-iron availability in iron balance. *Am. J. Clin. Nutr.* **54,** 717–722.

39. Trowbridge, F.L., Harris, S.S., Cook, J.D. Duan, J.T. Florentino, R.F., Kodyat, B.A., Venkatesh Mannar, M.G., Reddy, V., Tontisirin, K., Underwood, B. & Yip, R. (1993): Coordinated strategies for controlling micronutrient malnutrition: a technical workshop. *J. Nutr.* **123,** 775–787.

40. WHO/UNICEF/UNU Consultation. (1994): *Indicators and strategies for iron deficiency and anaemia programmes*. pp. 1–103. Geneva: World Health Organization.

Iron Nutrition in Health and Disease, edited by Leif Hallberg and Nils-Georg Asp
©1996 John Libbey & Company Ltd., pp. 339–347

Chapter 34

Role of the food industry in iron nutrition: Iron intake from industrial food products

R.F. Hurrell & S. Jacob

Swiss Federal Institute of Technology Zurich, Laboratory for Human Nutrition, P.O. Box 474, CH 8803 Rüschlikon, Switzerland

Summary

When evaluating the role of the food industry in iron nutrition in industrialized countries, we must consider that some population groups (infants, children, adolescents, adult women, pregnant women) are at risk of iron deficiency, whereas for other groups, such as adult men and post-menopausal women, there is some concern that too much iron may be detrimental to their health. The food industry should therefore increase the supply of absorbable iron to the groups at risk of iron deficiency but refrain where possible from providing extra iron to the groups who do not need it.

The amount of total iron (haem plus non-haem) coming from processed foods is high in industrialized countries. Studies in UK, USA, Denmark and France indicate that about 60–70 per cent of total iron intake is from processed foods and that about 30–40 per cent comes from fresh foods; in Spain and Italy this ratio is closer to 50:50. If we make an allowance for the greater absorption of haem iron, these ratios change only slightly; in the UK , for instance, the ratio of total iron from processed foods to fresh foods changes from about 65:35 to closer to 60:40 for absorbable iron. Depending on the country, cereals (bread, breakfast cereals), beverages (wine, chocolate drink) and meat make the greatest iron contribution from processed foods, whereas meat, vegetables and fruits contribute most of the iron intake from fresh foods. Meat (fresh and processed) is the largest single provider of absorbable iron in our diets.

Despite the high iron intake from processed foods, industry has little potential to influence iron nutrition through unfortified food products. Most meal combinations are selected by the consumer and only about 1 per cent of iron intake is from ready-prepared meals. Nevertheless, it is possible through a knowledge of the inhibitors (phytic acid, polyphenols) and enhancers (ascorbic acid, muscle tissue) of iron absorption to design meals of low, medium or high non-haem iron bioavailability. We have screened a series of commercial frozen dinners and found absorption in adult subjects to vary from 2.6 to 18.4 per cent. The high bioavailability meals would be ideal products that could be marketed specifically for consumption by adult or pregnant women.

The best approach for the food industry to improve iron nutrition, however, is to develop fortified food products targeted to the at-risk groups. This has proved successful with infant foods such as formulas and cereals. Fortification iron already accounts for some 20–25 per cent of iron intake in the USA, about 6 per cent in the UK, but far less in countries (Spain, France) where wheat flour is not fortified. There are technical problems, however, related to the addition of iron to food, especially with respect to unacceptable colour and flavour changes. The most bioavailable iron compounds usually generate the most organoleptic problems. Breakfast cereals and chocolate milk drinks are ideal fortification vehicles for children and adolescents, but they are often fortified with iron compounds of low availability such as reduced elemental iron or ferric pyrophosphate. Industry should ensure that iron added to foods is absorbable. This can be done by optimizing the iron compound used (ferrous fumarate and ferrous succinate are useful alternatives), adding absorption enhancers (ascorbic acid) and, where possible, removing absorption inhibitors (phytic acid).

Introduction

Although iron deficiency anaemia is mainly a problem in developing countries, it also affects millions of people in the industrialized world. According to DeMaeyer & Adiels-Tegman[1], 12 per cent of infants, 7 per cent of school children, 6 per cent of adolescents, 11 per cent of adult females and 14 per cent of pregnant women in Europe and North America are anaemic. At any one time, therefore, there are some 2 million pregnant women, 9 million school children, 10 million infants and 33 million adult women in these industrialized countries who would benefit from an extra supply of iron. This iron could be provided as a pharmaceutical preparation or it could come from the food supply, either from a better combination of foods or added to the food as fortification iron.

Iron fortification of foods, however, is not always regarded as positive. The fortification of widely consumed foods, such as wheat flour for example, provides extra iron to the whole population including adult men and post-menopausal women. These population groups do not require extra iron and it has been proposed that excess iron may even be detrimental to their health, leading to an increased incidence of atherosclerosis[2] and cancer[3] due to an increased oxidative stress.

This paper discusses the possible role of the food industry in influencing iron nutrition in industrialized countries. Iron intake from industrial food products is first reviewed and the potential of the food industry to influence iron nutrition through ready-prepared meals or fortified foods is discussed. Most of the information presented concerns adult foods, with some comments on foods for children and adolescents. Infant foods have not been considered in detail as most infant formulas and cereals are already fortified with iron[4]. Iron fortified formulas, in particular, are considered as the major factor responsible for the declining prevalence of anaemia in infants and pre-school children observed in the USA in the 1970s and 1980s[5].

Dietary iron intake from industrial food products

For our evaluation of the dietary energy and dietary iron intake from industrial food products in industrialized countries, we evaluated data from 6 countries; two in Northern Europe (United Kingdom (UK) and Denmark), two in Southern Europe (Spain and Italy), one in Central Europe (France) and one in North America (United States (USA)). We reviewed the following published national dietary intake data: UK on British adults[6]; US[7] based on the Second National Health and Nutrition Examination Survey (NHANES II); Denmark[8] and Spain[9]. For France, we used the dietary intake data from a recent survey of more than 1000 people aged from 6 months to 97 years living in the Paris area[10]. For Italy, we used a more restricted survey on some 1000 elderly Italians (>60 years) living in 14 centres throughout the country[11]. The British and Italian surveys used 7 day dietary records; the American the 24h recall method; the French the diet history method; and the Spanish and Danish evaluated total household consumption.

The surveys which were made in the UK, USA and Italy mostly gave sufficient detailed information to deduce whether a foodstuff had been industrially processed prior to purchase or whether it had been purchased fresh, later to be cooked at home or consumed raw. The information in the Spanish survey was also adequate, except for meat and fish products. We therefore assumed that 30 per cent of the meat consumed had been processed prior to purchase (hams, fermented sausages), and that 70 per cent of meat and 100 per cent of fish was purchased fresh. Less detailed information was given in the French and Danish surveys. We therefore assumed that 100 per cent of all beverages, cereals, fats and oils, sweets and desserts, milk and milk products were industrially processed, as was 30 per cent of meat, fish, eggs, fruits and vegetables. The remaining 70 per cent of these food groups were assumed to be purchased fresh. The estimations of iron and energy intake from processed foods obtained from the French and Danish data are therefore probably less accurate than those obtained for the UK, USA, Spain and Italy.

The energy intake data for five countries is shown in Table 1. For all countries, it can be seen that 74–80 per cent of energy consumed comes from foods which are industrially processed prior to purchase and that only 11–22 per cent of energy comes from foods that are purchased fresh and cooked at home. Only fruit and nuts (2–7 per cent of energy intake) would commonly be eaten raw. The main dietary energy components from fresh foods, as you would expect, are meat, fruits and vegetables. The main energy components from processed foods are cereals (23–30 per cent of energy intake), milk (11–16 per cent), oils and fats (4–23 per cent) and beverages (9–15 per cent). The beverages include soft drinks, chocolate drinks, tea, coffee and alcoholic beverages. The apparent wide variation in energy intake from fats and oils, 4–7 per cent in UK, USA and France compared to 21–23 per cent in Spain and Denmark is probably due to the different method of data collection.

The relative intake of total iron from processed and fresh foods is somewhat different (Table 2) since some major processed food groups, such as milk and milk products, and fats and oils, provide a significant energy contribution but contain little iron. In the UK, USA, Denmark and France some 60–70 per cent of the total iron intake would appear to come from processed foods, compared to around 50 per cent in Spain and Italy where people obtain more of their daily iron intake from fresh vegetables, pulses and fruits. The main processed food to provide iron is cereals which, depending on the country, provides from 13 to 50 per cent of the total iron intake. The relative contribution of cereal iron is greater in those countries (UK, USA, Denmark) where wheat flour is fortified with iron and in these countries it represents 33–50 per cent of total iron intake compared to 13–27 per cent in France, Spain and Italy. The next biggest contributors to iron intake from processed foods are processed meats (1–11 per cent) and beverages (4–19 per cent). In elderly Italians, 19 per cent of their total iron intake comes from red wine, whereas the Spanish people get 5 per cent of their iron from wine and 11 per cent of their iron from coffee, chocolate drinks and other beverages.

Most of the total iron intake from fresh foods comes from meats (13–19 per cent, Table 2).

Table 1. Percentage of energy intake in different countries from processed and fresh foods

Foods	UK		USA		Spain		Denmark		France	
	Fresh	Proc.	Fresh	Proc.	Fresh	Proc.	Fresh	Proc.	Fresh	Proc.
Beverages	–	9	–	11	–	10	–	NL	–	15
Cereal and cereal products	–	30	–	26	–	23	–	23	–	25
Eggs and egg dishes	2	–	3	–	2	–	2	1	1	1
Fruits and nuts	1	1	–	1	4	1	3	2	5[a]	2[a]
Fish and fish products	1	1	–	1	2	–	1	–	1	1
Milk and milk products	–	11	–	11	–	10	–	16	–	16
Meat and meat products	10	6	7	11	9	4	8	4	10	4
Vegetables and pulses	8	4	1	5	3	3	5	2	2[b]	1[b]
Fats and oils	–	6	–	4	–	23	–	21	–	7
Confectionery/ desserts	–	6	–	5	–	5	–	7	–	8
Subtotal	22	74	11	75	20	79	19	76	19	80
Total	96		86		99		95		99	

[a] includes fruit and vegetables. [b] pulses only. NL not listed.

This is an underestimation of the importance of meat, however, since meat contains haem iron which is absorbed to a far greater extent than the non-haem iron present in all other food groups. We have therefore attempted to account for haem iron absorption and to estimate the percentage of absorbable iron (as opposed to total iron) coming from processed and fresh foods. It was only possible to make the calculations for the UK and Spain since the surveys from these countries contained the most detailed information. For our calculations, we assumed that meat and meat products contained 50 per cent haem iron and 50 per cent non-haem iron, that haem iron was 25 per cent absorbed and that non-hacm iron was 7.5 per cent absorbed. Our results for absorbable iron from fresh and processed foods in the UK and Spain are shown in Table 3. Compared to the total iron intake from fresh meat, 15 per cent and 19 per cent in UK and Spain, respectively (Table 2), the percentage of absorbable iron intake from fresh meat increased to 25 per cent and 31 per cent respectively (Table 3). The percentage of iron intake from processed meats also increased from 8 per cent and 9 per cent for total iron (Table 2) to 13 per cent and 15 per cent for absorbable iron in Spain and UK respectively (Table 3). Despite these increases, however, other values of percentage iron intake changed only slightly. The percentage of absorbable iron coming from processed foods was 45 per cent in Spain and 60 per cent in the UK (Table 3), compared to values for total iron intake of 52 per cent and 65 per cent, respectively (Table 2). The percentage of absorbable iron coming from other individual food groups decreased slightly; however, the major providers of absorbable iron from processed foods were still cereals, processed meats and beverages, assuming of course that the fortification iron added to cereals and some beverages is absorbable.

Potential of the food industry to influence iron nutrition in industrialized countries

From the previous discussion, it is clear that consumers in industrialized countries receive some 50–70 per cent of their dietary iron intake from industrial food products. However, as most meal combinations are selected by the consumer, the food industry has little control or opportunity to influence the amount or bioavailability of iron in meals. Detailed information on the consumption of industrially prepared meals is lacking; however, in Spain, it is reported that only 0.6 per cent of the total dietary iron intake comes from these products[9]. In the USA, industrially prepared meals would appear to contribute around 1 per cent of the total iron

Table 2. Percentage of iron intake in different countries from processed and fresh foods

Foods	UK		US		Spain		Denmark		Italy		France	
	Fresh	Proc.	Fresh	Proc.	Fresh	Proc.	Fresh	Proc.	Fresh	Proc.	Fresh	Proc.
Beverages	–	4	–	4	–	16	–	NL	–	19[a]	–	5
Cereal and cereal products	–	42	–	33	–	13	–	50	–	22	–	27
Eggs and egg dishes	4	–	4	–	4	–	4	2	4	–	–	–
Fruits and nuts	1	1	1	2	7	2	1	2	5	–	18[b]	8[b]
Fish and fish products	2	1	1	1	3	–	1	–	2	–	2	1
Milk and milk products	–	2	–	2	–	1	–	3	–	2	6	–
Meat and meat products	15	9	17	11	19	8	13	6	15	1	18[c]	8[c]
Vegetables and pulses	11	4	5	7	13	10	8	4	16	3	–	1[d]
Fats and oils	–	–	–	–	–	1	–	–	–		–	1
Confectionary/ Desserts	–	2	–	–	–	1	–	4	–	–	–	5
Total	33	65	28	60	46	52	27	71	42	47	44	56

[a] From red wine only. [b] Includes fruit and vegetables. [3]Includes meat and eggs. [5]Pulses only. NL not listed.

Table 3. Percentage of absorbable iron from processed and fresh foods in the UK and Spain[a]

Foods	UK		Spain	
	Fresh	Proc.	Fresh	Proc.
Beverages	–	3	–	4[b] 8[c]
Cereal and cereal products	–	33	–	11
Eggs and egg dishes	3	–	3	–
Fruits and nuts	1	1	5	1
Fish and fish products	1	1	2	–
Milk and milk products	–	1	–	1
Meat and meat products	25	15	31	13
Vegetables and pulses	8	4	11	6
Fats and oils	–	–	–	1
Sweets	–	2	–	–
Total	**38**	**60**	**52**	**45**

[a] see text for explanation of calculations
[b] from wine and beer
[c] from chocolated drink

intake, at least during the NHANES II surveys in 1976–1980[7].

It would be possible, however, to industrially manufacture meals containing a definable amount of absorbable iron. It is necessary to know the haem iron content of the meal and the level of the major inhibitors (phytic acid, polyphenols) and enhancers (ascorbic acid, muscle tissue) of non-haem iron absorption. Hallberg & Rossander[12] designed 10 different meals whose absorbable iron content per 1000 kcal varied from 0.32 mg to 1.70 mg. As an example, details from five of these meals are shown in Table 4. All meals contained approximately 1000 kcal, but the non-haem iron content varied from 4.2 to 7.8 mg. Due to differences in the level of absorption inhibitors and enhancers, non-haem iron absorption ranged from 7.9 to 23.1 per cent. The lowest absorption was from the pizza meal. The meat-containing meals had the highest non-haem ion absorption, probably due to the enhancing effect of muscle tissue, and they also contained a further amount of absorbable iron from haem. They thus had the highest bioavailable iron density. We have recently screened the non-haem iron absorption in human subjects from a selection of commercial frozen low-calorie dinners marketed in the USA (Stouffers Lean Cuisine)[13]. We used the dual radioiron technique with ^{55}Fe and ^{59}Fe. We were able to select meals of low iron absorption (< 5 per cent), such as macaroni cheese and vegetable lasagne; meals of moderate iron absorption (5–10 per cent), such as Swedish meat balls and tuna noodle salad; and meals of high iron absorption (15–20 per cent), such as beef and bean enchiladas and stuffed bell-peppers. The meals of high iron absorption could clearly be targeted

Table 4. Development of meals with a definable iron density (Hallberg and Rossander[12])

Meal Composition	Kcal	Non-haem iron Content (mg)	Non-haem iron Abs.[a] (%)	Non-haem iron Abs (mg)	Calculated[b] haem Fe Abs. (mg)	Absorbed Fe per 1000 kcal (mg)
1. Pizza: *anchovy, tomatoes, cheese, beer*	1040	4.2	7.9	0.33	–	0.32
2. Spaghetti: *cheese, tomatoes, water*	1020	4.9	12.1	0.59	–	0.58
3. Boiled cod: *potatoes, bread, butter, cake*	1050	7.8	10.4	0.80	–	0.76
4. Chicken soup, steak and kidney pie: *peas, carrots, bread, butter, beer, jelly*	1010	5.7	18.9	1.08	0.23	1.30
5. Antipasta, Spaghetti: *meat, bread, wine, orange*	1150	7.8	23.1	1.80	0.15	1.70

[a] Corrected to 40% reference dose absorption.
[b] Haem Fe assumed to be 25% absorbed.

at pregnant women or adult women concerned about a low iron status.

Food fortification

Iron fortification of foods is the best way for the food industry to impact on iron nutrition and to provide extra iron to the population groups at risk of deficiency. This can take the form of fortification of a widely consumed product, such as wheat flour, which in many countries is mandatory, or the voluntary fortification of other foods.

Wheat flour enrichment is mandatory in the UK, USA and Denmark but not in Italy, France and Spain. The USA practices the highest level of enrichment and iron is added to white flour up to 44 mg/kg, or bread to 27.5 mg/kg, a similar level to the iron content of whole grain. In Denmark, the enrichment level for wheat flour is 30 mg/kg and in the UK only 16.5 mg/kg, as the iron level is brought back only to that of 80 per cent extraction flour[14]. As the level of native iron in 70 per cent extraction wheat flour is around 11–12 mg/kg, only 5mg of iron per kg is added to wheat flour in the UK. In the USA, corn meal, corn grits, rice and pasta products also have federal standards for voluntary iron enrichment and these commodities are mostly enriched as are other baked goods, such as crackers, rolls, cookies, doughnuts[14], but to a lesser extent. Other foods that are voluntarily fortified with iron in all countries include breakfast cereals and chocolate drink powders. These products are often fortified to contain 20–25 per cent of the iron Recommended Daily Allowance (RDA) in one serving.

The contribution of fortification iron to iron intake is thus highest in the USA where it amounts for 20–25 per cent of total iron intake. In the NHANES II survey[7], the iron contribution from foods that are normally fortified (white bread, rolls, crackers, corn flour, corn grits, pasta, breakfast cereals) was a little over 20 per cent. Lachance[15] has previously estimated that fortification iron represents 24 per cent of iron intake in the USA, whereas Subar and Bowering[16] reported that 25 per cent of the iron intake in US females comes from fortified foods (16 per cent from enriched cereals, 9 per cent from breakfast cereals and other voluntarily fortified foods).

The contribution of fortification iron to the iron intake in the UK would appear to be about 6 per cent, based on the survey of Gregory *et al.*[6], from which about 3 per cent comes from bread and 3 per cent from breakfast cereals. In British adolescents, however, intake of fortification iron from breakfast cereals may represent a much greater amount. Iron from breakfast cereals represented 15 per cent of the total iron intake in 11–12 year old boys and girls in northern England[17]. For those countries with no mandatory wheat flour enrichment, the iron intake from fortification iron would be expected to be relatively low. In Spain, however, a high proportion of total iron intake (11 per cent) comes from coffee, chocolate drinks and other beverages[9] and much of this could come from fortification iron added to chocolate drinks.

The fact that fortification iron is added to foods, however, does not necessarily mean that it can be absorbed, or that it will help prevent iron deficiency. Much fortification iron added to cereal foods today, particularly reduced elemental iron, is poorly absorbed. Table 5 shows the iron compounds commonly added to foods[4]. The freely water-soluble ferrous sulfate has a high relative absorption but often causes unacceptable colour and flavour changes and promotes fat oxidation in stored cereal flours. For this reason, it is commonly added only to infant formulas, and to bread and pasta products in the USA[18]. Most other iron fortified foods (except infant cereals) are fortified with poorly absorbable iron compounds. These compounds cause no organoleptic problems but are poorly soluble in the dilute acid of the gastric juice and thus have a low and variable absorption. Ferric pyrophosphate, commonly added to chocolate drinks, has a relative absorption in man of 20–70 per cent; carbonyl iron, sometimes added to wheat flour, has a relative absorption of 5–20 per cent[19]; and H-reduced elemental iron, commonly added to breakfast cereals and wheat flour, has not been adequately tested in man but from its poor solubility in dilute acid would be expected to have the lowest absorption of all. Alternative iron compounds exist, such as ferrous fumarate, ferrous succinate and electrolytic

Table 5: Iron compounds used in food fortification (Hurrell[4])

Compounds	Organoleptic problems	Relative absorption in man	Common fortified foods
Freely water soluble	often causes colour and flavour problems, and fat oxidation	100	infant formula, bread, pasta
Ferrous sulfate			
Insoluble in water/soluble in dilute acid			
Ferrous fumarate			
Ferrous succinate	usually no problems	90–100	infant cereals
Poorly soluble in dilute acid			
Ferric pyrophosphate		20–70	chocolate drinks
Elemental iron:			
Electrolytic	All inert organoleptically	75	infant cereals
Carbonyl		5–20	wheat flour
H-reduced		< carbonyl	wheat flour/breakfast cereals

iron, which are much better absorbed and do not usually cause organoleptic problems. So far, they are mainly used to fortify infant cereals.

The role of the food industry with respect to iron nutrition should be to develop food products, fortified with absorbable iron, which are targeted specifically at those population groups at risk of iron deficiency but which are not necessarily consumed by people who do not require extra iron. Breakfast cereals, chocolate drinks and other beverages would be ideal food vehicles to supply iron to children, adolescents and even adult and pregnant women; however, the poorly absorbed iron used in most of these products today should be replaced by iron compounds of high bioavailability. The food industry should optimize iron compounds in different products so as to obtain maximum absorption with no organoleptic problems; it should add absorption enhancers (ascorbic acid) to products together with the iron compound; and when possible remove the absorption inhibitors, such as phytic acid, from cereal and legume products[20].

We have attempted to optimize the iron compounds added to both infant cereals[21] and chocolate drink powders[22,23]. All studies were made in adult human subjects with radiolabelled iron compounds and ferrous sulfate was used as the standard (relative absorption 100) even though it could not be added commercially because of colour and flavour problems. In the infant cereal study, iron absorption from ferrous sulfate was 4.8 per cent (relative absorption 100). The relative absorption of ferrous fumarate was 100, ferrous succinate 92, ferric saccharate 74, and ferric pyrophosphate 39[21]. In the chocolate drink studies[22,23], iron absorption from ferrous sulfate was 3.5–5.7 per cent in three separate studies. The relative absorption of ferrous fumarate was 201, ferrous succinate 111, ferric saccharate 39, and ferric pyrophosphate 20. The optimum iron compound for infant cereals was ferrous fumarate, whereas ferrous succinate was optimum for chocolate drink powders, since fumarate on occasions caused colour changes.

Conclusions

In industrialized countries, 50–70 per cent of the daily iron intake comes from manufactured foods, but only about 1 per cent from industrially prepared meals. As the consumer chooses the meal combinations, the food industry has little real potential to influence iron nutrition with normal food products. It is possible to design meals with a defined absorbable iron density, by knowing the levels of absorption enhancers and inhibitors, and commercial frozen meals of high absorbable iron could be designed for adult or pregnant women. The best way for the food industry to influence iron nutrition, however, would be through fortification of specific foods targeted at groups at risk of iron deficiency and the greatest contribution that the food industry could make to improve iron nutrition would be to ensure that the iron added to foods is absorbable.

References

1. DeMaeyer, E. & Adiels-Tegman, M. (1985): The prevalence of anaemia in the world. *World Health Stat. Q.* **38,** 302–316.
2. Salonen, J.T., Nyyssönen, K., Korpela, H., Tuomilehto, J., Seppänen, R. & Salonen, R. (1992): High stored iron levels are associated with excess risk of myocardial infarction in Eastern Finnish men. *Circulation* **86,** 803–811.
3. Stevens, R.G., Jones, D.Y., Micozzi, M.S. & Taylor, P.R. (1988): Body iron stores and the risk of cancer. *N. Engl. J. Med.* **319,** 1047–1052.
4. Hurrell, R.F. (1992): Prospects for impoving the iron fortification of foods. In: *Nutritional anemias*, eds. S. Fomon & S. Zlotkin, pp. 193–208. New York: Raven Press.
5. Yip, R., Walsh, K.M., Goldfarb, M.G. & Binkin, N.J. (1987): Declining prevalence of anemia in childhood in a middle–class setting: a pediatric success story. *Pediatrics* **80,** 330–334.
6. Gregory, J., Foster, K., Tyler, H. & Wiseman, M. (1990): *The dietary and nutritional survey of British adults*. London: HMSO.
7. Block, G., Dresser, C.M., Hartman, A.M. & Carrol, M.D. (1985): Nutrient sources in the American diet: Quantitative data from the NHANES II survey. 1. Vitamins and minerals. *Am. J. Epidemiol.* **122,** 13–26.
8. Haraldsdottir, J., Holm, L., Höjmoerk-Jensen, J. & Müller, A. (1985): *Danskernes Kostvaner.* Kopenhagen: Ministry of Agriculture.
9. Dieta Alimentaria Espanola (1991): *Pesca y Alimentacion.* Madrid: Ministero de Agricultura.
10. Hercberg, S., Preziosi, P., Galán, P., Deheeger, M., Papoz, L. & Dupin, H. (1991): Apports nutritionnnels d'un échantillon représentatif de la population du Val-de-Marne: III. Les apports en minéraux et vitamines. *Rev. Epidém. et Santé Publ.* **39,** 245–261.
11. Krogh, V., Freudenheim, J.L., D'Amicis, A., Scaccini, C., Sette, S., Ferro-Luzzi, A. & Trevisan, M. (1993): Food Sources of Nutrients of the Diet of Elderly Italians: II. Micronutrients. *Int. J. Epidemiol.* **22,** 869–877.
12. Hallberg, L. & Rossander, L. (1982): Effect of different drinks on the absorption of non-heme iron from composite meals. *Hum. Nutr. Appl. Nutr.* **36,** 116–123.
13. Reddy, M., Hurrell, R.F. & Cook, J.D. (1995): unpublished results.
14. Bauernfiend, J.C., & DeRitter, E. (1991): Foods considered for nutrient addition: Cereal grain products. In: *Nutrient additions to foods*, eds. J.C. Bauernfiend & P.A. Lachance, pp. 143–209. Connecticut, USA: Food and Nutrition Press.
15. Lachance, P.A. (1989): Nutritional responsibilities of the food companies in the next century. *Food Technol.* **43,** 144–150.
16. Subar, A.F. & Bowering, J. (1988): The contribution of enrichment and fortification to the nutrient intake of women. *J. Am. Diet. Ass.* **88,** 1237–1245.
17. Moynihan, P.J., Anderson, C., Adamson, A.J., Rugg-Gunn, D.R., Appleton, D.R. & Butler, T.J. (1994): Dietary sources of iron in English adolescents. *J. Human Nutr. Diet.* **7,** 225–230.
18. Barret, F. & Ranum, P. (1985): Wheat and blended foods. In: *Iron fortification of foods*, eds. F.M. Clydesdale, K.L. Wiemer, pp. 75–109. Orlando: Academic Press.
19. Hallberg, L., Brune, M. & Rossander, L. (1986): Low availability of carbonyl iron in man: studies on iron fortification of wheat flour. *Am. J. Clin. Nutr.* **43,** 59–67.

20. Hurrell, R.F., Juillerat, M.A., Reddy, M.B., Lynch, S.R., Dassenko, S.A. & Cook, J.D. (1992): Soy protein, phytate and iron absorption an man. *Am. J. Clin. Nutr.* **56,** 573–578.

21. Hurrell, R.F., Furniss, D.E., Burri, J., Whittaker, P., Lynch, S.R. & Cook, J.D. (1989): Iron fortification of infant cereals: a proposal for the use of ferrous fumarate or ferrous succinate. *Am. J. Clin. Nutr.* ***49,*** *1274–1282.*

22. Hurrell, R.F., Reddy, M.B., Dassenko, S.A., Cook, J.D. & Shepherd, D. (1991): Ferrous fumarate fortification of a chocolate drink powder. *Brit. J. Nutr.* **65,** 271–283.

23. Hurrell, R.F. & Cook, J.D. (1995): unpublished results.

Iron Nutrition in Health and Disease, edited by Leif Hallberg and Nils-Georg Asp
©1996 John Libbey & Company Ltd., pp. 349–358

Chapter 35

Food processing influencing iron bioavailability

A.-S. Sandberg

Department of Food Science, Chalmers University of Technology, c/o SIK, P.O. Box 5401, S-40229, Göteborg, Sweden

Summary

The bioavailability of iron in cereals and legumes is strongly influenced by food processing because it affects the degradation and formation of inhibitors and enhancers of iron absorption. Also, the chemical form and solubility of iron can be altered by food processing, thereby influencing iron bioavailability. Furthermore, some food additives are inhibitors or enhancers of iron absorption.

Food processing of plant foods can lead to both positive and negative effects on iron availability; heat treatment often results in inactivation of the enzyme phytase which hydrolyses phytate, vitamin C can be destroyed during cooking and baking, and the structure of polyphenols can be altered. Other food processes activate the intrinsic phytase and polyphenol-oxidase of plant foods and, during lactic fermentation, factors stimulating iron absorption are produced. In meat products, haem iron can be degraded and converted to non-haem iron when the meat is cooked.

Examples of food bioprocesses activating the intrinsic enzymes of cereals and legumes are soaking, malting, hydrothermic processing and fermentation. During the germination step of the malting process, enzymes are synthesized or activated. Lactic fermentation leads to lowering of pH as a consequence of bacterial production of organic acids, mainly lactic acid, which is favourable for phytase activity, and some organic acids are also enhancers of iron absorption. The micro-organisms of the starter culture used in the fermentation can in some cases exert phytase activity. Phytase can also be added in the food process.

The utilization of iron and zinc and probably other minerals can be improved by bioprocesses which decrease the phytate content. Another possibility to increase the bioavailability of iron is the development of foods with a high microbial phytase activity, which would lead to phytate hydrolysis in the stomach. Fibre-rich cereals and legumes would then become good sources of iron and zinc as the content of these minerals is high. To increase the bioavailability of iron in tannin-rich foods, methods for the degradation of phenolic compounds inhibiting iron absorption must be developed. Formation of enhancers for absorption during bioprocessing is also important as well as their identification.

The increased knowledge of optimizing the bioprocesses to increase iron bioavailability can be used in food manufacturing of, for example, sourdough fermented bread, breakfast cereals made of malted flours or with the addition of phytase in the food process and weaning foods, malted or lactic fermented. Development of bioprocesses which optimally increase the intrinsic nutritional value of food products seems a possible way to reduce the risk for iron deficiency in vulnerable groups.

Introduction

Depending on the sedentary life style and the low energy expenditure of population groups in industrialized countries, it is difficult to meet the iron requirements. The bioavailability of iron in the diet is thus becoming increasingly important. In developing countries, the diet is usually based on cereals and legumes. Although the iron content of such staples is generally high, it has low bioavailability. This partly accounts for the high prevalence of iron deficiency anaemia in the population of those countries.

It is possible to increase the bioavailability of iron in the diet by altering the meal composition, i.e. by increasing foods containing enhancers of iron absorption (vitamin C, meat factor) and decreasing foods containing inhibitors of iron absorption (phytate, calcium, polyphenols). It is also possible to produce foods with high bioavailability of the naturally occurring iron, and this is a challenge for the food industry.

Food processing can have both positive and negative effects on iron bioavailability, because enhancers/inhibitors can be formed or degraded during the process. Food additives can also be inhibitors or enhancers of iron absorption. Also, the chemical form of iron can be altered during food processing and storage, such as the relative amounts of ferrous and ferric iron and the relative amounts of non-haem and haem iron can be altered, thereby affecting bioavailability. The bioavailability of iron is related to the solubility of iron. Poorly soluble forms of iron have a low bioavailability. Changes in solubility of iron during processing therefore can affect the bioavailability[1–4].

Food additives

A variety of substances are added to foods during processing for several purposes: to maintain freshness and safety; to help in processing or preparation, and; to make food more appealing.

Some of these additives have an effect on iron bioavailability because they are inhibitors or enhancers of iron absorption. Preservatives and antioxidants include substances such as calcium lactate, calcium sorbate, citric acid, EDTA, ascorbic acid, phytic acid. Calcium and phytic acid are well known inhibitors of iron absorption[5–6], wheeras ascorbic acid[7–8] and under certain conditions citric acid enhances iron absorption[9]. Iron is easily complexed by EDTA and iron(III) EDTA is well absorbed[10].

Other food additives are used as emulsifiers, stabilizers, leavening agents, pH control agents, hume-actants, dough conditioners and anti-caking agents. These include a number of calcium compounds, polysaccharides and organic acids. Food additives which affect appeal characteristics of foods include flavour enhancers, flavours, colours and sweeteners. Food dyes are complex organic molecules which have the potential of forming complexes with trace minerals[3].

Heat processing

There are a number of processes which may affect iron bioavailability, for example heat processes such as flaking, puffing, extrusion cooking, cooking, canning. Heat processing can lead to inactivation of enzymes or vitamins. Heat processing can inactivate the enzyme phytase, which hydrolyses phytate. Vitamin C can be destroyed during heat treatment and the structure of polyphenols can be altered. These effects are dependent on processing conditions, such as time, temperature, pH, moisture.

Both baking and microwave cooking increased non-haem iron in ground beef and a linear relationship was observed between non-haem iron in meat and the time of exposure to heat treatment[11]. The change was large enough to cause changes in absorbable iron in the meat. Nitrite added appeared to protect against heat induced changes in non-haem iron. Carpenter and Clark found a significant difference in the relative amounts of haem iron to non-haem iron in raw and cooked meat of different sources, which was cooked to an internal temperature of 71°C[12].

Changes in relative amounts of ferric and ferrous iron as a consequence of a wet-heat process, thermal processing in glass of spinach puree, were reported[13]. Thermal processing increased the percentage endogenous ferrous iron in raw spinach from baseline levels to 11 per cent. When different iron salts were added in the process, an increase in percentage of ferrous iron was also observed after processing.

Cooking in iron utensils can also considerably increase the iron content in food[14–16].

Physical processing

Physical processing, such as milling the grain and removing the outer layers of the grain, reduces the polyphenol and phytate content. Removing the outer layers of sorghum grains reduced the polyphenol and phytate contents by 96 per cent and 2 per cent, respectively, and resulted in an increase of iron absorption from 1.7 to 3.5 per cent[17].

Bioprocessing and bioavailability of iron

Bioprocessing can be defined as the use of microbial, animal or plant cells or enzymes to synthesize, degrade, transform or improve materials in foods and food ingredients. Bioprocessing of cereals and vegetables is a means to improve the bioavailability of minerals by degrading specific inhibitors that prevent the absorption from the food and by formation of promoting factors for the absorption. Phytate hydrolysis can occur in food production, either by phytase from plants, yeasts or micro-organisms. Examples of bioprocesses activating the intrinsic enzymes of cereals and legumes are soaking, malting and lactic fermentation. During the germination step of the malting process, enzymes are synthesized or activated. Lactic fermentation leads to lowering of pH as a consequence of bacterial production of organic acids, mainly lactic acid, which is favourable for phytase activity. Some organic acids formed during fermentation are enhancers of iron absorption. The microorganisms of the starter culture used in fermentation can in some cases exert phytase activity. Phytase can also be added in the food process.

Optimal conditions for phytase activity

To optimize the food process to increase iron bioavailability by phytate degradation, it is essential to know optimal conditions for phytase activity in cereals and legumes. Phytase activity is strongly dependent on pH and temperature and most phytases are active only in narrow pH and temperature ranges. There are differences in optimal conditions for phytase activity between different plant species. In 1953, Peers[18] showed that optimal conditions for wheat phytase were pH 5.1 and 55 °C and activity declines rapidly when changing pH. We recently found that the oat phytase has its optimal conditions at pH 4.3–4.5, 38 °C which thus differs from that of wheat[19]. These findings partly explain that oats was suggested to have a low phytase activity[20].

Scott[21] recently demonstrated an alkaline phytase activity of phytase extracted from different varieties of *Phaseolus vulgaris*. We found that brown beans have phytase activity at pH 4.5 and at pH 8 and 37 °C but the optimal activity was at pH 7.0 and 55 °C. In contrast to the acidic phytase, this neutral or alkaline enzyme is probably specific for inositol hexaphosphate and inositol pentaphosphate as inositol tetraphosphate and inositol triphosphate were accumulated when the enzyme was activated[22]. A pH optimum of yeast phytase was found at pH 3.5, but high activity occurs between 3.5 and 4.5[23]. Microbial phytase activity works in a broader pH area. Phytase produced by *Aspergillus niger* has one optimum at pH 5 and one at pH 2.5–3.0, probably due to additional acidic phosphatase activity[24], but activity occurs at all pH values between 1.0 and 7.5. We also found that this enzyme, when added to a meal, increased iron absorption, presumably by degrading phytate in the stomach[25].

Soaking and malting

Soaking of wheat bran, whole wheat flour and rye flour at optimal conditions for wheat phytase activity (pH 4.5–5, 55 °C) resulted in complete phytate hydrolysis[26,27] and to a marked increase in iron availability estimated *in vitro*[27]. We found that the inositol hexa- and pentaphosphate content must be reduced to levels beyond 0.5 µmol/g to give the strong increase in iron solubility at simulated physiological conditions, if no promoting factors were present.

Malting is a process during which the whole grain is soaked and then germinated. The amount of phytate in malted grains of wheat, rye and oats intended for the production of flour (germinated 3 days at 15 °C sprout length 10 mm) was only reduced slightly or not at all. However, when the malted cereals were ground and soaked at optimal conditions for wheat phytase there was a complete degradation of phytate[19], except for oats which under the conditions studied had a low phytase activity. By germination of oats for 5 days at 11 °C followed by incubation at 37–40 °C, it was possible to reduce phytate content of oats by 98 per cent (to < 0.5 μmol/g)[19]. This low level is desirable to greatly improve the bioavailability of iron from oats. It is of special importance to find methods of phytate reduction in oats. The high content of phytate in oats combined with a low phytase activity which is further decreased due to heat treatment of all commercial oat products, suggest that the negative effect on mineral absorption of oat products would be greater than that of other cereals. This assumption is confirmed in recent human absorption studies using radionuclide techniques, which demonstrated a low iron and zinc absorption from breakfast meals containing oat porridge and oat bran bread[28,29]. The iron and zinc absorption from oat porridge made of untreated flour was compared to that from oat porridge made of malted flour, with a phytate reduction of 77 per cent. Both iron and particularly zinc absorption was significantly improved from the porridge made of malted flour (Table 1)[30].

Fermentation

Lactic fermentation is an old method for food processing and preservation. Due to the production of lactic acid and other organic acids, the pH is lowered and the phytase activated. Lactic fermentation of maize, soya beans and sorghum reduces the phytate content[31,32]. We have shown that lactic fermentation of white sorghum and maize gruels can yield an almost complete degradation of phytate. At optimal conditions, the effect on *in vitro* estimation of iron availability was an almost tenfold increase[33].

Table 1. Iron and zinc absorption from oat porridge made of untreated flour and malted flour

Porridge meal	Zn absorption %	Fe absorption %	Phytate (μmol)
Untreated oat flour	11.8 ± 0.9	4.4 ± 1.2	435
Malted flour	18.3 ± 2.6 (*n*=10)	6.0 ± 1.2 (*n*=9)	107

The presence of tannins in sorghum not only decreased the availability of iron *per se*, but also seemed to inactivate the enzyme phytase. The use of lactic acid fermentation of high-tannin sorghum was therefore found to be less effective to reduce the phytate content[33]. Further studies are therefore needed in order to find methods to increase mineral availability in tannin rich-foods.

Sauerkraut, a lactic fermented vegetable, was found to markedly increase iron absorption from a meal[34]. Lactic acid-fermented vegetables added to a meal were found to increase the iron absorption in humans[35]. The fresh vegetables (carrots, turnips, onions) contained small amounts of phytate, which was hydrolysed during the fermentation. The amount of iron absorbed was increased when the fermented vegetables were added to a white wheat roll (the fractional absorption increased from 13.6 to 23.6), and also when added to phytate-rich meals, wholemeal rye and wheat rolls (the fractional absorption increased from 5.2 to 10.4). This indicates the formation of iron-promoting factors in lactic acid-fermented vegetables. No differences were found in zinc absorption between a meal containing raw or fermented vegetables.

During scalding and sourdough fermentation of bread the acidity of the dough is of great importance for phytate degradation[36–37]. We investi-

Table 2. Scalding and sourdough fermentation of bread containing rye bran - effect of acidity on phytate hydrolysis[38]

pH dough	pH bread	Phytate hydrolysis (%)
5.5	5.7	66
5.3	5.4	81
5.1	5.0	96
4.6	4.7	97
4.1	4.4	89
3.9	4.2	86

gated the phytate reduction in scalded bread and bread with varying amounts of sourdough baked with rye bran or oat bran addition (Table 2). The most marked phytate reduction of 96–97 per cent occurred in bread made with 10 per cent sourdough (pH 4.6) or in the breads in which the pH had been adjusted in the mild scalding with lactic acid, resulting in a pH between 4.4 and 5.1 in both dough and bread. The most effective phytate decomposition in bread with oat flour or oat bran occurred in bread made from scalded oat flour which had a sourdough content of 20–30 per cent. In these breads, with pH values between 4.3 and 4.6 in doughs and breads, the phytate was reduced from the initial content by 96 per cent[38]. Iron absorption from such sourdough fermented fibre-rich rye and wheat breads with a very low phytate content was investigated in humans using radionuclide technique[39]. We found that the percentage iron absorption was similar to that of white wheat bread not containing inhibitory factors. Consequently, the amounts of iron absorbed from wholemeal bread with its high content of iron, would be greater than from white bread, provided that the fermentation was optimized.

In another study of breadmaking we investigated the effect of different additives to the dough. Bread was made using whole wheat flour and flour of 60 per cent extraction rate; yeast was added and phytate degradation studied after different fermentation times[40]. Addition of milk to the dough inhibited enzymatic phytate hydrolysis resulting in depressed human iron absorption from the bread[41]. The results were considered an effect of formation of insoluble calcium phytate complexes. Fermented milk did not significantly affect enzymatic hydrolysis during fermentation, probably depending on the presence of lactic acid lowering the pH[40]. Addition of acetic acid or lingonberries to the dough increased the phytate reduction to 96 per cent and 83 per cent, respectively compared to 55 per cent in control bread without additives[23]. The pH of the doughs with 96 per cent reduction was between 4.5 and 5. The optimal phytate reduction would occur at a pH where the combined effect of the phytase of the flour and the yeast phytase is as high as possible.

Addition of enzymes

An alternative to activation of the intrinsic enzymes of foods is the addition of phytase during food processing. Microbial phytase enzyme preparations are now available commercially making their use in food processing technically feasible.

Bread was made using whole wheat flour and flour of 60 per cent extraction rate. Phytase from *A. niger* 1500 PU/g flour (one phytase unit, PU, is the amount of enzyme which liberates under standard conditions, pH 5.0, 37 °C, 1 nmol of inorganic phosphate from sodium phytate in 1 min) was added to the doughs. The phytate hydrolysis was, however, not complete (maximum 88 per cent hydrolysis), unless the pH was lowered to 3.5 which is close to the lower pH optimum[23]. Microbial *A. niger* phytase, therefore may be useful in the production of lactic acid fermented cereals and legumes (which normally have a low pH value) aimed at high mineral availability. A very effective phytate degradation was achieved by adding *A. niger* phytase to an oat-based nutrient solution fermented by *Lactobacillus plantarum*, but the added enzyme had a negative influence on the viable counts of *Lactobacilli* as well as the aroma[42].

The effect of reducing the phytate in soy-protein isolates on iron absorption was investigated in humans[43]. Addition of *A. niger* phytase in amounts which almost completely removed phytate in soy isolates increased iron absorption 4–5-fold.

Conclusions

Increased bioavailability of iron by food processing can be achieved by degradation of phytate to very low levels and by addition/formation of ascorbic and certain other organic acids. The bioavailability can also be improved by addition of microbial phytase, which can exert an effect in the stomach and small intestine. Much less is known about the degradation of polyphenols during food processing.

The utilization of iron and zinc and probably other minerals can be improved by bioprocesses which decrease the phytate content. Fibre-rich cereals and legumes would then become good sources of iron and zinc as the content of these minerals is high. To increase the bioavailability of iron in tannin-rich foods, methods for the degradation of phenolic compounds inhibiting iron absorption must be developed. Formation of enhancers for absorption during bioprocessing is also important as well as their identification.

The increased knowledge of optimizing the bioprocesses to increase mineral availability can be used in food manufacturing of, for example, sourdough fermented bread, breakfast cereals made of malted flours or with the addition of phytase in the food process, and weaning foods, malted or lactic fermented.

Another possibility to increase the bioavailability of minerals is the development of foods with a high phytase activity, which would lead to phytate hydrolysis in the stomach and small intestine. Bioprocessing which activates or synthesizes phytase combined with mild heat treatment is an example of minimal processing to keep phytase activity at high levels.

Development of bioprocesses which optimally increase the intrinsic nutritional value of food products seems a possible way to reduce the risk for iron deficiency in vulnerable groups and the need for fortification.

References

1. Clydesdale, F.M. (1982): The effects of physicochemical properties of food on the chemical status of iron. In: *Nutritional bioavailability of iron,* ed. C. Kies, pp. 55–84, ACS (American Chemical Society) Symposium Series 203.
2. Lee, K.M. (1982): Iron chemistry and bioavailability in food processing. In: *Nutritional bioavailability of iron,* ed. C. Kies, pp. 27–54, ACS Symposium Series 203.
3. Johnson, P.E. (1991): Effect of food processing and preparation on mineral utilization. In: *Nutritional and toxicological consequences of food processing. Advances in experimental medicine and biology*, ed. M. Friedman, pp. 483–498. New York: Plenum Press.
4. Sandberg, A.-S. (1991): The effect of food processing on phytate hydrolysis and availability of iron and zinc. In: *Nutritional and toxicological consequences of food processing*, ed. Friedman, pp. 499–508, New York: Plenum Press.
5. Hallberg, L., Rossander, L. & Skånberg, A.-B. (1987): Phytates and the inhibitory effect of bran on iron absorption in man. *Am. J. Clin. Nutr.* **45,** 988–996.
6. Hallberg, L., Brune, M., Erlandsson, M., Sandberg, A.-S. & Rossander-Hulthén, L. (1991): Calcium: effect of different amounts on nonheme and heme iron absorption in man. *Am. J. Clin. Nutr.* **53,** 112–119.
7. Sayers, M.H., Lynch, S.R., Jacobs, P. *et al.* (1973): The effect of ascorbic acid supplementation on the absorption of iron in maize, wheat and soya. *Br. J. Nutr.* **24,** 209–217.
8. Hallberg, L., Brune, M. & Rossander, L. (1986): Effect of ascorbic acid on iron absorption from different types of meals. Studies with ascorbic acid-rich foods and synthetic ascorbic acid given in different amounts with different meals. *Hum. Nutr. Appl. Nutr.* **40A,** 97–113.
9. Gillooly, M., Bothwell, T.H. & Torrance, J.D. (1983): The effects of organic acids, phytates and polyphenols on the absorption of iron from vegetables. *Br. J. Nutr.* **49,** 331–342.
10. MacPhail, A.P., Bothwell, T.H., Torrance, J.D., Derman, D.P., Bezwoda, W.R., Charlton, R.W. & Mayet, F. (1981): Factors affecting the absorption of iron from Fe(III) EDTA. *Br. J. Nutr.* **45,** 215–227.
11. Schricker, B.R. & Miller, D.D. (1983): Effects of cooking and chemical treatment on heme and nonheme iron in meat. *J. Food Sci.* **48,** 1340–1349.

12. Carpenter, C.E. & Clark, E. (1995): Evaluation of methods used in meat iron analysis and iron content of raw and cooked meats. *J. Agric. Food Chem.* **43,** 1824–1827.

13. Lee, K. & Clydesdale, F.M. (1981): Effect of thermal processing on endogenous and added iron in canned spinach. *J. Food Sci.* **46,** 1064–1068.

14. Burroughs, A.L. & Chan, J.J. (1972): Iron content of some Mexican-American foods. *J. Am. Diet. Assoc.* **60,** 123.

15. Brittin, H.C. & Nossaman, C.E. (1986): Iron content of food cooked in iron utensils. *J. Am. Diet. Assoc.* **86,** 897–901.

16. Mistry, A.N., Brittin, H.C. & Stoecker, B.J. (1988): Availability of iron from food cooked in an iron utensil determined by an *in vitro* method. *J. Food Sci.* **53,** 1546–1573.

17. Gillooly, M., Bothwell, T.H., Charlton, R.W., Torrance, J.D., Bezwoda, W.R., MacPhail, A.P., Derman, D.P., Novelli, L., Morrall, P. & Mayet, F. (1984): Factors affecting the absorption of iron from cereals. *Br. J. Nutr.* **51,** 37–46.

18. Peers, F.G. (1953): The phytase of wheat. *Biochem. J.* **53,** 102–110.

19. Larsson, M. & Sandberg, A.-S. (1992): Phytate reduction in oats during malting. *J. Food Sci.* **57,** 994–997.

20. Bartnik, M. & Szafranska, I. (1987): Changes in phytate content and phytase activity during the germination of some cereals. *J. Cer. Sci.* **5,** 23.

21. Scott, J.J. (1991): Alkaline phytase activity in non-ionic detergent extracts of legyme seeds. *Plant Physiol.* **95,** 1298.

22. Gustafsson, E.-L. & Sandberg, A.-S. (1995): Phytate reduction in brown beans (*Phaseolus vulgaris L.*). *J. Food Sci.* **60(1),** 149–152.

23. Türk, M., Carlsson, N.-G. & Sandberg, A.-S. (1996): Reduction in the levels of phytate during wholemeal breadmaking; effect of yeast and wheat phytases. *J. Cer. Sci.* **23**, 257–264.

24. Simell, M., Turunen, M., Piironen, J. & Vaara, T. (1990): In: *Proceedings of VIIth symposium 122 on bioconversion of plant raw materials - biotechnology advancement.* ed. Nikupaarela, M.L. pp. 145–161. Espoo, Finland.

25. Sandberg, A.-S., Rossander-Hultén, L. & Türk, M. (1996): Dietary Aspergillus niger phytase increases iron absorption in humans. *J. Nutr.* **126**, 476–480.

26. Mellanby, E. (1950): Some points in the chemistry and biochemistry of phytic acid and phytase. In: *A story of nutritional research*, pp. 248–282. Baltimore: Williams and Wilkins.

27. Sandberg, A.-S. & Svanberg, U. (1991): Phytate hydrolysis by phytase in cereals. Effects on *in vitro* estimation of iron availability. *J. Food Sci.* **56,** 1330–1333.

28. Sandström, B., Almgren, A., Kivistö, B. & Cederblad, A. (1987): Zinc absorption from meals based on rye, barley, oatmeal, triticale and whole-wheat. *J. Nutr.* **117,** 1898–1902.

29. Rossander-Hulthén, L., Gleerup, A. & Hallberg, L. (1990): Inhibitory effect of oat products on non-haem iron absorption in man. *Eur. J. Clin Nutr.* **44,** 783–791.

30. Larsson, M., Rossander-Hulthén, L., Sandström, B. & Sandberg, A.-S. (1996): Improved zinc and iron absorption from malted oats, with reduced phytate content. *Br. J. Nutr.* (in press).

31. Sudarmadji, S. & Markakis, P. (1977): The phytate and phytase of soybean tempeh. *J. Sci. Fd. Agric.* **28,** 381–383.

32. Lopez, Y., Gordon, D.T. & Fields, L. (1983): Release of phosphorus from phytate by natural lactic acid fermentation. *J. Food Sci.* **48,** 953–954.

33. Svanberg, U., Lorri, W. & Sandberg, A.-S. (1993): Lactic fermentation of non-tannin and high-tannin cereals: effect on *in vitro* estimation of iron availability and phytate hydrolysis. *J. Food Sci.* **58,** 408–412.

34. Hallberg, L. & Rossander, L. (1982): Absorption of iron from Western-type lunch and dinner meals. *Am. J. Clin. Nutr.* **35,** 502–509.

35. Rossander-Hultén, L., Sandberg, A.-S. & Sandström, B. (1992): The effect of dietary fibre on mineral absorption and utilization. In: *ILSI Human nutrition reviews. Dietary fibre- A component of food- nutritional function in health and disease*, ed. T. Schweizer & C. Edwards, pp. 197–216, London: Springer Verlag.

36. Salovaara, H. & Göransson, M. (1983): Nedbrytning av fytinsyra vid framställning av surt och osyrat rågbröd. *Näringsforskning* **27,** 97–101.

37. Bartnik, M. & Florysiak, J. (1988): Phytate hydrolysis during bread-making in several sorts of Polish bread. *Die Nahrung* **32,** 37–42.

38. Larsson, M. & Sandberg, A.-S. (1991): Phytate reduction in bread containing oat flour, oat bran or rye bran. *J. Cereal Sci.* **14,** 141–149.

39. Brune, M., Rossander-Hulthén, L., Hallberg, L., Gleerup, A. & Sandberg, A.-S. (1992): Human iron absorption from bread: inhibiting effects of cereal fiber, phytate and inositol phosphates with different numbers of phosphate groups. *J. Nutr.* **122,** 442–449.

40. Türk, M. & Sandberg, A.-S. (1992): Phytate hydrolysis during bread-making: effect of addition of phytase from *Aspergillus Niger*. *J. Cereal Sci.* **15,** 281–294.

41. Hallberg, L., Brune, M., Erlandsson, M., Sandberg, A.-S. & Rossander-Hultén, L. (1991): Calcium effect of different amounts on nonheme and heme iron absorption in humans. *Am. J. Clin. Nutr.* **53,** 112–119.

42. Marklinder, I.M., Larsson, M., Fredlund, K. & Sandberg, A.-S. (1995): Degradation of phytate by using varied sources of phytases in an oat-based nutrient solution fermented by *Lactobacillus plantarum* 2991. *Food Microbiol.* **12**, 487–495.

43. Hurrell, R.F., Juillerat, M.-A., Reddy, M.B., Lynch, S.R., Dassenko, S.A. & Cook, J.D. (1992): Soy protein, phytate, and iron absorption in humans. *Am. J. Clin. Nutr.* **56,** 573–578.

Index